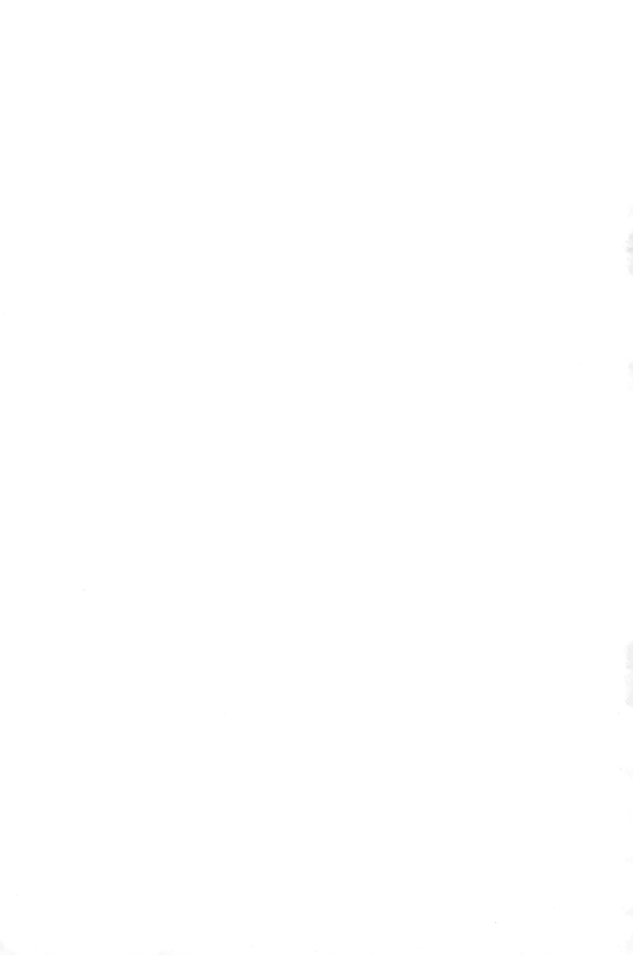

HANDBOOK OF DEPRESSION

HANDBOOK OF
DEPRESSION

THIRD EDITION

EDITED BY

IAN H. GOTLIB
CONSTANCE L. HAMMEN

THE GUILFORD PRESS
New York   London

© 2014 The Guilford Press
A Division of Guilford Publications, Inc.
72 Spring Street, New York, NY 10012
www.guilford.com

Printed in the United States of America

This book is printed on acid-free paper.

Last digit is print number: 9   8   7   6   5   4   3   2   1

The authors have checked with sources believed to be reliable in their efforts to provide information that is complete and generally in accord with the standards of practice that are accepted at the time of publication. However, in view of the possibility of human error or changes in behavioral, mental health, or medical sciences, neither the authors, nor the editors and publisher, nor any other party who has been involved in the preparation or publication of this work warrants that the information contained herein is in every respect accurate or complete, and they are not responsible for any errors or omissions or the results obtained from the use of such information. Readers are encouraged to confirm the information contained in this book with other sources.

Library of Congress Cataloging-in-Publication Data

Handbook of depression / edited by Ian H. Gotlib, Constance L. Hammen.—Third edition.
    pages cm
  Includes bibliographical references and index.
  ISBN 978-1-4625-0937-9 (hardcover)
  1. Depression, Mental—Handbooks, manuals, etc.   I. Gotlib, Ian H., editor of compilation.   II. Hammen, Constance L., editor of compilation.
  RC537.H3376 2014
  616.85′27—dc23
                                                                2013045288

About the Editors

Ian H. Gotlib, PhD, is the David Starr Jordan Professor and Chair of the Department of Psychology at Stanford University. His research examines cognitive, social, endocrinological, and neural factors and genetics in depressed individuals; mechanisms involved in the onset of depression in children at familial risk for developing this disorder; and the impact of innovative procedures to reduce young children's risk for depression. Dr. Gotlib has received the Distinguished Investigator Award from the National Alliance for Research on Schizophrenia and Depression (now the Brain and Behavior Research Foundation), the Joseph Zubin Award for outstanding lifetime contributions to the understanding of psychopathology from the Society for Research in Psychopathology (SRP), the Award for Distinguished Scientific Contributions from the American Psychological Association, and the Distinguished Scientist Award from the Society for a Science of Clinical Psychology (SSCP). He is a Fellow of the American Psychological Association and the Association for Psychological Science.

Constance L. Hammen, PhD, is Distinguished Professor in the Department of Psychology and the Department of Psychiatry and Biobehavioral Sciences at the University of California, Los Angeles. She served as chair of the Clinical Psychology Program at UCLA for 13 years. Her research focuses on risk factors for depression and bipolar disorder, stress processes and stress assessment, and the intergenerational transmission of depression. Dr. Hammen is a recipient of the Joseph Zubin Award from the SRP and the Distinguished Scientist Award from the SSCP. She serves on the board of directors of the Psychological Clinical Science Accreditation System and is a Founding Fellow of the Academy of Cognitive Therapy.

Contributors

Ashley Maehr Alexander, PsyD, private practice, Roswell, Georgia

Guillermo Perez Algorta, PhD, Department of Psychiatry, Ohio State University, Columbus, Ohio

Anna E. S. Allmann, MA, Department of Psychology, Stony Brook University, Stony Brook, New York

Kimberly Arditte, BA, Department of Psychology, University of Miami, Coral Gables, Florida

Alinne Z. Barrera, PhD, Clinical Psychology PhD Program, Palo Alto University, Palo Alto, California

Steven R. H. Beach, PhD, Owens Institute for Behavioral Research, University of Georgia, Athens, Georgia

Olivier Berton, PhD, Department of Psychiatry, Perelman School of Medicine, University of Pennsylvania, Philadelphia, Pennsylvania

Dan G. Blazer MD, PhD, Department of Psychiatry and Behavioral Sciences, Duke University Medical Center, Durham, North Carolina

Guy Bodenmann, PhD, Institute of Clinical Psychology and Department of Psychology, University of Zurich, Zurich, Switzerland

Lauren M. Bylsma, PhD, Childhood Depression Research Studies, University of Pittsburgh Medical Center, Pittsburgh, Pennsylvania

Robert M. Carney, PhD, Department of Psychiatry, Washington University School of Medicine, St. Louis, Missouri

Yulia E. Chentsova-Dutton, PhD, Department of Psychology, Georgetown University, Washington, DC

Natalie L. Colich, BA, Department of Psychology, Stanford University, Stanford, California

Amy K. Cuellar, PhD, Menninger Department of Psychiatry and Behavioral Sciences, Baylor College of Medicine, and Michael E. DeBakey VA Medical Center, Houston, Texas

Joanne Davila, PhD, Department of Psychology, Stony Brook University, Stony Brook, New York

Peter de Jonge, PhD, Department of Psychiatry, University Medical Center Groningen, University of Groningen, Groningen, Germany

Charlene A. Deming, EdM, Department of Psychology, Harvard University, Cambridge, Massachusetts

Sona Dimidjian, PhD, Department of Psychology and Neuroscience, University of Colorado Boulder, Boulder, Colorado

Thalia C. Eley, PhD, MRC Social, Genetic and Developmental Psychiatry Research Centre, Institute of Psychiatry, King's College London, London, United Kingdom

Megan Flynn, PhD, Department of Psychology, Bethel University, St. Paul, Minnesota

Kenneth E. Freedland, PhD, Department of Psychiatry, Washington University School of Medicine, St. Louis, Missouri

Katholiki Georgiades, PhD, Offord Centre for Child Studies, McMaster University, Hamilton, Ontario, Canada

Brandon E. Gibb, PhD, Department of Psychology, Binghamton University, Binghamton, New York

Michael J. Gitlin, MD, Department of Psychiatry and Biobehavioral Sciences, David Geffen School of Medicine, University of California, Los Angeles, Los Angeles, California

Catherine R. Glenn, PhD, Department of Psychology, Harvard University, Cambridge, Massachusetts

Sherryl H. Goodman, PhD, Department of Psychology, Emory University, Atlanta, Georgia

Ian H. Gotlib, PhD, Department of Psychology, Stanford University, Stanford, California

Chang-Gyu Hahn, MD, PhD, Center for Neurobiology and Behavior, Department of Psychiatry, Perelman School of Medicine, University of Pennsylvania, Philadelphia, Pennsylvania

Constance L. Hammen, PhD, Department of Psychology, University of California, Los Angeles, Los Angeles, California

Lori M. Hilt, PhD, Department of Psychology, Lawrence University, Appleton, Wisconsin

Karen Hodgson, MSc, MRC Social, Genetic and Developmental Psychiatry Research Centre, Institute of Psychiatry, King's College London, London, United Kingdom

Steven D. Hollon, PhD, Department of Psychology, Vanderbilt University, Nashville, Tennessee

Celia F. Hybels, PhD, Department of Psychiatry and Behavioral Sciences, Duke University Medical Center, Durham, North Carolina

Rick E. Ingram, PhD, Department of Psychology, University of Kansas, Lawrence, Kansas

Sheri L. Johnson, PhD, Department of Psychology, University of California, Berkeley, Berkeley, California

Jutta Joormann, PhD, Department of Psychology, Northwestern University, Evanston, Illinois

Nadine J. Kaslow, PhD, Department of Psychiatry and Behavioral Sciences, Emory University, Atlanta, Georgia

Ronald C. Kessler, PhD, Department of Health Care Policy, Harvard Medical School, Boston, Massachusetts

Daniel N. Klein, PhD, Department of Psychology, Stony Brook University, Stony Brook, New York

Jennifer Y. F. Lau, PhD, Department of Psychology, Institute of Psychiatry, King's College London, London, United Kingdom

Huynh-Nhu Le, PhD, Department of Psychology, George Washington University, Washington, DC

Minsun Lee, PhD, Department of Psychology, Drexel University, Philadelphia, Pennsylvania

Kathryn J. Lester, PhD, MRC Social, Genetic and Developmental Psychiatry Research Centre, Institute of Psychiatry, King's College London, London, United Kingdom

Cara M. Lusby, MA, Department of Psychology, Emory University, Atlanta, Georgia

David J. Miklowitz, PhD, Division of Child and Adolescent Psychiatry, Semel Institute for Neuroscience and Human Behavior, David Geffen School of Medicine, University of California, Los Angeles, Los Angeles, California

Alexander J. Millner, MA, Department of Psychology, Harvard University, Cambridge, Massachusetts

Susan Mineka, PhD, Department of Psychology, Northwestern University, Evanston, Illinois

Scott M. Monroe, PhD, Department of Psychology, University of Notre Dame, Notre Dame, Indiana

Ricardo F. Muñoz, PhD, Clinical Psychology PhD Program, Palo Alto University, Palo Alto, California, and Department of Psychiatry, San Francisco General Hospital, University of California, San Francisco, San Francisco, California

Arthur M. Nezu, PhD, Department of Psychology, Drexel University, Philadelphia, Pennsylvania

Christine Maguth Nezu, PhD, Department of Psychology, Drexel University, Philadelphia, Pennsylvania

Matthew K. Nock, PhD, Department of Psychology, Harvard University, Cambridge, Massachusetts

Susan Nolen-Hoeksema, PhD (deceased), Department of Psychology, Yale University, New Haven, Connecticut

Andrew D. Peckham, BA, Department of Psychology, University of California, Berkeley, Berkeley, California

Marissa N. Petersen-Coleman, PsyD, private practice, Atlanta, Georgia

Diego A. Pizzagalli, PhD, Department of Psychiatry, McLean Hospital, Harvard Medical School, Belmont, Massachusetts

Jonathan Rottenberg, PhD, Department of Psychology, University of South Florida, Tampa, Florida

Karen D. Rudolph, PhD, Department of Psychology, University of Illinois at Urbana–Champaign, Champaign, Illinois

Andrew G. Ryder, PhD, Department of Psychology, Concordia University, Montreal, Quebec, Canada

Stephen M. Schueller, PhD, Department of Preventive Medicine, Feinberg School of Medicine, Northwestern University, Chicago, Illinois

Victoria Shahly, PhD, Department of Health Care Policy, Harvard Medical School, Boston, Massachusetts

Josephine Shih, PhD, Department of Psychology, Saint Joseph's University, Philadelphia, Pennsylvania

Greg J. Siegle, PhD, Department of Psychiatry, Western Psychiatric Institute and Clinic, University of Pittsburgh, Pittsburgh, Pennsylvania

George M. Slavich, PhD, Cousins Center for Psychoneuroimmunology, University of California, Los Angeles, Los Angeles, California

Lisa R. Starr, PhD, Department of Clinical and Social Sciences in Psychology, University of Rochester, Rochester, New York

Dana Steidtmann, PhD, Department of Psychiatry and Behavioral Sciences, Stanford University, Stanford, California

Jessica B. Stern, BA, Department of Psychology, Drexel University, Philadelphia, Pennsylvania

Catherine B. Stroud, PhD, Department of Psychology, Williams College, Williamstown, Massachusetts

Michael E. Thase, MD, Department of Psychiatry, Perelman School of Medicine, University of Pennsylvania, Philadelphia, Pennsylvania

Leandro D. Torres, PhD, Department of Psychology, San Francisco General Hospital, University of California, San Francisco, San Francisco, California

Michael T. Treadway, PhD, Center for Depression, Anxiety and Stress Research, McLean Hospital, Harvard Medical School, Belmont, Massachusetts

Jeanne Tsai, PhD, Department of Psychology, Stanford University, Stanford, California

Hanna M. van Loo, MD, Department of Psychiatry, University Medical Center Groningen, University of Groningen, Groningen, Germany

Suzanne Vrshek-Schallhorn, PhD, Department of Psychology, University of North Carolina at Greensboro, Greensboro, North Carolina

Philip S.-E. Wang, MD, DrPH, National Institute of Mental Health, National Institutes of Health, Bethesda, Maryland

Mark A. Whisman, PhD, Department of Psychology and Neuroscience, University of Colorado Boulder, Boulder, Colorado

Marsha A. Wilcox, EdD, ScD, Janssen Research & Development LLC, Titusville, New Jersey

Eric Youngstrom, PhD, Department of Psychology, University of North Carolina at Chapel Hill, Chapel Hill, North Carolina

Contents

Introduction

IAN H. GOTLIB *and* CONSTANCE L. HAMMEN

Depression is among the most prevalent of all psychiatric disorders. Recent estimates indicate that over 15% of the American population, primarily women, will experience a clinically significant episode of depression at some point in their lives. In fact, Whiteford and colleagues (2013) recently reported data from the World Health Organization (WHO) Global Burden of Disease Study (2010) indicating that depressive disorders accounted for almost half of all disability-adjusted life years, three times more burdensome than anxiety disorders. In epidemiological studies, depression has been found to be associated with poor physical health, in particular with fibromyalgia, high rates of cardiac problems, and higher rates of smoking (e.g., Nicholson, Kuper, & Hemingway, 2006; Patten et al., 2005). There is also a significant economic cost of depression. In an analysis of depression in the workplace, Kessler and colleagues (2006) estimated that the annual salary-equivalent costs of depression-related lost productivity in the United States exceed $36 billion. And because this figure does not take into account the impact of depression on factors such as the performance of coworkers, turnover, and industrial accidents, it is likely to be an underestimate.

In addition to these findings concerning the impact of depression on health and workplace productivity, there is now mounting evidence that depression adversely affects the quality of interpersonal relationships and, in particular, relationships with spouses and children. Not only does depression predict subsequent divorce (Breslau et al., 2001), but also children of parents with depression are themselves at elevated risk for psychopathology (Hammen, Brennan, & Shih, 2004). Finally, the personal cost of depression in terms of death by suicide is alarmingly high (Nordentoft, Mortensen, & Pedersen, 2011).

Many individuals with depression also experience recurrences of the disorder. About half of patients with depression will have more than one depressive episode (Hardeveld, Spijker, De Graaf, Nolen, & Beekman, 2013). This high recurrence rate in depression suggests that specific factors serve to increase people's risk for developing repeated episodes of this disorder. In this context, therefore, in trying to understand mechanisms that increase risk for depression, investigators have examined biological and genetic factors

1

and psychological and environmental characteristics that may lead individuals to experience depressive episodes.

The enormous costs of depression, combined with the recent documentation of increasing rates of depressive disorders, have led to an exponential increase in research examining factors involved in the onset, course, and maintenance of depression, as well as the effectiveness of psychological and biological treatments for depression; this research has resulted in significant advances in our understanding of virtually all aspects of this disorder. Because there was not a single source to which scientists and other interested readers could turn to learn about recent important developments in different areas of depression research, we began to assemble the first edition of this *Handbook* in 2000, and we published the second edition in 2009. The continuing rapid development of research and theory in depression since then provided the impetus for us to update and expand the *Handbook*. In particular, we have increased our coverage of bipolar disorders, with three chapters covering clinical features, risk and etiological factors, and treatment. In addition, we have added chapters on the comorbidity of depression and anxiety and on emotional functioning in depression. We are fortunate that most of the senior authors who contributed to the previous edition of the *Handbook* continued to participate in this edition; moreover, we were able to add a stellar group of new contributors to the *Handbook*.

Reflecting changes in the field, the authors of the chapters in this edition of the *Handbook* have strengthened their focus on important methodological issues and advances, including discussions of the results of longitudinal research, of investigations that integrate diverse domains of functioning, and of international and large-scale multisite studies of depression. The chapters also reflect a growing focus on biological aspects of depression, including neuroimaging and genetics (and their interaction), affective neuroscience in adults and children, and the relation between depression and inflammatory processes. At the same time, the authors do not lose sight of the importance of social and emotional functioning in depressive disorders. Indeed, we believe that the authors who have contributed to this edition of the *Handbook* have ensured that this is the strongest possible compendium of contemporary research and theory in the depressive disorders.

We have organized this book into four broad sections; we believe that these domains are the major areas of depression research in which significant advances are being made and in which research will continue to increase our understanding of the nature of this disorder. The authors of the chapters in the first section discuss descriptive and definitional aspects of depression, including epidemiology, assessment, methodological issues in the study of depression, chronicity, comorbidity, emotional functioning, health, and the course and features of bipolar disorder. The second section contains chapters dealing with vulnerability, risk, and models of depression. In this section the authors describe advances in the genetics, biology, and neurobiology of depression, arguably the three areas of research in depression that have experienced the greatest growth over the past few years. Authors also discuss developments in our understanding of cognitive and interpersonal aspects of depression, the functioning of the offspring of depressed parents, the importance of stress and of early adverse experiences, and the etiology and risk factors for bipolar disorder. The third section of this *Handbook* describes advances in our understanding of depression as it occurs in specific populations. The authors of these chapters discuss the presentation of depression in different cultures, depression in couples and families, gender differences in depression, depression in children, adolescents, and older adults, and the relation between depression and suicide. The final section of the volume is devoted to issues involving the prevention and treatment of depression. Here the authors describe recent developments in the prevention of major depression and advances in pharmacotherapy, cognitive-behavioral therapy, marital and family therapy, and interpersonal therapy for depression. This section also includes important chapters describing pharmacological and psychosocial interventions for bipolar disorder and innovations in the treatment of depression in children and adolescents. As in previous editions, we asked all of the authors in this edition of the *Handbook* to conclude their chapters with a section describing what they think are the most important directions for future research in this field. These comments give the reader a sense of not only the advances that have been made in each area of research in depression but also the important issues that are likely to take center stage over the next few years. We discuss these directions in more detail in the concluding chapter of the *Handbook*. As you will see from the chapters in this *Handbook*, we have clearly made significant progress over the past decade in our quest to understand, treat, and prevent the onset of depression. And, more important, the coming decade promises to be even more exciting than the last.

REFERENCES

Breslau, J., Miller, E., Jin, R., Sampson, N. A., Alonso, J., Andrade, L. H., et al. (2011). A multinational study of mental disorders, marriage, and divorce. *Acta Psychiatrica Scandinavica, 124*, 474–486.

Hammen, C., Brennan, P., & Shih, J. (2004). Family discord and stress predictors of depression and other disorders in adolescent children of depressed and nondepressed women. *Journal of the American Academy of Child and Adolescent Psychiatry, 43*, 994–1002.

Hardeveld, F., Spijker, J., De Graaf, R., Nolen, W. A., & Beekman, A. T. (2013). Recurrence of major depressive disorder and its predictors in the general population: Results from the Netherlands Mental Health Survey and Incidence Study (NEMESIS). *Psychological Medicine, 43*, 39–48.

Kessler, R. C., Akiskal, H. S., Ames, M., Birnbaum, H., Greenberg, P., Hirschfeld, R. M., et al. (2006). Prevalence and effects of mood disorders on work performance in a nationally representative sample of U.S. workers. *American Journal of Psychiatry, 163*, 1561–1568.

Nicholson, A., Kuper, H., & Hemingway, H. (2006). Depression as an aetiologic and prognostic factor in coronary heart disease: A meta-analysis of 6362 events among 146,538 participants in 54 observational studies. *European Heart Journal, 27*, 2763–2774.

Nordentoft, M., Mortensen, P. B., & Pedersen, C. B. (2011). Absolute risk of suicide after first hospital contact in mental disorder. *Archives of General Psychiatry, 68*(10), 1058–1064.

Patten, S. B., Beck, C. A., Kassam, A., Williams, J. V., Barbui, C., & Metz, L. M. (2005). Long-term medical conditions and major depression: Strength of association for specific conditions in the general population. *Canadian Journal of Psychiatry, 50*, 195–202.

Whiteford, H. A., Degenhardt, L., Rehm, J., Baxter, A. J., Ferrari, A. J., Erskine, H. E., et al. (2013). Global burden of disease attributable to mental and substance use disorders: Findings from the Global Burden of Disease Study 2010. *Lancet, 382*, 1575–1586.

PART I

DESCRIPTIVE ASPECTS OF DEPRESSION

Depression is one of the most common psychiatric disorders and, from a societal perspective, is among the most costly. Of the eight chapters in this section, four are new to this volume, added to more fully characterize new directions that are informing the entire field. The authors discuss issues concerning the onset and course of depression, its prevalence and societal costs, and important conceptual and methodological factors involved in studying this disorder. The features and course of bipolar disorder are also discussed in this section. Kessler, de Jonge, Shahly, van Loo, Wang, and Wilcox (Chapter 1) describe epidemiological aspects of depression—its prevalence and its economic cost and issues of severity that define its public health significance. Nezu, Nezu, Lee, and Stern (Chapter 2) describe the most widely used interview-based and self-report measures of depression and discuss important issues involved in the assessment of this disorder. Extending this discussion, Ingram, Siegle, and Steidtmann (Chapter 3) describe a number of methodological issues in the study of depressive disorders and make several noteworthy recommendations concerning how research in this area might proceed most fruitfully, including a discussion of the Research Domain Criteria framework. Klein and Allmann (Chapter 4) present a chapter that is new to this volume, examining the course of depression and featuring the altered DSM-5 characterization of chronic, persistent depression. Mineka and Vrshek-Schallhorn (Chapter 5) also present a new chapter for the volume on the comorbidity between depression and anxiety and strategies for disentangling their common and specific features. Rottenberg and Bylsma (Chapter 6) add a new chapter on emotional functioning in depression. Freedland and Carney (Chapter 7) examine links between depression and medical illness and delineate controversies and challenges in the assessment and treatment of depression in medically ill individuals. The single chapter on features of bipolar disorder in the second edition is now divided into two chapters to more fully represent new developments in the field. In the first of these chapters, Youngstrom and Algorta (Chapter 8) discuss unresolved definitional and diagnostic and course features of bipolar disorder.

CHAPTER 1

Epidemiology of Depression

RONALD C. KESSLER, PETER DE JONGE, VICTORIA SHAHLY,
HANNA M. VAN LOO, PHILIP S.-E. WANG, *and* MARSHA A. WILCOX

The first modern epidemiological surveys including information about depression were carried out in the late 1950s in the Midtown Manhattan (Srole, Langner, Michael, Opler, & Rennie, 1962) and the Stirling County (Leighton, Harding, & Macklin, 1963) studies. These studies used dimensional screening scales of nonspecific psychological distress to pinpoint respondents likely to have mental disorders and then administered clinical follow-up interviews to them. The outcome was a global measure of mental disorder rather than individual diagnoses, although the screening scales included questions that could subsequently be interpreted as part of the depressive syndrome to make rough post hoc estimates about prevalence and correlates of depressive disorders (Murphy, Laird, Monson, Sobol, & Leighton, 2000).

Later surveys up through the 1980s used variants on the Midtown Manhattan and Stirling County screening scales, but generally without clinical follow-up (see Link & Dohrenwend, 1980, for a review). Scale scores were sometimes dichotomized to define "cases" based on some standard clinical cut point, but there was controversy about the appropriate decision rules for defining cases (Seiler, 1973). To resolve this controversy, structured diagnostic interviews were developed for use in community surveys. The Diagnostic Interview Schedule (DIS; Robins, Helzer, Croughan, Williams, & Spitzer, 1981) was the first such instrument. Dimensional screening scales continued to be used to screen for mental illness in primary care (Goldberg, 1972) and to assess symptom severity and treatment effectiveness among patients in treatment for mental disorders (Derogatis, 1977). However, psychiatric epidemiologists, influenced by the widely published results of the first study to use the DIS, the Epidemiologic Catchment Area (ECA) study (Robins & Regier, 1991), largely abandoned dimensional distress measures in favor of dichotomous interview-based case classifications in general population surveys beginning in the late 1980s.

We now have over three decades of experience using fully structured diagnostic interviews such as the DIS and the more recently developed Composite International Diagnostic Interview (CIDI; Robins et al., 1988), the Primary Care Evaluation of Mental

Disorders (PRIME-MD; Spitzer et al., 1994), and Mini-International Neuropsychiatric Interview (MINI; Sheehan et al., 1998). It is clear from this experience that fully structured diagnostic interviews, although useful, are inadequate to provide complete information about the magnitude of the problem of mental illness, as DSM and ICD criteria are so broad that close to one-half of people in the general population receive one or more lifetime diagnoses (Kessler et al., 2007) and close to one-fifth carry a current diagnosis (Kessler et al., 2008). With prevalence estimates as high as these, the dichotomous case data provided in diagnostic interviews need to be supplemented with dimensional information on severity to be useful to health policy planners.

Only the most recent epidemiological data on the prevalence of major depression include dimensional measures of severity. This is an important expansion of previous research in light of the suggestion by some commentators that most untreated community cases of major depression are fairly mild cases (Regier, Narrow, Rupp, Rae, & Kaelber, 2000). The first part of this chapter presents the main findings in the literature on the descriptive epidemiology of major depression, including the most recent evidence on clinical severity. The second part of the chapter expands the discussion of severity by reviewing available data on the consequences of depression as assessed in community surveys.

DESCRIPTIVE EPIDEMIOLOGY

Point Prevalence

Community surveys find that up to 20% of adults and up to 50% of children and adolescents report depressive symptoms during recall periods between 1 week and 6 months (Kessler & Bromet, 2013). Point prevalence estimates for DSM major depressive disorder (MDD) in surveys that use structured diagnostic interviews are considerably lower, with rates of current MDD typically less than 1% among children (reviewed by Merikangas & Angst, 1995), up to 6% among adolescents (reviewed by Kessler, Avenevoli, & Merikangas, 2001), and 2–4% among adults (reviewed by Kessler & Bromet, 2013).

The discrepancy between the high symptom prevalence and lower depressive disorder prevalence means that many people have subsyndromal depressive symptoms. Epidemiological studies investigating these symptoms have been hampered by inconsistent definitions of subsyndromal depression (Rodriguez, Nuevo, Chatterji, & Ayuso-Mateos, 2012) but have documented rates among both adolescents (Kessler & Walters, 1998) and adults (Judd, Akiskal, & Paulus, 1997) as high as, if not higher than, rates of MDD, with especially high relative rates among older adults (Meeks, Vahia, Lavretsky, Kulkarni, & Jeste, 2011). Longitudinal research shows that subsyndromal depression is a powerful predictor of subsequent MDD (Klein et al., 2013) and an important contributor to the persistence and severity of MDD (Altamura et al., 2011). The World Health Organization's (WHO) World Health Survey found that subsyndromal depression is quite common throughout the world, is associated with similar risk factors to MDD, and is associated with substantial decrements in health (Ayuso-Mateos, Nuevo, Verdes, Naidoo, & Chatterji, 2010).

12-Month Prevalence

Many community surveys focus on 12-month prevalence of MDD (i.e., the percentage of people with MDD at some time in the 12 months before interview) based on the fact that public health planning is typically made on an annual basis. The most recent such data come from the WHO World Mental Health (WMH) surveys, which are large national general population epidemiological surveys in 18 countries with a combined sample of 89,037 respondents (Bromet et al., 2011). The average 12-month prevalence estimate of DSM-IV major depressive episodes is 5.5% in the 10 WMH surveys in high-income countries and 5.9% in the 8 surveys in low- to middle-income countries. These estimates are somewhat higher than the 3.2% 12-month prevalence of major depressive episodes *alone* found among 245,404 respondents in 60 countries in the World Health Surveys (Moussavi et al., 2007), but the World Health Surveys also showed that 9.3–23.0% of respondents with chronic physical conditions had *comorbid* major depressive episodes. The World Health Surveys also found that the impact of MDD on decrements in functioning is higher than that of virtually any other condition studied.

Lifetime Prevalence

Epidemiological surveys generally use retrospective reports to assess lifetime prevalence and age-of-onset (AOO) of MDD. Lifetime prevalence estimates in U.S. surveys have ranged widely, from as low as 6% (Weissman, Livingston, Leaf, Florio, & Holzer, 1991) to as high as 25% (Lewinsohn, Rohde, Seeley, & Fischer, 1991). The estimate in the National Comorbidity Survey Replication (NCS-R), the most recent validated U.S. epidemiological study, was 16.6% (Kessler, Berglund, Demler, Jin, & Walters, 2005). Clinical reappraisal data confirm the validity of the NCS-R estimate (Haro et al., 2006), suggesting that more than 30 million U.S. adults have met criteria for MDD at some time in their lives. The WMH surveys, which used the same diagnostic assessment as the NCS-R, estimated that lifetime prevalence of MDD was 14.6% in the 10 high-income and 11.1% in the 8 low- to middle-income countries studied (Bromet et al., 2011).

Age of Onset

Lifetime prevalence estimates represent cumulative prevalence *to date*. Some survey respondents who have never yet had MDD will have it later. Lifetime *risk* (as opposed to lifetime *prevalence*) can be estimated with actuarial methods that use retrospective AOO reports to predict subsequent risk for respondents who have not yet passed through the risk period. This type of analysis was carried out in the WMH surveys (Kessler et al., 2007). Median AOO of mood disorders across countries was in the age range of 29–43, with the AOO distributions across countries showing consistently low risk through the early teens, a roughly linear increase thereafter through late middle age, and a more gradual increase later in life. Projected lifetime risk by age 75 was 40–170% greater than the proportion of respondents with lifetime-to-date MDD at the time of interview.

In considering these results, it is important to recognize that the WMH lifetime risk projections assumed that conditional risk is constant across cohorts. This assumption is clearly incorrect, as shown by the fact that AOO curves differ substantially by cohort, with estimated risk successively higher in each younger cohort. This pattern of intercohort variation could be due to the risk of depression increasing in successively more recent cohorts, to various methodological possibilities involving cohort-related differences in willingness to admit depression or to recall past episodes of depression (Giuffra & Risch, 1994), or to some combination of substantive and methodological influences.

There is no way to adjudicate among these contending interpretations definitively with cross-sectional data of the sort available in the WMH surveys. Longitudinal data are needed. One published report with such data made a comparison of depression prevalence estimates in two U.S. national surveys administered in 1991–1992 and 2001–2002 that used similar (but not identical) assessments of 12-month MDD (Compton, Conway, Stinson, & Grant, 2006). The comparison suggested that the prevalence of MDD increased significantly over the decade. However, this result can be called into question based on the baseline prevalence estimate (3.3%) being implausibly low due to methodological limitations in the assessment method. These limitations were corrected in the second survey, which would be expected to increase the prevalence estimate. However, the researchers failed to take this into consideration in their interpretation of the result, leading to the incorrect conclusion that prevalence increased substantially over time. Other longitudinal studies in the United States (Kessler, Demler, et al., 2005) and the Netherlands (de Graaf, ten Have, van Gool, & van Dorsselaer, 2012) failed to find evidence of significant time trends in prevalence.

Subtypes

A number of proposals have been made to subtype MDD based on symptom profiles (reviewed by Baumeister & Parker, 2012). The most consistent suggestion concerns a distinction between melancholic symptoms (e.g., weight loss, insomnia, appetite loss) and atypical symptoms (e.g., weight gain, hypersomnia, appetite increase), although many other distinctions have been proposed. A recent meta-analysis found little empirical support for these symptom-based subtyping distinctions (van Loo, de Jonge, Romeijn, Kessler, & Schoevers, 2012). That meta-analysis identified 34 studies of dimensions underlying depressive symptoms using cluster analysis, factor analysis, or latent class analysis to define subtypes. No symptom clusters emerged consistently across those studies other than a broad dimension for overall symptom severity.

Another way to define MDD symptom subtypes is in terms of synergistic effects among symptoms and/or comorbidities in predicting some outcome, such as differential treatment response or differential persistence and severity. Synergistic effects are typically examined by using some type of regression tree method (Berk, 2008; Breiman, Friedman, Olshen, & Stone, 1984; Hastie, Tibshirani, & Friedman, 2009). Although much less widely used than the internal-consistency subtyping approach described in the preceding paragraph, the few depression subtype studies using regression tree methods have yielded promising results (Joel et al., 2014; McKenzie et al., 2011; Nelson et al., 2012). However, these studies are too few and too inconsistent in outcomes to warrant synthesis. Given the high risks of overfitting in the stepwise data mining methods used in these analyses, it is especially important for future studies of this sort to use internal cross-validation methods and replication across multiple datasets before accepting results as reliable.

Another important subtyping distinction concerns cyclical depression. Two cycling MDD subtypes have been identified exclusive of those associated with bipolar disorder: seasonal affective disorder (SAD; Rosenthal et al., 1984) and premenstrual dysphoric disorder (PMDD; Halbreich, 1997). Community surveys find that 10% or more of people in the general population report seasonal variations in depressed mood and related symptoms (e.g., Booker & Hellekson, 1992). Seasonal depression is typically most common in the winter months and more prevalent in northern than in southern latitudes. However, the prevalence of DSM-5 SAD, which requires a lifetime diagnosis of recurrent episodes of mood disorder with regular onsets and offsets in particular times of the year, is much less common. Indeed, Blazer, Kessler, and Swartz (1998) found that only 1% of the population met narrowly defined criteria for MDD with a seasonal pattern, representing only about 5% of all people with MDD.

Community surveys show that most women report symptom changes associated with the menstrual cycle (Campagne & Campagne, 2007; Winer & Rapkin, 2006). Only between 4 and 6% of women, however, report what appears to be DSM-5 PMDD (Di Giulio & Reissing, 2006), which requires a clear recurring pattern of onset and offset of five or more mood and related symptoms at specific points in the majority of menstrual cycles over the course of a full year. Assessments with daily mood diaries over two or more menstrual cycles typically show only about half of women who report cyclical mood problems actually have PMDD, the others having more chronic syndromal or subsyndromal mood disorders that are exacerbated by menstrual symptoms (Freeman, DeRubeis, & Rickels, 1996). There is great interest in PMDD based on evidence of family aggregation with MDD and responsiveness to selective serotonin reuptake inhibitors but not tricyclic antidepressants (Freeman, Rickels, Sondheimer, & Polansky, 1999). There is also controversy, though, regarding appropriate diagnostic and assessment criteria (Campagne & Campagne, 2007). Community epidemiological data on PMDD are scant due to logistic complications in assessment. Given the existence of so many uncertainties about PMDD, a large, representative epidemiological survey using diary data would be very valuable.

Course

Little longitudinal research has studied the course of MDD in general population samples (but for important exceptions, see Gamma, Angst, Ajdacic, Eich, & Rossler, 2007; Yaroslavsky, Pettit, Lewinsohn, Seeley, & Roberts, 2013). However, cross-sectional surveys consistently find the ratio of 12-month to lifetime MDD to be in the range .5–.6 (Bromet et al., 2011), suggesting that between one-half and two-thirds of people with lifetime MDD will be in episode in any given year in the remainder of their lives. At least three separate processes contribute to the size of this ratio: probability of first episode chronicity, the probability of episode recurrence among people with a history of nonchronic MDD, and speed of episode recovery.

Epidemiological studies show the first of these three processes is quite small, with only a small fraction of people reporting a single lifetime depressive episode persisting for many years. Prevalence of dysthymia and chronic minor depression are somewhat higher but still only in the range of 3–4% of the population (Kessler & Bromet, 2013). Episode recurrence, in contrast, is very common, with the vast majority of people with lifetime MDD having recurrent episodes (Hardeveld, Spijker, De Graaf, Nolen, & Beekman, 2013; Pettit, Hartley, Lewinsohn, Seeley, & Klein, 2013). Finally, speed of episode recovery appears to be highly variable, although the epidemiological evidence on this issue is slim (Kendler, Walters, & Kessler, 1997; McLeod, Kessler, & Landis, 1992).

Comorbidity

Studies of diagnostic patterns in community samples document substantial comorbidity between MDD and other mental disorders (Kessler, Ormel, et al., 2011). Indeed, lifetime comorbidity is the norm among people with MDD. In the NCS-R, for example, nearly three-fourths of respondents with lifetime MDD also had at least one other lifetime DSM-IV disorder (Kessler et al., 2003), including 59% with anxiety disorders, 31.9% with impulse control disorders, and 24.0% with substance use disorders. Lifetime comorbidity is even higher among respondents with 12-month MDD, implying that comorbid MDD is more persistent. Comparison of retrospective AOO reports in the NCS-R showed that MDD was reported to have started at an earlier age than all other comorbid disorders in only 12.4% of lifetime cases and 12.2% of 12-month cases, although temporal priority was much more common in cases of comorbidity with substance use disorders (41.3–49.2%) than with either anxiety disorders (13.7–14.6%) or impulse control disorders (17.9–20.9%).

Controversy exists about the extent to which this high comorbidity is an artifact of changes in the diagnostic systems used in almost all recent studies of comorbidity (Frances et al., 1992). Beginning with DSM-III, these systems dramatically increased the number of diagnostic categories and reduced the number of exclusion criteria so that many people who would have received only a single diagnosis in previous systems now receive multiple diagnoses. The intention was to retain potentially important differentiating information that could be useful in refining understanding of etiology, course, and likely treatment response (First, Spitzer, & Williams, 1990). However, it can also be argued that this had the unintended negative consequence of artificially inflating estimates of comorbidity. This uncertainty might be resolved in future attempts to determine the validity of diagnostic distinctions, based on the new National Institute of Mental Health (NIMH) Research Domain Criteria (RDoC) initiative (*www.nimh.nih. gov/research-priorities/rdoc/index.shtml*). The RDoC initiative will break down DSM diagnoses, which are currently based only on observable symptoms, into their underlying neural circuit-based domains and constructs. Identifying the common domains and constructs in which dysfunction is occurring may ultimately help to explain the high diagnostic overlap and comorbidity between depression and other DSM disorders. Until that time, though, we are left with a situation in which MDD appears to be highly comorbid with a number of other disorders.

As noted earlier, the majority of comorbid MDD is temporally secondary in the sense that first onset of MDD occurs subsequent to first onset of other comorbid disorders. Survival analysis of cross-sectional data in the WMH surveys using retrospective AOO reports to determine temporal priority shows that a wide range of temporally primary disorders predict subsequent MDD onset (Kessler, Ormel, et al., 2011). Most of these associations are confined to active, as opposed to remitted, primary disorders. The fact that remitted disorders generally do not predict MDD suggests indirectly that earlier disorders are (variable) risk factors rather than (fixed) risk markers (Kraemer et al., 1997).

The structure of comorbidity has been the subject of considerable interest over the past decade, beginning with an influential paper by Krueger (1999) that led to many other researchers using factor analysis to document associations among hierarchy-free anxiety, mood, behavior, and substance disorders associated with latent internalizing and externalizing disorders. The internalizing dimension is sometimes further divided into secondary dimensions of fear (e.g., panic, phobia) and distress (e.g., major depressive episode, generalized anxiety disorder) (Beesdo et al., 2009; Cox & Swinson, 2002; Krueger & Markon, 2006a; Lahey et al., 2008; Slade & Watson, 2006; Vollebergh et al., 2001). These results have been used to argue for a reorganization of the classification of mental disorders in the DSM and ICD diagnostic systems (Andrews et al., 2009; Goldberg, Krueger, Andrews, & Hobbs, 2009; Krueger & Markon, 2006b; Watson, 2005; Wittchen, Beesdo, & Gloster, 2009), although other data suggest that this theoretical structure might be insufficiently robust to serve as the basis for such a reorganization (Beesdo et al., 2009; Wittchen et al., 2009). For example, the distinction between fear and distress disorders does not emerge in all studies (Beesdo et al., 2009; Krueger, Caspi, Moffitt, & Silva, 1998; Krueger & Finger, 2001; Wittchen, Beesdo-Baum, et al., 2009), and model fit deteriorates when additional disorders are added or when the model is estimated separately among people at different life-course stages (Watson, 2005; Wittchen, Beesdo-Baum et al., 2009).

Despite these inconsistencies, the general finding of strong comorbidity within the internalizing and externalizing domains has raised the question of whether common risk factors exist for disorders in these domains and, if so, whether risk factors for individual disorders in previous studies are actually risk factors for broader predispositions. This issue of specificity versus generality of risk factors is of considerable importance, as a number of hypotheses about causal pathways posit very specific associations between particular risk factors and particular outcomes. These interpretations would be called into question if empirical research showed that risk factors have less specific predictive effects (Green et al., 2010). In addition, evidence that a risk factor has a broad effect on a wide range of disorders would increase interest in that risk factor as an intervention target (Mrazek & Haggerty, 1994). It is noteworthy that not only environmental risk factors but also genes might be generalized risk targets of this sort, as recent studies suggest that some genes have pleiotropic effects that confer risk for a range of psychiatric disorders (Cross-Disorder Group of the Psychiatric Genomics Consortium, 2013).

Although use of latent variable models to study risk factor specificity is only in its infancy, research already has shown considerable value. For example, Kramer, Krueger, and Hicks (2008) found that the widely observed association of gender with MDD became insignificant when controls were included for latent internalizing and externalizing dimensions, arguing that gender is more directly associated with these overall latent dimensions than with MDD or any other disorder within these dimensions. In another example, Kessler and colleagues (2010) found that the effects of childhood adversities on onset of MDD and other individual mental disorders were largely mediated by more direct effects on predispositions for internalizing and externalizing disorders.

One special class of latent variable risk factor studies uses samples of twins to estimate effects of genetic factors on comorbidity. These studies suggest that much of the comorbidity between particular pairs of mental disorders in epidemiological samples, such as eating disorders and substance use disorders (Baker, Mitchell, Neale, & Kendler, 2010) or nicotine dependence and major depression (Lyons et al., 2008), can be explained by a latent variable model that assumes the existence of genetic influences. More elaborate studies have shown that much of the comorbidity among anxiety disorders (Tambs et al., 2009) and among personality disorders (Kendler et al., 2008) can be explained by similar models. Other studies have shown that intergenerational continuity of childhood-onset externalizing disorders can be explained by a similar genetic model (Bornovalova, Hicks, Iacono, & McGue, 2010) and that decomposition of factor analyses into separate additive genetic and environmental components results in stable internalizing and externalizing factors only for genetic, not environmental, influences (Kendler et al., 2011; Kendler, Prescott, Myers, & Neale, 2003).

It is important to note that the findings of strong genetic influences on comorbidity are constrained by the additivity (i.e., no interactions between genetic and environmental effects) and equal environment (i.e., comparability of environmental similarity between identical and nonidentical twins) assumptions needed to identify standard behavior genetic models. These assumptions have long been the subject of controversy. Caution is consequently needed in interpreting these results (Molenaar, 2010). An additional important implication is that the term *genetic* has a much broader meaning than typically appreciated. For example, as noted by Lewontin in 1974, a genetic effect on tryptophan metabolism mediated through "melatin deposition to skin color to hiring discrimination to lower income" would emerge in a standard twin analysis as documenting strong "heritability for 'economic success,'" even if the true driving force behind the association was hiring discrimination based on skin color.

The risk factor studies described above treated latent measures of internalizing and externalizing predispositions as independent variables in causal models that predict individual disorders. Most of these studies used cross-sectional data assessing comorbidity at a point in time, although several studies used longitudinal data to determine whether the structure of internalizing and externalizing disorders is stable over time (Krueger et al., 1998). Other longitudinal studies examined temporal progression (Stein et al., 2001) or sequencing (Newman et al., 1996) between earlier and later disorders and documented strong persistence of disorders over time and predictive associations between some, but not other temporally, primary and later disorders. However, none of these studies investigated the extent to which associations of earlier disorders with later disorders were explained by latent internalizing or externalizing variables. For example, Fergusson, Horwood, and Ridder (2007) found that childhood conduct disorder but not attention-deficit/hyperactivity disorder (ADHD) predicted subsequent onset of substance disorders, whereas Beesdo and colleagues (2007) found that temporally primary social anxiety disorder predicted subsequent onset and persistence of MDD. However, they did not study whether these associations were due to effects of latent internalizing or externalizing predispositions.

More recent studies have examined the extent to which latent internalizing and externalizing predispositions might account for development of lifetime comorbidity between MDD and other disorders based on analysis of large-scale community epidemiological surveys that assess lifetime prevalence of mental disorders and use retrospectively reported information on AOO to study time-lagged associations (Kessler, Cox, et al., 2011; Kessler, Ormel, et al., 2011; Kessler, Petukhova, & Zaslavsky, 2011). These analyses find good fit of a latent variable model, suggesting that common causal pathways account for most comorbidities of MDD with other disorders, although evidence exists that MDD and generalized anxiety disorder (GAD) have significant residual associations. The latter might be due to symptom overlap between MDD and GAD (Cramer, Waldorp, van der Maas, & Borsboom, 2010). Thus far, though, all of these analyses have focused on predicting lifetime first onset of MDD using retrospective analyses. A new study based on a large multiwave longitudinal study is currently under way to determine whether the retrospective results can be replicated and extended to study onset and persistence of disorders over time (Beesdo et al., 2009; Beesdo, Pine, Lieb, & Wittchen, 2010).

Clinical Severity

The NCS-R is the only large U.S. national survey that assessed MDD clinical severity. Respondents who met criteria for 12-month MDD were administered the Quick Inventory of Depressive Symptomatology Self-Report (QIDS-SR; Rush, Carmody, & Reimitz, 2000) to assess symptom severity in the worst month of the past year. The QIDS-SR is strongly related to the Hamilton Rating Scale for Depression (HAM-D; Hamilton, 1960). Transformation rules converted QIDS-SR scores into clinical severity categories mapped to conventional HAM-D ranges of *none* (i.e., not clinically depressed), *mild, moderate, severe*, and *very severe*. Over 99% of respondents with 12-month MDD were independently classified by the QIDS-SR as being clinically depressed during the worst month of the year, with 10.4% having mild, 38.6% moderate, 38.0% severe, and 12.9% very severe depression. QIDS-SR mild through severe cases had average episode durations of

13.8–16.6 weeks, whereas very severe cases had average episode duration of 23.1 weeks during the year. Symptom severity was strongly related to role impairment and comorbidity. These results speak directly to the concern that prevalence estimates in community surveys might be upwardly biased due to the inclusion of clinically insignificant cases (Narrow, Rae, Robins, & Regier, 2002). The NCS-R results show this concern is not warranted with respect to MDD.

CONSEQUENCES OF DEPRESSION

Psychiatric epidemiologists have traditionally been much more interested in discovering modifiable risk factors (Eaton & Weil, 1955) than in documenting adverse consequences of mental illness (Faris & Dunham, 1939). This situation has changed in recent years, though, because the rise of evidence-based medicine has made it necessary to document societal costs of illness (Gold, Siegel, Russell, & Weinstein, 1996). MDD has emerged as an important disorder in this new work because MDD has been ranked as one of the most burdensome diseases in the world in terms of total disability-adjusted life years (Murray et al., 2012). This high ranking is due to a combination of high lifetime prevalence, early AOO, high chronicity, and high role impairment. Only a brief overview of the studies of impairment in MDD is presented here, with a focus on effects on role incumbency, role performance, morbidity, and mortality. A more detailed review is presented elsewhere (Kessler, 2012).

Life-Course Role Incumbency, Timing, and Transitions

Given its typically early AOO, MDD might be expected to have adverse effects on critical developmental transitions such as educational attainment and timing of marriage. Numerous epidemiological studies have examined these effects. These studies show that MDD and other early-onset mental disorders predict termination of education (Breslau, Lane, Sampson, & Kessler, 2008) and difficulties becoming married (Breslau et al., 2011). Other studies show that premarital MDD predicts divorce. Other studies have examined associations of MDD with employment emphasizing the impact of job loss on MDD rather than MDD as a risk factor for job loss (Dooley, Fielding, & Levi, 1996). However, a recent analysis from the WMH surveys documented the latter association by showing that history of MDD as of the age of completing schooling predicted current (at the time of interview) unemployment and work disability (Kawakami et al., 2012).

Role Performance

A considerable body of research shows that MDD predicts impaired role performance, with a special focus on marital quality and work performance. It has long been known that marital dissatisfaction and discord are strongly related to depressive symptoms (Culp & Beach, 1998; Whisman, 1999). Fewer studies have considered the effects of MDD (Coyne, Thompson, & Palmer, 2002), but the latter studies consistently document significant adverse effects. Considerable research documents that physical violence perpetration and victimization in marital relationships are both significantly associated with MDD (Stith, Smith, Penn, Ward, & Tritt, 2004). Although these studies have generally focused on adverse mental health *consequences* of relationship violence (Afifi et al., 2009), a growing body of research has more recently suggested that marital violence is partly a consequence of preexisting mental disorders (Kessler, Molnar, Feurer, & Appelbaum, 2001). Indeed, longitudinal studies consistently find that premarital history of MDD predicts subsequent marital violence perpetration (Fang, Massetti, Ouyang, Grosse, & Mercy, 2010) and victimization (Stith et al., 2004).

Considerable research has examined days out of role associated with various physical and mental disorders (Alonso et al., 2004). These studies typically find MDD associated with one of the highest numbers of days out of role at the societal level of any physical or mental disorder due to its combination of high prevalence and strong individual-level effects. In the WMH surveys, for example, 62,971 respondents across 24 countries were assessed for a wide range of common physical and mental disorders, as well as for days out of role in the 30 days before interview (Alonso et al., 2011). MDD was associated with 5.1% of all days out of role, the fourth highest population attributable risk proportion of all disorders considered (exceeded only by headache/migraine, other chronic pain conditions, and cardiovascular disorders) and by far the largest among the mental disorders. A number of epidemiological surveys in the United States have estimated the workplace costs of MDD in absenteeism and low work performance (often referred to as *presenteeism*; Greenberg et al., 2003). These studies found that MDD significantly predicts overall lost work performance. Several studies attempted to estimate the annual salary-equivalent human capital value of these losses. These estimates were in the range of $30.1 billion (Stewart, Ricci, Chee, Hahn, & Morganstein, 2003) to $51.5 billion (Greenberg et al., 2003).

A number of community surveys, most of them carried out in the United States, examined comparative effects of diverse illnesses on various aspects of role functioning (Merikangas et al., 2007). Results typically showed that musculoskeletal disorders and MDD were associated with the highest levels of disability at the societal level among all commonly occurring disorders assessed. The most compelling study of this sort outside the United States was based on 15 national surveys carried out as part of the WMH surveys (Ormel et al., 2008). Disorder-specific disability scores were compared across people who experienced each of 10 chronic physical disorders and 10 mental disorders in the year before the interview. MDD and bipolar disorder were the mental disorders most often rated as severely impairing in both developed and developing countries. None of the physical disorders considered had impairment levels as high as these mood disorders despite the fact that the physical disorders included severe conditions such as cancer, diabetes, and heart disease. Nearly all the higher mental than physical ratings were statistically significant at the .05 level. Another set of surveys examined comparative decrements in perceived health associated with a wide range of disorders (Moussavi et al., 2007). MDD was one of the three disorders associated with the highest decrements in perceived health in these studies.

Morbidity and Mortality

It is well established that MDD is significantly associated with many chronic physical disorders, including arthritis, asthma, cancer, cardiovascular disease, diabetes, hypertension, chronic respiratory disorders, and a variety of chronic pain conditions (Baxter, Charlson, Somerville, & Whiteford, 2011). Although most data documenting these associations come from clinical samples, similar data exist in community epidemiological surveys. These associations have considerable individual and public health significance and can be thought of as representing costs of MDD in at least two ways. First, to the extent that MDD is a causal risk factor, it leads to increased prevalence of physical disorders. Evidence about MDD as a cause is spotty, though, although we know from meta-analyses of longitudinal studies that MDD is a consistent predictor of subsequent first onset of coronary artery disease, stroke, diabetes, heart attacks, and certain types of cancer. A number of biologically plausible mechanisms have been proposed to explain the prospective associations of MDD with these disorders (de Jonge et al., 2010). Second, even if MDD is a consequence rather than a cause of chronic physical disorders, comorbid MDD is often associated with a worse course of the physical disorder (Gillen, Tennen, McKee, Gernert-Dott, & Affleck, 2001), possibly through nonadherence to treatment regimens (Ziegelstein et al., 2000). Based on these considerations, it is not surprising that MDD is associated with elevated risk of early death (Carney, Freedland, Miller, & Jaffe, 2002). This is true not only because people with MDD have high suicide risk but also because MDD is associated with elevated risk of many types of disorders and with elevated mortality risk among people with certain kinds of disorders.

CONCLUSIONS AND FUTURE DIRECTIONS

Epidemiological evidence shows that MDD is a commonly occurring, seriously impairing, and often undertreated disorder. MDD occurs in the context of a very high prevalence of depressed mood and a high prevalence of subsyndromal depressive episodes. MDD is often recurrent and is typically comorbid with other mental disorders that are usually temporally primary in the sense that first lifetime onset of MDD usually occurs after the onset of at least one other lifetime comorbid disorder. Future efforts such as the NIMH RDoC initiative will be needed to identify the neural circuitry, disease mechanisms, and critical periods underlying depression—information essential to improving our current diagnostic, therapeutic, and prevention strategies. Progress in these areas is sorely needed, as evidenced by the structural impairments that occur subsequent to the onset of MDD, including low educational attainment, poor marital outcomes, and poor socioeconomic outcomes. The day-to-day role impairments that occur in conjunction with MDD include poor performance in both productive and social roles. Increased efforts are needed to document the cost-effectiveness of expanded depression treatment and of treatment-quality improvement initiatives. Because employers play such a large part in driving health insurance benefit design in the United States, it is especially important to document the return on investment of expanded depression outreach and treatment from the employer perspective. We also need to expand research on modifiable barriers to help seeking for depression and to evaluate the effectiveness of systematic depression screening and outreach programs designed to increase the proportion of people with depression who seek treatment.

ACKNOWLEDGMENTS

Preparation of this chapter was supported in part by Janssen Pharmaceutical Research and Development and the U.S. Public Health Service (Grant Nos. MH46376, MH49098, MH528611, MH061941, U01-MH060220, and R01-MH070884). Peter de Jonge is supported by a VICI grant (No. 91812607) from the Netherlands Research Foundation (NWO-ZonMW). Marsha A. Wilcox is an employee of Janssen. Portions of this chapter have appeared previously in Kessler et al. (2003), copyright 2003 by the American Medical Association; Kessler, Cox, et al. (2011), copyright 2011 by Wiley Periodicals, Inc.; and Kessler (2012), copyright 2012 by Elsevier. All used with permission. We appreciate the helpful comments of the editors.

REFERENCES

Afifi, T. O., MacMillan, H., Cox, B. J., Asmundson, G. J., Stein, M. B., & Sareen, J. (2009). Mental health correlates of intimate partner violence in marital relationships in a nationally representative sample of males and females. *Journal of Interpersonal Violence, 24*(8), 1398–1417.

Alonso, J., Angermeyer, M. C., Bernert, S., Bruffaerts, R., Brugha, T. S., Bryson, H., et al. (2004). Disability and quality of life impact of mental disorders in Europe: Results from the European Study of the Epidemiology of Mental Disorders (ESEMeD) project. *Acta Psychiatrica Scandinavica Supplementum* (420), 38–46.

Alonso, J., Petukhova, M., Vilagut, G., Chatterji, S., Heeringa, S., Üstün, T. B., et al. (2011). Days out of role due to common physical and mental conditions: Results from the WHO World Mental Health surveys. *Molecular Psychiatry, 16*(12), 1234–1246.

Altamura, A. C., Buoli, M., Dell'osso, B., Albano, A., Serati, M., Colombo, F., et al. (2011). The impact of brief depressive episodes on the outcome of bipolar disorder and major depressive disorder: A 1-year prospective study. *Journal of Affective Disorders, 134*(1–3), 133–137.

Andrews, G., Goldberg, D. P., Krueger, R. F., Carpenter, W. T., Hyman, S. E., Sachdev, P., et al. (2009). Exploring the feasibility of a meta-structure for DSM-IV and ICD-11: Could it improve utility and validity? *Psychological Medicine, 39*, 1993–2000.

Ayuso-Mateos, J. L., Nuevo, R., Verdes, E., Naidoo, N., & Chatterji, S. (2010). From depressive symptoms to depressive disorders: The relevance of thresholds. *British Journal of Psychiatry, 196*(5), 365–371.

Baker, J. H., Mitchell, K. S., Neale, M. C., & Kendler, K. S. (2010). Eating disorder symptomatology and substance use disorders: Prevalence and shared risk in a population based twin sample. *International Journal of Eating Disorders, 43*(7), 648–658.

Baumeister, H., & Parker, G. (2012). Meta-review of depressive subtyping models. *Journal of Affective Disorders, 139*(2), 126–140.

Baxter, A. J., Charlson, F. J., Somerville, A. J., & Whiteford, H. A. (2011). Mental disorders as risk factors: Assessing the evidence for the Global Burden of Disease Study. *BMC Medicine, 9*, 134.

Beesdo, K., Bittner, A., Pine, D. S., Stein, M. B., Hofler, M., Lieb, R., et al. (2007). Incidence of social anxiety disorder and the consistent risk for secondary depression in the first three decades of life. *Archives of General Psychiatry, 64*(8), 903–912.

Beesdo, K., Hofler, M., Gloster, A., Klotsche, J., Lieb, R., Beauducel, A., et al. (2009). The structure of common mental disorders: A replication study in a community sample of adolescents and young adults. *International Journal of Methods in Psychiatric Research, 18*(4), 204–220.

Beesdo, K., Pine, D. S., Lieb, R., & Wittchen, H. U. (2010). Incidence and risk patterns of anxiety and depressive disorders and categorization of generalized anxiety disorder. *Archives of General Psychiatry, 67*(1), 47–57.

Berk, R. (2008). *Statistical learning from a regression perspective.* New York: Springer-Verlag.

Blazer, D. G., Kessler, R. C., & Swartz, M. S. (1998). Epidemiology of recurrent major and minor depression with a seasonal pattern: The National Comorbidity Survey. *British Journal of Psychiatry, 172*, 164–167.

Booker, J. M., & Hellekson, C. J. (1992). Prevalence of seasonal affective disorder in Alaska. *American Journal of Psychiatry, 149*(9), 1176–1182.

Bornovalova, M. A., Hicks, B. M., Iacono, W. G., & McGue, M. (2010). Familial transmission and heritability of childhood disruptive disorders. *American Journal of Psychiatry, 167*(9), 1066–1074.

Breiman, L., Friedman, J., Olshen, R., & Stone, C. (1984). *Classification and regression trees.* Belmont, CA: Wadsworth.

Breslau, J., Lane, M., Sampson, N., & Kessler, R. C. (2008). Mental disorders and subsequent educational attainment in a U.S. national sample. *Journal of Psychiatric Research, 42*(9), 708–716.

Breslau, J., Miller, E., Jin, R., Sampson, N. A., Alonso, J., Andrade, L. H., et al. (2011). A multinational study of mental disorders, marriage, and divorce. *Acta Psychiatrica Scandinavica, 124*(6), 474–486.

Bromet, E., Andrade, L. H., Hwang, I., Sampson, N. A., Alonso, J., de Girolamo, G., et al. (2011). Cross-national epidemiology of DSM-IV major depressive episode. *BMC Medicine, 9,* 90.

Campagne, D. M., & Campagne, G. (2007). The premenstrual syndrome revisited. *European Journal of Obstetrics, Gynecology, and Reproductive Biology, 130*(1), 4–17.

Carney, R. M., Freedland, K. E., Miller, G. E., & Jaffe, A. S. (2002). Depression as a risk factor for cardiac mortality and morbidity: A review of potential mechanisms. *Journal of Psychosomatic Research, 53*(4), 897–902.

Compton, W. M., Conway, K. P., Stinson, F. S., & Grant, B. F. (2006). Changes in the prevalence of major depression and comorbid substance use disorders in the United States between 1991–1992 and 2001–2002. *American Journal of Psychiatry, 163*(12), 2141–2147.

Cox, B. J., & Swinson, R. P. (2002). Instrument to assess depersonalization–derealization in panic disorder. *Depression and Anxiety, 15*(4), 172–175.

Coyne, J. C., Thompson, R., & Palmer, S. C. (2002). Marital quality, coping with conflict, marital complaints, and affection in couples with a depressed wife. *Journal of Family Psychology, 16*(1), 26–37.

Cramer, A. O., Waldorp, L. J., van der Maas, H. L., & Borsboom, D. (2010). Comorbidity: A network perspective. *Behavioral and Brain Sciences, 33*(2–3), 137–150; discussion, 150–193.

Cross-Disorder Group of the Psychiatric Genomics Consortium. (2013). Identification of risk loci with shared effects on five major psychiatric disorders: A genome-wide analysis. *Lancet, 381,* 1371–1379.

Culp, L. N., & Beach, S. R. H. (1998). Marriage and depressive symptoms: The role and bases of self-esteem differ by gender. *Psychology of Women Quarterly, 22*(4), 647–663.

de Graaf, R., ten Have, M., van Gool, C., & van Dorsselaer, S. (2012). Prevalence of mental disorders and trends from 1996 to 2009: Results from the Netherlands Mental Health Survey and Incidence Study-2. *Social Psychiatry and Psychiatric Epidemiology, 47*(2), 203–213.

de Jonge, P., Rosmalen, J. G., Kema, I. P., Doornbos, B., van Melle, J. P., Pouwer, F., et al. (2010). Psychophysiological biomarkers explaining the association between depression and prognosis in coronary artery patients: A critical review of the literature. *Neuroscience and Biobehavioral Reviews, 35*(1), 84–90.

Derogatis, L. R. (1977). *SCL-90 administration, scoring and procedures manual for the revised version.* Baltimore: Johns Hopkins University.

Di Giulio, G., & Reissing, E. D. (2006). Premenstrual dysphoric disorder: Prevalence, diagnostic considerations, and controversies. *Journal of Psychosomatic Obstetrics and Gynecology, 27*(4), 201–210.

Dooley, D., Fielding, J., & Levi, L. (1996). Health and unemployment. *Annual Review of Public Health, 17,* 449–465.

Eaton, J. W., & Weil, R. J. (1955). *Culture and mental disorders.* Glencoe, IL: Free Press.

Fang, X., Massetti, G. M., Ouyang, L., Grosse, S. D., & Mercy, J. A. (2010). Attention-deficit/hyperactivity disorder, conduct disorder, and young adult intimate partner violence. *Archives of General Psychiatry, 67*(11), 1179–1186.

Faris, R., & Dunham, H. (1939). *Mental disorders in urban areas.* Chicago: University of Chicago Press.

Fergusson, D. M., Horwood, L. J., & Ridder, E. M. (2007). Conduct and attentional problems in childhood and adolescence and later substance use, abuse and dependence: Results of a 25-year longitudinal study. *Drug and Alcohol Dependence, 88*(Suppl. 1), S14–26.

First, M. B., Spitzer, R. L., & Williams, J. B. W. (1990). Exclusionary principles and the comorbidity of psychiatric diagnoses: A historical review and implications for the future. In J. D. Maser & C. R. Cloninger (Eds.), *Comorbidity of mood and anxiety disorders* (pp. 83–109). Washington, DC: American Psychiatric Press.

Frances, A., Manning, D., Marin, D., Kocsis, J., McKinney, K., Hall, W., et al. (1992). Relationship of anxiety and depression. *Psychopharmacology, 106*(Suppl.), S82–86.

Freeman, E. W., DeRubeis, R. J., & Rickels, K. (1996). Reliability and validity of a daily diary for premenstrual syndrome. *Psychiatry Research, 65*(2), 97–106.

Freeman, E. W., Rickels, K., Sondheimer, S. J., & Polansky, M. (1999). Differential response to antidepressants in women with premenstrual syndrome/premenstrual dysphoric disorder: A randomized controlled trial. *Archives of General Psychiatry, 56*(10), 932–939.

Gamma, A., Angst, J., Ajdacic, V., Eich, D., & Rossler, W. (2007). The spectra of neurasthenia and depression: Course, stability and transitions. *European Archives of Psychiatry and Clinical Neuroscience, 257*(2), 120–127.

Gillen, R., Tennen, H., McKee, T. E., Gernert-Dott, P., & Affleck, G. (2001). Depressive symptoms and history of depression predict rehabilitation efficiency in stroke patients. *Archives of Physical Medicine and Rehabilitation, 82*(12), 1645–1649.

Giuffra, L. A., & Risch, N. (1994). Diminished recall and the cohort effect of major depression: A stimulation study. *Psychological Medicine, 24*(2), 375–383.

Gold, M. R., Siegel, J. E., Russell, L. B., & Weinstein, M. C. (1996). *Cost-effectiveness in health and medicine.* New York: Oxford University Press.

Goldberg, D. P. (1972). *The detection of psychiatric illness by questionnaire: A technique for the identification and assessment of non-psychotic psychiatric illness.* London: Oxford University Press.

Goldberg, D. P., Krueger, R. F., Andrews, G., & Hobbs, M. J. (2009). Emotional disorders: Cluster 4 of the proposed meta-structure for DSM-IV and ICD-11. *Psychological Medicine, 39,* 2043–2059.

Green, J. G., McLaughlin, K. A., Berglund, P. A., Gruber, M. J., Sampson, N. A., Zaslavsky, A. M., et al. (2010). Childhood adversities and adult psychiatric disorders in the National Comorbidity Survey replication I: Associations with first onset of DSM-IV disorders. *Archives of General Psychiatry, 67*(2), 113–123.

Greenberg, P. E., Kessler, R. C., Birnbaum, H. G., Leong, S. A., Lowe, S. W., Berglund, P. A., et al. (2003). The economic burden of depression in the United States: How did it change between 1990 and 2000? *Journal of Clinical Psychiatry, 64*(12), 1465–1475.

Halbreich, U. (1997). Premenstrual dysphoric disorders: A diversified cluster of vulnerability traits to depression. *Acta Psychiatrica Scandinavica, 95*(3), 169–176.

Hamilton, M. (1960). A rating scale for depression. *Journal of Neurology, Neurosurgery and Psychiatry, 23,* 56–62.

Hardeveld, F., Spijker, J., De Graaf, R., Nolen, W. A., & Beekman, A. T. (2013). Recurrence of major depressive disorder and its predictors in the general population: Results from the Netherlands Mental Health Survey and Incidence Study (NEMESIS). *Psychological Medicine, 43*(1), 39–48.

Haro, J. M., Arbabzadeh-Bouchez, S., Brugha, T. S., de Girolamo, G., Guyer, M. E., Jin, R., et al. (2006). Concordance of the Composite International Diagnostic Interview Version 3.0 (CIDI 3.0) with standardized clinical assessments in the WHO World Mental Health surveys. *International Journal of Methods in Psychiatric Research, 15*(4), 167–180.

Hastie, T., Tibshirani, R., & Friedman, J. (2009). *The elements of statistical learning: Data mining, inference, and prediction* (2nd ed.). New York: Springer-Verlag.

Joel, I., Begley, A. E., Mulsant, B. H., Lenze, E. J., Mazumdar, S., Dew, M. A., et al. (2014). Dynamic prediction of treatment response in late-life depression. *American Journal of Geriatric Psychiatry, 22*(2), 167–176.

Judd, L. L., Akiskal, H. S., & Paulus, M. P. (1997). The role and clinical significance of subsyndromal depressive symptoms (SSD) in unipolar major depressive disorder. *Journal of Affective Disorders, 45*(1–2), 5–17; discussion, 17–18.

Kawakami, N., Abdulghani, E. A., Alonso, J., Bromet, E., Bruffaerts, R., & Caldas de Almeida, J. M. (2012). Early-life mental disorders and adult household income in the World Mental Health Surveys. *Biological Psychiatry, 72*(3), 228–237.

Kendler, K. S., Aggen, S. H., Czajkowski, N., Roysamb, E., Tambs, K., Torgersen, S., et al. (2008). The structure of genetic and environmental risk factors for DSM-IV personality disorders: A multivariate twin study. *Archives of General Psychiatry, 65*(12), 1438–1446.

Kendler, K. S., Aggen, S. H., Knudsen, G. P., Roysamb, E., Neale, M. C., & Reichborn-Kjennerud, T. (2011). The structure of genetic and environmental risk factors for syndromal and subsyndromal common DSM-IV axis I and all axis II disorders. *American Journal of Psychiatry, 168*(1), 29–39.

Kendler, K. S., Prescott, C. A., Myers, J., & Neale, M. C. (2003). The structure of genetic and environmental risk factors for common psychiatric and substance use disorders in men and women. *Archives of General Psychiatry, 60*(9), 929–937.

Kendler, K. S., Walters, E. E., & Kessler, R. C. (1997). The prediction of length of major depressive episodes: Results from an epidemiological sample of female twins. *Psychological Medicine, 27*(1), 107–117.

Kessler, R. C. (2012). The costs of depression. *Psychiatric Clinics of North America, 35*(1), 1–14.

Kessler, R. C., Aguilar-Gaxiola, S., Alonso, J., Angermeyer, M. C., Anthony, J. C., Brugha, T. S., et al. (2008). Prevalence and severity of mental disorders in the World Mental Health Survey Initiative. In R. C. Kessler & T. B. Üstün (Eds.), *The WHO World Mental Health Surveys: Global perspectives on the epidemiology of mental disorders* (pp. 534–540). New York: Cambridge University Press.

Kessler, R. C., Angermeyer, M., Anthony, J. C., De Graaf, R., Demyttenaere, K., Gasquet, I., et al. (2007). Lifetime prevalence and age-of-onset distributions of mental disorders in the World Health Organization's World Mental Health Survey Initiative. *World Psychiatry, 6*(3), 168–176.

Kessler, R. C., Avenevoli, S., & Merikangas, K. (2001). Mood disorders in children and adolescents: An epidemiologic perspective. *Biological Psychiatry, 49*(12), 1002–1014.

Kessler, R. C., Berglund, P., Demler, O., Jin, R., Koretz, D., Merikangas, K. R., et al. (2003). The epidemiology of major depressive disorder: Results from the National Comorbidity Survey Replication (NCS-R). *Journal of the American Medical Association, 289*, 3095–3105.

Kessler, R. C., Berglund, P., Demler, O., Jin, R., & Walters, E. E. (2005). Lifetime prevalence and age-of-onset distributions of DSM-IV disorders in the National Comorbidity Survey Replication. *Archives of General Psychiatry, 62*(6), 593–602.

Kessler, R. C., & Bromet, E. J. (2013). The epidemiology of depression across cultures. *Annual Review of Public Health, 34*, 119–138.

Kessler, R. C., Cox, B. J., Green, J. G., Ormel, J., McLaughlin, K. A., Merikangas, K. R., et al. (2011). The effects of latent variables in the development of comorbidity among common mental disorders. *Depression and Anxiety, 28*(1), 29–39.

Kessler, R. C., Demler, O., Frank, R. G., Olfson, M., Pincus, H. A., Walters, E. E., et al. (2005). Prevalence and treatment of mental disorders, 1990 to 2003. *New England Journal of Medicine, 352*, 2515–2523.

Kessler, R. C., McLaughlin, K. A., Green, J. G., Gruber, M. J., Sampson, N. A., Zaslavsky, A. M., et al. (2010). Childhood adversities and adult psychopathology in the WHO World Mental Health Surveys. *British Journal of Psychiatry, 197*(5), 378–385.

Kessler, R. C., Molnar, B. E., Feurer, I. D., & Appelbaum, M. (2001). Patterns and mental health predictors of domestic violence in the United States: Results from the National Comorbidity Survey. *International Journal of Law and Psychiatry, 24*(4–5), 487–508.

Kessler, R. C., Ormel, J., Petukhova, M., McLaughlin, K. A., Green, J. G., Russo, L. J., et al. (2011). Development of lifetime comorbidity in the World Health Organization World Mental Health Surveys. *Archives of General Psychiatry, 68*(1), 90–100.

Kessler, R. C., Petukhova, M., & Zaslavsky, A. M. (2011). The role of latent internalizing and externalizing predispositions in accounting for the development of comorbidity among common mental disorders. *Current Opinion in Psychiatry, 24*(4), 307–312.

Kessler, R. C., & Walters, E. E. (1998). Epidemiology of DSM-III-R major depression and minor depression among adolescents and young adults in the National Comorbidity Survey. *Depression and Anxiety, 7*(1), 3–14.

Klein, D. N., Glenn, C. R., Kosty, D. B., Seeley, J. R., Rohde, P., & Lewinsohn, P. M. (2013). Predictors of first lifetime onset of major depressive disorder in young adulthood. *Journal of Abnormal Psychology, 122*(1), 1–6.

Kraemer, H. C., Kazdin, A. E., Offord, D. R., Kessler, R. C., Jensen, P. S., & Kupfer, D. J. (1997). Coming to terms with the terms of risk. *Archives of General Psychiatry, 54*(4), 337–343.

Kramer, M. D., Krueger, R. F., & Hicks, B. M. (2008). The role of internalizing and externalizing liability factors in accounting for gender differences in the prevalence of common psychopathological syndromes. *Psychological Medicine, 38*(1), 51–61.

Krueger, R. F. (1999). The structure of common mental disorders. *Archives of General Psychiatry, 56*(10), 921–926.

Krueger, R. F., Caspi, A., Moffitt, T. E., & Silva, P. A. (1998). The structure and stability of common mental disorders (DSM-III-R): A longitudinal-epidemiological study. *Journal of Abnormal Psychology, 107*(2), 216–227.

Krueger, R. F., & Finger, M. S. (2001). Using item response theory to understand comorbidity among anxiety and unipolar mood disorders. *Psychological Assessment, 13*(1), 140–151.

Krueger, R. F., & Markon, K. E. (2006a). Reinterpreting comorbidity: A model-based approach to understanding and classifying psychopathology. *Annual Review of Clinical Psychology, 2*, 111–133.

Krueger, R. F., & Markon, K. E. (2006b). Understanding psychopathology: Melding behavior genetics, personality, and quantitative psychology to develop an empirically based model. *Current Directions in Psychological Science, 15*(3), 113–117.

Lahey, B. B., Rathouz, P. J., Van Hulle, C., Urbano, R. C., Krueger, R. F., Applegate, B., et al. (2008). Testing structural models of DSM-IV symptoms of common forms of child and adolescent psychopathology. *Journal of Abnormal Child Psychology, 36*(2), 187–206.

Leighton, D. C., Harding, J. S., & Macklin, D. B. (1963). *The Stirling County Study: Vol. 3. The character of danger.* New York: Basic Books.

Lewinsohn, P. M., Rohde, P., Seeley, J. R., & Fischer, S. A. (1991). Age and depression: Unique and shared effects. *Psychology and Aging, 6*(2), 247–260.

Lewontin, R. C. (1974). Annotation: The analysis of variance and the analysis of causes. *American Journal of Human Genetics, 26*(3), 400–411.

Link, B. G., & Dohrenwend, B. P. (1980). Formulation of hypotheses about the true relevance of demoralization in the United States. In B. P. Dohrenwend, B. S. Dohrenwend, M. Schwarz-Gould, B. Link, R. Neugebauer & R. Wunsch-Hitzig (Eds.), *Mental illness in the United States: Epidemiological estimates* (pp. 114–132). New York: Praeger.

Lyons, M., Hitsman, B., Xian, H., Panizzon, M. S., Jerskey, B. A., Santangelo, S., et al. (2008). A twin study of smoking, nicotine dependence, and major depression in men. *Nicotine and Tobacco Research, 10*(1), 97–108.

McKenzie, D. P., Toumbourou, J. W., Forbes, A. B., Mackinnon, A. J., McMorris, B. J., Catalano, R. F., et al. (2011). Predicting future depression in adolescents using the Short Mood and Feelings Questionnaire: A two-nation study. *Journal of Affective Disorders, 134*(1–3), 151–159.

McLeod, J. D., Kessler, R. C., & Landis, K. R. (1992). Speed of recovery from major depressive episodes in a community sample of married men and women. *Journal of Abnormal Psychology, 101*(2), 277–286.

Meeks, T. W., Vahia, I. V., Lavretsky, H., Kulkarni, G., & Jeste, D. V. (2011). A tune in "a minor" can "b major": A review of epidemiology, illness course, and public health implications of subthreshold depression in older adults. *Journal of Affective Disorders, 129*(1–3), 126–142.

Merikangas, K. R., Ames, M., Cui, L., Stang, P. E., Üstün, T. B., Von Korff, M., et al. (2007). The impact of comorbidity of mental and physical conditions on role disability in the U.S. adult household population. *Archives of General Psychiatry, 64*(10), 1180–1188.

Merikangas, K. R., & Angst, J. (1995). The challenge of depressive disorders in adolescence. In M. Rutter (Ed.), *Psychosocial disturbances in young people: Challenges for prevention* (pp. 131–165). Cambridge, UK: Cambridge University Press.

Molenaar, P. C. M. (2010). On the limits of standard quantitative genetic modeling of inter-individual variation: Extensions, ergodic conditions and a new genetic factor model of intra-individual variation. In K. E. Hood, C. T. Halpern, G. Greenberg, & R. M. Lerner (Eds.), *Handbook of developmental science, behavior, and genetics.* (pp. 626–648). Malden, MA: Blackwell.

Moussavi, S., Chatterji, S., Verdes, E., Tandon, A., Patel, V., & Üstün, T. B. (2007). Depression, chronic diseases, and decrements in health: Results from the World Health Surveys. *Lancet, 370*, 851–858.

Mrazek, P. J., & Haggerty, R. J. (1994). *Reducing risks for mental disorders: Frontiers for preventive intervention research.* Washington, DC: National Academy Press.

Murphy, J. M., Laird, N. M., Monson, R. R., Sobol, A. M., & Leighton, A. H. (2000). A 40-year perspective on the prevalence of depression: The Stirling County Study. *Archives of General Psychiatry, 57*(3), 209–215.

Murray, C. J., Vos, T., Lozano, R., Naghavi, M., Flaxman, A. D., Michaud, C., et al. (2012). Disability-adjusted life years (DALYs) for 291 diseases and injuries in 21 regions, 1990–2010: A systematic analysis for the Global Burden of Disease Study 2010. *Lancet, 380*, 2197–2223.

Narrow, W. E., Rae, D. S., Robins, L. N., & Regier, D. A. (2002). Revised prevalence estimates of mental disorders in the United States: Using a clinical significance criterion to reconcile 2 surveys' estimates. *Archives of General Psychiatry, 59*(2), 115–123.

Nelson, J. C., Zhang, Q., Deberdt, W., Marangell, L. B., Karamustafalioglu, O., & Lipkovich, I. A. (2012). Predictors of remission with placebo using an integrated study database from patients with major depressive disorder. *Current Medical Research and Opinion, 28*(3), 325–334.

Newman, D. L., Moffitt, T. E., Caspi, A., Magdol, L., Silva, P. A., & Stanton, W. R. (1996). Psychiatric disorder in a birth cohort of young adults: Prevalence, comorbidity, clinical significance, and new case incidence from ages 11 to 21. *Journal of Consulting and Clinical Psychology, 64*(3), 552–562.

Ormel, J., Petukhova, M., Chatterji, S., Aguilar-Gaxiola, S., Alonso, J., Angermeyer, M. C., et al.(2008). Disability and treatment of specific mental and physical disorders across the world. *British Journal of Psychiatry, 192*(5), 368–375.

Pettit, J. W., Hartley, C., Lewinsohn, P. M., Seeley, J. R., & Klein, D. N. (2013). Is liability to recurrent major depressive disorder present before first episode onset in adolescence or acquired after the initial episode? *Journal of Abnormal Psychology, 122*(2), 353–358.

Regier, D. A., Narrow, W. E., Rupp, A., Rae, D. S., & Kaelber, C. T. (2000). The epidemiology of mental disorder treatment need: Community estimates of "medical necessity." In G. Andrews & S. Henderson (Eds.), *Unmet need in psychiatry: Problems, resources, responses* (pp. 41–58). Cambridge, UK: Cambridge University Press.

Robins, L. N., Helzer, J. E., Croughan, J., Williams, J. B. W., & Spitzer, R. L. (1981). *NIMH Diagnostic Interview Schedule: Version III.* Rockville, MD: National Institute of Mental Health.

Robins, L. N., & Regier, D. A. (Eds.). (1991). *Psychiatric disorders in America: The Epidemiologic Catchment Area Study.* New York: Free Press.

Robins, L. N., Wing, J., Wittchen, H.-U., Helzer, J. E., Babor, T. F., Burke, J. D., et al. (1988). The Composite International Diagnostic Interview: An epidemiologic instrument suitable for use in conjunction with different diagnostic systems and in different cultures. *Archives of General Psychiatry, 45*(12), 1069–1077.

Rodriguez, M. R., Nuevo, R., Chatterji, S., & Ayuso-Mateos, J. L. (2012). Definitions and factors associated with subthreshold depressive conditions: A systematic review. *BMC Psychiatry, 12*, 181.

Rosenthal, N. E., Sack, D. A., Gillin, J. C., Lewy, A. J., Goodwin, F. K., Davenport, Y., et al. (1984). Seasonal affective disorder. A description of the syndrome and preliminary findings with light therapy. *Archives of General Psychiatry, 41*(1), 72–80.

Rush, A. J., Carmody, T., & Reimitz, P.-E. (2000). The Inventory of Depressive Symptomatology (IDS): Clinician (IDS-C) and Self-Report (IDS-SR) ratings of depressive symptoms. *International Journal of Methods in Psychiatric Research, 9*, 45–59.

Seiler, L. H. (1973). The 22-item scale used in field studies of mental illness: A question of method, a question of substance, and a question of theory. *Journal of Health and Social Behavior, 14*(3), 252–264.

Sheehan, D. V., Lecrubier, Y., Sheehan, K. H., Amorim, P., Janavs, J., Weiller, E., et al. (1998). The Mini-International Neuropsychiatric Interview (M.I.N.I.): The development and validation of a structured diagnostic psychiatric interview for DSM-IV and ICD-10. *Journal of Clinical Psychiatry, 59*(Suppl. 20), 22–33; quiz, 34–57.

Slade, T., & Watson, D. (2006). The structure of common DSM-IV and ICD-10 mental disorders in the Australian general population. *Psychological Medicine, 36*(11), 1593–1600.

Spitzer, R. L., Williams, J. B., Kroenke, K., Linzer, M., deGruy, F. V., III, Hahn, S. R., et al. (1994). Utility of a new procedure for diagnosing mental disorders in primary care: The PRIME-MD 1000 study. *Journal of the American Medical Association, 272,* 1749–1756.

Srole, L., Langner, T. S., Michael, S. T., Opler, M. K., & Rennie, T. A. C. (1962). *Mental health in the metropolis: The Midtown Manhattan Study.* New York: McGraw-Hill.

Stein, M. B., Fuetsch, M., Muller, N., Hofler, M., Lieb, R., & Wittchen, H. U. (2001). Social anxiety disorder and the risk of depression: A prospective community study of adolescents and young adults. *Archives of General Psychiatry, 58*(3), 251–256.

Stewart, W. F., Ricci, J. A., Chee, E., Hahn, S. R., & Morganstein, D. (2003). Cost of lost productive work time among U.S. workers with depression. *Journal of the American Medical Association, 289,* 3135–3144.

Stith, S. M., Smith, D. B., Penn, C. E., Ward, D. B., & Tritt, D. (2004). Intimate partner physical abuse perpetration and victimization risk factors: A meta-analytic review. *Aggression and Violent Behavior, 10*(1), 65–98.

Tambs, K., Czajkowsky, N., Roysamb, E., Neale, M. C., Reichborn-Kjennerud, T., Aggen, S. H., et al. (2009). Structure of genetic and environmental risk factors for dimensional representations of DSM-IV anxiety disorders. *British Journal of Psychiatry, 195*(4), 301–307.

van Loo, H. M., de Jonge, P., Romeijn, J. W., Kessler, R. C., & Schoevers, R. A. (2012). Data-driven subtypes of major depressive disorder: A systematic review. *BMC Medicine, 10,* 156.

Vollebergh, W. A., Iedema, J., Bijl, R. V., de Graaf, R., Smit, F., & Ormel, J. (2001). The structure and stability of common mental disorders: The NEMESIS study. *Archives of General Psychiatry, 58*(6), 597–603.

Wang, P. S., & Kessler, R. C. (2005). Global burden of mood disorders. In D. Stein, D. Kupfer, & A. Schatzberg (Eds.), *Textbook of mood disorders* (pp. 55–67). Washington, DC: American Psychiatric Publishing.

Watson, D. (2005). Rethinking the mood and anxiety disorders: A quantitative hierarchical model for DSM-V. *Journal of Abnormal Psychology, 114*(4), 522–536.

Weissman, M. M., Livingston, B. M., Leaf, P. J., Florio, L. P., & Holzer, C. I. (1991). Affective disorders. In L. N. Robins & D. A. Regier (Eds.), *Psychiatric disorders in America: The Epidemiologic Catchment Area Study* (pp. 53–80). New York: Free Press.

Whisman, M. A. (1999). Marital dissatisfaction and psychiatric disorders: Results from the National Comorbidity Survey. *Journal of Abnormal Psychology, 108*(4), 701–706.

Winer, S. A., & Rapkin, A. J. (2006). Premenstrual disorders: Prevalence, etiology and impact. *Journal of Reproductive Medicine, 51*(Suppl. 4), 339–347.

Wittchen, H. U., Beesdo, K., & Gloster, A. T. (2009). A new meta-structure of mental disorders: A helpful step into the future or a harmful step back to the past? *Psychological Medicine, 39*(12), 2083–2089.

Wittchen, H. U., Beesdo-Baum, K., Gloster, A., Hofler, M., Klotsche, J., Lieb, R., et al. (2009). The structure of mental disorders re-examined: Is it developmentally stable and robust against additions? *International Journal of Methods in Psychiatric Research, 18*(4), 189–203.

Yaroslavsky, I., Pettit, J. W., Lewinsohn, P. M., Seeley, J. R., & Roberts, R. E. (2013). Heterogeneous trajectories of depressive symptoms: Adolescent predictors and adult outcomes. *Journal of Affective Disorders, 148*(2–3), 391–399.

Ziegelstein, R. C., Fauerbach, J. A., Stevens, S. S., Romanelli, J., Richter, D. P., & Bush, D. E. (2000). Patients with depression are less likely to follow recommendations to reduce cardiac risk during recovery from a myocardial infarction. *Archives of Internal Medicine, 160*(12), 1818–1823.

CHAPTER 2

Assessment of Depression

Arthur M. Nezu, Christine Maguth Nezu, Minsun Lee, *and* Jessica B. Stern

We begin this chapter by providing an overview of several depression measures, listed in alphabetical order and divided into two categories—clinician ratings and self-report inventories. Some measures were chosen based on their widespread usage, whereas others were included because of their focus on a specific population (e.g., patients with bipolar disorder or cardiac illness). Due to space limitations, we focus on fewer measures than we did in previous versions of this chapter (e.g., Nezu, Nezu, Friedman, & Lee, 2009), including only those for which we have significantly updated information. We conclude with a final section highlighting important future directions.

CLINICIAN RATINGS

Hamilton Rating Scale for Depression

The Hamilton Rating Scale for Depression (HAMD; Hamilton, 1960) was originally designed to evaluate the severity of depressive symptoms among patients previously diagnosed with a depressive disorder. Historically, the HAMD is the most widely used clinician rating of depression and is often viewed as the "gold standard." The HAMD contains 21 items, only 17 of which are typically scored. It takes approximately 20 minutes to complete based on information gleaned from a semistructured interview. Despite its continued popularity, problems have been identified regarding the reliability and validity of the HAMD (Santor & Coyne, 2001). For example, based on an evaluation of 70 studies that were published subsequent to a major review by Hedlund and Viewig (1979), Bagby, Ryder, Schuller, and Marshall (2004) voiced serious concerns about the status of the HAMD as a gold standard. They examined three major psychometric properties: reliability, item response, and validity. In general, internal, interrater, and retest reliabilities at the *scale* level were acceptable; at the *item* level, however, interrater and retest reliabilities were inconsistent and questionable. Low correlations between the HAMD and the Structured Clinical Interview for DSM-IV (SCID; First, Spitzer, Gibbon, & Williams, 1997) were considered to be problematic. Important features of the DSM-IV definition of depression were not fully captured by the HAMD, and some symptoms were not assessed at all. Although convergent and discriminant validity coefficients were adequate, the multidimensional nature of the HAMD was noted to lead to difficulties in interpreting the meaning of the total score. Bagby and colleagues argued further that because the HAMD was developed several decades ago, many symptoms of depression currently thought to be important (e.g., feelings of worthlessness, concentration difficulties, reverse vegetative symptoms) are not contained in this inventory. They suggested that a substantial revision or complete rejection of the HAMD should be considered based on a contemporary definition of depression.

Despite such controversy, the HAMD has remained a popular instrument and is used with a variety of populations. The advocates for the instrument argue that the HAMD should not be compared with DSM-IV criteria because the two measures have different objectives; whereas the HAMD assesses depression *severity* in patients with depression, DSM-IV defines a *diagnosis* of depression (Corruble & Hardy, 2005). In addition, it has been emphasized that the long-term wide usage of the HAMD can provide continuity in assessment methodology, which allows comparison across decades of studies (Zimmerman, Posternak, & Chelminski, 2005).

A recent meta-analysis, conducted by Trajković and colleagues (2011) and based on 409 articles, examined internal consistency, interrater reliability, and test–retest reliability of the HAMD. The analysis showed that although some studies found low coefficients of reliability, the HAMD exhibits good internal consistency. In addition, this analysis showed that interrater reliability has been increasing throughout the years, as demonstrated by a chronological review of the literature. In an attempt to address the uncertainty over interrater reliability, Kobak, Williams, and Engelhardt (2008) conducted a study comparing the interrater reliability obtained by video conferencing versus that obtained by face-to-face interviews. They found no significant differences between the two methods.

GRID-HAMD

The GRID-HAMD (Kalali et al., 2002) was developed by the Depression Rating Scale Standardization Team (DRSST), formed in 1999 to address concerns regarding the lack of standardization in administering and scoring the HAMD. The DRSST is composed of researchers from academia, the pharmaceutical industry, clinical practice, and government and is sponsored by the International Society for CNS Drug Development. This group presented its recommendations at the 2001 New Clinical Drug Evaluation Unit (NCDEU) conference, sponsored by the National Institute of Mental Health (NIMH), where a new approach to administering and scoring the HAMD was advocated. The GRID-HAMD consists of three components: (1) the GRID scoring structure that operationalizes the intensity and frequency of each item while allowing these to be rated simultaneously; (2) a semistructured guide; and (3) a scoring manual.

Based on studies that examined usability, reliability, and validity of the GRID-HAMD, Williams and colleagues (2008) found the overall interrater reliability and concurrent validity to be high. Specifically, they reported that interrater reliability was .95 and that internal consistency reliability was .78 when the GRID-HAMD was administered to a total of 150 patients with major depressive disorder (MDD) by 29 raters from 10 U.S. investigative sites. With regard to its usability, they reported that 75% of the raters found the GRID-HAMD "very easy" or "easy" to use and that no one rated it "very difficult."

Depression Interview and Structured Hamilton

The Depression Interview and Structured Hamilton (DISH; Freedland et al., 2002) is a semistructured interview developed specifically for the Enhancing Recovery in Coronary Heart Disease (ENRICHD; ENRICHD Investigators, 2000) study, which was a multi-center clinical trial for patients who suffered myocardial infarction. The purpose of the DISH is to (1) screen medical patients for depression; (2) diagnose MDD, dysthymia, and minor depression according to DSM-IV criteria; (3) assess depressive severity using the 17-item HAMD; and (4) document the history and course of a patient's depression.

An initial validity study found that a SCID diagnosis made by either a clinical social worker or a clinical psychologist agreed with a DISH diagnosis (made by a trained nurse or lay interviewer) on 88% of the interviews. In the ENRICHD trial, clinicians agreed with 93% of research nurses' DISH diagnoses. Based on such initial findings, a National Heart, Lung, and Blood Institute (NHLBI) Working Group regarding the assessment and treatment of patients with cardiovascular disease recommended the use of the DISH for "diagnostic ascertainment" with regard to clinical trials (Davidson et al., 2006).

Structured Clinical Interview for DSM-IV Axis I Disorders

The SCID (First et al., 1997) provides a standardized clinical interview to determine DSM-IV (American Psychiatric Association, 1994) differential diagnoses. Six scores are derived for Mood Episodes, Psychotic Symptoms, Psychotic Disorders, Mood Disorders, Substance Use Disorders, and Anxiety and Other Disorders. Although this instrument is structured to match specific DSM-IV diagnostic criteria, it utilizes the skills of trained clinicians by allowing them to probe, restate questions, challenge respondents, and ask for clarification. Administration of the entire SCID ranges from 45 to 90 minutes. In certain cases, however, it is possible to administer specific modules, such as the Mood Disorder module, if time is a factor.

The SCID was first published in 1983 and has evolved along with the revisions of the DSM-III, DSM-III-R, DSM-IV, and DSM-IV-TR. A recent assessment of the interrater reliability of the SCID by Lobbestael, Leurgans, and Arntz (2011) revealed moderate to excellent agreement for the Axis I disorders, and the majority of the categorically and dimensionally measured Axis II disorders were represented by excellent interrater agreement. The actual κ value for a mixed sample of 151 inpatients and outpatients yielded a κ value of 0.66 for major depression and 0.81 for dysthymia.

There are two versions of the SCID: (1) SCID—Clinician Version (SCID-CV; First et al., 1997); and (2) SCID—Research Version (SCID-RV; First, Gibbon, Spitzer, & Williams, 1996). The SCID-RV is longer than the SCID-CV because it contains more disorders, subtypes, severity, and course specifiers. In order to include participants who have limited resources (e.g., lowered income levels, persons with concomitant medical illnesses), the SCID has been conducted over the telephone to overcome transportation or mobility problems. However, one study found that participants were more likely to receive a lifetime diagnosis of MDD after an in-person interview than after a telephone interview (Cacciola, Alterman, Rutherford, McKay, & May, 1999). The SCID has also been administered and evaluated in studies screening for depression in medically ill populations, such as primary care patients (Vuorilehto, Melartin, & Isometsa, 2006).

Screening Assessment of Depression—Polarity

Because patients with bipolar disorder are frequently misdiagnosed with MDD (Hirschfeld, Lewis, & Vornik, 2003), researchers have created procedures to differentiate these diagnostic categories. The Screening Assessment of Depression—Polarity (SAD-P; Solomon et al., 2006) was developed in the NIMH Collaborative Program on the Psychobiology of Depression longitudinal study, which followed individuals with a variety of mood disorders for a median length of 16 years. It is a rating scale composed of three items: The first pertains to the number of prior episodes of major depression; the second item focuses on family history of depression or mania; and the third item addresses the presence of delusions during the current depressive episode. A total score of 2 or greater indicates that the individual's current depressive episode may be part of bipolar illness and that a more in-depth assessment is warranted. Data from the Collaborative Program indicated that the overall sensitivity in accurately identifying patients with bipolar disorder was found to be .82, .72 in the bipolar I cross-validation sample, and .58 in the bipolar II cross-validation sample.

SELF-REPORT MEASURES

Beck Depression Inventory

The Beck Depression Inventory (BDI; Beck, Ward, Mendelson, Mock, & Erbaugh, 1961) is one of the most widely used self-report measures of depressive symptomatology across a variety of patient and nonpatient populations. The original BDI was developed as a clinician rating scale and published by Beck and colleagues in 1961, revised as a self-report instrument in 1971, and revised again (BDI-II) in order to make its symptom content more reflective of DSM-IV criteria (Beck, Steer, & Brown, 1996). Although still composed of 21 items, in contrast to its predecessor, the BDI-II contains four new symptoms—agitation, worthlessness, concentration difficulty, and loss of energy—and now inquires about sleep and appetite *increases*, rather than only decreases. In addition, the time frame for the BDI-II is 2 weeks.

The BDI-II has strong psychometric properties. For example, when the BDI-II was administered to individuals with psychiatric diagnoses and to other populations, such as college students, the measure yielded high internal consistency coefficients ($\alpha = .92$ and .93, respectively) with a test–retest reliability of $r = .93$ (Beck et al., 1996). The BDI-II has been found to consist of two factors—cognitive symptoms (e.g., pessimism, guilt, suicidal thoughts) and somatic–affective symptoms (e.g., sadness, loss of pleasure, crying, agitation). Comparisons between the BDI and the BDI-II suggest that the BDI-II is a stronger instrument in terms of its factor structure (Dozois, Ahnberg, & Dobson, 1998). The BDI-II has also been validated in a primary care setting (Arnau, Meagher, Norris, & Bramson, 2001), as well as in a sample of southern rural African American women (Gary & Yarandi, 2004). Use of the BDI-II as an online measure showed that psychometric properties of the assessment were not lost in the Internet-based approach compared with the in-person method (Holländare, Askerlund, Nieminen, & Engstrom, 2008).

Beck Depression Inventory for Primary Care

The BDI for Primary Care (BDI-PC; Beck, Guth, Steer, & Ball, 1997) is a seven-item screening instrument developed to be a primary care modification of the BDI-II. To avoid confounding between the symptoms of a medical condition that may be due to biological, medical, or substance abuse disorders, the somatic and behavioral symptoms of depression were not included. Thus the BDI-PC minimizes the possibility of yielding spuriously high estimates of depression for patients with medical problems by focusing on psychological/cognitive symptoms, such as sadness, pessimism, past failure, loss of pleasure, self-dislike, self-criticism, and suicidal thoughts or wishes. These seven items were chosen because they loaded strongly ($\geq .35$) on the cognitive dimension of BDI-II scores.

Beck Depression Inventory—Fast Screen

The BDI—Fast Screen (BDI-FS; Beck, Steer, & Brown, 2000) is the most recent version of the BDI-PC and is an abbreviated self-report inventory that was designed to rapidly screen medical patients for depression using criteria from the DSM-IV (American Psychiatric Association, 1994). This measure is composed primarily of the cognitive items of depression, which are included because they are considered to reflect the archetypal mood state of depression independent of medical illness features. Items assessing sadness and loss of interest or pleasure in activities, as well as suicidal thoughts, are also included. The BDI-FS has been found to be a psychometrically sound screening measure for depression in a variety of medical populations, including patients with sickle cell disease (Jenerette, Funk, & Murdaugh, 2005) and individuals diagnosed with multiple sclerosis (Benedict, Fishman, McClellan, Bakshi, & Weinstock-Guttman, 2003).

Cardiac Depression Scale

Research has increasingly documented the high prevalence and incidence of MDD among various cardiac patient populations (Nezu, Nezu, & Jain, 2005; see Freedland & Carney, Chapter 7, this volume). In light of this research, cardiac researchers have sought to develop measures of depression specifically validated on cardiac patient samples. The Cardiac Depression Scale (CDS) represents such a measure and was originally developed and validated in Australia (Hare & Davis, 1996). It consists of 26 items representing symptoms specific to cardiac patients with depression and uses a 7-point Likert-type scale. The CDS has demonstrated high internal consistency, test–retest reliability, and concurrent validity (King, Colella, Faris, & Thompson, 2009; Wise, Harris, & Carter, 2006). A brief, visual analog version of the scale has also been developed for rapid or repeated assessments (Di Benedetto, Lindner, Hare, & Kent, 2005).

According to its authors, the CDS has advantages over other depression scales that have been used for medical populations. For example, it was developed and validated specifically for cardiac patients, whereas other measures were developed and validated in psychiatric populations. Thus the CDS can be more sensitive in detecting the type of depression specific to cardiac patients, which is often characterized as subclinical or "reactive" (Di Benedetto, Lindner, Hare, & Kent, 2006). In addition, the CDS is posited to have psychometric advantages over the BDI, which typically produces a positively skewed distribution; in contrast, CDS scores have a normal distribution, enabling differentiation among scores in the lower range (Hare & Davis, 1996).

The CDS has also been translated into other languages and has been found to have acceptable psychometric properties. For example, Gholizadeh and colleagues (2010) found the Iranian version of the CDS to be a valid and reliable measure of depression in people with heart disease. In addition, Wang, Ski, Thompson, and Hare (2011) evaluated the validity and reliability of the Chinese version of the short form of the CDS as a screening tool and found it to have strong properties, as well as being user-friendly for monitoring depressed mood in Chinese-speaking patients with cardiac disease.

Center for Epidemiologic Studies Depression Scale

The Center for Epidemiologic Studies developed a 20-item self-report scale of depressive symptomatology specifically for the general population (Radloff, 1977). The CES-D has frequently been used in epidemiological studies of depression, as a screening tool for treatment studies, and for measuring change over time in symptom severity. Scale items were originally chosen from previously developed scales in order to represent the major symptoms of clinical depression. The instrument was designed to be brief and takes less than 10 minutes to complete. Based on a principal-components analysis of data from general population samples, four major factors have been identified: depressed affect, positive affect, somatic and retarded activity, and an interpersonal factor (Radloff, 1977).

The CES-D has been used in many countries and has also been adapted to be utilized in computer-assisted and telephone interviews. Studies have indicated that the psychometric properties of the computerized version are equivalent to that of the paper-and-pencil format (Ogles, France, Lunnen, Bell, & Goldfarb, 1998). Furthermore, using the CES-D for voice recognition computer-assisted interviews has been found to be advantageous for overcoming language barriers and disabilities and for educating underserved populations (Muñoz, McQuaid, González, Dimas, & Rosales, 1999).

CES-D-10

This 10-item version was derived from the original CES-D in order to more closely correspond with DSM-IV criteria for depression (Irwin, Artin, & Oxman, 1999). It was also revised to accommodate the needs of older respondents, who may find the response format confusing, the questions emotionally stressful, and the time to complete it burdensome. Another stated purpose for this revision was to retain the advantageous qualities of a measure that has been valuable to community-based researchers while increasing its generalizability to current psychiatric understanding. The CES-D-10 has demonstrated high internal consistency ($\alpha = .87$; Turvey, Wallace, & Herzog, 1999), as well as good specificity (81–93%) and sensitivity (79–100%) when using a cutoff score of ≥ 4 (Irwin et al., 1999). It has been translated into Chinese and found to be a valid measure of depression in both clinical and nonclinical populations (Yu, Lin, & Hsu, 2013).

Hospital Anxiety and Depression Scale

The Hospital Anxiety and Depression Scale (HADS) was initially developed to identify caseness of anxiety and depressive disorders among medical, nonpsychiatric patients (Zigmond & Snaith, 1983). Fourteen items are equally distributed into two subscales—Anxiety and Depression. To prevent overlap and inflated associations with somatic disorders, all symptoms of either anxiety or depression also relating to physical disorders (e.g., headaches, fatigue) were excluded.

In a review of over 200 studies that used the HADS, Herrmann (1997) concluded that it is a clinically meaningful screening tool that is also sensitive to changes related to the natural course of depression, as well as to responses due to both psychological and pharmacological interventions. In their review of an additional 747 studies published since that review, Bjelland, Dahl, Haug, and Neckelmann (2002) reported that the Cronbach's α for the depression scale ranged between .67 and .90, and that a score of 8 and above on the depression scale yielded a sensitivity and specificity of .80. Overall, these authors concluded that the HADS was effective in identifying depression caseness across somatic, psychiatric, primary care, and nonpatient populations. The HADS has also been administered and evaluated in studies to screen individuals with depression in a variety of medical populations, including individuals with cancer (Mitchell, Meader, & Symonds, 2010) and diabetes (Sultan, Luminet, & Hartemann, 2010).

Although the HADS has demonstrated satisfactory reliability, sensitivity, and specificity, considerable controversy has arisen regarding the bidimensional (i.e., anxiety and depression) factor structure. In particular, Cosco and colleagues (Cosco, Doyle, Ward, & McGee, 2012) found in a systematic review of the latent structure of the HADS that 25 of the 50 reviewed studies reported a two-factor structure, but the other 25 studies yielded solutions ranging from one to four factors. They concluded that the latent structure of the HADS is highly dependent on the statistical methods employed. More specifically, exploratory factor analysis studies reported two-factor structures, confirmatory factor analysis studies revealed three-factor structures, and item response theory studies produced unidimensional structures.

Mood Disorder Questionnaire

The Mood Disorder Questionnaire (MDQ; Hirschfeld et al., 2000) is a 13-item self-report inventory developed to help screen for individuals who are potentially experiencing bipolar spectrum disorder. These items address whether several of any reported manic or hypomanic symptoms or behaviors (e.g., elevated energy levels) were experienced during the same period of time. In addition, respondents are asked to indicate the severity of impairment such symptoms engendered on a 4-point scale.

The MDQ has been administered in different populations, including psychiatric outpatients, primary care outpatients, and general populations. The sensitivity of the MDQ in psychiatric outpatient settings ranged from .63 to .76 and the specificity from .85 to .90 (Hirschfeld, 2010). The overall sensitivity was higher in bipolar I disorder than in bipolar II disorder. In primary care settings, the MDQ has been demonstrated to identify individuals with bipolar disorder among patients with depression (Hirschfeld, Cass, Holt, & Carlson, 2005; Olfson et al., 2005). However, the sensitivity of the MDQ in a general population was as low as .28, although the specificity was .97 (Hirschfeld et al., 2003). It has also been noted that the MDQ has limitations for detecting bipolar disorder, in particular bipolar II disorder, in nonclinical populations (Dodd et al., 2009). A factor analysis of the MDQ identified a 2-factor structure— an elevated mood overactivity factor and an irritable behavior factor (Mangelli, Benazzi, & Fava, 2005). Despite the recency of this instrument, the MDQ has already been widely used in research and clinical settings and has been translated into 16 languages. However, it has not fared equally well in all countries. For example, Hu and colleagues (2012) recently evaluated the usefulness of the MDQ to identify bipolar patients in 13 mental health centers in China. They concluded that the routine use of the MDQ as a screening scale for bipolar disorder among Chinese patients being treated for MDD was not justified, as the maximum sensitivity metric identified between bipolar disorder and MDD was only 0.31.

Patient Health Questionnaire Depression Scale

The Patient Health Questionnaire Depression Scale (PHQ-9; Kroenke & Spitzer, 2002) is a self-report measure that generally takes less than 10 minutes to complete. Items come directly from the nine signs and symptoms of major depression as delineated in DSM-IV.

Major depression is diagnosed if five or more of these nine criteria have been present at least *more than half the days* during the preceding 2 weeks and if one of the symptoms is depressed mood or anhedonia. One of the nine symptom criteria (*thoughts that you would be better off dead or of hurting yourself in some way*) counts if present at all, regardless of duration.

PHQ-9 scores range from 0 to 27. Cutoff points of 5, 10, 15, and 20 represent the thresholds for mild, moderate, moderately severe, and severe depression, respectively. For a single screening cut point, a PHQ-9 score of 10 or greater was initially recommended (Kroenke, Spitzer, & Williams, 2001). Internal consistency (Cronbach's α ranging from .86 to .89) and test–retest reliability (intraclass correlations range from .81 to .96) of the PHQ-9 have been found to be adequate (Kroenke et al., 2001). In addition, the PHQ has been validly applied to various medical populations, such as patients with dialysis (Watnick, Wang, Demadura, & Ganzini, 2005), individuals suffering from traumatic brain injury (Fann et al., 2005), and patients with heart failure (Hammash et al., 2013).

In addition, the PHQ-9 has been translated and validated in many languages, including Spanish (Diez-Quevedo, Rangil, Sanchez-Planell, Kroenke, & Spitzer, 2001), German (Löwe, Gräfe, et al., 2004; Löwe, Spitzer, et al., 2004), and Nigerian (Adewuya, Ola, & Afolabi, 2006). Moreover, Huang, Chung, Kroenke, Delucchi, and Spitzer (2006) found the PHQ-9 to measure a common construct of depression across various diverse population samples (i.e., African American, Chinese American, Latino, and non-Hispanic white patient groups).

PHQ-2

The PHQ-2 (Kroenke, Spitzer, & Williams, 2003) was developed as a two-item version of the PHQ-9 to address the need for briefer measures to be used in busy clinical settings. This version inquires only about depressed mood and anhedonia. Kroenke and colleagues (2003) evaluated the criterion validity of the PHQ-2 with reference to the structured interview conducted by independent mental health professionals. They reported that the PHQ-2 was able to detect MDD with a sensitivity of 83% and a specificity of 92% using an optimal cutoff score of 3 (Kroenke et al., 2003). However, among a sample of 2,642 patients attending family practices in New Zealand, when using this same cutoff score, sensitivity was found to be only .61 with a specificity of .92. Based on these results, the New Zealand researchers suggest that if a patient scores 2 or more on the PHQ-2, he or she should be asked to complete the PHQ-9 in order to obtain a more accurate detection of depression.

Zung Self-Rating Depression Scale

The Zung Self-Rating Depression Scale (SDS; Zung, 1965) is among the most popular self-rating depression scales. This 20-item questionnaire was developed to quickly assess the cognitive, behavioral, and affective symptoms of depression. The psychometric properties of the SDS have been examined in a number of different cultures, including Dutch, Finnish, and Japanese populations. One study of 85 patients with and 28 patients without depression in a Dutch day clinic found the internal consistency to be .82 and the split-half reliability to be .79 (de Jonghe & Baneke, 1989). A study that examined the concurrent validity of the SDS in relation to the Depression (D) scale of the Minnesota Multiphasic Personality Inventory (MMPI-2) found zero-order correlation of .77 between the SDS and D scales. The study also reported the sensitivity of SDS to be .57 and specificity to be .83 (Thurber, Snow, & Honts, 2002).

Factor analyses of the SDS have been conducted and have produced somewhat inconsistent results. For example, Sakamoto, Kijima, Tomoda, and Kambara (1998) reported three factors: Cognitive, Affective, and Somatic Symptoms. The analysis was conducted based on a sample of 2,187 Japanese college students, which resulted in a goodness-of-fit index (GFI) of .94. It was further supported by a confirmatory factor analysis in a sample of 597 Japanese undergraduates (GFI = .92). In a more recent study with 28,588 first-year university students in Japan, the confirmatory factor analysis yielded the same three factors of SDS with a GFI of .98 (Kitamura, Hirano, Chen, & Hirata, 2004). On the other hand, Kivelae and Pahkala (1987) reported three factors—labeled as Depressed Mood, Loss of Self-Esteem, and Irritability and Agitation after conducting a principal-components factor analysis with a sample of 290 adults with depression ages 60 and older in Finland. Furthermore, Romera, Delgado-Cohen, Perez, Caballero, and Gilaberte (2008) reported a four-factor solution consisting of a Core Depressive factor, a Cognitive factor, an Anxiety factor, and a Somatic factor in their study with 1,049 patients with MDD in the primary care setting. It is possible that age, symptom severity, or culturally related factors contributed to differences among these factors.

The Zung SDS has also been translated into multiple languages. For example, Mammadova, Sultanov, Hajiyeva, Aichberger, and Heinz (2012) recently translated this measure into Azerbaijani and evaluated its psychometric properties, finding it to be reliable, with high degrees of sensitivity and specificity. Chagas and colleagues (2010) recently found the Brazilian version of the SDS to be a valid tool for screening depression among patients with Parkinson's disease.

GUIDELINES FOR SELECTING DEPRESSION MEASURES

Given the plethora of psychometrically sound measures of depression, the question arises—"Which one do I choose?" Moreover, because each individual is unique, no textbook strategy is readily apparent (Nezu & Nezu, 1993), thus requiring decision-making guidelines. In this context, we recommend that the following questions be considered when choosing assessment tools:

1. What are the goals of assessment?
2. Who is to be assessed?
3. What is the value of a given measure?
4. Who is the source of the information?

What Are the Assessment Goals?

With regard to assessing depression, the following are potential assessment objectives: (1) screening; (2) diagnosis and classification; (3) description of problem areas and symptoms; (4) prediction of behavior; and (5) outcome evaluation.

Screening

In clinical settings, screening can indicate whether further assessment is warranted. For research purposes, it is often helpful to determine whether a given individual might meet initial inclusion criteria. To be useful, screening instrument scores should be correlated with scores provided by a more comprehensive assessment regarding the presence or absence of the disorder being assessed. Cutoff scores are often required when using screening instruments, along with information about its sensitivity and specificity. Examples include the PHQ and HADS.

Diagnosis and Classification

Measures that are designed specifically for formulating diagnoses should contain content that clearly corresponds to the criteria required for diagnosis by a formal diagnostic system, such as the DSM. The diagnosis that the instrument points to should be reliable over time and, when clinical judgment is involved, should demonstrate good interrater agreement when the system is implemented by independent evaluators assessing the same individual. Furthermore, such a measure should also lead to an accurate differential diagnosis; that is, it should correctly denote not only what diagnosis a person qualified for but also which diagnoses he or she does *not* qualify for, especially when there is symptom overlap across diagnoses. Examples of such assessment procedures described earlier include the DISH, SAD-P, and SCID.

Description of Symptoms and Symptom Severity

Many assessment tools measure various dimensions of depression, such as the topography, range, severity, and/or frequency of symptoms. Such measures often provide specific idiographic information for persons within a specific diagnostic group (e.g., sleep difficulties, suicidal ideation, difficulties in concentration). Severity of depressive symptomatology is the most frequent assessment goal in both clinical and research settings, given that such evaluations are important with regard to treatment success. To be useful in providing such information, measures of symptom severity especially need to be documented to be reliable over time. Most of the measures previously described, such as the BDI, CES-D, and PHQ-9, assess depressive severity.

Treatment Outcome

Depression measures can also help to monitor therapeutic progress. It is important that the measure be stable in the absence of conditions that produce change and also be sufficiently sensitive to detect change. Investigations of whether changes in scores on the measure following treatment correlate significantly with changes in scores on other measures of the same construct provide further evidence of treatment sensitivity, as well as convergent validity. With respect to depression, measures that assess symptom severity can serve as instruments that provide information concerning the effects of treatment (e.g., a decrease in symptom severity).

Whom Are We Assessing?

People suffering from depression represent a heterogeneous group (see Ingram, Siegle, & Steidtmann, Chapter 3, this volume). Therefore, it is important to use measures that were developed specifically for the particular subgroup of depressed people that the investigator is interested in examining.

Age Differences

One variable of consequence is age. For example, adult measures of depression would be potentially inappropriate for children not only because of language differences but also because of potential differences in the overall constellation of symptoms and their behavioral expression. As such, various depression measures have been developed specifically for differing age groups, such as the Children's Depression Inventory (CDI; Kovacs, 1992) for children and the Geriatric Depression Scale (Yesavage et al., 1983) for adults 65 years and older.

Concomitant Diagnoses

Another individual-difference variable is the presence of additional psychiatric or medical diagnoses. In certain cases, these concomitant problems can limit the validity of depression measures that do not take these disorders into account. An example includes the Calgary Depression Scale for Schizophrenia (Addington, Addington, & Maticka-Tyndale, 1993), a clinician-rated protocol that was developed in response to the observation that other assessment instruments for depression did not accurately represent depressive symptoms or syndromes in persons with schizophrenia. Examples of measures specifically developed to assess depression in medical populations previously described include the BDI-FS, CDS, HADS, and PHQ-9.

Cultural Differences

Of particular importance regarding interindividual differences is the potential influence of ethnic and cultural backgrounds. It is not enough to ensure that a self-report measure has been competently translated into another language; it is critical to also demonstrate that it actually addresses constructs that have meaning within a given culture. Research has shown that although some similarities are evident in the expression of depression across various cultures, differences do exist (Kaiser, Katz, & Shaw, 1998; see Chentsova-Dutton, Ryder, & Tsai, Chapter 18, this volume). Such differences (e.g., headaches and "nerves" in Latino and Mediterranean cultures, fatigue and "imbalance" among Asian cultures) may be a function of varying values among cultures or in the manner in which Western society interprets these values. Various measures of depression, initially developed in Western cultures, have been demonstrated to be applicable across a variety of cultures and have been translated into numerous languages, such as the BDI, PHQ-9, HADS, and CES-D. In recent years, these newly translated measures have shown high levels of reliability and validity in many new cultural groups and countries, thereby allowing researchers to compare symptomology and epidemiology in these new groups with those for whom these measures were initially developed. For example, in a study conducted in Greece (Michopoulos et al., 2008), the HADS presented high internal consistency and stability across Greek hospitalized patients.

In addition to the adaptation of Western measures to new cultures, certain measures of depression have been specifically developed for non-Western cultures. One such measure is the Lee and Rhee Depression Scale (LRDS; Hwang et al., 2012), which was constructed to develop a culturally sensitive measure of depression in Korea that would detect symptomology that can be overlooked by Western depression scales.

What Is the Value of a Given Measure?

We define the "value" of a measure as the joint function of the psychometric properties of a measure and the cost–benefit ratio regarding various practical concerns. In describing the various measures, we highlighted the strength of their psychometric properties. A cost–benefit analysis of practical issues should address: (1) the amount of time required by both the patient and the assessor; (2) potential risks or dangers associated with a given assessment procedure; (3) potential ethical violations associated with a given measure; (4) the effects of a given procedure on others involved (e.g., family members); (5) short-term versus long-term benefits or liabilities related to a given assessment procedure; and (6) the incremental utility of the measure (e.g., how much unique information does this measure offer?).

One additional practical issue to be considered is the cognitive complexity (e.g., length and number of individual items, readability, linguistic problems) of a measure. Shumway, Sentell, Unick, and Bamberg (2004) assessed the cognitive complexity of 15 self-administered depression measures and found considerable variability among them. With regard to measures described in this chapter, the BDI was found to be one of the most complex, whereas the Zung was among the least complex. Consequently, when one is concerned about the ability of a given patient or research participant to understand and respond accurately to a given depression measure because of limited educational background, levels of cognitive complexity should be considered.

Who Is the Source of the Information?

Depression measures can be divided into two categories based on the source of the information: self-report and clinician-rated measures. Each method has its advantages and disadvantages. For example, although self-report questionnaires are relatively brief and require less time to complete than do clinician-rated measures, they are more susceptible to respondent bias (e.g., individuals may not be truthful or may wish to present themselves in a particularly "good" or "bad" light). Clinician-rated measures are likely to produce more reliable results than are self-report inventories, but they often require special training in the structured interviews that can accompany such procedures. All else being equal, a combination of both procedures will likely yield the most valid and comprehensive picture of a given person. It is important, however, that the reader consider all the questions posed in this section when choosing among the various depression measures.

CONCLUSIONS AND FUTURE DIRECTIONS

Despite the plethora of current depression measures, it is important that researchers and clinicians continue to develop new measures and engage in major revisions of existing instruments. We argue this point in order to address (1) the changing definition of depression (i.e., changes in diagnostic criteria) and the need to have measures that are consistent with contemporary thinking; (2) the changing nature of how depression is experienced and expressed by various cultures and subcultures of individuals who will be acculturated during the next several decades into mainstream Western society in varying degrees; (3) the improved understanding of how depression is expressed concomitantly with other mental health (e.g., anxiety disorders, bipolar disorder) and medical or physical health (e.g., cardiovascular disease, cancer, diabetes) diagnoses; and (4) the need to have psychometrically sound but user-friendly (e.g., brief, physically accessible, cognitively understandable) measures to accommodate a variety of patient needs. We end this chapter by highlighting important areas of future research and conceptual focus regarding the assessment of depression, including (1) definitional issues, (2) diversity issues, and (3) advances in technology.

Definitional Issues

As we noted earlier in describing the various measures of depression, new inventories have been developed or existing measures have been revised in order to be more consistent and current with changes in the definition of depression that have occurred over the past several decades (e.g., changes in DSM diagnostic criteria). Measures of depression must continue to be current, especially in light of such controversies regarding the appropriateness of the "gold standard" status that certain measures currently enjoy as a function of tradition rather than of validity, such as the HAMD. The construction of the GRID-HAMD and work by the DRSST to improve the HAMD are excellent examples of such efforts. In addition, not only do older measures need to be revised, but basic research on the psychometric properties of such revisions must continue as well.

A related issue involves differences in what various researchers believe constitutes "core symptoms" of depression. For example, some measures were specifically developed to assess all nine DSM-IV diagnostic criteria dimensions, whereas others were constructed that deliberately exclude certain criteria, such as suicidal ideation. Because it is unlikely that any one study will be conducted to compare simultaneously the psychometric properties of a large number of measures, it will be difficult to ascertain which assessment tool is more reliable and valid across different populations and testing settings. One major divarication that appears currently unresolved is the definition of depression as it is experienced by samples of medical patients. As we noted earlier, whereas several measures of depression were developed specifically for such individuals with the notion of deliberately excluding somatic symptoms, such as fatigue and sleep disturbances (e.g., BDI-FS, BDI-PC, HADS), other measures were not (e.g., CDS, PHQ-9). In fact, the CDS, which was developed specifically for patients with cardiovascular disease, contains items addressing somatic symptoms, such as fatigue, with the notion that fatigue in heart patients with depression is related more strongly to mood disturbance than to cardiovascular problems. Interestingly, the NHLBI Working Group recommended that the first edition of the BDI be used as the measure of choice for both epidemiological and treatment outcome research due to its widespread usage and extensive database, with the caveat that in the future the BDI-II may accumulate additional psychometric properties to support its use (Davidson et al., 2006). It is important to note, however, that if cardiac researchers follow this recommendation, assuming that several measures of depression are not likely to be administered in the same study, the goal of collecting additional evidence for other inventories that do not have the history of the BDI, including the BDI-II, appears limited. Given that fatigue is a highly prevalent symptom of various cardiovascular disorders, particularly of heart failure, it is critical that future research focus on establishing a more valid definition of depression in medical patient populations, such as individuals with heart disease, in order to obtain a more comprehensive understanding of the experience and impact of this mood disorder.

Diversity Issues

As we mentioned earlier in this chapter, the phenomenology and expression of depression can vary across different ethnically based cultures, thus calling into question the validity of measures that were originally developed using samples of white, middle-class adults. In addition, because of their minority status, various ethnically diverse populations in the United States may have had limited access to traditional mental health services, thus creating further obstacles to this validation process.

In general, we need to gain a better understanding of how depression is conceptualized in both its experience and expression across different cultures and then to develop psychometrically sound measures to better assess depression among such ethnically diverse populations. For example, Gloria, Castellanos, Kanagui-Muñoz, and Rico (2012) recently found that, when asked to complete three commonly used depression scales (i.e., BDI-II, CES-D, Zung), many Latina/o undergraduate students did not respond to specific items on each scale that addressed personal feelings (e.g., sexuality, feelings of worthlessness), thus compromising the utility of these measures.

As immigrant populations increase in the United States, so does acculturation, making this endeavor particularly difficult. For example, Lin (1989) noted that, whereas a review of the literature continues to support the hypothesis that Chinese individuals tend to deny depression or express it somatically rather than psychologically, Western influences in China have actually modified this behavioral pattern. Thus currently relevant and valid measures of depression in various cultures today may become outdated in the near future.

Future research also should focus on improving the assessment of depression among (1) individuals residing in rural areas, (2) individuals who have lower economic status and literacy rates, (3) older adults, and (4) those with a disability. Increasing the number of valid and reliable assessment modalities for such populations can lead to two important outcomes: first, the degree and amount of treatment interventions aimed at reducing depression for these groups will expand; and, second, the accuracy of the estimate of the incidence and prevalence of depression in the general population will also be improved.

Advances in Technology

After considering the varied populations in need of further study and some of the obstacles faced by clinicians, it is not surprising that research efforts over the past decade have been aimed at reducing such barriers by expanding beyond the traditional paper-and-pencil or interview techniques. As researchers have recognized the advancement of technology and the potential of the Internet as a source of data collection, computer- and/or Internet-based measurements of depression have been developed. Examples include the computerized adaptive version of the BDI (Gardner et al., 2004), the Interactive Voice Response Hamilton Depression Rating Scale (IVR HAMD; Kobak, Mundt, Greist, Katzelnick, & Jefferson, 2000), the short Web-based version of the CES-D (Herrero & Meneses, 2006), and the interactive voice response version of the PHQ-9 (Turvey, Sheeran, Dindo, Wakefield, & Klein, 2012). In general, these computerized versions of standard measurements of depression have been reported to be equivalent to paper-and-pencil formats.

Computerized voice recognition programs have the capability to evaluate depression among non-English-speaking persons, patients with disabilities, low literacy populations, and geriatric samples (González et al., 2000). In addition, they can record and chart a patient's weekly assessment, increase the public's awareness of depression, improve the detection and treatment of depression in the general population, and objectify assessments, while being cost- and time-efficient (Ogles et al., 1998). Mundt and colleagues (2007) established the feasibility of obtaining voice acoustic measures reflecting depression severity; they found that several voice acoustic measures correlated significantly with depression severity measured by standard measures of depression severity (e.g., HAMD) during a 6-week observation.

Electronic momentary assessment techniques provide precise and prospective information of emotional experiences in a daily life context (Ebner-Priemer & Trull, 2009) and have been used with individuals diagnosed with MDD (Thompson et al., 2012). Momentary assessment methodology has advantages in that it offers real-time assessment and reveals repetitive and relevant patterns of emotional expression hard to detect by depression questionnaires. In particular, momentary assessment using an electronic device enables person-tailored feedback on dynamic patterns of emotions, as well as the collection of real-time data (Heron & Smyth, 2010).

Nevertheless, such technologically advanced protocols are not without problems. For example, it has been suggested that state anxiety can increase as a result of the computerized testing situation and can potentially confound results (Merten & Ruch, 1996). Furthermore, computerized screening poses the dilemma of treating patients who are suicidal or have acute crises (Ogles et al., 1998). In addition, Cacciola and colleagues (1999) found that participants were more likely to receive a lifetime diagnosis of MDD when they were administered an in-person SCID than a telephone-based SCID. In recent years, increased familiarity with technology due to the rapid growth of residential computing has been used to argue against potential confounding effects of computerized assessment (Herrero & Meneses, 2006). In fact, Weisband and Kiesler (1996) reported in their meta-analysis that the impact of computer administration on self-disclosure from 1964 to 1994 has declined over the years. Nevertheless, substantial research may still be needed to improve upon this technology, as well as to identify, and subsequently resolve, important ethical dilemmas.

REFERENCES

Addington, D., Addington, J., & Maticka-Tyndale, E. (1993). Rating depression in schizophrenia: A comparison of a self-report and an observer report scale. *Journal of Nervous and Mental Disease, 181*, 561–565.

Adewuya, A. O., Ola, B. A., & Afolabi, O. O. (2006). Validity of the patient health questionnaire (PHQ-9) as a screening tool for depression amongst Nigerian university students. *Journal of Affective Disorders, 96*, 89–93.

American Psychiatric Association. (1994). *Diagnostic and statistical manual of mental disorders* (4th ed.). Washington, DC: Author.

Arnau, R. C., Meagher, M. W., Norris, M. P., & Bramson, R. (2001). Psychometric evaluation of the Beck Depression Inventory—II with primary care medical patients. *Health Psychology, 20*, 112–119.

Bagby, R. M., Ryder, A. G., Schuller, D. R., & Marshall, M. B. (2004). The Hamilton Depression Rating Scale: Has the gold standard become a lead weight? *American Journal of Psychiatry, 161*, 2163–2177.

Beck, A. T., Guth, D., Steer, R. A., & Ball, R. A. (1997). Screening for major depression disorders in medical inpatients with the Beck Depression Inventory for Primary Care. *Behaviour Research, and Therapy, 35*, 785–791.

Beck, A. T., Steer, R. A., & Brown, G. K. (1996). *Manual for the BDI-II*. San Antonio, TX: Psychological Corporation.

Beck, A. T., Steer, R. A., & Brown, G. K. (2000). *Manual for the Beck Depression Inventory—Fast Screen for Medical Patients*. San Antonio, TX: Psychological Corporation.

Beck, A. T., Ward, C. H., Mendelson, M., Mock, J., & Erbaugh, J. (1961). An inventory for measuring depression. *Archives of General Psychiatry, 4*, 561–571.

Benedict, R. H. B., Fishman, I., McClellan, M. M., Bakshi, R., & Weinstock-Guttman, B. (2003). Validity of the Beck Depression Inventory—Fast Screen in multiple sclerosis. *Multiple Sclerosis, 9*, 393–396.

Bjelland, I., Dahl, A. A., Haug, T. T., & Neckelmann, D. (2002). The validity of the Hospital

Anxiety and Depression Scale: An updated review. *Journal of Psychosomatic Research, 52,* 69–77.

Cacciola, J. S., Alterman, A. I., Rutherford, M. J., McKay, J. R., & May, D. J. (1999). Comparability of telephone and in-person structured clinical interview for DSM-III-R (SCID) diagnoses. *Assessment, 6,* 235–242.

Chagas, M. H., Tumas, V., Loureiro, S. R., Hallck, J. E. C., Trzesneak, C., de Sousa, J. P. M., et al. (2010).Validity of a Brazilian version of the Zung Self-Rating Depression Scale for screening of depression in patients with Parkinson's disease. *Parkinsonism and Related Disorders, 16,* 42–45.

Corruble, E., & Hardy, P. (2005). Why the Hamilton Depression Rating Scale endures. *American Journal of Psychiatry, 162,* 2394.

Cosco, T. D., Doyle, F., Ward, M., & McGee, H. (2012). Latent structure of the Hospital Anxiety and Depression Scale: A 10-year systematic review. *Journal of Psychosomatic Research, 72,* 180–184.

Davidson, K. W., Kupfer, D. J., Bigger, J. T., Califf, R. M., Carney, R. M., Coyne, J. C., et al. (2006). Assessment and treatment of depression in patients with cardiovascular disease: National Heart, Lung, and Blood Institute Working Group Report. *Annals of Behavioral Medicine, 32,* 121–126.

de Jonghe, J. F., & Baneke, J. J. (1989). The Zung Self-Rating Depression Scale: A replication study on reliability, validity and prediction. *Psychological Reports, 64,* 833–834.

Di Benedetto, M., Lindner, H., Hare, D. L., & Kent, S. (2005). A Cardiac Depression Visual Analogue Scale for the brief and rapid assessment of depression following acute coronary syndromes. *Journal of Psychosomatic Research, 59,* 223–229.

Di Benedetto, M., Lindner, H., Hare, D. L., & Kent, S. (2006). Depression following acute coronary syndromes: A comparison between the Cardiac Depression Scale and the Beck Depression Inventory— II. *Journal of Psychosomatic Research, 60,* 13–20.

Diez-Quevedo, C., Rangil, T., Sanchez-Planell, L., Kroenke, K., & Spitzer, R. L. (2001). Validation and utility of the patient health questionnaire in diagnosing mental disorders in 1003 general hospital Spanish inpatients. *Psychosomatic Medicine, 63,* 679–686.

Dodd, S., Williams, L. J., Jacka, F. N., Pasco, J. A., Bjerkeset, O., & Berk, M. (2009). Reliability of the Mood Disorder Questionnaire: Comparison with the Structured Clinical Interview for the DSM-IV-TR in a population sample. *Australian and New Zealand Journal of Psychiatry, 43,* 526–530.

Dozois, D. J. A., Ahnberg, J. L., & Dobson, K. S. (1998). A psychometric evaluation of the Beck Depression Inventory—II. *Psychological Assessment, 10,* 83–89.

Ebner-Priemer, U. W., & Trull, T. J. (2009). Ecological momentary assessment of mood disorders and mood dysregulation. *Psychological Assessment, 21,* 463–475.

ENRICHD Investigators. (2000). Enhancing Recovery in Coronary Heart Disease Patients (ENRICHD): Study design and methods. *American Heart Journal, 139,* 1–9.

Fann, J. R., Bombardier, C. H., Dikmen, S., Esselman, P., Warms, C., Pelzer, E., et al. (2005). Validity of the Patient Health Questionnaire–9 in assessing depression following traumatic brain injury. *Journal of Head Trauma Rehabilitation, 20,* 501–511.

First, M. B., Gibbon, M., Spitzer, R. L., & Williams, J. B. (1996). *Structured Clinical Interview for DSM-IV Axis I Disorders–Nonpatient Edition (SCID-I/NP, Version 2.0).* New York: New York State Psychiatric Institute, Biometrics Research Department.

First, M. B., Spitzer, R. L., Gibbon, M., & Williams, J. B. (1997). *User's guide for the Structured Clinical Interview for DSM-IV Axis I Disorders.* Washington, DC: American Psychiatric Press.

Freedland, K. E., Skala, J. A., Carney, R. M., Raczynski, J. M., Taylor, C. B., Mendes de Leon, C. F., et al. (2002). The Depression Interview and Structured Hamilton (DISH): Rationale, development, characteristics, and clinical validity. *Psychosomatic Medicine, 64,* 897–905.

Gardner, W., Shear, K., Kelleher, K. J., Pajer, K. A., Mammen, O., Buysse, D., et al. (2004). Computerized adaptive measurement of depression: A simulation study. *BMC Psychiatry, 4,* 13.

Gary, F. A., & Yarandi, H. N. (2004). Depression among southern rural African American women: A factor analysis of the Beck Depression Inventory—II. *Nursing Research, 53,* 251–259.

Gholizadeh, L., Salamonson, Y., Davidson, P. M., Parvan, K., Frost, S. A., Chang, S., et al. (2010). Cross-cultural validation of the Cardiac Depression Scale in Iran. *British Journal of Clinical Psychology, 49,* 517–528.

Gloria, A. M., Castellanos, J., Kanagui-Muñoz, M., & Rico, M. A. (2012). Assessing Latina/o undergraduates' depressive symptomatology: Comparisons of the Beck Depression Inventory—II, the Center for Epidemiological Studies—Depression Scale, and the Self-Report Depression Scale. *Hispanic Journal of Behavioral Sciences, 34,* 160–181.

González, G. M., Winfrey, J., Sertic, M., Salcedo, J., Parker, C., & Mendoza, S. (2000). A bilingual telephone-enabled speech recognition application for screening depression symptoms. *Professional Psychology: Research and Practice, 31,* 398–403.

Hamilton, M. (1960). Development of a rating scale for depression. *Journal of Neurology, Neurosurgery and Psychiatry, 23,* 56–62.

Hammash, M. H., Hall, L. A., Lennie, T. A., Heo, S., Chung, M. L., Lee, K. S., et al. (2013). Psychometrics of the PHQ-9 as a measure of depressive symptoms in patients with heart failure. *European Journal of Cardiovascular Nursing, 12*(5), 446–453.

Hare, D. L., & Davis, C. R. (1996). Cardiac Depression Scale: Validation of a new depression scale for cardiac patients. *Journal of Psychosomatic Research, 40,* 379–386.

Hedlund, J. L., & Vieweg, B. W. (1979). The Hamilton Rating Scale for Depression: A comprehensive review. *Journal of Operational Psychiatry, 10,* 149–165.

Heron, K. E., & Smyth, J. M. (2010). Ecological momentary interventions: Incorporating mobile technology into psychosocial and health behaviour treatments. *British Journal of Health Psychology, 15,* 1–39.

Herrero, J., & Meneses, J. (2006). Short Web-based versions of the Perceived Stress (PSS) and Center for Epidemiological Studies—Depression (CESD) Scales: A comparison to pencil and paper responses among Internet users. *Computers in Human Behavior, 22,* 830–836.

Herrmann, C. (1997). International experiences with the Hospital Anxiety and Depression Scale: A review of validation data and clinical results. *Journal of Psychosomatic Research, 42,* 17–41.

Hirschfeld, R. M. A. (2010). Mood Disorder Questionnaire: It's impact on the field. *Depression and Anxiety, 27,* 627–630.

Hirschfeld, R. M., Calabrese, J. R., Weissman, M. M., Reed, M., Davies, M. A., Frye, M. A., et al. (2003). Screening for bipolar disorder in the community. *Journal of Clinical Psychiatry, 64,* 53–59.

Hirschfeld, R. M., Cass, A. R., Holt, D. C., & Carlson, C. A. (2005). Screening for bipolar disorder in patients treated for depression in a family medicine clinic. *Journal of the American Board of Family Practice, 18,* 233–239.

Hirschfeld, R. M. A., Lewis, L., & Vornik, L. A. (2003). Perceptions and impact of bipolar disorder: How far have we really come?: Results of the National Depressive and Manic-Depressive Association 2000 survey of individuals with bipolar disorder. *Journal of Clinical Psychiatry, 64,* 161–174.

Hirschfeld, R. M. A., Williams, J. B. W., Spitzer, R. L., Calabrese, J. R., Flynn, L., Keck, P. E., Jr., et al. (2000). Development and validation of a screening instrument for bipolar spectrum disorder: The Mood Disorder Questionnaire. *American Journal of Psychiatry, 157,* 1873–1875.

Holländare, F., Askerlund, A., Nieminen, A., & Engström, I. (2008). Can the BDI-II and MADRS-S be transferred to online use without affecting their psychometric properties? *Electronic Journal of Applied Psychology, 4,* 63–65.

Hu, C., Xiang, Y. T., Wang, G., Ungvari, G. S., Dickerson, F. B., Kilbourne, A. M., et al. (2012). Screening for bipolar disorder with the Mood Disorders Questionnaire in patients diagnosed as major depressive disorder: The experience in China. *Journal of Affective Disorders, 141,* 40–46.

Huang, F. Y., Chung, H., Kroenke, K., Delucchi, K. L., & Spitzer, R. L. (2006). Using the Patient

Health Questionnaire—9 to measure depression among racially and ethnically diverse primary care patients. *Journal of General Internal Medicine, 21,* 547–552.

Hwang, S. H., Rhee, M. K., Kang, R. H., Lee, H. Y. Ham, B. J., Lee, Y. S., et al. (2012). Development and validation of a screening scale for depression in Korea: The Lee and Rhee Depression Scale. *Psychiatric Investigations, 9,* 36–44.

Irwin, M., Artin, K., & Oxman, M. N. (1999). Screening for depression in the older adult. *Archives of Internal Medicine, 159,* 1701–1704.

Jenerette, C., Funk, M., & Murdaugh, C. (2005). Sickle cell disease: A stigmatizing condition that may lead to depression. *Issues in Mental Health Nursing, 26,* 1081–1101.

Kaiser, A. S., Katz, R., & Shaw, B. F. (1998). Cultural issues in the management of depression. In S. S. Kazarian & D. E. Evans (Eds.), *Cultural clinical psychology: Theory, research, and practice* (pp. 177–214). New York: Oxford University Press.

Kalali, A., Bech, P., Williams, J., Kobak, K., Lipsitz, J., Engelhardt, N., et al. (2002). The New GRID-HAM-D: Results from field trials. *European Neuropsychopharmacology, 12*(Suppl. 3), 239.

King, K. M., Colella, T. J., Faris, P., & Thompson, D. R. (2009). Using the cardiac depression scale in men recovering from coronary artery bypass surgery. *Journal of Clinical Nursing, 18,* 1617–1624.

Kitamura, T., Hirano, H., Chen, Z., & Hirata, M. (2004). Factor structure of the Zung Self-Rating Depression Scale in first-year university students in Japan. *Psychiatry Research, 128,* 281–287.

Kivelae, S., & Pahkala, K. (1987). Factor structure of the Zung Self-Rating Depression Scale among a depressed elderly population. *International Journal of Psychology, 22,* 289–300.

Kobak, K. A., Mundt, J. C., Greist, J. H., Katzelnick, D. J., & Jefferson, J. W. (2000). Computer assessment of depression: Automating the Hamilton Depression Rating Scale. *Drug Information Journal, 34,* 145–156.

Kobak, K. A., Williams, J. B., & Engelhardt, N. (2008). A comparison of face-to-face and remote assessment of inter-rater reliability on the Hamilton Depression Rating Scale via videoconferencing. *Psychiatry Research, 158,* 99–103.

Kovacs, M. (1992). *Children's Depression Inventory manual.* North Tonawanda, NY: Multi-Health Systems.

Kroenke, K., & Spitzer, R. L. (2002). The PHQ-9: A new depression diagnostic and severity measure. *Psychiatry Annals, 32,* 1–7.

Kroenke, K., Spitzer, R. L., & Williams, J. B. (2003). The Patient Health Questionnaire–2: Validity of a two-item depression screener. *Medical Care, 41,* 1284–1292.

Kroenke, K., Spitzer, R. L., & Williams, J. B. W. (2001). The PHQ-9: Validity of a brief depression severity measure. *Journal of General Internal Medicine, 16,* 606–613.

Lin, N. (1989). Measuring depressive symptomatology in China. *Journal of Nervous and Mental Disorders, 177,* 121–131.

Lobbestael, J., Leurgans, M., & Arntz, A. (2011). Inter-rater reliability of the Structured Clinical Interview for DSM-IV Axis I Disorders (SCID I) and Axis II Disorders (SCID II). *Clinical Psychology and Psychotherapy, 18,* 75–79.

Löwe, B., Gräfe, K., Zipfel, S., Witte, S., Loerch, B., & Herzog, W. (2004). Diagnosing ICD-10 depressive episodes: Superior criterion validity of the Patient Health Questionnaire. *Psychotherapy and Psychosomatics, 73,* 386–390.

Löwe, B., Spitzer, R. L., Gräfe, K., Kroenke, K., Quenter, A., Zipfel, S., et al. (2004). Comparative validity of three screening questionnaires for DSM-IV depressive disorders and physicians' diagnoses. *Journal of Affective Disorders, 78,* 131–140.

Mammadova, F., Sultanov, M., Hajiyeva, A., Aichberger, M., & Heinz, A. (2012). Translation and adaptation of the Zung Self- Rating Depression Scale for application in the bilingual Azerbaijani population. *European Psychiatry, 27,* S27–S31.

Mangelli, L., Benazzi, F., & Fava, G. A. (2005). Assessing the community prevalence of bipolar spectrum symptoms by the Mood Disorder Questionnaire. *Psychotherapy and Psychosomatics, 74*, 120–122.

Merten, T., & Ruch, W. (1996). A comparison of computerized and conventional administration of the German versions of the Eysenck Personality Questionnaire and the Carroll Rating Scale for Depression. *Personality and Individual Differences, 20*, 281–291.

Michopoulos, I., Douzenis, A., Kalkavoura, C., Christodoulou, C., Michalopoulou, P., Kalemi, G., et al. (2008). Hospital Anxiety and Depression Scale (HADS): Validation in a Greek general hospital sample. *Annals of General Psychiatry, 7*, 4.

Mitchell, A. J., Meader, N., & Symonds, P. (2010). Diagnostic validity of the Hospital Anxiety and Depression Scale (HADS) in cancer and palliative settings: A meta-analysis. *Journal of Affective Disorders, 126*, 335–348.

Mundt, J. C., Snyder, P. C., Cannizzaro, M. S., Kara Chappie, K., & Geralts, D. S. (2007). Voice acoustic measures of depression severity and treatment response collected via interactive voice response (IVR) technology. *Journal of Neurolinguistics, 20*, 50–64.

Muñoz, R. F., McQuaid, J. R., González, G. M., Dimas, J., & Rosales, V. A. (1999). Depression screening in a women's clinic: Using automated Spanish- and English-language voice recognition. *Journal of Consulting and Clinical Psychology, 67*, 502–510.

Nezu, A. M., & Nezu, C. M. (1993). Identifying and selecting target problems for clinical interventions: A problem-solving model. *Psychological Assessment, 5*, 254–263.

Nezu, A. M., Nezu, C. M., Friedman, J., & Lee, M. (2009). Assessment of depression. In I. H. Gotlib & C. L. Hammen (Eds.), *Handbook of depression* (2nd ed., pp. 44–68). New York: Guilford Press.

Nezu, A. M., Nezu, C. M., & Jain, D. (2005). *The emotional wellness way to cardiac health: How letting go of depression, anxiety, and anger can heal your heart.* Oakland, CA: New Harbinger.

Ogles, B. M., France, C. R., Lunnen, K. M., Bell, M. T., & Goldfarb, M. (1998). Computerized depression screening and awareness. *Community Mental Health Journal, 34*, 27–38.

Olfson, M., Das, A. K., Gameroff, M. J., Pilowsky, D., Feder, A., Gross, R., et al. (2005). Bipolar depression in a low-income primary care clinic. *American Journal of Psychiatry, 162*, 2146–2151.

Radloff, L. S. (1977). The CES-D Scale: A self-report depression scale for research in the general population. *Applied Psychological Measurement, 1*, 385–401.

Romera, I., Delgado-Cohen, H., Perez, T., Caballero, L., & Gilaberte, I. (2008). Factor analysis of the Zung Self-Rating Depression Scale in a large sample of patients with major depressive disorder in primary care. *BMC Psychiatry, 8*, 4.

Sakamoto, S., Kijima, N., Tomoda, A., & Kambara, M. (1998). Factor structures of the Zung Self-Rating Depression Scale (SDS) for undergraduates. *Journal of Clinical Psychology, 54*, 477–487.

Santor, D. A., & Coyne, J. C. (2001). Examining symptom expression as a function of symptom severity: Item performance on the Hamilton Rating Scale for Depression. *Psychological Assessment, 13*, 127–139.

Shumway, M., Sentell, T., Unick, G., & Bamberg, W. (2004). Cognitive complexity of self-administered depression measures. *Journal of Affective Disorders, 83*, 191–198.

Solomon, D. A., Leon, A. C., Maser, J. D., Truman, C. J., Coryell, W., Endicott, J., et al. (2006). Distinguishing bipolar major depression from unipolar major depression with the screening assessment of depression-polarity (SAD-P). *Journal of Clinical Psychiatry, 67*, 434–442.

Sultan, S., Luminet, O., & Hartemann, A. (2010). Cognitive and anxiety symptoms in screening for clinical depression in diabetes: A systematic examination of diagnostic performances of the HADS and BDI-SF. *Journal of Affective Disorders, 123*, 332–336.

Thompson, R. J., Mata, J., Jaeggi, S. M., Buschkuehl, M., Jonides, J., & Gotlib, I. H. (2012). The everyday emotional experience of adults with major depressive disorder: Examining emotional instability, inertia, and reactivity. *Journal of Abnormal Psychology, 121*, 819–829.

Thurber, S., Snow, M., & Honts, C. R. (2002). The Zung Self-Rating Depression Scale: Convergent validity and diagnostic discrimination. *Assessment, 9*, 401–405.

Trajković, G., Starčević, V., Latas, M., Leštarević, M., Ille, T., Bukumirić, Z., et al. (2011). Reliability of the Hamilton Rating Scale for Depression: A meta-analysis over a period of 49 years. *Psychiatry Research, 189*, 1–9.

Turvey, C. L., Sheeran, T., Dindo, L., Wakefield, B., & Klein, D. (2012). Validity of the Patient Health Questionnaire, PHQ-9, administered through interactive-voice-response technology. *Journal of Telemedicine and Telecare, 18*, 348–351.

Turvey, C. L., Wallace, R. B., & Herzog, R. (1999). A revised CES-D measure of depressive symptoms and DSM-based measure of major depressive episode in the elderly. *International Journal of Psychogeriatrics, 11*, 139–148.

Vuorilehto, M., Melartin, T., & Isometsa, E. (2006). Depressive disorders in primary care: Recurrent, chronic, and co-morbid. *Psychological Medicine, 35*, 673–682.

Wang, W., Ski, C. F., Thompson, D. R., & Hare, D. L. (2011). A psychometric evaluation of the Chinese version of the Short-Form Cardiac Depression Scale. *Psychosomatics, 52*, 450–454.

Watnick, S., Wang, P. L., Demadura, T., & Ganzini, L. (2005). Validation of 2 depression screening tools in dialysis patients. *American Journal of Kidney Disease, 46*, 919–924.

Weisband, S., & Kiesler, S. (1996). Self-disclosure on computer forms: Meta-analysis and implications. *Proceedings of the SIGCHI Conference on Human Factors in Computing Systems* (pp. 3–10). New York: Association for Computing Machinery.

Williams, J. B. W., Kobak, K. A., Bech, P., Engelhardt, N., Evans, K., Lipsitz, J., et al. (2008). The GRID-HAMD: Standardization of the Hamilton Depression Rating Scale. *International Clinical Psychopharmacology, 23*, 120–129.

Wise, F. M., Harris, D. W., & Carter, L. M. (2006). Validation of the Cardiac Depression Scale in a cardiac rehabilitation population. *Journal of Psychosomatic Research, 60*, 177–183.

Yesavage, J. A., Brink, T. L., Rose, T. L., Lum, O., Huang, V., Adey, M., et al. (1983). Development and validation of a geriatric depression screening scale: A preliminary report. *Journal of Psychiatric Research, 17*, 37–49.

Yu, S., Lin, Y., & Hsu, W. (2013). Applying structural equation modeling to report psychometric properties of Chinese version 10-item CES-D depression scale. *Quality and Quantity, 47*, 1511–1518.

Zigmond, A. S., & Snaith, R. P. (1983). The Hospital Anxiety and Depression Scale. *Acta Psychiatrica Scandinavica, 67*, 361–370.

Zimmerman, M., Posternak, M. A., & Chelminski, I. (2005). Is it time to replace the Hamilton Depression Rating Scale as the primary outcome measure in treatment studies of depression? *Journal of Clinical Psychopharmacology, 25*, 105–110.

Zung, W. W. K. (1965). A self-rating depression scale. *Archives of General Psychiatry, 12*, 63–70.

CHAPTER 3

Methodological Issues in the Study of Depression

RICK E. INGRAM, GREG J. SIEGLE, *and* DANA STEIDTMANN

The appearance of the third edition of this *Handbook* underscores the enormous interest in understanding depression. Whether from a research or a clinical practice perspective, knowledge of depression is arguably necessary for all mental health professionals and students. It is simply not possible to comprehend depression meaningfully in the absence of methodologically sound research. Thus our purpose in this chapter is to examine relevant issues and strategies for conducting research on depression. No single chapter can examine all of the basic methodological issues that must guide the conduct of scientific research (issues such as random selection and internal and external validity). Nor can a single chapter articulate all of the important details to consider in every study of depression. In this chapter, therefore, we focus on several major issues that are broadly important for research efforts on depression. We assume that sound general methodological techniques are well understood by researchers; consequently, we do not comment on these unless they are particularly germane to a topic of depression research.

DEFINING THE CONSTRUCT FOR RESEARCH: WHAT IS DEPRESSION?

It is imperative that investigators begin with a clear definition of the type of depression in which they are interested. There is arguably no more important procedure in depression research than to decide whether a "syndrome" of depression is to be examined and, if so, to define who is depressed and by what criteria.

The Depression Spectrum as a Theoretical Construct

Disorders within the depression spectrum have historically been conceived of as encompassing states that range from emotional distress to despondency to melancholia. For example, major depressive disorder (MDD) is conceptualized within the medical model as a group of related symptoms, some of which are seen as criteria for a disorder (e.g., sad mood) and others of which are not (e.g., being discouraged about the future). According to DSM-5 (American Psychiatric Association, 2013), a certain number, but not a certain constellation, of symptoms must be present for a diagnosis. Consequently, very different conditions can receive the same diagnostic label of *depression*. The fact that some symptoms are recognized for a disorder whereas others are not underscores the idea that what is defined as *depression* is constructed from a group of symptoms that the clinical community has collectively termed to constitute MDD. Thus MDD, as well as the other depression spectrum disorders, are constructs that are part of a broader class of psychological ideas. Should the scientific and clinical communities decide that these disorders are characterized by different groups of symptoms (e.g., that suicidal ideation rather than sad mood is the defining feature of depression), the nature of the depression spectrum itself would change, the characteristics of people diagnosed with these disorders would be different, and epidemiological data concerning the prevalence of depression spectrum disorders would be transformed. Thus we define a construct such as "depression" by a consensus of the scientific and clinical communities.

The Depression Spectrum as Clinical Syndromes

DSM-5 is one classification system that defines depression for clinical and research purposes; other classifications that do not presuppose the existence of such syndromic entities, such as the National Institute of Mental Health (NIMH) Research Domain Criteria (RDoC), simply lay out related symptoms (e.g., loss) that may or may not be part of a syndromic picture. Given the historical popularity of the DSM, we first consider this scheme. In something of a departure from previous editions, DSM-5 uses a joint categorical and dimensional approach to psychological disorders; "Axis III" of the DSM specifically regards specifying disorder severity on a continuum. In addition, MDD is conceptualized explicitly as existing within a broader framework of related symptomatology. For example, chronic MDD is now classified as "persistent depressive disorder." Specifiers for having features of anxiety, suicidality, and mania are also codable. Thus the DSM affords considerable freedom in research on the construct of depression. For example, an investigator who assumes that depression is continuous can still study depression by selecting participants who meet DSM-IV-TR criteria for depression.

On the other hand, if an investigator assumes a broader, dimensional view of depression in which subclinical depressive states can be used as proxies to understand clinically significant depression, this assumption can have a dramatic impact on the nature of participant samples, on the obtained results, and on the conclusions that are drawn. A number of researchers have questioned the advisability of attempting to understand clinical depression using such subclinical samples (Kendall & Flannery-Schroeder, 1995; Tennen, Hall, & Affleck, 1995), with some suggesting that doing so runs the risk not only of trivializing depression research but also of diminishing the contributions of psychology in the view of science in general and of psychiatry in particular (Coyne, 1994). Several researchers have offered methodological suggestions for dealing with some of these issues (Ingram & Hamilton, 1999; Kendall, Hollon, Beck, Hammen, & Ingram, 1987); NIMH has taken the position that depression and other disorders are so nested within broader collections of symptoms that the entire notion of disorders is premature (Simpson, 2012). Thus only dimensions corresponding to traditional symptoms, such as feelings of loss or a lack of pleasure, are recognized.

Thus there is considerable interest in the relations of subclinical states and associated continua with a syndromic conception of MDD. Synthesizing these notions is clearly a challenge for the next generation of depression research, particularly as a large traditional literature relies on a discrete conception of depression as a disorder. Some challenges include, but are not limited to, the following. First, questions of continuity focus on addressing depressive syndromes of differing severity, but, as we note later in this chapter, symptom-focused methodologies may still have a place in psychiatric research. Second, it is unclear whether variation in features of depression at low severity can be treated the same way as variation in high-severity conditions. As a very simple illustration, an investigator interested in how depression is related to interpersonal disturbance might find little interpersonal disturbance when studying mild depressive states. However, given the widespread recognition that clinically significant depression is accompanied by problematic interpersonal functioning (see Hammen & Shih, Chapter 15, this volume), generalization of such a subclinical finding to severe depression would be inappropriate and misleading. Finally, and in a somewhat related fashion, dimensional features of depression may potentiate categorical processes at the severe end of the spectrum. Consider an example of sleep disturbances, which are common in depressive disorders (Hamilton, Karlson, Luxton, Nelson, & Stevens, 2009). Consistent with the RDoC, if sleep disturbances are themselves dimensional, it may be the case that mild sleep disturbances are observed in mild forms of the depression syndrome and that serious sleep disturbances are observed in severe versions of the syndrome. However, if serious, but not mild, sleep disturbances disrupt biological regulation, then this may also cause problems in MDD that are absent in subclinical depression. Thus, studying sleep in subclinically depressed participants to understand the implications of sleep disturbances in clinical depression would be misguided, even if the research demonstrated that sleep disturbances do vary on a continuum.

Depression as a Subclinical Syndrome

Another approach is to use the syndromic features of depression as heuristics to define a low-grade phenomenon that is representative of the clinical state but that does not meet all relevant criteria for a diagnosis. There are several reasons for which an investigator might choose this route. Subclinical states may represent risk factors for diagnostic syndromes and thus may be conceptualized as one way to study risk (Cuijpers & Smit, 2004). Another reason is that such mild states often represent more than just ordinary unhappiness, sad mood, or simply having a bad-mood day (Gotlib, Lewinsohn, & Seeley, 1995). Indeed, it is possible for these states to be accompanied by at least some clear depressive symptoms (mild to moderate levels of motivational and cognitive deficits, vegetative signs, disruptions in interpersonal relationships, etc.). The symptoms of mild depression, though less serious than those of their clinical counterparts, may also interfere with significant aspects of individuals' lives. Thus the emotionally problematic, disruptive, and common nature of mild or subclinical depressive states would appear to justify their study, and clearly the study of subclinical states deserves equal attention to methodological soundness as does consideration of syndromic conditions. We therefore turn to a brief discussion of several approaches to this problem, each of which has received some research attention and presents some unique methodological issues.

Subclinical Depression Defined by Elevated Scores on Depression Questionnaires

One common approach to studying subclinical depression is to select individuals on the basis of scores that are elevated above some cutoff on a depression questionnaire (see

Nezu et al., Chapter 2, this volume). We illustrate several points with the Beck Depression Inventory (BDI), which is arguably the most widely used self-report measure in depression research. Thus, aside from the validity concerns regarding self-report measures such as the BDI (Beck, Steer, & Garbin, 1988), there are additional issues for recruitment, particularly regarding the specification of cutoff points. It is unclear what aspects of the clinical disorder are captured by cutoff points. There is also no universal standard for a "sufficiently" depressed subclinical sample.

Assuming that investigators are interested in studying individuals who are experiencing specific features of depression, common cutoff scores of 10 or 14 are not guaranteed to preserve these features. Rather, Tennen and colleagues (1995) have argued that such scores may be obtained even though the essential features of sad mood or loss of interest may not be endorsed by many respondents. A related consideration is the intensity of the endorsed critical symptoms. For instance, to count as endorsing a critical symptom, does one only need to check "I feel sad" on the BDI rather than the other available options, such as "I am so sad or unhappy that I can't stand it"? Clearly, on a measure with scores that can range as high as 63, a score of 10 or 14 may be obtained by individuals who are not experiencing cardinal symptoms with much intensity. Fortunately, the solution for this problem is relatively straightforward: Investigators can select only participants who, depending on the investigator's interest, endorse the critical diagnostic features of interest. Investigators interested in more problematic subclinical states may want to require not only the endorsement of these items but, furthermore, that they be endorsed at the higher levels available on the BDI. Such a strategy is strongly consistent with the RDoC initiative in that specific symptoms of interest can be targeted (e.g., cognitive disruptions) in combination with the use of overall thresholds to ensure clinical impact.

Alternatives to Studying the Depression Syndrome

Symptom Profile Research Strategies and Subtype Strategies

NIMH's RDoC initiative is founded on the idea that syndromic notions of disorders are premature. The initiative argues that the collections of symptoms that currently compose syndromes do not have strong empirical support as syndrome clusters. There are likely enough subtypes to suggest that any current syndromic conception is noisy to the point of invalidity and that syndromes are not rooted in understandable mechanisms. In contrast, features of depression, such as "loss" or "inattention," may be easier to quantify and understand at a biological level. The hope is that, eventually, when the biological substrates of symptoms are better understood, their covariance at a mechanistic level can be explained and new, mechanistically grounded symptom clusters can be considered. Perhaps these will look like the current MDD diagnosis. Or perhaps the constructs will be far different—for example, allowing negative affect–specific diagnoses such as the mixed anxiety–depression syndrome, which was not adopted in DSM-5 because of a lack of buy-in from clinicians. This conception gives rise to the utility of assessing specific theoretically guided subtypes of depression rather than depression writ large.

Symptom Profiles

One approach, which is consistent with the RDoC initiative, is the idea of assessing individuals who exhibit some constellation of depressive symptoms posited to represent a specific syndrome or depression subtype (e.g., *anhedonia*, or the inability to take pleasure in activities). Several investigators have pointed out the limitations of the traditional diagnostic syndrome-based approach (Ingram, Miranda, & Segal, 1998; Kendall & Brady, 1995; Persons, 1986). These limitations stem from the fact that this approach implicitly assumes that individuals with the same syndrome are equivalent in all, or most important, in psychological ways—an assumption that is clearly not correct. For example, Kendall and Brady (1995) note that the symptoms of psychological disorders are so diverse that two people could be diagnosed with the same disorder but actually have very few symptoms in common. In the specific case of depression, only five of the nine criteria detailed in DSM-5 are necessary for a diagnosis; thus, it is possible that two depressed individuals could have only one common symptom, and even the nature and experience of that one symptom could vary. Indeed, except for a diagnosis of depression, these two individuals could have virtually nothing in common, including the variables that caused the disorder and that determine its course. Moreover, relying solely on the concept of a syndrome to study a problem such as depression may miss important information (Persons, 1986). Thus, a sample of "depressed" individuals, selected only because they have enough symptoms to qualify as depressed, represents a phenotypically heterogeneous group.

It seems likely that different causal processes give rise to various symptom patterns that are clustered under the label of *depression*. Few clinical scientists would dispute at least some causal heterogeneity, yet few empirical data are available to help sort out the parameters of the different causal pathways that are both possible and potentially numerous. Indeed, although the possible subtypes of depression may not be endless, they are potentially so diverse that they may functionally defy conceptual classification and empirical scrutiny. Nevertheless, to disregard conceptually the possibility of different subtypes or to acquiesce methodologically to the complexity of possible causal heterogeneity by ignoring the implications of lumping together various subtypes in research studies likely hinders efforts to understand the nature of depression. Given this state of affairs, at least two broad sets of assumptions can guide methodological decision making: conceptual proposals for various subtypes and a more empirically derived approach focused on the examination of different subsets of symptoms.

Depending on the precise conceptual questions posed by investigators, a symptom-based conceptualization may be a viable alternative to the traditional diagnostic syndrome-based approach. Rather than grouping all individuals together because they have met some threshold of depressive symptoms, a symptom profile approach targets specific symptoms that are considered important. For example, negative affect is a variable that is critical to the definition of depression, and it is also thought to play a significant role in determining psychological and social functioning of depressed people. Investigators who are interested in negative affect might choose to study this variable in the context of a depressive state, yet it is important to realize that people with depression (clinical, subclinical, dysthymia), anxiety (general anxiety states, as well as more specific anxious states such as phobia and obsessive–compulsive problems), and physical illnesses (acute and chronic) all experience negative affect. If negative affect is studied only in the context of a depressive syndrome, then important aspects of this phenomenon may be missed. Alternatively, a focus on negative affect rather than on the syndrome of depression permits the study of individuals who share this state and are similar in important respects.

Using symptom clusters, or even one symptom, to select research participants does not rule out obtaining other information from participants. For instance, if a specific measure of negative affect is used, a depression syndrome can still be assessed. Indeed, in the case of a variable such as negative affect, this procedure allows investigators to determine whether a depressive syndrome (or other syndromes) or some pattern of depressive (or other) symptoms contributes to explaining variance over and above that associated with negative affect. Hence, a specific focus on negative affect allows investigators to determine the correlates and possible causes of a process that may be fundamental to many types of psychopathology and also to examine how this variable is associated with other symptoms and behaviors. Negative affect is, of course, merely an example. Investigators may decide to focus on other target symptoms or on clusters of similar symptoms.

It may therefore be worthwhile for researchers to consider examining depressive symptom profiles or clusters rather than (or perhaps in addition to) the aggregation of symptoms represented by classifying people as having depression. Of course, if researchers are interested in a depression construct characterized by the experience of a variety of symptoms (and are not interested in specific subtypes), then the syndrome approach is warranted. Clearly, though, the symptom profile approach encompasses a high degree of flexibility and potentially addresses a number of questions that are simply not possible when participants are selected only for high versus low scores on a depression self-report measure or when they exceed some clinical threshold of depressive symptoms. It also allows researchers to investigate more precise conceptual questions.

Subtypes

Virtually all investigators operate from a theoretical framework that specifies at least some idea about causal processes. Unless they propose that all cases that meet the criteria for depression are caused by the same factors, it is possible conceptually to stipulate different subtypes and then proceed to test the subtypes based on the predictions derived from a given model. These predictions presumably involve proposals about the symptoms and features that should follow from the proposed causal process, along with implications for prevention and treatment. Thus it should be possible to identify empirically those individuals who exhibit the proposed subtype and then determine whether they become depressed when the "right" circumstances occur as specified by the particular subtype model (e.g., certain life events).

Selective Depressive Symptoms

There are a variety of reasons for investigators to study symptomatology in depression. In particular, in conjunction with subtype- or symptom-profile approaches, symptom-threshold models allow assessment of clinical relevance and permit investigators to examine the relation between the degree or severity of depressive symptoms and some other construct. To advance toward eventual syndromic conceptions, investigators may wish to examine the relations among a few select symptoms or even between one symptom and another construct or a constellation of symptoms that cluster together (e.g., vegetative symptoms) and some other variable. For example, investigators may wish to understand specific mechanisms of depression that they believe to be independent of other aspects of depression, in which case the most appropriate strategy may be to examine individuals who are not experiencing the entire depressive syndrome. This strategy has advantages and disadvantages, as described later.

Studying Symptoms in Unselected Samples: Assessing Calculus Interests among Preschoolers

One strategy that researchers have adopted to assess the association between depression symptoms and variables of some theoretical interest is to examine the correlation between these variables in an unselected sample. Studies employing this strategy are based on assumptions that both symptoms and their association with some other variable are continuous, relatively normally distributed, and meaningful at both the high and low ends of the symptom spectrum and that the associations between these variables are linear.

We argue that such assumptions are flawed. The majority of participants in an unselected sample will likely have very a low proportion of the symptoms of interest. Thus studies that adopt this correlational strategy are assessing the relation between symptoms and some other variable in a sample in which the symptom is largely absent. Such a strategy is akin to studying interest in learning calculus among preschoolers. Because preschoolers have no such interest, correlations between scores on a questionnaire measuring this interest (undoubtedly randomly distributed) and some other measure would be meaningless, as, we argue, is research that attempts to study the relation between a construct and depressive symptoms in a sample relatively without depression.

There are several appropriate ways to examine relations involving depressive symptomatology. One approach is to study only individuals who score above some cutoff point on symptoms of interest. A sample composed of research participants who score above some value on items on the BDI-II is more appropriate for answering questions about relations between degree of symptomatology and other variables. Indeed, it has been demonstrated that results can vary in important ways depending on whether associations are examined in the entire sample or in those who exceed the cutoff for a subsample with depression (Ingram & Hamilton, 1999).

Another strategy is to ensure that the full range of depressive symptoms of interest is represented in the sample. For example, the researcher interested in this type of question could adopt a stratified sampling approach. This would involve selecting equal numbers of participants who fall within equal intervals on the depression symptoms of interest (e.g., on the BDI, selecting the same number of participants who score a 0, 1, 2, etc., up to some cutoff on the full inventory or a subscale). Such a strategy creates an artificial sample, but it does so in a way that allows investigators to examine the genuine associations between depressive symptoms, even at the very low end, and other variables.

Assessing Depression Mechanisms

A final strategy, consistent with the RDoC initiative, is to abandon traditional notions of depression and, instead, rebuild the study of the depression spectrum from mechanisms on up to eventual symptoms and symptom clusters. Here, the ideas of "independent" and "dependent" variables are confounded, with a stronger emphasis on integrating across domains of measurement from self-report to biological and cognitive mechanisms. So, for example, transdiagnostic mechanisms common in depression, such as decreased executive control, identified with prefrontal cortex deficits, may be of primary interest. Thus researchers may elect to study prefrontal deficits. This strategy could involve stratifying recruitment on prefrontal function, rather than aspects of depression per se, and assessing the impact of prefrontal function on phenomena of interest such as how people process emotional information. Analyses could later involve understanding the extent to which prefrontal function or prefrontal impact on emotional information processing explains variance in aspects of depression.

Methodological Issues and Challenges Related to the Study of Depression

Having now presented some of the issues involved in defining depression or aspects of depression operationally, we turn to a consideration of methodological issues for the purposes of adequately studying one of these depressive states (or patterns of symptoms). In particular, we examine some common problems in depression research and suggest possible solutions to these difficulties.

Third Variables: Broad and Specific Perspectives

Both broad and more specific ways to consider third-variable confounding can be considered; either or both are applicable depending on the particular questions being asked. The broader perspective focuses on the idea of "nuisance variables" (Meehl, 1978) and is a concern not only in depression studies but also in all studies that examine individual-difference variables (Campbell & Stanley, 1966). This represents a problem for research regardless of whether the focus is on MDD, subclinical depression, or symptom profiles. One specific area of concern for depression is reflected in comorbidity, which presents more of an issue for studies of MDD than for research on subclinical depression or symptom-driven approaches. It is well known that depression is correlated with other emotionally dysfunctional states, thus making it difficult to know whether results are largely a function of depression alone, of some correlated state, or of a combination of depression and other states. As focus shifts toward transdiagnostic mechanisms, this concern is multiplied in that many disease mechanisms tend to occur together; separating what is unique versus independent about them will be a primary research challenge.

In a similar fashion, consideration of physical comorbidities has become increasingly important in recent years. To illustrate one example, mortality associated with the aftermath of myocardial infarction (MI) is greatly increased in the presence of depression; the extent to which post-MI depression represents a unique subtype is unclear. Moreover, physical and mental comorbidities may interact. For instance, nearly all patients with depression after MI have significant anxiety (Denollet, Strik, Lousberg, & Honig, 2006). Another reason to consider physical comorbidities is that physical conditions and their associated treatments may induce depressions that are different in character from most naturally occurring depressions: Steroid- and cytokine-induced depressions, postpartum depressions, and lesion and psychoactive drug-induced depressions also have unique characteristics, highlighting the potential utility of attending to these features in more general studies of depression.

Statistical solutions to the presence of nuisance variables have often been proposed (Locascio, Lee, & Meltzer, 1988). For example, a researcher interested in depression could assess possibly correlated nuisance variables, such as anxiety, then statistically control for them in subsequent results. But such techniques frequently introduce interpretative problems associated more strongly with the covariates than with the research questions at hand, leading to well-rehearsed cautions regarding careless adjustments for covariates (Alemayehu, 2011; Miller & Chapman, 2001). A second method also involves assessing the nuisance variable, then selecting only research participants who endorse depressive symptoms but do not endorse more than an average value on the nuisance variable, for example, anxiety symptoms. However, even when investigators adhere to exclusion criteria that rule out comorbid diagnoses or problems, a subclinical comorbid state may still exist, as might the existence of other unassessed problems. Also, if depression strongly covaries with "nuisance variable," this strategy could yield a biased understanding of depression; for example, if the nuisance variable is anxiety, examining only individuals with depression but without anxiety would be unrepresentative of the population at large.

There are occasions on which covariation is not necessarily a problem and may, in fact, lead to a more precise description of the causes and correlates of depression, as well as other symptom patterns. For example, Tennen and colleagues (1995) noted a growing body of research that has demonstrated important distinctions in the correlates of depression and anxiety despite their high correlation (Kendall & Watson, 1989). But these are often mitigated by poor accounting for the effects of covariation. Thus, although solutions to the problem of third (and fourth, fifth, etc.) variables tend to fall into the broad categories of statistical control (if the third variable can be adequately measured) or exclusionary criteria (if a third variable can be identified), there is no "one size fits all" solution to nuisance-variable issues. How to deal with these confounds is ultimately up to the investigator. Researchers who are interested in assessing "pure" depression will make different decisions than will the investigators who are interested in depression as it occurs more naturally.

Interacting and Mechanistically Common Comorbidity

Comorbid states may interact with depression or associated features, for example, by increasing the severity of depression or by changing the nature of depression in the presence of the comorbid condition. In this context, attempts to decouple naturally co-occurring affective states may create an artificial condition. Hence this situation would represent not simple nuisance covariation but a condition in need of more subtle decomposition because the comorbidity is part and parcel of the depressed state. For instance, the nature of the association between depression and anxiety is still a matter of debate. Whereas some investigators maintain that depression and anxiety lie on a continuum, others contend that depression and anxiety represent orthogonal dimensions, for which particular combinations (e.g., mixed anxiety–depression) represent a qualitatively different disorder than having just one condition (e.g., Angst & Merikangas, 1998; see Mineka & Vrshek-Schallhorn, Chapter 5, this volume, for a more detailed discussion of this issue). This consideration is particularly important because over half of adults with depression report significant anxiety (Fawcett & Howard, 1983). Because patients with comorbid conditions take longer to recover than do people with "pure" depression (Angst, 1997), this distinction is particularly important. Thus, at the very least, it is likely not appropriate to statistically adjust for anxiety in depression; statistical models involving depression–anxiety interactions may be more appropriate. Similarly, if a there are common transdiagnostic processes underlying depression and anxiety—for example, associated with negative affect (Watson, Clark, & Carey, 1988)—understanding these common processes may prove more interesting than trying to differentiate depression and anxiety at all.

Regardless of whether comorbidity is conceptualized as a nuisance variable to be controlled, as an important part of depression, or as an interactive moderator or mediator, investigators would be well advised to be aware of the issues of third variables and to develop a plan for dealing with them. In virtually all cases, investigators may wish to attempt to assess systematically those states that are known or suspected to be associated with depression or the features of depression being examined. What they do with this assessment is then a function of the particular question being addressed.

Stability Considerations

Issues concerning stability of depression and its features have important methodological implications. One of the most significant effects of depressive states is that they endure over some period of time, and, just like a headache that gets better after a few hours as opposed to a migraine that lasts for days, it could be argued that the endurance of a disorder rather than its "mere" onset is what confers both emotional misery and significantly impaired function. Thus focusing research efforts on stable aspects of those states may be of interest, particularly if the researcher's interest is in what is maintaining the disorder. This is especially important in studies of subclinical depression because the milder nature of these states suggests that they will be less stable than the fully diagnosable clinical syndrome, particularly in its chronic variant. Potentially, then, the meaningfulness of research on subclinical features of depression will be enhanced by showing that the features endure over some period of time rather than remitting quickly.

Stability considerations bring with them some important methodological requirements. Most research on depression is pragmatically a two-step process, the first of which involves measuring the presence of depressive features on one occasion and the second conducting the research on a second occasion with individuals who meet the initial criteria. However, evidence of depression such as scores on depression measures can change over even relatively short periods of time. Thus a group of individuals initially selected for high levels of depression may include a substantial number of people who no longer fall in a depressed range when experimental testing commences. Functionally, and as per our discussion of preschool calculus, such research constitutes testing hypotheses in a "depressed" sample in which not everyone has depression. The best-case scenario in such a situation is that error variance increases, rendering detection of differences more difficult; a worst-case scenario is that such a procedure may produce misleading or erroneous results.

Studying depression as a clinical syndrome raises a potentially different set of stability issues. Some individuals will continue to meet criteria for depression at the time of experimental testing if the testing occurs a short time after diagnostic assessments; that said, if other tests are performed even a few weeks from initial assessments, it is wise to verify the depressed state given the temporally variable nature of the unstable syndrome. For example, if an individual needs to meet five of nine criteria to be diagnosed and one symptom (e.g., eating disturbance) is unstable, the diagnostic picture can vary from day to day. The severity of depression (e.g., the number and intensity of symptoms) can also vary, sometimes substantially, over the course of days or weeks. Such variability is commonly assessed in treatment studies (e.g., Jarrett, Vittengl, Doyle, & Clark, 2007) and could be useful in nontreatment studies as well. In addition, the *pattern* of symptoms may change over time. For example, as the stability of symptoms and severity across depressive episodes is notoriously low (Lewinsohn, Pettit, Joiner, & Seeley, 2003), the same individual's "depression" may look different when assessed at different times. Beyond continuing to meet criteria, researchers' conclusions should thus take into account the symptom patterns and intensities at the time of experimental testing rather than those present at the time of selection into the study.

To establish the stability of the depressive state or features in which investigators are interested, Kendall and colleagues (1987) and Tennen and colleagues (1995) have argued for the use of multiple-gating procedures in which researchers establish appropriate depression scores or criteria at selection, readminister the depression measure at testing, and then analyze data from only those individuals who score in the specified range or who meet criteria on both occasions. This helps to at least ensure that this phenomenon has been stable over some period of time and that participants are actually experiencing depression at the time of testing.

Developmental Considerations

The extent to which depression in adults and in children represents the same disorder is the subject of debate (e.g., Kaufman, Martin, King, & Charney, 2001; see Gibb, Chapter 20, this volume). Diagnostic criteria for child and adult depression are similar, yet diagnosis in children is often more difficult because children may have trouble reporting symptoms and may experience different patterns of symptoms. Thus clinicians often rely on observations, such as tearfulness or academic problems, to make an early-onset diagnosis (Ryan, 2001). Symptom measures also suggest that depression and other disorders, such as anxiety and attention-deficit/hyperactivity disorder (ADHD), may overlap considerably at early ages (Angold, Costello, & Erkanli, 1999). Also, biological mechanisms associated with adult depression may not generalize to children (Kaufman et al., 2001). For example, event-related brain potentials suggest that adults with depression display greater brain responses to errors than do healthy adults (Tucker, Luu, Frishkoff, Quiring, & Poulsen, 2003). The event-related potential is late to develop and is not easily detectable in children (Ladouceur, Dahl, & Carter, 2007). Similarly, hypofrontality is a key biological measure in adult depression (Siegle, Thompson, Carter, Steinhauer, & Thase, 2007). Because the prefrontal cortex is still developing through adolescence, it is unclear what the effects of hypofrontality would be in the developing brain.

These issues become more complicated when we consider developmental factors. For example, studies examining depression in samples that range from ages 4 to 14 years will, at best, find enormous variance; there is little in common between a 4-year-old and a 14-year-old, except that they are both children. Even the definition of childhood is unclear; whereas some federal entities (e.g., the draft board) recognize childhood as ending at age 18, others, such as NIMH, make the distinction at age 21. Studies of childhood depression variables need to consider carefully the pros and cons of various age cutoff points for samples.

Race, Ethnicity, and Culture Considerations

Projections based on the 2010 United States census suggest that the next 50 years will bring an increasingly ethnically diverse nation (see the 2012 U.S. Census Bureau Population Projections, *www.census.gov/population/projections/data/national/2012.html*). By 2043, no single ethnic group will constitute a majority in the United States, thus making the United States a "majority–minority" country; similarly, the Hispanic population is projected to more than double by 2060, with approximately one in three U.S. residents being of Hispanic ethnicity (vs. one in six in the 2010 census). Indeed, the complexity of cultural considerations in research makes the difficult, age-related concerns we have just discussed seem straightforward and simple. In the past, culture was commonly seen, at least implicitly, as synonymous with race. Although race is a well-established biological construct (Bonham, Warshauer-Baker, & Collins, 2005), political considerations have created a controversy over its existence and meaning that, misguided or not, may prove to be a benefit to the extent that it forces research to focus on shared cultural experiences as important variables.

In addition, research is increasingly focusing on measurement of ethnic identification as a construct distinct from race and worthy of study. For example, federal research guidelines, including those from NIMH, require assessing race and ethnicity as separate constructs, and researchers must make attempts to recruit underrepresented racial and ethnic groups. In addition, clinically relevant American Psychological Association journals (e.g., *Journal of Abnormal Psychology, Journal of Consulting and Clinical Psychology*) strongly encourage investigators to report the racial and ethnic composition of their samples. Even in those cases in which samples are relatively ethnically and/or racially homogenous, detailed reporting of racial and ethnic composition, rather than collapsing across cells, can facilitate meta-analytic studies that take into consideration race and ethnicity.

Although race and ethnicity are but two facets of the complex construct of culture, they have tended to be the focus of research into cultural constructs. However, researchers have begun examining culture in more nuanced ways. For example, there are multiple self-report measures designed to measure acculturation (see Thomson & Hoffman-Goetz, 2009, for a review of measures in Latino/Hispanic populations; see Unger et al., 2002, for a review of measures in middle-school children). These measures are recognized as imperfect in that they tend to focus on proxies of acculturation and have not typically been theoretically derived. However, scales such as this provide a start to assessing cultural constructs in new ways. In addition, although socioeconomic status has long been recognized as a potent variable of interest with regard to many health outcomes, including depression (e.g., Everson, Lynch, & Kaplan, 2002), researchers have also begun exploring relations between more granular but related cultural variables such as employment satisfaction and financial strain and depression (Zimmerman & Katon, 2005). Ultimately, these finer-grained approaches are likely to prove more useful in understanding depression causation.

In addition, as increasing numbers of studies have been aimed at investigating questions related to culture, evidence for the association of cultural variables with depression outcomes of interest has begun to accumulate. As an example, researchers using meta-analysis have found that treatments for depression that are specifically adapted for clients of color were moderately more effective than nonadapted traditional treatments (Smith, Rodrigues, & Bernal, 2011). Findings such as this, combined with projections for an increasingly ethnically diverse population, highlight the importance of continuing to refine research methodologies for assessing ethnic and cultural variables and their relations to depression constructs of interest.

ISSUES IN UNDERSTANDING CAUSALITY

Understanding causal issues is important, if not essential, for many research efforts. Yet, what is *causality*? The simplest view refers to the onset of depression, the transition from a relatively normal state into a state of psychological disorder. However, because depression can develop over time, is not static after its onset, and recurs in many cases, a causal cycle may be a better formulation of this idea.

The Causal Cycle of Depression

Vulnerability

One cause of depression involves vulnerability to disorder. Definitions of vulnerability vary, but Ingram and colleagues (Ingram et al., 1998; Ingram, Atchley, & Segal, 2011) suggest several core features that characterize most accounts of vulnerability to depression. A core feature is that vulnerability is a trait as opposed to a state that characterizes the actual appearance of the depression. Depending on the level of analysis used, vulnerability can be seen as residing in genetic factors, biological substrates, or psychological variables. In addition, vulnerability is usually conceptualized as a latent endogenous process that is reactive to the effects of stress. Vulnerability is synonymous with the diathesis in the diathesis–stress approach that is common among current models of depression.

Onset

Following vulnerability, onset of the disorder is the next stage of the causal sequence. Onset is perhaps the most easily conceptualized aspect of causality because it tends to be treated as synonymous with causality. However, *onset* is more precisely defined as the appearance of depressive symptoms. If the type of MDD specified by DSM-5 is of interest, then *onset* is defined as the appearance of at least five out of nine symptoms, one of which must be sad mood or loss of pleasure, and all of which persist for at least 2 weeks.

Maintenance of Depression

Another aspect of the causal sequence is maintenance of the depressed state. By virtually all estimates, depression is a persistent disorder with symptoms lasting many months (sometimes even with effective treatment), and even years in some cases. There is some consensus among investigators that untreated depression lasts between 6 months and 1 year, although the disorder may last up to 2 years in more severe cases (Keller, Shapiro, Lavori, & Wolfe, 1982). In fact, symptoms that endure for an extended period of time are most likely linked to the disruption and personal turmoil that accompany depression. Thus the factors involved in the perpetuation of depression can be considered to be causal.

Response, Remission, and Recovery

Rush, Kraemer, and colleagues (2006) recommend that *response* be defined as a clinically significant reduction in symptoms. Although a reduction in clinical significance has typically been described as a 50% reduction in symptoms (Frank et al., 1991), Rush and colleagues suggest that, rather than use a universal definition, investigators should determine response rates in reference to specific patient characteristics. For example, they argue that rather than a 50% symptom reduction for all patients, a 25% reduction is a reasonable criterion for cases of treatment-resistant depression. In relation to response, *remission* is defined as the complete, or near complete, disappearance of all criterion symptoms, accompanied by the assumption that variables underlying the disorder may still be present. This is particularly the case when some symptoms, although diminished beyond clinical significance, are still present. On the other hand, *recovery* suggests the disappearance of symptom criteria *and* the underlying processes. Rush and colleagues suggest that *remission* be defined as the lack of sufficient symptoms for a period of at least 3 consecutive weeks and that *recovery* be defined as the lack of sufficient symptoms for a 4-month period.

TREATMENT EFFECTS

The current "gold standard" in treatment research is the randomized controlled design in which participants are assigned to a treatment or to either a placebo, waiting-list, or alternative treatment condition. More complex designs involving selective applications of adjunctive treatments or algorithmic interventions (e.g., starting with a single treatment, then augmenting or switching between or among treatments) are also gaining popularity. Indeed, algorithmic treatments have been most widely studied with respect to pharmacotherapy interventions such as the Texas Medication Algorithm Project (Crismon et al., 1999) and the Sequenced Treatment Alternatives to Relieve Depression study (STAR*D; Rush et al., 2004; Rush, Trivedi, et al., 2006). More recently, however, researchers are also focusing on these methods in the context of psychotherapy treatments (e.g., Weisz et al., 2012) including psychotherapy for depression (e.g., Steidtmann et al., 2013). These designs can increase our understanding of the extent to which specific treatments affect specific mechanisms of disorder, as well as enhancing treatment outcomes for depression.

Arguably, the power of treatment designs lies in the nature of assessments before, during, and after treatment. Assessment of symptoms alone helps us to understand the time course of recovery. Additional assessment of cognitive, social, and biological mechanisms can provide insights concerning the mechanisms of recovery. The more frequently investigators perform such assessments, the more likely it is that they can begin to make claims regarding mediation and moderation of recovery by assessed factors (Kraemer, Stice, Kazdin, Offord, & Kupfer, 2001). For example, treatments such as antidepressant medications are designed to affect brain mechanisms proximally associated with symptoms, presumably leaving trait-vulnerability mechanisms in place (DeRubeis, Siegle, & Hollon, 2008). Assessment of cognitive and biological mechanisms before, during, and after antidepressant treatment can help us understand the extent to which changes in these mechanisms are addressed by medications. In contrast, an intervention such as cognitive therapy nominally focuses on changing underlying vulnerabilities and is associated with reduction of future risk for depression (Hollon, Stewart, & Strunk, 2006). Designs that examine and contrast such interventions, along with pre- and postassessments, can allow examination of differential mechanisms of change and their effects on underlying vulnerability factors across interventions. Recent work in this regard has proven powerful and unintuitive. For example, antidepressants appear to affect information processing long before symptoms are affected, suggesting they might share more common mechanisms with interventions such as cognitive therapy than previously believed (Harmer, Goodwin, & Cowen, 2009; McCabe, Mishor, Cowen, & Harmer, 2010).

Thus, inferring that specific aspects of a treatment are directly associated with remission or recovery is difficult in that multiple, nonspecific factors may also contribute to symptom change. As another example, momentary symptom reduction due to antidepressants may lead to lifestyle changes that promote continued risk reduction. Comparison with placebo treatments can help us understand the extent to which specific aspects of recovery are uniquely associated with treatment mechanisms. Possibly, then, adjunctive application of interventions that specifically target circumscribed mechanisms (e.g., Siegle, Ghinassi, & Thase, 2007) may be particularly revealing in this regard because such interventions can suggest which aspects of depression are dependent on specific brain or cognitive mechanisms. Such mechanistically targeted treatments—for example, to address specific biases in information processing (Bar-Haim, 2010)—are increasingly popular. Prospective interventions, such as those employed with vulnerable youth who do not yet have depression, may also be revealing, providing evidence of whether, if specific vulnerability mechanisms are addressed, depression will develop (see Gotlib & Colich, Chapter 13, this volume, for a more detailed discussion of this point). Assessments of specific changes in brain and behavioral functioning associated with symptom reduction (e.g., as afforded by neuroimaging, information processing, and ecological momentary assessments) can also aid in this regard.

CONCLUSIONS, FUTURE DIRECTIONS, AND A CAUTIONARY NOTE ON DEMONSTRATING CAUSALITY

It is important to consider that none of the designs we have described are generally considered to be causal tests. Rather, like most clinical research, the designs we have described are often inherently quasi-experimental, with the potential exception of treatment designs in which depression status may, to some extent, be experimentally manipulated. Recall that longitudinal designs are uniquely equipped to demonstrate temporal antecedence, which is necessary but not sufficient to show causality. As a prerequisite to showing that a variable is causal, data must demonstrate that the variable in question predicts depressive symptomatology (e.g., Segal et al., 2006). Satisfying this prerequisite, however, is also not enough; showing that a variable predicts the occurrence of depression is an important step, but in and of itself it does not establish a cause and effect. For example, even if a longitudinal design shows that certain responses predict subsequent depression, other processes that are correlated with the variables in question may serve as the actual causative factors for depression. As such, third-variable causality is extremely difficult to rule out.

Importantly, new technologies are on the horizon that may better afford the potential for causal tests that have not been possible in the past. Causal investigations of depression are traditionally elusive, as it has been unethical to willfully make a person depressed. But new, targeted, reversible treatments for depression may permit single-subject designs that break this barrier. For example, consider treatments involving deep-brain stimulation, in which stimulating electrodes are placed in a brain structure thought to be causal to an individual's depression (Holtzheimer et al., 2012; Lozano et al., 2012). In these treatments it is the norm to do "single-subject experiments" in which, after the electrodes are placed and before the system is turned on, depressive affect is assessed. The electrodes are turned on, and the system is adjusted dynamically until depressive symptoms lift. The system is turned off, and symptoms are observed to return. At this point the system is turned on again, with the causal inference that affecting a single brain region indeed affects depressive affect. Of course, the operationalization of depression, relevant variables to be measured in association with brain function, and so forth are all subject to the same considerations described throughout this chapter.

We end this chapter with a point that we have noted a number of times throughout the various issues we discuss but that nevertheless warrants repeated emphasis. The appropriateness of many of the strategies and tactics that we and others have discussed relative to depression research depends on the precise conceptual questions and hypotheses proposed. Some tactics may be perfectly appropriate for one type of question concerning depression but grossly inappropriate for another. Far too infrequently, however, do investigators elaborate the specific conceptual question in which they are interested with precise reference to a given population with depression. As we have noted, for example, we think there are legitimate reasons to study subclinical depression; nevertheless, the field would be well served if investigators always stated exactly why the questions they address using this particular group are important. Similarly, investigators interested in a "pure" major depressive state that is not associated with the conditions that typically co-occur with clinical depression would serve the field well by explicitly addressing why this particular type of sample is of interest. Overall, therefore, precise conceptual and empirical questions will guide a more precise choice of research procedures and samples that ultimately increase our understanding of depression (Ingram & Hamilton, 1999).

In a general sense, we believe that the field has labored implicitly for too long under a uniformity myth wherein depression is a single phenomenon that can always, or virtually always, be investigated with a few straightforward research strategies. This uniformity myth is giving way to a much more complex understanding of depression and, with it, the need to utilize complex research strategies. Although depression research was simpler when the field adhered implicitly to this uniformity myth, more sophisticated strategies are beginning to reveal important aspects of the processes that underlie depression in ways that earlier and simpler studies could not. To continue this progress, we must appreciate the complexity of the specific phenomena that characterize what we broadly call *depression*; state very clearly our theoretical questions, with precise reference to the depression type and phenomena to which they are to be applied; then select a research strategy that matches the type of depression we want to understand. We must confront both the complexity of depression and the methodological strategies that can be used to investigate it, then make the best choices possible.

Certainly, some researchers may yearn for a return to an earlier time when depression research was simply a matter of comparing groups with and without depression, as assessed by a questionnaire. In the version of this chapter that appeared in the first edition of this *Handbook* (Ingram & Siegle, 2002) we made reference to a television commercial that at the time attempted to entice people to buy the new Oldsmobile by noting that it was "not your father's Oldsmobile." That commercial, thankfully, has disappeared, but the analogy still applies. Contemporary research on depression is no longer our father's Oldsmobile. That car was cheaper and easy to service but not all that reliable. New cars are more expensive to buy and to operate and much more complicated and difficult to service. Yet the ride is better and more reliable, and we are more assured of getting to our ultimate destination. It is time to trade up.

REFERENCES

Alemayehu, D. (2011). Current issues with covariate adjustment in the analysis of data from randomized controlled trials. *American Journal of Therapeutics, 18,* 153–157.

American Psychiatric Association. (2013). *Diagnostic and statistical manual of mental disorders* (5th ed.). Arlington, VA: Author.

Angold, A., Costello, J. E., & Erkanli, A. (1999). Comorbidity. *Journal of Child Psychology and Psychiatry, 40,* 57–87

Angst, J. (1997). Depression and anxiety: Implications for nosology, course, and treatment. *Journal of Clinical Psychiatry, 58,* 3–5.

Angst, J., & Merikangas, K. R. (1998). Mixed anxiety depression. *Psychiatria Hungarica, 3,* 263–268.

Bar-Haim, Y. (2010). Research review: Attention bias modification (ABM): A novel treatment for anxiety disorders. *Journal of Child Psychology and Psychiatry, 51,* 859–870.

Beck, A. T., Steer, R. A., & Garbin, M. G. (1988). Psychometric properties of the Beck Depression Inventory: Twenty-five years of evaluation. *Clinical Psychology Review, 8,* 77–100.

Bonham, V. L., Warshauer-Baker, E., & Collins, F. S. (2005). Race and ethnicity in the genome era: The complexity of the constructs. *American Psychologist, 60,* 9–15.

Campbell, D. T., & Stanley, J. C. (1966). *Experimental and quasi-experimental designs for research.* Chicago: Rand McNally.

Coyne, J. C. (1994). Self-reported distress: Analog or ersatz depression? *Psychological Bulletin, 116,* 29–45.

Crismon, M. L., Trivedi, M., Pigott, T. A, Rush, A. J., Hirschfeld, M. A., Kahn, D. A., et al. (1999). The Texas Medication Algorithm Project: Report of the Texas Consensus Conference Panel on Medication Treatment of Major Depressive Disorder. *Journal of Clinical Psychiatry, 60,* 142–156.

Cuijpers, P., & Smit, F. (2004). Subthreshold depression as a risk indicator for major depressive disorder: A systematic review of prospective studies. *Acta Psychiatrica Scandinavica, 109,* 325–331.

Denollet, J., Strik, J. J., Lousberg, R., & Honig, A. (2006). Recognizing increased risk of depressive comorbidity after myocardial infarction: Looking for 4 symptoms of anxiety–depression. *Psychotherapy and Psychosomatics, 75,* 346–352.

DeRubeis, R. J., Siegle, G. J., & Hollon, S. D. (2008). Cognitive therapy versus medication for depression: Treatment outcomes and neural mechanisms. *Nature Reviews Neuroscience, 9,* 788–796.

Everson, S. A., Lynch, J. W., & Kaplan, G. A. (2002). Epidemiologic evidence for the relation between socioeconomic status and depression, obesity, and diabetes. *Journal of Psychosomatic Research, 53,* 891–895.

Fawcett, J., & Howard, M. (1983). Anxiety syndromes and their relationship to depressive illness. *Journal of Clinical Psychiatry, 444,* 8–11.

Frank, E., Prien, R. F., Jarret, R. B., Keller, M. B., Kupfer, D. J., Lavori, P. W., et al. (1991). Conceptualization and rationale for consensus definitions of terms in major depressive disorder: Remission, recovery, relapse, and recurrence. *Archives of General Psychiatry, 48,* 851–855.

Gotlib, I. H., Lewinsohn, P. M., & Seeley, J. R. (1995). Symptoms versus a diagnosis of depression: Differences in psychosocial functioning. *Journal of Consulting and Clinical Psychology, 63,* 90–100.

Hamilton, N. A., Karlson, C., Luxton, D., Nelson, C., & Stevens, N. R. (2009). Insomnia. In R. E. Ingram (Ed.), *International encyclopedia of depression* (pp. 343–348). New York: Springer.

Harmer, C. J., Goodwin, G. M., & Cowen, P. J. (2009). Why do antidepressants take so long to work?: A cognitive neuropsychological model of antidepressant drug action. *British Journal of Psychiatry, 195,* 102–108.

Hollon, S. D., Stewart, M., & Strunk, D. (2006). Enduring effects for cognitive behavior therapy in the treatment of depression and anxiety. *Annual Review of Psychology, 57,* 285–315.

Holtzheimer, P. E., Kelley, M. E., Gross, R. E., Filkowski, M. M., Garlow, S. J., Barrocas, A., et al. (2012). Subcallosal cingulate deep brain stimulation for treatment-resistant unipolar and bipolar depression. *Archives of General Psychiatry, 69,* 150–158.

Ingram, R. E., Atchley, R. A., & Segal, Z. V. (2011). *Vulnerability to depression: From cognitive neuroscience to prevention and treatment.* New York: Guilford Press.

Ingram, R. E., & Hamilton, N. A. (1999). Evaluating precision in the social psychological assessment of depression: Methodological considerations, issues, and recommendations. *Journal of Social and Clinical Psychology, 18,* 160–180.

Ingram, R. E., Miranda, J., & Segal, Z. V. (1998). *Cognitive vulnerability to depression.* New York: Guilford Press.

Ingram, R. E., & Siegle, G. J. (2002). Methodological issues in depression research: Not your father's Oldsmobile. In I. H. Gotlib & C. L. Hammen (Eds.), *Handbook of depression* (pp. 86–114). New York: Guilford Press.

Jarrett, R. B., Vittengl, J. R., Doyle, K., & Clark, L. A. (2007). Changes in cognitive content during and following cognitive therapy for recurrent depression: Substantial and enduring but not predictive of change in depressive symptoms. *Journal of Consulting and Clinical Psychology, 75,* 432–446.

Kaufman, J., Martin, A., King, R., & Charney, D. (2001). Are child-, adolescent-, and adult-onset depression one and the same disorder? *Biological Psychiatry, 49,* 980–1001.

Keller, M. B., Shapiro, R. W., Lavori, P. W., & Wolfe, N. (1982). Relapse in RDC major depressive disorders: Analysis with the life table. *Archives of General Psychiatry, 39,* 911–915.

Kendall, P. C., & Brady, E. U. (1995). Comorbidity in the anxiety disorders of childhood: Implications for validity and clinical significance. In K. D. Craig & K. S. Dobson (Eds.), *Anxiety and depression in adults and children* (pp. 3–35). Thousand Oaks, CA: Sage.

Kendall, P. C., & Flannery-Schroeder, E. C. (1995). Rigor, but not rigor mortis, in depression research. *Journal of Personality and Social Psychology, 68,* 892–894.

Kendall, P. C., Hollon, S. D., Beck, A. T., Hammen, C. L., & Ingram, R. E. (1987). Issues and recommendations regarding use of the Beck Depression Inventory. *Cognitive Therapy and Research, 11,* 289–299.

Kendall, P. C., & Watson, D. (Eds.). (1989). *Anxiety and depression: Distinctive and overlapping features.* San Diego, CA: Academic Press.

Kraemer, H. C., Stice, E., Kazdin, A., Offord, D., & Kupfer, D. (2001). How do risk factors work together?: Mediators, moderators, and independent, overlapping, and proxy risk factors. *American Journal of Psychiatry, 158,* 848–856.

Ladouceur, C. D., Dahl, R. E., & Carter, C. S. (2007). The development of action monitoring through adolescence into adulthood: ERP and source localization. *Developmental Science, 10,* 874–891.

Lewinsohn, P. M., Pettit, J. W., Joiner, T. E., Jr., & Seeley, J. R. (2003). The symptomatic expression of major depressive disorder in adolescents and young adults. *Journal of Abnormal Psychology, 112,* 244–252.

Locascio, J. J., Lee, J., & Meltzer, H. Y. (1988). Importance of adjusting for correlated concomitant variables in psychiatric research. *Psychiatry Research, 23,* 311–327.

Lozano, A. M., Giacobbe, P., Hamani, C., Rizvi, S. J., Kennedy, S. H., Kolivakis, T. T., et al (2012). A multicenter pilot study of subcallosal cingulate area deep brain stimulation for treatment-resistant depression. *Journal of Neurosurgery, 116,* 315–322.

McCabe, C., Mishor, Z., Cowen, P. J., & Harmer, C. J. (2010). Diminished neural processing of aversive and rewarding stimuli during selective serotonin reuptake inhibitor treatment. *Biological Psychiatry, 67,* 439–445.

Meehl, P. E. (1978). Theoretical risks and tabular asterisks: Sir Karl, Sir Ronald, and the slow progress of soft psychology. *Journal of Consulting and Clinical Psychology, 46,* 806–834.

Miller, G. A., & Chapman, J. P. (2001). Misunderstanding analysis of covariance. *Journal of Abnormal Psychology, 110,* 40–48.

Persons, J. B. (1986). The advantages of studying psychological phenomena rather than psychiatric diagnoses. *American Psychologist, 41,* 1252–1260.

Rush, A. J., Fava, M., Wisniewski, S. R., Trivedi, M., Sackeim, H. A., Thase, M. E., et al. (2004). Sequenced treatment alternatives to relieve depression (STAR*D): Rationale and design. *Controlled Clinical Trials, 25,* 119–142.

Rush, A. J., Kraemer, H. C., Sackeim, H. A., Fava, M., Trivedi, M. H., Frank, E., et al. (2006). Report by the ACNP Task Force on Response and Remission in Major Depressive Disorder. *Neuropsychopharmacology, 31,* 1841–1853.

Rush, A. J., Trivedi, M. H., Wisniewski, S. R., Nierenberg, A. A., Stewart, J. W., Warden, D., et al. (2006). Acute and longer-term outcomes in depressed outpatients requiring one or several treatment steps: A STAR*D report. *American Journal of Psychiatry, 163,* 1905–1917.

Ryan, D. (2001). Diagnosing pediatric depression. *Biological Psychiatry, 49,* 1050–1054.

Segal, Z. V., Kennedy, M. D., Gemar, M., Hood, K., Pedersen, R., & Buis, T. (2006). Cognitive reactivity to sad mood provocation and the prediction of depressive relapse. *Archives of General Psychiatry, 63,* 749–755.

Siegle, G. J., Ghinassi, F., & Thase, M. E. (2007). Neurobehavioral therapies in the 21st century: Summary of an emerging field and an extended example of Cognitive Control Training for depression. *Cognitive Therapy and Research, 31*, 235–262.

Siegle, G. J., Thompson, W., Carter, C. S., Steinhauer, S. R., & Thase, M. E. (2007). Increased amygdala and decreased dorsolateral prefrontal BOLD responses in unipolar depression: Related and independent features. *Biological Psychiatry, 61*, 198–209.

Simpson, H. B. (2012). The RDoC project: A new paradigm for investigating the pathophysiology of anxiety. *Depression and Anxiety, 29*, 251–252.

Smith, T. B., Rodríguez, M., & Bernal, G. (2011). Culture. *Journal of Clinical Psychology, 67*, 166–175.

Steidtmann, D., Manber, R., Blasey, C., Markowitz, J. C., & Klein, D. N. (2013). Detecting critical decision points in psychotherapy and psychotherapy + medication for chronic depression. *Journal of Consulting and Clinical Psychology, 81*, 783–792.

Tennen, H., Hall, J. A., & Affleck, G. (1995). Depression research methodologies in the *Journal of Personality and Social Psychology*: A review and critique. *Journal of Personality and Social Psychology, 68*, 870–884.

Thomson, M. D., & Hoffman-Goetz, L. (2009). Defining and measuring acculturation: A systematic review of public health studies with Hispanic populations in the United States. *Social Science and Medicine, 69*, 983–991.

Tucker, D. M., Luu, P., Frishkoff, G., Quiring, J., & Poulsen, C. (2003). Frontolimbic response to negative feedback in clinical depression. *Journal of Abnormal Psychology, 112*, 667–678.

Unger, J. B., Gallaher, P., Shakib, S., Ritt-Olson, A., Palmer, P. H., & Johnson, C. (2002). The AHIMSA Acculturation Scale: A new measure of acculturation for adolescents in a multicultural society. *Journal of Early Adolescence, 22*, 225–251.

Watson, D., Clark, L. A., & Carey, G. (1988). Positive and negative affectivity and their relation to anxiety and depressive disorders. *Journal of Abnormal Psychology, 97*, 346–353.

Weisz, J. R., Chorpita, B. F., Palinkas, L. A., Schoenwald, S. K., Miranda, J., & Bearman, S. K., (2012). Testing standard and modular designs for psychotherapy treating depression, anxiety, and conduct problems in youth: A randomized effectiveness trial. *Archives of General Psychiatry, 69*, 274–282.

Zimmerman, F. J., & Katon, W. (2005). Socioeconomic status, depression disparities, and financial strain: What lies behind the income-depression relationship? *Health Economics, 14*, 1197–1215.

CHAPTER 4

Course of Depression
Persistence and Recurrence

DANIEL N. KLEIN *and* ANNA E. S. ALLMANN

Traditionally, depressive disorders have been viewed as acute and time-limited. However, in recent decades, depression has been reconceptualized as a highly recurrent or chronic and often lifelong condition (Andrews, 2001). Neither view is completely accurate (Monroe & Harkness, 2012). Rather, the course of depression is markedly heterogeneous and includes single brief episodes that remit and never recur, multiple acute episodes interspersed with periods of complete recovery, acute episodes followed by long periods of residual symptoms, and chronic episodes that may fluctuate in severity but persist for decades. This fact raises significant challenges for clinicians, patients, and family members trying to forecast the course of the disorder and formulate appropriate treatment plans, but it may also provide some leverage in understanding the etiological and pathophysiological heterogeneity of depression.

In this chapter, we (1) discuss the concepts of recovery, chronicity, and recurrence; (2) summarize data on the rates of recovery, chronicity, and recurrence in major depressive disorder (MDD) and dysthymic disorder; (3) note a number of conceptual and methodological issues that underlie the research literature; (4) review the classification, correlates, and predictors of persistent/chronic depression; (5) summarize correlates and predictors of recurrent depression; and (6) consider the concept of a chronic/recurrent spectrum.

RECOVERY, CHRONICITY, AND RECURRENCE

The terms *recovery, chronic*, and *recurrence* have been used in a variety of ways in the literature (see Rush et al., 2006, for a recent attempt to standardize terminology). Unfortunately, almost no studies have compared the validity of alternative definitions. Recurrent and chronic depression depend on the prior recovery or failure to recover, respectively, from an episode of depression. *Recovery* refers to attaining a period of no or few symptoms after an episode of depression. Investigators differ in how long this period is required to last, with most definitions ranging from 2 to 6 months. They also differ on the symptom threshold required (e.g., no symptoms, one or two symptoms, or falling beneath the diagnostic threshold). The criteria used to define recovery have important implications not just for the rates of recovery but also for rates of chronicity and recurrence (Monroe & Harkness, 2011). Stricter definitions of recovery produce lower estimates of recovery and recurrence and higher estimates of chronicity (Furukawa et al., 2008).

Chronicity refers to episodes that persist for an extended period of time. Most investigators (and the third through fifth editions of the *Diagnostic and Statistical Manual of Mental Disorders* [DSM]; American Psychiatric Association, 1980, 1994, 2013) require that episodes last at least 2 years to be considered chronic, although shorter (e.g., 1-year) and longer (5-year) periods have been used. Investigators also differ on whether full criteria for depression must be met for the entire time or whether periods of subthreshold symptomatology or brief remissions (e.g., up to 2 months) are permitted.

Recurrence refers to the onset of a new episode of depression following a period of recovery. New episodes are typically defined as meeting DSM criteria for a depressive disorder (although these thresholds are themselves somewhat arbitrary). The recurrent subtype, or specifier, refers to individuals who have had more than one lifetime episode. As noted subsequently, rates of recurrence are highly dependent on the length of the follow-up period since recovery.

NATURALISTIC COURSE OF MDD

There are numerous follow-up studies of the course of depression. Unfortunately, very few (e.g., Eaton et al., 2008) trace course trajectories from the initial episode; such studies are important to reduce sampling bias for more chronic and recurrent cases and provide a comprehensive prospective picture. The data summarized in this section stem from naturalistic studies (as opposed to clinical trials) of clinical and community samples; participants were not treated by the investigators, but they may or may not have received treatment during the course of the study. In most cases, the studies are prospective, but some of the data we cite are retrospective.

Most individuals who experience a major depressive episode (MDE) recover. The average duration of an MDE is 20–30 weeks in clinical (Keller et al., 2013) and nonclinical (Rohde, Lewinsohn, Klein, Seeley, & Gau, 2013) samples. The longer the duration of the episode, the lower the probability of recovery (Keller et al., 2013). For 10–20% of individuals with an MDE, the episode becomes chronic. In the Collaborative Depression Study (CDS), Keller and colleagues (2013) followed a large clinical sample for 30 years. They reported that after 2 years, 20% of patients had not recovered from their first prospectively observed MDE; after 5 years, 12% had not recovered; after 10 years, 8% had not recovered; and after 15 years, 6% still had not recovered. In long-term follow-up of a community sample of participants experiencing their first lifetime MDE, Eaton and colleagues (2008) found that 15% had not recovered after a 13- to 23-year period. With respect to dysthymic disorder, in a 10-year follow-up of a clinical sample, Klein, Shankman, and Rose (2006) reported a recovery rate of 74%, with a median time to recovery of 52 months.

In individuals who recover from an MDE, the risk of recurrence varies considerably depending on length of follow-up and the nature of the sample. In the first year after recovery, 25–35% of psychiatric and primary care patients experience a recurrence (e.g.,

Gopinath, Katon, Russo, & Ludman, 2007; Maj, Veltro, Pirozzi, & Lobrace, 1992). The CDS reported recurrence rates of 40% at a 5-year follow-up; 60% at 10 years; 85% at 20 years; and 91% at 30 years (Keller et al., 2013). However, MDD recurrence rates are only 40–50% in long-term follow-ups of community samples (Eaton et al., 2008; Hardeveld, Spijker, De Graaf, Nolen, & Beekman, 2013; Rohde et al., 2013). In Klein and colleagues' (2006) sample of dysthymic patients, the estimated risk of recurrence into another period of chronic depression was 71%.

With each recurrence of MDD, the risk of further recurrences increases. Although the duration of episodes is similar across recurrences, the interval between episodes grows progressively shorter with each recurrence (Eaton et al., 2008; Keller et al., 2013). Individuals with MDD have an average of five to nine episodes over the course of their lives (Burcusa & Iacono, 2007).

CONCEPTUAL AND METHODOLOGICAL ISSUES

Persistence and recurrence are nonmutually exclusive aspects of the course of depression and can exist in different combinations within a given individual. Recurrence implies remission, which should build in a negative correlation with chronicity. On the other hand, a greater number of episodes increases the chance that at least one episode is persistent. In addition, persons with double depression (discussed later) have many more MDEs than those with nonchronic depression (Klein et al., 2006), and residual symptoms are probably the strongest predictor of recurrence (e.g., Judd, Schettler, Akiskal, & Keller, 2013). Furthermore, most patients with chronic depression eventually recover, and the majority subsequently experience a recurrence (Klein et al., 2006). Thus it is likely that there are a substantial number of individuals with both chronic/persistent and recurrent depression.

We can identify three approaches to the topics of chronicity and recurrence in the literature. The first two approaches concern the goals of classification and prognosis, respectively. From a classification perspective, recurrence and chronicity can be viewed as markers of distinct forms, or subtypes, of depression. In contrast, the prognostic perspective seeks to identify factors that predict whether individuals in an episode of depression will develop chronic depression or experience a recurrence. Classification studies generally combine individuals in second and all subsequent episodes together and contrast them with individuals with only one episode. Prognostic studies typically include individuals with any number of episodes and focus on predicting the next recurrence, regardless of its number (Monroe & Harkness, 2011).

The third approach is concerned with whether recurrence and chronicity reflect factors that are evident before the onset of depression or whether they emerge after onset as an effect of the episode itself or other processes associated with the episode. These have been referred to as the liability and scar models, respectively (Burcusa & Iacono, 2007; Pettit, Hartley, Lewinsohn, Seeley, & Klein, 2013). As the liability model assumes a preexisting disposition to chronic or recurrent depressions, it is consistent with the subtype view of depression discussed earlier, which views the disorder as heterogeneous and hypothesizes that persistent and/or recurrent depressions differ qualitatively or quantitatively from nonpersistent and/or nonrecurrent depressions. The scar model, in contrast, holds that processes emerge during the course of depressive episodes that increase the risk of persistence or future episodes. A number of such processes have been posited, including rumination (Nolen-Hoeksema & Wisco, 2008), mood-related differential activation of negative cognitions (Teasdale, 1988), increasing linkage of serotonergic function with depressed mood (Robinson & Sahakian, 2008), excessive reassurance seeking (Joiner, 2000), stress sensitization/kindling (Post, 1992), and stress generation (Hammen, 2006).

Few studies have directly compared the liability and scar models. In a 14-year longitudinal study of a community sample of adolescents, Pettit and colleagues (2013) reported evidence supporting both models. Prior to first onset of MDD, subthreshold depression and parental history of recurrent MDD distinguished individuals who went on to have recurrent MDE episodes from those with a single episode. However, consistent with the stress-generation model, after their first MDE, individuals who later had a recurrence experienced a greater number of life stressors than individuals who did not have another MDE during the rest of the follow-up.

As these data suggest, the liability and scar models may not be mutually exclusive, as both might apply to different factors. In addition, the distinction between the two models could be complex and subtle; for example, subthreshold symptoms prior to the first episode may set other processes/consequences into motion before onset of the full episode; thus what appear to be liability effects may really be scars (Wichers et al., 2010).

Finally, it is important to consider some of the methodological problems that plague this literature. First, many studies examining predictors of the persistent/chronic-episodic and recurrent-single episode distinctions rely on cross-sectional and retrospective comparisons. Moreover, of prospective studies, few focus on individuals in a first episode of MDD, and even fewer begin prior to the onset of MDD (Monroe & Harkness, 2011). This creates a number of problems. First, studies beginning after the onset of MDD cannot distinguish features that preceded onset (the liability model) from those that emerged during or after the first episode (the scar model).

Second, in cross-sectional and retrospective studies of individuals who are currently in an episode, it is impossible to determine how long the episode will persist or whether individuals in their first episode will have a recurrence in the future. Hence, some individuals in the nonchronic and single-episode groups will later change groups, adding error to the comparisons. This problem is particularly acute for distinguishing single-episode from recurrent depression, as recurrence is common, whereas the odds of someone presenting with an acute episode that subsequently persists for several years is lower, although not negligible. To reduce the likelihood of misclassification, the sample should be prospectively followed for an extended period of time to monitor recovery and recurrence. Again, this is likely to be a more successful strategy for persistence than recurrence, as the duration of follow-up required to rule out chronicity is 2 years after episode onset, whereas a recurrence can occur at any point in the individual's life.

Finally, as Monroe and Harkness (2011) have noted, most prospective studies of the recurrence of depressive episodes combine individuals with first and with multiple episodes. As indicated previously, these studies are best suited to addressing the question of prediction: Which variables forecast whether an individual with depression will develop another episode in the future? However, they are not appropriate for answering the classification question of whether there are meaningful differences between single-episode and recurrent depression, as predictors may forecast a third or fourth episode among those with recurrent depression rather than distinguishing the single episode from recurrent subgroup. This is important, as factors predicting a first episode may differ from those predicting subsequent episodes (Lewinsohn, Allen, Seeley, & Gotlib, 1999; Post, 1992).

PERSISTENT (OR CHRONIC) DEPRESSION

Classification of Chronic Depression

Chronic depressions can take a number of forms that vary in their pattern of severity over time. The two major categories of chronic depression in the fourth edition of the DSM (DSM-IV; American Psychiatric Association, 1994) were dysthymic disorder and MDE, chronic. These two categories were recently combined under the rubric of persistent depression in the fifth edition of the DSM (DSM-5; American Psychiatric Association, 2013).

First introduced in DSM-III (American Psychiatric Association, 1980), dysthymic disorder was defined in DSM-IV by a chronic course (depressed most of the day, more days than not, for at least 2 years), persistent symptoms (no symptom-free periods of longer than 2 months), an insidious onset (no MDE within the first 2 years of the disturbance), and at least two of a list of six associated depressive symptoms (appetite disturbance, sleep disturbance, low energy/fatigue, low self-esteem, problems with concentration/decisions, hopelessness). Most persons with dysthymic disorder experience exacerbations that meet criteria for an MDE (Klein et al., 2006), which is often referred to as "double depression" (Keller & Shapiro, 1982).

In DSM-IV, the chronic specifier for an MDE referred to episodes that met full criteria continuously for a minimum of 2 years. Approximately 20% of patients with an MDE meet these criteria (Gilmer et al., 2005).

Based on the lack of evidence for differences between dysthymic disorder, double depression, and chronic MDD discussed in the next subsection, DSM-5 combined these various forms of chronic depression in the new category of "persistent depressive disorders." MDE specifiers reflecting persisting residual symptoms (i.e., MDE in partial remission, or recurrent MDE with incomplete recovery between episodes) also fall under this rubric if there are at least 2 years of continuous depressive symptoms.

The DSM-5 criteria for persistent depressive disorder are the same as those for DSM-IV dysthymic disorder, except that the requirement of insidious onset was dropped to allow for chronic MDE episodes with an acute onset and MDE episodes with chronic residual symptoms. This broader category also includes specifiers that mirror and permit the re-creation of the DSM-IV classification: with pure dysthymic syndrome, with persistent MDE, and with intermittent MDEs with and without the current episode. Other specifiers include severity (mild, moderate, severe); particular symptom patterns (e.g., anxious distress, melancholic features, atypical features, mood-congruent and incongruent psychotic features); remission status (full, partial); and age of onset (early [< 21], late [≥ 21]).

DSM-IV symptom criteria for MDD and dysthymic disorder differed. Because the latter were retained in DSM-5 persistent depression, it created the possibility of "diagnostic orphans" who would have met DSM-IV criteria for chronic MDE but do not meet DSM-5 criteria for persistent depression. The extent of this problem remains to be determined.

There are few data on the prevalence of DSM-5 persistent depression in the general population, as most epidemiological studies have examined only a subset of chronic depressive conditions. Recently, however, Murphy and Byrne (2012) reported that, in a nationally representative Australian sample, the lifetime prevalence of all forms of chronic depression combined was 4.6%. Cases of chronic depression constitute almost

30% of cases of depressive disorder in the community and close to half of cases of mood disorders in outpatient mental health settings (Benazzi, 1998, Murphy & Byrne, 2012).

Do the Various Forms of Chronic Depression Differ?

The various categories and specifiers for chronic depression in DSM-IV (dysthymic disorder; MDE, chronic; MDE in partial remission; recurrent MDEs without full interepisode recovery) enhanced descriptive validity by reflecting the variation of the longitudinal course of depression. However, research comparing different forms of chronic depression indicates that there are virtually no differences between patients with dysthymic disorder and those with double depression on comorbidity, personality, childhood adversity, familial psychopathology, and course (Klein et al., 1995, 2006; Lizardi et al., 1995; Pepper et al., 1995; Rhebergen et al., 2009). Similarly, most studies comparing patients with dysthymic disorder with those with chronic MDD report negligible differences (Blanco et al., 2010; Yang & Dunner, 2001). Finally, two large studies found virtually no differences between patients with double depression, patients with chronic MDD, and patients with chronic MDEs superimposed on dysthymic disorder (a more chronic form of double depression) on comorbidity, psychosocial functioning, depressive cognitions, coping style, early adversity, family history, and treatment response (McCullough et al., 2000, 2003).

The lack of differences between the various forms of chronic depression is also supported by within-subject longitudinal data. As noted previously, almost all patients with dysthymic disorder experience exacerbations that meet criteria for MDEs, suggesting that dysthymic disorder and double depression are different phases of the same condition. In addition, in a 10-year follow-up study, Klein and colleagues (2006) found that although patients with dysthymic disorder and double depression often experienced recurrences of chronic depression, the forms of chronic depression varied, suggesting that they were varying expressions of a single condition.

These data support DSM-5's consolidation of the various forms of DSM-IV chronic depression under the single rubric of persistent depression. However, in sharp contrast to the lack of differences among the various forms of chronic depression, there appear to be important distinctions between chronic and nonchronic forms of depression, as reviewed later (Klein, 2008). Moreover, the chronic versus nonchronic distinction appears to be relatively stable over time. Thus, in their 10-year follow-up, Klein and colleagues (2006) found that patients with dysthymic disorder and double depression were 14 times more likely to exhibit a chronic course than patients with nonchronic major depression. Conversely, patients with nonchronic major depression were 12 times more likely to exhibit a nonchronic depressive course than patients with dysthymic disorder and double depression.

Predictors and Correlates of Persistent/Chronic Depression

In this subsection, we review clinical, etiological, psychopathological, and pathophysiological correlates and predictors of chronic depression from both cross-sectional and longitudinal studies. We emphasize variables that distinguish persistent/chronic depression from episodic/acute depression, although we selectively include some comparisons between persons with chronic depression and those with no history of depression.

Comorbidity

Chronic depressions are frequently accompanied by nonaffective disorders, particularly anxiety, substance use, and personality disorders (Blanco et al., 2010; Murphy & Byrne, 2012). For example, Pepper and colleagues (1995) reported that 60% of patients with dysthymic disorder met criteria for a personality disorder. Rates of comorbid anxiety, substance use, and personality disorders are consistently reported to be higher among persons with chronic depression than among those with episodic depression (e.g., Blanco et al., 2010; Murphy & Byrne, 2012; Pepper et al., 1995).

Early Maltreatment

Adults with chronic depression report experiencing high levels of maltreatment and adversity in childhood and have significantly higher levels than persons with episodic depression (Klein, Arnow, et al., 2009; Wiersma et al., 2009). These findings are consistent with a number of longitudinal studies reporting that various forms of childhood maltreatment predict persistence of depressive episodes (Nanni, Uher, & Danese, 2012). Most longitudinal studies rely on retrospective assessments of childhood events conducted many years later, raising concerns about recall biases. However, studies using official records of childhood maltreatment have reported similar findings (Horwitz, Widom, McLaughlin, & White, 2001; Scott, McLaughlin, Smith, & Ellis, 2012).

Childhood maltreatment is a risk factor for many other mental disorders, and this may contribute to the high comorbidity between chronic depression and other forms of psychopathology. The often considerable interval between the occurrence of maltreatment and the onset of chronic depression raises the question of which factors mediate this link. Possible pathways include the development of maladaptive interpersonal styles, depressogenic cognitive schemas, abnormalities in neurobiological stress response systems, and stress generation, all of which may increase risk for chronic depression (Dougherty, Klein, & Davila, 2004; Hammen, Hazel, Brennan, & Najman, 2012).

Familial Transmission and Genetics

Family studies are the first line of evidence in testing the role of genetic factors in a disorder. First-degree relatives of probands with chronic depression exhibit higher rates of both chronic and nonchronic depressive disorders than relatives of healthy controls (Klein et al., 1995; Klein, Shankman, Lewinsohn, Rohde, & Seeley, 2004). There is also some specificity of familial transmission, as first-degree relatives of probands with chronic depressions have higher rates of chronic depression than relatives of probands with nonchronic MDD (Klein et al., 1995, 2004; Mondimore et al., 2006). However, studies conflict on whether relatives of probands with chronic depression also have a higher rate of nonchronic MDD than relatives of probands with nonchronic depression.

These studies are consistent with several models of the relationship between chronic and nonchronic depressions: (1) chronic depression is qualitatively similar to, but more severe than, nonchronic major depression with respect to familial liability; (2) chronic depression is associated with a qualitatively distinct familial liability; and (3) chronic depression is associated with a general familial liability for mood disorders, as well as a more specific familial liability to chronic depression. Unfortunately, the data are insufficient to choose among these models at the present time.

To distinguish genetic and environmental effects, it is necessary to conduct twin and adoption studies. Unfortunately, there are no twin or adoption studies of chronic depression with reasonable sample sizes.

Few genetic linkage and association studies have specifically examined chronic depression phenotypes. However, several recent studies have suggested that childhood maltreatment may moderate the association between a polymorphism in the promoter region of the serotonin transporter gene (*5-HTTLPR*) and chronic depression. In two independent samples, Uher and colleagues (2011) found that individuals with two short *5-HTTLPR* alleles who also had histories of childhood maltreatment had particularly heightened risk for "persistent depression." In contrast, there was no effect for single-episode depression. "Persistent depression" was defined as meeting criteria for MDD during the preceding year in at least two of four assessments conducted over 7–14 years; hence, this category could also include some recurrent depressions. However, two other studies suggest that the effect may be specific to chronic depression. Brown and colleagues (2013) found a significant interaction between *5-HTTLPR* genotype and childhood maltreatment for chronic depression, but not new depressive onsets. Moreover, Fisher and colleagues (2012) failed to find a *5-HTTLPR*-by-childhood-maltreatment interaction in a large sample of individuals with recurrent MDD or no history of psychopathology. Taken together, these findings suggest that chronic depression is characterized by a specific set of interacting genetic and environmental processes that are distinct from single-episode and recurrent depression.

Personality/Temperament

In their influential model, Watson and Clark (1995) proposed that depression is associated with high levels of negative emotionality (NE) and low levels of positive emotionality (PE). NE, which is analogous to neuroticism, reflects sensitivity to negative stimuli resulting in a range of negative moods, such as sadness, fear, anxiety, and anger. PE, which is closely related to extroversion, includes exuberance, reward sensitivity, and sociability. PE and NE may play particularly important roles in chronic depression. Thus patients with dysthymia and double depression report higher levels of NE and lower levels of PE than patients with nonchronic MDD and healthy controls (Klein, Taylor, Dickstein, & Harding, 1988; Sang et al., 2011; Wiersma et al., 2011). Moreover, Hirschfeld (1990) found that even after recovery, individuals with a history of dysthymic disorder exhibited significantly greater NE and significantly lower PE than individuals with a history of MDD and individuals with no history of psychopathology.

There is suggestive evidence that personality/temperament differences may be evident prior to the development of chronic depression. Using examiner's ratings of the laboratory behavior of a large cohort of 3-year-olds, Caspi, Moffitt, Newman, and Silva (1996) identified a cluster of "inhibited" children who were characterized by a combination of low PE and high NE behaviors, including sluggishness, low approach, social reticence, and fearfulness. Children in this cluster had significantly higher levels of parent-rated internalizing behavior problems at ages 13 and 15 (Caspi, 2000), and elevated rates of interview-assessed depressive disorders and suicide attempts (but not anxiety disorders, alcoholism, or antisocial behavior) at age 21 (Caspi et al., 1996). Although the investigators have not reported whether the same children exhibited these problems at each time point, many of these youths may have had depressive symptoms that persisted from adolescence to young adulthood.

Cognitive Factors

In light of the central role of cognitive theories in depression, there has been surprisingly little research on the role of cognitive factors in chronic depression. McCullough and colleagues (1994) found that a nonclinical sample with chronic depression exhibited more stable and global attributions for negative events and less stable attributions for positive events than healthy controls. Similarly, Riso and colleagues (2003) reported that patients with chronic depression exhibited more stable and global attributions for negative events, a higher level of dysfunctional attitudes, a more ruminative response style, and higher levels of maladaptive schemas and core beliefs than healthy controls.

Few prospective studies have examined whether cognitive variables precede the development of chronicity, whether they are a consequence of persistent depression, or whether depressive cognitions and symptoms are both caused by third variables. In addition, studies of cognitive factors in chronic depression have relied exclusively on self-report measures. As a result, little is known about the role of automatic and implicit processes in chronic depression, such as the attentional and memory biases that are associated with depression in general.

Interpersonal Factors

Coyne (1976) proposed that individuals with depression have a negative impact on others by excessively seeking reassurance. These demands eventually become aversive and begin to erode relationships, serving to perpetuate depressive episodes. Joiner (2000) extended this model by describing a variety of other self-propagating interpersonal processes that might serve to maintain depression, including negative feedback seeking, interpersonal conflict avoidance, and blame maintenance.

Numerous studies have reported that low social support, conflicted family and marital relationships, and interpersonal difficulties are associated with a poorer course and outcome of depression (Hölzel, Härter, Reese, & Kriston, 2011). Klein and colleagues (1988) and Hays and colleagues (1997) found that patients with chronic depression reported having less social support than patients with nonchronic depression. In addition, Brown and colleagues have found that interpersonal difficulties predict chronic depression in prospective studies with clinical and community samples (e.g., Brown, Craig, Harris, Handley, & Harvey, 2007).

Individuals with chronic depression continue to experience greater interpersonal difficulties after recovery than individuals who have recovered from MDD and controls who were never mentally ill (Klein, Lewinsohn, & Seeley, 1997; Rhebergen et al., 2010), suggesting that these deficits are not simply due to the depressed state. However, longitudinal studies are required to untangle the complex, and most likely reciprocal and transactional, associations between chronic depression and dysfunctional interpersonal relationships.

Chronic Stress

Although depressive episodes are frequently preceded by stressful life events, chronic and nonchronic depressions do not differ in this respect. However, chronic depression is associated with a higher level of chronic stress and daily hassles than nonchronic depression (Moerk & Klein, 2000).

The direction of this relationship is difficult to determine: Chronic stress may cause or maintain depression, but chronic depression can also generate long-term difficulties. However, there is some evidence that chronic stress contributes to the maintenance of chronic depression. In a multiwave longitudinal study of dysthymia and double depression, Dougherty and colleagues (2004) found that after controlling for prior level of depression, chronic stress predicted the subsequent level of depression at each follow-up assessment. In contrast, depressive symptoms did not predict subsequent chronic stress.

Neurobiology

Despite the voluminous literature on the neurobiology of mood disorders, research on the biological correlates of chronic depression is surprisingly sparse. There has been extensive documentation of neuroendocrine dysregulation in the major mood disorders, particularly involving the hypothalamic–pituitary–adrenal (HPA) axis. However, evidence for HPA-axis abnormalities in chronic depression is weaker. A common index of HPA-axis dysregulation is failure to suppress the production of cortisol after ingestion of the synthetic corticosteroid dexamethasone (referred to as the dexamethasone suppression test, or DST). Patients with chronic depression tend to have rates of DST nonsuppression that are lower than those of depressed comparison groups (Ravindran, Bialik, & Lapierre, 1994; Szádóczky, Fazekas, Rihmer, & Arato, 1994), and similar to healthy controls (Watson et al., 2002). Watson, Gallagher, Ferrier, and Young (2006) hypothesized that if chronic depression is associated with tonic, as opposed to phasic, elevations in glucocorticoids, then arginine vasopressin (AVP) may play a greater role in regulating the HPA axis. Consistent with this hypothesis, they found that patients with chronic depression exhibited significantly higher levels of post-DST AVP than healthy controls. Finally, using another index of HPA axis dysregulation, Vreeburg and colleagues (2013) found that a diminished cortisol awakening response predicted a chronic course in a large sample of patients with depressive and anxiety disorders. Interestingly, this was evident in patients with both depression and anxiety.

Structural and functional neuroimaging studies have identified a variety of structural and functional abnormalities in a number of brain regions in patients with MDD, including the dorsolateral and orbital prefrontal cortex, anterior cingulate cortex, striatum, amygdala, and hippocampus. However, there have been few neuroimaging studies of chronic depression. Using magnetic resonance imaging (MRI), Shah and colleagues (Shah, Ebmeier, Glabus, & Goodwin, 1998; Shah, Glabus, Goodwin, & Ebmeier, 2002) reported that patients with chronic MDD exhibited right frontal-striatal atrophy and reduced gray matter density in the left temporal cortex, including the hippocampus, compared with patients who had recovered from an MDD episode and healthy controls.

Using functional MRI, Ravindran and colleagues (2009) examined neural responses to negative, positive, and neutral scenes in patients with dysthymia and in healthy controls. Contrasting negative to neutral stimuli, patients with dysthymia exhibited greater activation in the left posterior cingulate and right amygdala than the control group. In the positive versus neutral contrast, patients with dysthymia showed reduced dorsolateral prefrontal cortex and greater left anterior cingulate activation.

Finally, Posner and colleagues (2013) compared resting-state functional connectivity in the default mode network (DMN), a set of brain regions that deactivate during goal-directed behavior, in patients with dysthymic disorder and in healthy controls. Consistent with the notion that dysthymia is associated with internally focused mental activity such as rumination, patients exhibited greater DMN connectivity than controls, a difference that disappeared after successful treatment.

There is a pressing need for more systematic research on the neurobiological correlates of persistent depression. Furthermore, such work needs to begin to distinguish abnormalities that precede and may play a causal role in persistent depression from those that are concomitants or consequences of chronicity.

PREDICTORS AND CORRELATES OF RECURRENCE AND RECURRENT DEPRESSION

In this section we briefly summarize the results of cross-sectional and longitudinal studies comparing individuals with depression with one versus multiple episodes and predicting recurrence (for reviews, see Burcusa & Iacono, 2007; Hardeveld, Spijker, De Graaf, Nolen, & Beekman, 2010). As noted earlier, most of the latter studies do not distinguish between first and subsequent recurrences; hence it is unclear whether the results apply to the single-episode versus recurrent distinction.

Clinical Features

This is the most frequently studied domain of predictors. Greater severity of the index episode and the presence of comorbid anxiety, substance use, and personality disorders consistently predict recurrence and are associated with the recurrent subtype (Burcusa & Iacono, 2007; Hardeveld et al., 2010; Keller et al., 2013). Residual symptoms after the episode are also consistent predictors of recurrence (Burcusa & Iacono, 2007; Hardeveld et al., 2010; Judd et al., 2013). Number of prior episodes is another consistent predictor of recurrence (Burcusa & Iacono, 2007; Hardeveld et al., 2010; Keller et al., 2013), although it is not useful in distinguishing first onset from recurrent MDD. Findings on age of onset are mixed, and the duration of the index episode (including the first lifetime episode) is not related to recurrence (Burcusa & Iacono, 2007; Hardeveld et al., 2010). This latter finding suggests that persistence and recurrence are somewhat independent.

Childhood Maltreatment

A number of prospective longitudinal studies have reported that various forms of childhood maltreatment are associated with recurrence, although the evidence is not as strong as it is for chronicity (Burcusa & Iacono, 2007; Nanni et al., 2012).

Family History and Genetics

Family history of depression predicts recurrence and is more common in the recurrent subtype (Burcusa & Iacono, 2007; Sullivan, Neale & Kendler, 2000). Recurrence itself runs in families (Klein, Lewinsohn, Rohde, Seeley, & Durbin, 2002), and family history of recurrent depression is particularly strongly associated with a greater risk of recurrence (Lewinsohn, Rohde, Seeley, Klein, & Gotlib, 2000). There have been several large linkage and genomewide association studies of recurrent depression; however, findings have been inconclusive (e.g., Lewis et al., 2010).

Personality

A number of studies have reported that neuroticism predicts recurrence and is associated with the recurrent subtype (Burcusa & Iacono, 2007; Klein, Kotov, & Bufferd, 2011).

Cognitive and Interpersonal Factors

A negative cognitive style, including rumination (Spasojević & Alloy, 2001) and dysfunctional attitudes and depressotypic attributions (Iacovello, Alloy, Abramson, Whitehouse, & Hogan, 2006; Lewinsohn et al., 1999), predict recurrence. In addition, patients with depression and with a history of recurrent episodes report more overgeneral autobiographical memories than first-episode patients (Nandrino, Pezard, Posté, Revéillère, & Beaune, 2002). Evidence for an association between low social support and recurrence is mixed (Burcusa & Iacono, 2007; Hardeveld et al., 2010).

Stress

Stressful life events commonly precede the onset of depressive episodes; in many cases, life events are dependent on an individual's behavior, suggesting that the individual with depression may, at least in part, be responsible for "generating" the stressors that precipitate recurrence (Hammen, 2006). Indeed, individuals with depression and with a history of prior episodes report more dependent life events than individuals with a single episode (Harkness, Monroe, Simons, & Thase, 1999). However, there is also evidence that severe life events are more common before the first episode than before subsequent episodes (Post, 1992; Stroud, Davila, & Moyer, 2008). It remains unclear whether the reason is that repeated episodes become increasingly autonomous from the environment or whether there is a process of sensitization in which increasingly minor events that are not included in most life stress assessments are capable of precipitating subsequent episodes (Monroe & Harkness, 2005).

Neurobiology

Research on neurobiological predictors of recurrence is limited. However, there is evidence that recurrence is associated with decreased delta sleep and rapid eye movement latency (e.g., Hatzinger, Hemmeter, Brand, Ising, & Holsboer-Trachsler, 2004), abnormally high levels of cortisol on the dexamethasone suppression–corticotopin releasing hormone test after remission (e.g., Appelhof et al., 2006), and reduced amygdala and hippocampal volume (Lorenzetti, Allen, Fornito, & Yücel, 2009).

IS THERE A CHRONIC/RECURRENT SPECTRUM?

As noted earlier, there is probably some overlap between chronic/persistent and recurrent depression, although data on its extent are limited and primarily cross-sectional/retrospective. As both of these constructs unfold over time, a longitudinal perspective is critical, as some individuals with one of these forms/subtypes may develop the other over the course of their lives (Monroe & Harkness, 2011). As indicated previously, many of the correlates and predictors of persistence and recurrence are similar, including greater familial liability for mood disorders, higher rates of childhood maltreatment, more psychiatric comorbidity, and higher levels of neuroticism and depressotypic cognitive biases. As few studies have attempted to separate chronicity from recurrence, however, it is unclear whether these effects are driven primarily by one of these two subtypes/dimensions or whether both make independent contributions.

Given the overlap in correlates/predictors, it is worth considering whether persistent and recurrent depression should be viewed as belonging on the same spectrum (Klein, 2008; Monroe & Harkness, 2011). This spectrum is independent of severity, as it includes both severe (e.g., chronic MDE) and mild (e.g., dysthymia) conditions. Moreover, there is evidence that some trait-based conditions, such as DSM-IV depressive personality, belong on this spectrum (Akiskal, 1989). For example, the first-degree relatives of patients with chronic depression exhibit elevated levels of depressive personality traits (Klein, 1999), and individuals with depressive personality disorder are at increased risk for developing dysthymic disorder over time (Kwon et al., 2000).

Delineating a chronic/recurrent depression spectrum could have important implications for parsing the heterogeneity of depression, including selecting phenotypes for studies of etiology, pathophysiology, and treatment response, as well as clinical implications for treatment planning. However, current definitions of the persistent and recurrent subtypes may not be optimal for capturing this spectrum. Persistent depression is defined by having an episode lasting at least 2 years at some point in the course of the disorder. This includes a wide variety of individuals, ranging from those with a pediatric onset and decades of unrelenting depression to individuals with an isolated episode that persisted for 24 months in middle age that was associated with a major life event or transition but who were euthymic for decades before the episode and achieved full remission after the episode. Likewise, recurrent depression is defined as having two or more episodes, which can include individuals who regularly experience episodes every year or two for decades to persons with a brief episode in young adulthood that was associated with a major life event or transition and a second episode many decades later, also associated with a major life stressor. It is likely that the first in each of these pairs of examples is more likely to be part of a "chronic/recurrent spectrum" than the second.

Age of onset is another dimension that may play a role in a chronic/recurrent spectrum. An earlier onset provides greater "opportunity" for chronicity and multiple episodes and shares many of the same correlates as persistent and recurring depressions. DSM-III through DSM-5 include early–late onset as subtypes of dysthymia/persistent depression. However, there is evidence that these subtypes are valid for depression in general. An earlier onset (< age 21 by convention, but with few data supporting this particular cutoff) is associated with higher rates of mood disorders in relatives, greater childhood adversity, and more psychiatric comorbidity across many forms of depression (e.g., Klein et al., 1999; Korten, Comijs, Lamers, & Penninx, 2012). Moreover, the combination of early onset and recurrence appears to have particularly pernicious consequences (Hammen, Brennan, Keenan-Miller, & Herr, 2008).

The most comprehensive approach is a life-course perspective (Klein, 2008; Monroe & Harkness, 2011). A life-course-based approach should take into account the number and duration of episodes and the duration and extent of remissions as a function of the individual's age or the time since the onset of the disorder. In addition, it should consider preexisting depressive traits (Akiskal, 1989) and chronic subthreshold symptoms (Klein, Shankman, Lewinsohn, & Seeley, 2009). There is support for a limited version of a life-course approach in chronic depression. Mondimore and colleagues (2007) compared a definition of chronicity based on course since onset with DSM–IV criteria for chronic MDD and dysthymic disorder and found that the former approach yielded a stronger association with rates of chronic depression in relatives.

CONCLUSIONS AND FUTURE DIRECTIONS

Traditionally, depression has been conceptualized as acute and remitting. However, it is now clear that the course of depression is markedly heterogeneous; 10–20% of MDEs are chronic, and approximately half of individuals with a first MDE in community samples (but nearly all in clinical samples) eventually experience a recurrence. The various manifestations of chronic depression have been grouped under the rubric of persistent depressive disorder in DSM-5. Persistent depression differs from nonchronic depression in numerous respects, including comorbidity, personality/cognitive style, history of childhood maltreatment, and family history of mood disorders and chronic depression, in particular. In addition, the chronic/nonchronic distinction is stable over time. Research on recurrence is less conclusive, as classification and prediction studies are not always clearly distinguished and much of this literature combines individuals in a first episode with those who have had multiple episodes. However, the recurrent subtype and the risk of recurring episodes are associated with many of the same factors that are linked to persistent depression. This suggests that there may be a chronic/recurrent spectrum that could be useful in parsing the etiological, psychopathological, and pathophysiological heterogeneity of depression.

Further work is needed in a number of areas. First, compared with some other disorders, such as schizophrenia, there are surprisingly few longitudinal studies of first-episode samples. This may be because the majority of first depressive episodes are untreated; hence case identification is challenging. Nonetheless, such studies are needed to avoid sampling biases and to accurately distinguish individuals who will have only one episode from those who will go on to have multiple episodes (Monroe & Harkness, 2011). Ideally, these investigations should begin prior to the first episode to distinguish liability factors from scars.

The cognitive–affective neuroscience and genetics of persistent and recurrent depression are understudied topics, particularly in light of the large literature in these areas on depression in general. As the many inconsistent findings in the neurobiology and genetics of depression are often attributed to the heterogeneity of the disorder, it is surprising that course-based subtypes and dimensions have not received greater attention.

Most research has examined chronicity/persistence and recurrence separately. Thus we know surprisingly little about the relationship between these two subtypes, and few studies have distinguished the effects of chronicity from those of recurrence on predictors and correlates. Future work should incorporate both of these features and examine their unique and joint influences.

Finally, there is a need to develop a life-course taxonomy of depression that provides greater resolution in mapping the boundaries of a chronic/recurrent spectrum. This will be challenging due to the variety and complexity of the course configurations evident in depression. However, diagnostic and etiological heterogeneity are arguably the greatest obstacle to progress in understanding, treating, and preventing depression. As course-based subtypes and dimensions may provide leverage in parsing this heterogeneity, this should be a priority for future research.

REFERENCES

Akiskal, H. S. (1989). Validating affective personality types. In L. Robins & J. Barrett (Eds.), *The validity of psychiatric diagnosis* (pp. 217–227). New York: Raven Press.

American Psychiatric Association. (1980). *Diagnostic and statistical manual of mental disorders* (3rd ed.). Washington, DC: Author.

American Psychiatric Association. (1994). *Diagnostic and statistical manual of mental disorders* (4th ed.). Washington, DC: Author.

American Psychiatric Association. (2013). *Diagnostic and statistical manual of mental disorders* (5th ed.). Arlington, VA: Author.

Andrews, G. (2001). Should depression be managed as a chronic disease? *British Medical Journal, 322*, 419.

Appelhof, B. C., Huyser, J., Verweij, M., Brouwer, J. P., van Dyck R., Fliers, E., et al. (2006). Glucocorticoids and relapse of major depression (dexamethasone/corticotropin-releasing hormone test in relation to relapse of major depression). *Biological Psychiatry, 59*, 696–701.

Benazzi, F. (1998). Chronic depression: A case series of 203 outpatients treated at a private practice. *Journal of Psychiatry and Neuroscience, 23*, 51–55.

Blanco, C., Okuda, M., Markowitz, J. C., Liu, S. M., Grant, B. F., & Hasin, D. S. (2010). The epidemiology of chronic major depressive disorder and dysthymic disorder: Results from the National Epidemiologic Survey on Alcohol and Related Conditions. *Journal of Clinical Psychiatry, 71*, 1645–1656.

Brown, G. W., Ban, M., Craig, T. K., Harris, T. O., Herbert, J., & Uher, R. (2013). Serotonin transporter length polymorphism, childhood maltreatment, and chronic depression: A specific gene–environment interaction. *Depression and Anxiety, 30*, 5–13.

Brown, G. W., Craig, T. K. J., Harris, T. O., Handley, R. V., & Harvey, A. L. (2007). Validity of retrospective measures of early maltreatment and depressive episodes using the Childhood Experience of Care and Abuse (CECA) instrument: A life-course study of adult chronic depression: 2. *Journal of Affective Disorders, 103*, 217–224.

Burcusa, S. L., & Iacono, W. G. (2007). Risk for recurrence in depression. *Clinical Psychology Review, 27*, 959–985.

Caspi, A. (2000). The child is father of the man: Personality continuities from childhood to adulthood. *Journal of Personality and Social Psychology, 78*, 158–172.

Caspi, A., Moffitt, T. E., Newman, D. L., & Silva, P. A. (1996). Behavioral observations at age 3 years predict adult psychiatric disorders: Longitudinal evidence from a birth cohort. *Archives of General Psychiatry, 53*, 1033.

Coyne, J. C. (1976). Depression and the response of others. *Journal of Abnormal Psychology, 85*, 186.

Dougherty, L. R., Klein, D. N., & Davila, J. (2004). A growth curve analysis of the course of dysthymic disorder: The effects of chronic stress and moderation by adverse parent–child relationships and family history. *Journal of Consulting and Clinical Psychology, 72*, 1012.

Eaton, W. W., Shao, H., Nestadt, G., Lee, B. H., Bienvenu, O. J., & Zandi, P. (2008). Population-based study of first onset and chronicity in major depressive disorder. *Archives of General Psychiatry, 65*, 513.

Fisher, H. L., Cohen-Woods, S., Hosang, G. M., Uher, R., Powell-Smith, G., Keers, R., et al. (2012). Stressful life events and the serotonin transporter gene 5-HTTLPR in recurrent clinical depression. *Journal of Affective Disorders, 136*, 189–193.

Furukawa, T. A., Fujita, A., Harai, H., Yoshimura, R., Kitamura, T., & Takahashi, K. (2008). Definitions of recovery and outcomes of major depression: results from a 10-year follow-up. *Acta Psychiatrica Scandinavica, 117*, 35–40.

Gilmer, W. S., Trivedi, M. H., Rush, A. J., Wisniewski, S. R., Luther, J., Howland, R. H., et al. (2005). Factors associated with chronic depressive episodes: A preliminary report from the STAR*D project. *Acta Psychiatrica Scandinavica, 112*, 425–433.

Gopinath, S., Katon, W. J., Russo, J. E., & Ludman, E. J. (2007). Clinical factors associated with relapse in primary care patients with chronic or recurrent depression. *Journal of Affective Disorders, 101,* 57–63.

Hammen, C., Brennan, P. A., Keenan-Miller, D., & Herr, N. R. (2008). Early onset recurrent subtype of adolescent depression: Clinical and psychosocial correlates. *Journal of Child Psychology and Psychiatry, 49,* 433–440.

Hammen, C., Hazel, N., Brennan, P., & Najman, J. (2012). Intergenerational transmission and continuity of stress and depression: Depressed women and their offspring in 20 years of follow-up. *Psychological Medicine, 42,* 931–942.

Hammen, C. L. (2006). Stress generation in depressions: Reflections on origins, research, and future directions. *Journal of Clinical Psychology, 62,* 1065–1082.

Hardeveld, F., Spijker, J., De Graaf, R., Nolen, W. A., & Beekman, A. T. F. (2010). Prevalence and predictors of recurrence of major depressive disorder in the adult population. *Acta Psychiatrica Scandinavica, 122,* 184–191.

Hardeveld, F., Spijker, J., De Graaf, R., Nolen, W. A., & Beekman, A. T. F. (2013). Recurrence of major depressive disorder and its predictors in the general population: Results from the Netherlands Mental Health Survey and Incidence Study (NEMESIS). *Psychological Medicine, 43,* 39–48.

Harkness, K. L., Monroe, S. M., Simons, A. D., & Thase, M. (1999). The generation of life events in recurrent and nonrecurrent depression. *Psychological Medicine, 29,* 135–144.

Hatzinger, M., Hemmeter, U. M., Brand, S., Ising, M., & Holsboer-Trachsler, E. (2004). Electroencephalographic sleep profiles in treatment course and long-term outcome of major depression: Association with DEX/CRH-test response. *Journal of Psychiatric Research, 38,* 453–465.

Hays, J. C., Krishnan, K. R. R., George, L. K., Pieper, C. F., Flint, E. P., & Blazer, D. G. (1997). Psychosocial and physical correlates of chronic depression. *Psychiatry Research, 72,* 149–159.

Hirschfeld, R. M. A. (1990) Personality and dysthymia. In S. W. Burton & H. S. Akiskal (Eds.), *Dysthymic disorder* (pp. 69–77). London: Gaskell.

Hölzel, L., Härter, M., Reese, C., & Kriston, L. (2011). Risk factors for chronic depression: A systematic review. *Journal of Affective Disorders, 129,* 1–13.

Horwitz, A. V., Widom, C. S., McLaughlin, J., & White, H. R. (2001). The impact of childhood abuse and neglect on adult mental health: A prospective study. *Journal of Health and Social Behavior, 42,* 184–201.

Iacoviello, B. M., Alloy, L. B., Abramson, L. Y., Whitehouse, W. G., & Hogan, M. E. (2006). The course of depression in persons at high and low cognitive risk for depression: A prospective study. *Journal of Affective Disorders, 93,* 61–69.

Joiner, T. E. (2000). Depression's vicious scree: Self-propagating and erosive processes in depression chronicity. *Clinical Psychology: Science and Practice, 7,* 203–218.

Judd, L. L., Schettler, P. J., Akiskal, H. S., & Keller, M. B. (2013). Dimensional symptomatic structure of the long-term course of unipolar major depressive disorder. In M. B. Keller, W. H. Coryell, J. Endicott, J. D. Maser, & P. J. Schettler (Eds.), *Clinical guide to depression and bipolar disorder* (pp. 27–46). Washington, DC: American Psychiatric Press.

Keller, M. B., Boland, R., Leon, A., Solomon, D., Endicott, J., & Li, C. (2013). Clinical course and outcome of unipolar major depression. In M. B. Keller, W. H. Coryell, J. Endicott, J. D. Maser, & P. J. Schettler (Eds.), *Clinical guide to depression and bipolar disorder* (pp. 155–173). Washington, DC: American Psychiatric Press.

Keller, M. B., & Shapiro, R. W. (1982). "Double depression": Superimposition of acute depressive episodes on chronic depressive disorders. *American Journal of Psychiatry, 139,* 438–442.

Klein, D. N. (1999). Depressive personality in the relatives of outpatients with dysthymic disorder and episodic major depressive disorder and normal controls. *Journal of Affective Disorders, 55,* 19–27.

Klein, D. N. (2008). Classification of depressive disorders in the DSM-V: Proposal for a two-dimension system. *Journal of Abnormal Psychology, 117,* 552–560.

Klein, D. N., Arnow, B. A., Barkin, J. L., Dowling, F., Kocsis, J. H., Leon, A. C., et al. (2009).

Early adversity in chronic depression: Clinical correlates and response to pharmacotherapy. *Depression and Anxiety, 26*, 701–710.

Klein, D. N., Kotov, R., & Bufferd, S. J. (2011). Personality and depression: Explanatory models and review of the evidence. *Annual Review of Clinical Psychology, 7*, 269–295.

Klein, D. N., Lewinsohn, P. M., Rohde, P., Seeley, J. R., & Durbin, E. C. (2002). Clinical features of major depressive disorder in adolescents and their relatives: Impact on familial aggregation, implications for phenotype definition, and specificity of transmission. *Journal of Abnormal Psychology, 111*, 98–106.

Klein, D. N., Lewinsohn, P. M., & Seeley, J. R. (1997). Psychosocial characteristics of adolescents with a past history of dysthymic disorder: Comparison with adolescents with past histories of major depressive and non-affective disorders, and never mentally ill controls. *Journal of Affective Disorders, 42*, 127–135.

Klein, D. N., Riso, L. P., Donaldson, S. K., Schwartz, J. E., Anderson, R. L., Ouimette, P. C., et al. (1995). Family study of early-onset dysthymia: Mood and personality disorders in relatives of outpatients with dysthymia and episodic major depression and normal controls. *Archives of General Psychiatry, 52*, 487–496.

Klein, D. N., Schatzberg, A. F., McCullough, J. P., Dowling, F., Goodman, D., Howland, R. H., et al. (1999). Age of onset in chronic major depression: Relation to demographic and clinical variables, family history, and treatment response. *Journal of Affective Disorders, 55*, 149–157.

Klein, D. N., Shankman, S. A., Lewinsohn, P. M., Rohde, P., & Seeley, J. R. (2004). Family study of chronic depression in a community sample of young adults. *American Journal of Psychiatry, 161*, 646–653.

Klein, D. N., Shankman, S. A., Lewinsohn, P. M., & Seeley, J. R. (2009). Subthreshold depressive disorder in adolescents: Predictors of escalation to full syndrome depressive disorders. *Journal of the American Academy of Child and Adolescent Psychiatry, 48*, 703–710.

Klein, D. N., Shankman, S. A., & Rose, S. (2006). Ten-year prospective follow-up study of the naturalistic course of dysthymic disorder and double depression. *American Journal of Psychiatry, 163*, 872–880.

Klein, D. N., Taylor, E. B., Dickstein, S., & Harding, K. (1988). Primary early-onset dysthymia: Comparison with primary non-bipolar, non-chronic major depression on demographic, clinical, familial, personality, and socioenvironmental characteristics and short-term outcome. *Journal of Abnormal Psychology, 97*, 387–398.

Korten, N., Comijs, H. C., Lamers, F., & Penninx, B. W. (2012). Early and late onset depression in young and middle aged adults: Differential symptomatology, characteristics and risk factors? *Journal of Affective Disorders, 138*, 259–267.

Kwon, J. S., Kim, Y. M., Chang, C. G., Park, B. J., Kim, L., Yoon, D. J., et al. (2000). Three-year follow-up of women with the sole diagnosis of depressive personality disorder: Subsequent development of dysthymia and major depression. *American Journal of Psychiatry, 157*, 1966–1972.

Lewinsohn, P. M., Allen, N. B., Seeley, J. R., & Gotlib, I. H. (1999). First-onset versus recurrence of depression: Differential processes of psychosocial risk. *Journal of Abnormal Psychology, 108*, 483–489.

Lewinsohn, P. M., Rohde, P., Seeley, J. R., Klein, D. N., & Gotlib, I. H. (2000). The natural course of adolescent major depressive disorder: II. Predictors of depression recurrence in young adults. *American Journal of Psychiatry, 157*, 1584–1591.

Lewis, C. M., Ng, N. Y., Butler, A. W., Cohen-Woods, S., Uher, R., Pirlo, K, et al. (2010) Genome-wide association study of major recurrent depression in the U.K. population. *American Journal of Psychiatry, 167*, 949–957.

Lizardi, H., Klein, D. N., Ouimette, P. C., Riso, L. P., Anderson, R. L., & Donaldson, S. K. (1995). Reports of the childhood home environment in early-onset dysthymia and episodic major depression. *Journal of Abnormal Psychology, 104*, 132–139.

Lorenzetti, V., Allen, N. B., Fornito, A., & Yücel, M. (2009). Structural brain abnormalities in major depressive disorder: A selective review of recent MRI studies. *Journal of Affective Disorders, 117,* 1–17.

Maj, M., Veltro, F., Pirozzi, R., & Lobrace, S. (1992). Pattern of recurrence of illness after recovery from an episode of major depression: A prospective study. *American Journal of Psychiatry, 149,* 795–800.

McCullough, J. P., Klein, D. N., Borian, F. E., Howland, R. H., Riso, L. P., Keller, M. B., et al. (2003). Group comparisons of DSM-IV subtypes of chronic depression: Validity of the distinctions: Part 2. *Journal of Abnormal Psychology, 112,* 614–622.

McCullough, J. P., Klein, D. N., Keller, M. B., Holzer, C. E., Davis, S. M., Kornstein, S. G., et al. (2000). Comparison of DSM-III-R chronic major depression and major depression superimposed on dysthymia (double depression): A study of the validity and value of differential diagnosis. *Journal of Abnormal Psychology, 109,* 419–427.

McCullough, J. M., McCune, K. J., Kaye, A. L., Braith, J. A., Friend, R., Roberts, W. C., et al. (1994). One-year prospective replication study of an untreated sample of community dysthymia subjects. *Journal of Nervous and Mental Disease, 182,* 396–401.

Moerk, K. C., & Klein, D. N. (2000). The development of major depressive episodes during the course of dysthymic and episodic major depressive disorders: A retrospective examination of life events. *Journal of Affective Disorders, 58,* 117–123.

Mondimore, F., Zandi, P., MacKinnon, D., McInnis, M., Miller, E., Crowe, R., et al. (2006). Familial aggregation of illness chronicity in recurrent, early-onset major depression pedigrees. *American Journal of Psychiatry, 163,* 1554–1560.

Mondimore, F. M., Zandi, P. P., MacKinnon, D. F., McInnis, M. G., Miller, E. B., Schweizer, B., et al. (2007). Comparison of the familiality of chronic depression in recurrent early-onset depression pedigrees using different definitions of chronicity. *Journal of Affective Disorders, 100,* 171–177.

Monroe, S. M., & Harkness, K. L. (2005). Life stress, the "kindling" hypothesis, and the recurrence of depression: Considerations from a life stress perspective. *Psychological Review, 112,* 417–445.

Monroe, S. M., & Harkness, K. L. (2011). Recurrence in major depression: A conceptual analysis. *Psychological Review, 118,* 655.

Monroe, S. M., & Harkness, K. L. (2012). Is depression a chronic mental illness? *Psychological Medicine, 42,* 899.

Murphy, J. A., & Byrne, G. J. (2012). Prevalence and correlates of the proposed DSM-5 diagnosis of Chronic Depressive Disorder. *Journal of Affective Disorders, 139,* 172–180.

Nandrino, J.-L., Pezard, L., Posté, A., Revéillère, C., & Beaune, D. (2002). Autobiographical memory in major depression: A comparison between first-episode and recurrent patients. *Psychopathology, 35,* 335–340.

Nanni, V., Uher, R., & Danese, A. (2012). Childhood maltreatment predicts unfavorable course of illness and treatment outcome in depression: A meta-analysis. *American Journal of Psychiatry, 169,* 141–151.

Nolen-Hoeksema, S., Wisco, B. E., & Lyubomirsky, S. (2008). Rethinking rumination. *Perspectives on Psychological Science, 3,* 400–424.

Pepper, C. M., Klein, D. N., Anderson, R. L., Riso, L. P., Ouimette, P. C., & Lizardi, H. (1995). DSM-III-R Axis II comorbidity in dysthymia and major depression. *American Journal of Psychiatry, 152,* 239–247.

Pettit, J. W., Hartley, C., Lewinsohn, P. M., Seeley, J. R., & Klein, D. N. (2013). Is liability to recurrent major depressive disorder present before first episode onset in adolescence or acquired after the initial episode? *Journal of Abnormal Psychology, 122,* 353–358.

Posner, J., Hellerstein, D. J., Gat, I., Mechling, A., Klahr, K., Wang, Z., et al. (2013). Antidepressants normalize the default mode network in patients with dysthymia antidepressants and the default mode network. *JAMA Psychiatry, 70,* 373–382.

Post, R. M. (1992). Transduction of psychosocial stress into the neurobiology of recurrent affective disorder. *American Journal of Psychiatry, 149,* 999–1010.

Ravindran, A. V., Bialik, R. J., & Lapierre, Y. D. (1994). Primary early onset dysthymia, biochemical correlates of the therapeutic response to fluoxetine: I. Platelet monoamine oxidase activity and the dexamethasone suppression test. *Journal of Affective Disorders, 31,* 111–117.

Ravindran, A. V., Smith, A., Cameron, C., Bhatla, R., Cameron, I., Georgescu, T. M., et al. (2009). Toward a functional neuroanatomy of dysthymia: A functional magnetic resonance imaging study. *Journal of Affective Disorders, 119,* 9–15.

Rhebergen, D., Beekman, A. T., Graaf, R. D., Nolen, W. A., Spijker, J., Hoogendijk, W. J., et al. (2009). The three-year naturalistic course of major depressive disorder, dysthymic disorder and double depression. *Journal of Affective Disorders, 115,* 450–459.

Rhebergen, D., Beekman, A. T., de Graaf, R., Nolen, W. A., Spijker, J., Hoogendijk, W. J., et al. (2010). Trajectories of recovery of social and physical functioning in major depression, dysthymic disorder and double depression: A 3-year follow-up. *Journal of Affective Disorders, 124,* 148–156.

Riso, L. P., Du Toit, P. L., Blandino, J. A., Penna, S., Dacey, S., Duin, J. S., et al. (2003). Cognitive aspects of chronic depression. *Journal of Abnormal Psychology, 112,* 72.

Robinson, O. J., & Sahakian, B. J. (2008). Recurrence in major depressive disorder: A neurocognitive perspective. *Psychological Medicine, 38,* 315–318.

Rohde, P., Lewinsohn, P. M., Klein, D. N., Seeley, J. R., & Gau, J. M. (2013). Key characteristics of major depressive disorder occurring in childhood, adolescence, emerging adulthood, and adulthood. *Clinical Psychological Science, 1,* 41–53.

Rush, A. J., Kraemer, H. C., Sackeim, H. A., Fava, M., Trivedi, M. H., Frank, E., et al. (2006). Report by the ACNP Task Force on response and remission in major depressive disorder. *Neuropsychopharmacology, 31,* 1841–1853.

Sang, W., Li, Y., Su, L., Yang, F., Wu, W., Shang, X., et al. (2011). A comparison of the clinical characteristics of Chinese patients with recurrent major depressive disorder with and without dysthymia. *Journal of Affective Disorders, 135,* 106–110.

Scott, K. M., McLaughlin, K. A., Smith, D. A. R., & Ellis, P. M. (2012). Childhood maltreatment and DSM-IV adult mental disorders: Comparison of prospective and retrospective findings. *British Journal of Psychiatry, 200,* 469–475.

Shah, P. J., Ebmeier, K. P., Glabus, M. F., & Goodwin, G. M. (1998). Cortical grey matter reductions associated with treatment-resistant chronic unipolar depression: Controlled magnetic resonance imaging study. *British Journal of Psychiatry, 172,* 527–532.

Shah, P. J., Glabus, M. F., Goodwin, G. M., & Ebmeier, K. P. (2002). Chronic, treatment-resistant depression and right fronto-striatal atrophy. *British Journal of Psychiatry, 180,* 434–440.

Spasojević, J., & Alloy, L. B. (2001). Rumination as a common mechanism relating depressive risk factors to depression. *Emotion, 1,* 25–57.

Stroud, C. B., Davila, J., & Moyer, A. (2008). The relationship between stress and depression in first onsets versus recurrences: A meta-analytic review. *Journal of Abnormal Psychology, 117,* 206–213.

Sullivan, P. F., Neale, M. C., & Kendler, K. S. (2000). Genetic epidemiology of major depression: Review and meta-analysis. *American Journal of Psychiatry, 157,* 1552–1562.

Szádóczky, E., Fazekas, I., Rihmer, Z., & Arató, M. (1994). The role of psychosocial and biological variables in separating chronic and non-chronic major depression and early-late-onset dysthymia. *Journal of Affective Disorders, 32,* 1–11.

Teasdale, J. D. (1988). Cognitive vulnerability to persistent depression. *Cognition and Emotion, 2,* 247–274.

Uher, R., Caspi, A., Houts, R., Sugden, K., Williams, B., Poulton, R., et al. (2011). Serotonin transporter gene moderates childhood maltreatment's effects on persistent but not single-episode depression: Replications and implications for resolving inconsistent results. *Journal of Affective Disorders, 135,* 56–65.

Vreeburg, S. A., Hoogendijk, W. J. G., DeRijk, R. H., van Dyck, R., Smit, J. H., Zitman, F. G., et al. (2013). Salivary cortisol levels and the 2-year course of depressive and anxiety disorders. *Psychoneuroendocrinology, 38,* 1494–1502.

Watson, D., & Clark, L. A. (1995). Depression and the melancholic temperament. *European Journal of Personality, 9,* 351–366.

Watson, S., Gallagher, P., Del-Estal, D., Hearn, A., Ferrier, I. N., & Young, A. H. (2002). Hypothalamic–pituitary–adrenal axis function in patients with chronic depression. *Psychological Medicine, 32,* 1021–1028.

Watson, S., Gallagher, P., Ferrier, I. N., & Young, A. H. (2006). Post-dexamethasone arginine vasopressin levels in patients with severe mood disorders. *Journal of Psychiatric Research, 40,* 353–359.

Wichers, M., Peeters, F., Geschwind, N., Jacobs, N., Simons, C. J. P., Derom, C., et al. (2010). Unveiling patterns of affective responses in daily life may improve outcome prediction in depression: A momentary assessment study. *Journal of Affective Disorders, 124,* 191–195.

Wiersma, J. E., Hovens, J. G. F. M., van Oppen, P., Giltay, E. J., van Schaik, D. J. F., Beekman, A. T. F., et al. (2009). The importance of childhood trauma and childhood life events for chronicity of depression in adults. *Journal of Clinical Psychiatry, 70,* 983–989.

Wiersma, J. E., van Oppen, P., van Schaik, D. J., van der Does, A. J., Beekman, A. T., & Penninx, B. W. (2011). Psychological characteristics of chronic depression: A longitudinal cohort study. *Journal of Clinical Psychiatry, 72,* 288–294.

Yang, T., & Dunner, D. L. (2001). Differential subtyping of depression. *Depression and Anxiety, 13,* 11–17.

CHAPTER 5

Comorbidity of Unipolar Depressive and Anxiety Disorders

Susan Mineka *and* Suzanne Vrshek-Schallhorn

The overlap or comorbidity of anxiety and depressive disorders has been a topic of great interest to psychologists and psychiatrists for at least the past 30 years. Numerous epidemiological and clinical studies have documented that people who have one of these disorders are at greatly elevated risk of having one or more other anxiety or depressive disorders (often known as the emotional or internalizing disorders). This co-occurrence is more common with certain anxiety disorders than with others, and the disorders can occur either concurrently or at different points in a person's life (e.g., Brown, Campbell, Lehman, Grisham, & Mancill, 2001; Kessler, Nelson, McGonagle, & Liu, 1996). This comorbidity is especially important because disorders from both of these categories can be highly debilitating and are associated with an enormous cost (disease burden) to society (e.g., Üstün, Ayuso-Mateos, Chatterji, Mathers, & Murray, 2004). Because of high rates of comorbidity and because both anxiety and depressive disorders are also very common classes of disorders (among the U.S. population, lifetime prevalence of anxiety disorders is about 25–29%, and lifetime prevalence for unipolar major depression alone is about 17%; see Kessler et al., Chapter 1, this volume), comorbid anxiety and depression may affect millions of individuals. It is not surprising, therefore, that psychopathologists have been interested in elucidating the nature of the overlap, the factors that cause the overlap, and how best to treat the millions of people who have these comorbid disorders.

In this chapter, we first briefly review some of the already well-documented evidence for comorbidity between depression and the anxiety disorders. Second, we review the major structural models of relations between these disorders in order to gain a better understanding of the nature of their overlap. Next, we examine evidence for similarities and differences in the risk factors for these classes of disorders, with a focus on genetic, personality, and environmental (i.e., life stress) risk factors. We also present additional highlights from several types of research that help to illuminate these issues—including research on cognitive biases, neuroendocrine functioning, and psychophysiology—and we conclude with what we see as important directions for future research on the comorbidity between depressive and anxiety disorders.

Throughout this chapter, we make the case that one key to understanding the comorbidity of depressive and anxiety disorders—thereby hopefully elucidating their etiologies—is delineating common and specific risk factors for these disorders. By common risk factors, we are referring to constructs that increase risk for both types of disorders. Conversely, by specific risk factors, we are referring to constructs that increase risk for only one or a few disorders from this group. Delineating common risk factors for the set of these disorders could suggest novel treatment targets and also could suggest approaches to preventive interventions that may reduce risk for this spectrum of disorders in a maximally efficient manner. Understanding specific risk factors is also valuable. For example, a treatment developed to address common features of these emotional disorders could be augmented to address an aspect of dysfunction specific to a certain disorder.

Understanding the comorbidity between depressive and anxiety disorders is also important because, relative to noncomorbid disorders, comorbidity is associated with greater distress and disability (e.g., Andrews, Slade, & Issakidis, 2002), higher rates of help seeking (e.g., Roness, Mykletun, & Dahl, 2005), poorer prognosis in treatment (e.g., Curry et al., 2006), and greater risk for suicidal ideation and attempts (e.g., Sareen et al., 2005; also see Mineka, Watson, & Clark, 1998, for an early review). Thus it is important that we study comorbidity, both to gain a better understanding of the etiology of the emotional disorders and to inform treatment for comorbid manifestations of these disorders.

DEFINITIONS AND DIFFERENT TYPES OF COMORBIDITY

In this area, comorbidity generally refers to the co-occurrence of two different disorders (as defined by the current diagnostic system, such as DSM-IV or DSM-5). However, it is also sometimes used to refer to the co-occurrence of symptoms that are central to the definitions of different disorders.[1] When self-ratings (as opposed to clinician ratings) of anxious or depressive symptoms are used, research has shown that individuals are far less discriminating between these two types of symptoms than are clinicians (e.g., Clark, 1989; Mineka et al., 1998). As these earlier reviews indicated, the same seems to be true about diagnosing different syndromes, with self-ratings showing less discriminating power than clinician ratings. We focus here almost entirely on syndromal comorbidity.

Comorbidity of two or more disorders can manifest itself in three different forms—cross-sectional, cumulative (lifetime), and sequential—depending on the different time courses considered. *Cross-sectional comorbidity* occurs when different disorders manifest themselves either at the same time or within some limited time frame (e.g., the past year). Many published studies on this topic use the term *comorbidity* in this way. However, multiple disorders can occur at different points in an individual's life rather than at the same time, and this phenomenon is labeled *cumulative* or *lifetime* comorbidity—also a topic of considerable interest. Finally, some researchers have been interested in determining whether there is any pattern regarding which disorder(s) tends to precede which other disorders in terms of co-occurrence; this pattern is called *sequential comorbidity*.

---

[1]See Mineka et al. (1998) for a discussion of findings that anxiety symptoms tend to precede depressive symptoms when both are present in a given period. See also Starr and Davila (2012) for a recent 3-week daily diary study of 55 participants who met criteria for current GAD and had a history of at least one to two cardinal symptoms of MDD; this study found that daily anxious mood predicted later depressed mood at a variety of time lags, but not vice versa.

THE EXTENT AND NATURE OF COMORBIDITY BETWEEN DEPRESSIVE AND ANXIETY DISORDERS

Epidemiological Evidence for Comorbidity

At this point at least three major epidemiological studies have been conducted in the United States over the past 35 years: the Epidemiologic Catchment Area (ECA) study from the early 1980s; the National Comorbidity Survey (NCS) from the early 1990s and its follow-up from the early 2000s; and the National Comorbidity Survey—Replication (NCS-R) from the early 2000s. A number of similar studies have also been conducted in various other countries around the world, such as, for example, the Netherlands (e.g., de Graaf, Bijl, Ravelli, Smit, & Vollebergh, 2002); the general patterns of results seem to be similar in different Western countries, although the details obviously differ. Importantly, similar patterns of results to those observed in adults also occur in children and adolescents (e.g., Kessler, Avenevoli, & Merikangas, 2001; Merikangas et al., 2010) and older adults (e.g., Byers, Yaffe, Covinsky, Friedman, & Bruce, 2010). It is also noteworthy that nearly all studies on this topic have focused only on comorbidity of anxiety disorders with *unipolar depressive disorders*, even though several studies have revealed, if anything, higher comorbidity rates for *bipolar disorder* with anxiety disorders, with anxiety symptoms occurring during both manic and depressive episodes (Merikangas et al., 2007; Provencher, Guimond, & Hawke, 2012). This is an important and interesting topic that has unfortunately not been carefully studied and so is not discussed here.

One major point that has emerged about comorbidity is that not only are rates of comorbidity of depression with a considerable number of other disorders high, but also, in most cases, the depression was secondary to the occurrence of another disorder (see Kessler et al., 1996, for a review of such findings). For example, in the ECA study, 75% of the cases of depression were secondary to another disorder (Robins, Locke, & Regier, 1991), and in the original NCS, 62% of those with major depressive disorder (MDD) had experienced another disorder first. Moreover, in the NCS, 58% of those with lifetime depression also had a lifetime anxiety disorder diagnosis, and of those with MDD in the past 12 months, 51% also had an anxiety disorder (see Kessler et al., 1996, for a review of such findings). MDD was also more strongly related to anxiety disorders than to any other category of disorders studied in the NCS. Finally, 68% of the cases of secondary depression were associated with a primary anxiety disorder (vs. 19% with a primary substance use disorder, for example). Among the anxiety disorders, depression comorbidity with generalized anxiety disorder (GAD) was highest, followed by panic disorder and posttraumatic stress disorder (PTSD) (odds ratios [ORs] were 6.0, 4.0 and 4.0, respectively). Comorbidity with agoraphobia, specific phobia, and social phobia was also quite common but slightly less so (ORs were 3.4, 3.1, and 2.9, respectively).[2]

Although much less has been written on this topic as it pertains to children, adolescents, and older adults, the available research suggests a similar pattern as in adults. (One exception is that certain disorders such as panic disorder have an average age of onset in the 20s; therefore, one would not expect to see, for example, comorbidity between depression and panic disorder in adolescents.) For example, Kessler and colleagues (2001) reported in an epidemiological study of children and adolescents that 75% of participants with depression had a history of at least one anxiety disorder. For older adults, results

---

[2]Comparable figures from the NCS-R are not publicly available, so we present only these results from the NCS (Kessler, Berglund, et al., 2005).

from the NCS-R revealed that, although 12-month prevalence of these emotional disorders declined substantially from ages 55 to 85, the relative rates of anxiety and mood disorders remained similar (12 and 5%, respectively; Byers et al., 2010). The percentage of this population receiving comorbid depressive and anxiety disorder diagnoses also declined over this time period, from 4.8% at ages 55–64 to only 1% at ages 85 and older.

Structural Models Characterizing the Nature of Comorbidity

Characterizing the structure of relations between depressive and anxiety disorders has long been of interest as one important means to understanding comorbidity. Clark and Watson (1991) proposed one of the first structural models of the emotional disorders, the tripartite model, which suggested that these disorders share in common a general distress dimension but also have syndrome-specific features. Others proposed similar structural models with three factors, such as fear, anxiety, and depression (Chorpita, Albano, & Barlow, 1998). The tripartite model posited that low positive affect was specific to depression, whereas elevated physiological arousal was specific to anxiety syndromes. Initial support emerged in that, as hypothesized, scales developed to assess anxious arousal and anhedonia differentiated anxiety and depressive syndromes (Watson, Weber, et al., 1995), and factor analyses of a variety of anxious and depressive symptoms supported the tripartite structure (Watson, Clark, et al., 1995). However, as reviewed by Mineka and colleagues (1998), substantial heterogeneity among the anxiety disorders made such a model less plausible than originally hoped. For example, physiological arousal was shown to be elevated only in panic disorder (Brown, Chorpita, & Barlow, 1998) and perhaps also in PTSD (Brown et al., 2001), but not in other anxiety disorders. Furthermore, low positive affect does not appear to be specific to depression as initially proposed because social phobia is also associated with low positive affect (e.g., Brown et al., 1998).

Watson (2009) later proposed a revision, the quadripartite model, which in essence suggested that there are additional disorder-specific factors beyond the two articulated in the original tripartite model and that disorders will vary in the extent to which they load on the various common and specific risk factors. This model thus derived its name from the four possible combinations from the 2×2 matrix of relatively high versus low loading on general distress and specific factors. Although few empirical examples of the new quadripartite approach are yet available, Watson provided several illustrations. For example, the four symptom clusters of PTSD demonstrate high loading on general distress and low specificity to depression versus anxiety.

As support for the original tripartite model began to wane, a body of research emerged using confirmatory factor analysis (CFA) to examine the structural relations between unipolar depression and the anxiety disorders. This research has examined which disorders tend to cluster together and which higher-order dimensions characterize them. The first such study used CFA to examine comorbidity patterns in more than 900 participants (18–21 years old) from the Dunedin Multidisciplinary Health and Development Study (Krueger, Caspi, Moffitt, & Silva, 1998). The DSM-III-R diagnoses included two depressive disorders (MDD, dysthymia), five anxiety disorders (GAD, agoraphobia, social phobia, simple phobia, and obsessive–compulsive disorder [OCD]), and three additional disorders (conduct disorder/antisocial personality disorder, marijuana dependence, and alcohol dependence).

A model in which all depressive and anxiety disorders grouped together as internalizing disorders (cf. emotional disorders), distinct from but correlated with the externalizing disorders (e.g., conduct disorder), was supported (Krueger et al., 1998). Later replications and extensions identified this same internalizing factor but also provided evidence that the internalizing factor acts as a second-order factor in a hierarchy above two lower-order factors: anxious–misery (or distress) and fear (e.g., Krueger, 1999b; Slade & Watson, 2006). Although the specific loadings and the disorders examined vary slightly across reports, results generally indicate that anxious–misery disorders (sometimes called "distress disorders") include major depression, dysthymia, GAD, and PTSD. Fear disorders include specific phobia, social phobia, panic disorder, agoraphobia, and possibly OCD.

Although the extent of replication of these findings is remarkable, a few studies have yielded divergent results—one notably so. Because comorbidity patterns for 19 disorders studied in the NCS-R violated certain assumptions of CFA used in prior studies, exploratory latent class analysis was used to characterize the most common profiles of comorbidity (Kessler, Chiu, Demler, & Walters, 2005). Four of seven latent classes that were identified involved depression and anxiety disorders: (1) "pure" internalizing disorders, notable for showing a lack of comorbidity, with one diagnosis per person (14.5% of the sample); (2) cases with comorbidity between depression and the full range of anxiety disorders, with approximately three diagnoses per person (5%); (3) mixed comorbid internalizing and externalizing disorders, with two diagnoses on average (2.3%)—often social phobia and attention-deficit/hyperactive disorder; and (4) severely comorbid depression, characterized by MDD comorbid with, on average, four other internalizing and externalizing disorders (1.6%). These results illustrate that although the lower-order dimensions anxious–misery and fear are statistically differentiable, they are so highly correlated that they do not appear to translate into separate patterns of comorbidity.

Finally, several studies have also examined the relation of personality measures to the internalizing dimension. In one study, the latent internalizing dimension was strongly positively correlated with negative emotionality (cf. neuroticism) in both males and females and was negatively correlated with positive emotionality in females, but not in males (Krueger, McGue, & Iacono, 2001). Similarly, the Youth Emotion Project, a study of a diverse sample of more than 600 older adolescents/young adults, examined the relation between the latent internalizing dimension and a latent neuroticism variable (but not other personality traits) in older adolescents and found a correlation of .98 between the two constructs (Griffith et al., 2010).

IMPLICATIONS OF GENETIC, PERSONALITY, AND LIFE-STRESS RESEARCH FOR EMOTIONAL DISORDER COMORBIDITY

Evidence on Genetic Risk Factors

Research on genetic aspects of comorbidity between depressive and anxiety disorders can be considered at two levels—behavioral genetics and molecular genetics. Behavioral genetic research regarding comorbidity that employs twin studies is much more well established than is molecular genetic research (i.e., examination of specific genetic polymorphisms). The latter area, in its relative infancy, has to date focused mostly on depression alone.

Behavioral genetic work in twin samples has provided evidence for the degree of genetic contributions to individual disorders and has also provided evidence for the structure of the overlap in genetic factors between disorders. First, meta-analyses have indicated that genetic factors make modest to moderate contributions to liability to depression (with a point estimate for heritability of 0.37; Sullivan, Neale, & Kendler, 2000) and several anxiety disorders (heritability of 0.32 for GAD, 0.43 for panic disorder; Hettema, Neale, & Kendler, 2001). Individual twin studies support similarly modest to moderate genetic contributions for other anxiety disorders (e.g., 0.35 for specific phobias; Kendler et al., 1995; see Lau et al., Chapter 9, this volume, for a more detailed review of this literature).

Second, studies examining the latent structure of these genetic contributions not only support the results of factor analytic structural comorbidity models but also show that genetic factors help to account for comorbidity patterns among the emotional disorders much more than do environmental factors. For example, in more than 5,600 twins from the Virginia Twin Registry, structural equation modeling of five emotional disorder diagnoses (MDD, GAD, panic disorder, animal phobias, situational phobias) revealed two latent genetic subfactors (Kendler, Prescott, Myers, & Neale, 2003). One subfactor loaded primarily on MDD (0.53) and GAD (0.52), representing an anxious–misery genetic factor, and a second loaded primarily on the two types of phobias examined (0.45–0.49), representing a fear genetic factor. (However, contrary to expectations, both genetic factors loaded at low levels on panic disorder, 0.31 and 0.09, respectively.) Of particular interest, only genetic and not environmental factors formed a structure consistent with patterns of comorbidity, supporting the formulation that comorbidity is heavily due to common genetic factors. Specifically, loadings for *unshared environmental* factors that were unique to each disorder ranged from 0.44 to 0.80, whereas such disorder-specific loadings for genetic factors ranged from 0.00 to 0.20. Thus latent modeling indicated that environmental factors tended to load on disorders individually and that genetic factors loaded broadly across disorders. Although this study did not examine specific combinations of disorders, its evidence for common (and not for specific) genetic factors strongly suggests a largely genetic basis for comorbidity.

Latent models like these describing differentiable genetic factors for anxious–misery and fear disorders are consistent with a quantitative review by Middeldorp, Cath, Van Dyck, and Boomsma (2005), who tabulated genetic correlations between disorders from the results reported in 23 individual twin studies. Correlations between the respective genetic contributions to MDD and GAD were high, ranging from 0.86 to 1.0—nearly total overlap (see Mineka, Anand, & Sumner, 2014, for a review). By contrast, correlations between genetic contributions to MDD and other anxiety disorders were lower on average (panic disorder, 0.59–0.71; specific phobias, 0.07–0.31; agoraphobia, 0.16; social phobia, 0.11–1.0).

Furthermore, in a study of more than 9,000 twins from the Virginia Adult Twin Study of Psychiatric and Substance Use Disorders, Hettema, Neale, Myers, Prescott, and Kendler (2006) modeled the latent genetic variance as: (1) common across depression and six anxiety disorders and shared with neuroticism, (2) common but unshared with neuroticism, or (3) specific to individual disorders. Results indicated that over one-third to one-half of the genetic variance contributing to MDD and the anxiety disorders is shared with neuroticism. A second latent genetic factor unshared with neuroticism loaded primarily on MDD, GAD, and panic disorder. Specific phobias, agoraphobia, and social phobia demonstrated disorder-specific latent genetic loadings that these researchers speculated might have formed a third latent (fear) genetic factor if it had been possible to test for one.

As noted earlier, at this time limited conclusions can be drawn about molecular genetic polymorphisms (relatively frequent individual differences in the genetic code) and comorbidity. However, one set of findings worth mentioning pertains to the serotonin transporter-linked polymorphic region, 5-HTTLPR, which was first reported to interact with stressful life events to increase risk for depression and several related outcomes such as depressive symptoms by Caspi and colleagues (2003). Caspi and colleagues' findings have generated both replications and nonreplications—as well as much controversy. However, their finding that the short (or S) allele (version) of this polymorphism is significantly associated with depression in interaction with various forms of life stress was supported by the most recent and comprehensive meta-analysis conducted (Karg, Burmeister, Shedden, & Sen, 2011). Meta-analyses also support a significant but small main effect (rather than an interaction with stress) of 5-HTTLPR on neuroticism level (e.g., Sen, Burmeister, & Ghosh, 2004).

Although gene–environment interactions of 5-HTTLPR for anxiety disorders have rarely been examined, one such study indicated that the S/S genotype interacts with childhood adversity to predict anxiety sensitivity, which is a marker of risk for several anxiety disorders (Stein, Schork, & Gelernter, 2007). In addition, several studies have linked the 5-HTTLPR polymorphism with onsets of PTSD in interaction with traumatic events (for a review, see Mehta & Binder, 2012). Thus there is good evidence of the involvement of 5-HTTLPR in depression and neuroticism and some early evidence of its involvement in at least one anxiety disorder, suggesting that it may well behave as a common risk factor for the emotional disorders, rather than a factor that is specific to depression.

Evidence on Personality Risk Factors

Personality variables have also been studied as possible risk factors for comorbid anxiety and depressive disorders. In the literature on comorbidity of anxiety and depressive disorders, only neuroticism and extraversion seem to have been examined in multiple studies. It is also unfortunate that few studies on this topic are prospective in nature; therefore, conclusions about which personality variables truly serve as risk factors (as opposed to mere correlates) are premature at this time. Nevertheless, there are numerous studies suggesting that higher levels of neuroticism are more associated with comorbid mood and anxiety disorders than with either anxiety or mood disorders alone, which are themselves associated with elevated levels of neuroticism. For example, Weinstock and Whisman (2006) used data on DSM-III-R diagnoses from the NCS ($n = 5,847$) conducted in the early 1990s and found that neuroticism was elevated (comparably) in pure depressive and in pure anxiety disorders. However, they also found that individuals with comorbid disorders showed even greater elevations of neuroticism. In a large study of participants from the Virginia twin registry ($n > 7,000$), Khan, Jacobson, Gardner, Prescott, and Kendler (2005) also found that, of several personality dimensions examined, neuroticism accounted for the highest proportion (20–45%) of comorbidity within the emotional disorders.

Relatedly, as mentioned previously, Griffith and colleagues (2010) found that a single internalizing factor among the mood and anxiety disorders was virtually identical to latent neuroticism ($r = .98$) in a sample of 621 ethnically diverse adolescents participating in a longitudinal prospective study of common and specific risk factors for emotional disorders (the Youth Emotion Project; see Zinbarg et al., 2010, for background; see also Krueger, 1999a, for related findings.) Finally, in a sample of 640 adult outpatients with one or more emotional disorders, Cuijpers, van Straten, and Donker (2005) found that neuroticism was significantly higher in participants with two diagnoses than in those with one and highest in those with three or four diagnoses. These cross-sectional findings are not particularly surprising given content overlap between items for neuroticism and depressive and anxiety symptoms (see Zinbarg et al., 2010, for discussion).

Supporting strong hypotheses that elevated neuroticism is a significant predictor of comorbidity, one prospective study has recently found that elevated neuroticism is indeed a strong predictor of comorbid anxiety and mood disorders (Zinbarg et al., 2014). Specifically, this study of a diverse sample of more than 500 older adolescents/young adults from the Youth Emotion Project used a latent general neuroticism factor assessed at baseline (when participants were an average of 17 years old) to predict the onset of anxiety and depressive disorders at a 3-year follow-up. Over this 3-year period, latent neuroticism predicted cumulative comorbidity of anxiety and depressive disorders significantly more strongly than it did onset of anxiety or depressive disorders alone.

As noted earlier, the only other Big Five personality trait that has received some attention in the study of comorbidity of anxiety and mood disorders is extraversion. Bienvenu and colleagues (2001) found that low extraversion was associated with both social phobia and agoraphobia, but surprisingly, not with major depression (an association that has been found in several other studies, e.g., Krueger, Caspi, Moffitt, Silva, & McGee, 1996; Watson, Gamez, & Simms, 2005). Therefore, one might expect that low extraversion would predict comorbidity of social phobia (or perhaps agoraphobia) and depression, but no studies appear to have examined this hypothesis.

In addition to studying personality variables as risk factors, more cognitively oriented researchers have studied the role of cognitive constructs such as negative *attributional (explanatory) style* and *dysfunctional attitudes* as risk factors for onsets of depressive and (to a lesser extent) anxiety disorders. For example, a depressogenic attributional style and dysfunctional attitudes have been shown to predict the onset of both mood and anxiety disorders (e.g., Zinbarg et al., 2014). However, at least one large study found that these constructs did not predict onset of anxiety disorders alone (Alloy et al., 2006), although the effect sizes were in the predicted direction. In addition, both Zinbarg and colleagues (2014) and Alloy and colleagues (2006) found that negative cognitive styles also predicted onset of comorbid anxiety and depressive disorders (cumulatively). Importantly, however, Zinbarg and colleagues also showed that negative cognitive styles lose their predictive power when neuroticism is entered into the equation, suggesting that these negative cognitive style variables are primarily cognitive facets of the broader concept of neuroticism.

Environmental Precipitants as Risk Factors

Stressful life events have long been known to be associated with precipitating the onset of depressive disorders (especially the first episode); much less is known, however, about their role in precipitating the onset of anxiety disorders or comorbid anxiety and depressive disorders. For example, Monroe and Harkness (2005) and Monroe, Slavich, and Georgiades (2009) estimated that about 70% of people with a first onset of depression have had a recent major stressful life event (in the past few months) but that only about 40% of people with a recurrent episode have had a recent major life event (see Monroe, Slavich, & Georgiades, Chapter 16, this volume, for a more detailed discussion of this research). However, in contrast to the wealth of evidence on this topic for depression, relatively few studies have examined the role of stressful life events in the onset of anxiety disorders. One early study compared the role of stressful life events in the onset of depression versus anxiety versus mixed anxiety–depression. In a sample of 164 young women,

Finlay-Jones and Brown (1981) reported that severe loss events were likely to have precipitated onset of a depressive disorder (within 1 year) and that severe danger events were the likely precipitants in the onset of anxiety states. For cases of comorbid depression and anxiety, the precipitant was most likely to be both a severe loss event and a severe danger event (see Monroe, 1990, for an early review).

Although this level of specificity for environmental precipitants is consistent with the behavioral genetic findings described previously (see Kendler, Prescott, et al., 2003), there have also been noteworthy nonreplications. In a much larger study on this topic, Kendler, Hettema, Butera, Gardner, and Prescott (2003) studied more than 7,000 twin pairs, assessing the occurrence of MDD, a generalized anxiety syndrome (with a 2-week minimum duration), and a mixed anxiety–depression syndrome. Stressful life events were rated on dimensions of loss, humiliation, entrapment, and danger. Kendler, Hettema, and colleagues found that loss events within 1 month prior to onset significantly predicted all three syndromes and that humiliation events significantly predicted depression and mixed anxiety–depression episodes. Entrapment and danger events were also associated with mixed episodes within 2 months prior to the onset of the episode. Thus, in this much larger and more generalizable sample, the level of specificity of event type to syndrome that the earlier, smaller study had reported was not replicated.

In discussing the role of stress in precipitating anxiety and/or depressive disorders, no researchers seem to have distinguished among the different kinds of stress that might be involved in precipitating comorbid disorders. For example, it is possible that stressful life events are involved in the onset of panic disorder per se but that the stress involved in the onset of future comorbid depression is not necessarily in the form of a stressful life event as traditionally defined. Instead, it might be that, for some people, it is the chronic stress of living with panic disorder (including its uncontrollable and unpredictable panic attacks that are often terrifying) that leads to the depressive episode. Several theorists have discussed this as a likely possibility, but we are not aware of any research directly addressing the issue (e.g., Alloy, Kelly, Mineka, & Clements, 1990; see Akiskal, 1990, for a related argument).

Early life stress and adversity have also been shown in numerous studies to play a role in increasing vulnerability for the subsequent onset of mood and anxiety disorders and probably their comorbidity, although the latter has only rarely been examined. For example, Green and colleagues (2010) used data from the large NCS-R to show that there was little specificity in terms of which childhood adversities were associated with which specific disorders in adolescence and adulthood. They found that childhood adversities were involved in 32% of cases of anxiety disorders and 26% of depressive disorders, but unfortunately they did not present results on comorbidity. The authors were careful to note that they were not claiming these were causal effects because numerous third variables could not be ruled out as playing the true causal role. In a somewhat similar Canadian study of more than 6,500 individuals, Levitan, Rector, Sheldon, and Goering (2003) reported that early sexual abuse was associated with comorbid anxiety and mood disorders (but not with pure disorders). Until these findings are replicated, however, these results should be viewed cautiously given other studies such as the NCS-R that suggest more nonspecific effects. (It is unfortunate that Green et al., 2010, did not present results on comorbidity in their very large NCS-R sample.) Heim and Nemeroff (2001) also presented evidence that early life stress induces a long-lived hyperreactivity of the corticotropin-releasing factor system, which in turn increases stress responsiveness that should increase risk for both mood and anxiety disorders and, quite likely, their comorbidity.

OTHER EXAMPLES OF COMMON AND SPECIFIC FEATURES AND RISK FACTORS FROM VARIOUS RESEARCH METHODOLOGIES

Examples from Cognitive Bias Research

The past 20 years have seen a great deal of research on the cognitive processing of emotion-relevant material and how it is related to depressive and anxiety disorders (a topic commonly known as cognitive biases in the emotional disorders; e.g., Mathews & MacLeod, 2005). (By the term *bias* we mean nonveridical processing of emotion-relevant material, mostly in attention or memory; see Joormann & Arditte, Chapter 14, this volume.) Moreover, in recent years much attention has been devoted both to the role that such biases may play in the origins and maintenance of these disorders and to how altering such cognitive biases may be useful in treating these disorders (see MacLeod & Mathews, 2012; Mathews & MacLeod, 2005). Given the extensive comorbidity between these categories of disorders, it may seem surprising that we do not know more about the effects of comorbidity on cognitive biases. However, enough is known to be confident that this is an important topic for future research because, as we illustrate, comorbidity can have substantial effects on cognitive biases, and risk factors vary to some extent across disorders.

First, let us briefly summarize some of the major differences in findings on cognitive biases for depression and anxiety disorders when they are considered separately. Most anxiety (but not depressive) disorders seem to be characterized by an automatic, unconscious *attentional bias* toward threatening information, even when that information is presented very briefly (e.g., 30–500 msec) or sometimes even subliminally. In contrast, MDD seems to be characterized by a bias toward certain types of negative information only when that information is presented for longer stimulus intervals, such as 1000–1500 msec. This finding is thought to reflect biased elaborative processing of negative information in depression, which might indicate difficulty updating the contents of working memory for negative stimuli. On the other hand, *memory biases* for emotion-relevant information are much more readily observed in individuals with depression than in those with anxiety (e.g., see Mathews & MacLeod, 2005, for an earlier review). Finally, both depression and anxiety disorders seem to be associated with *interpretive biases*, reflected by a tendency to interpret ambiguous information in a negative manner.

Progress on the topic of comorbidity in this realm has been hampered by several unfortunate factors, which are not unique to cognitive bias research. For example, many researchers studying people with potentially comorbid diagnoses have not been careful to first document potential comorbidity by conducting careful assessments for multiple disorders. In addition, many investigators have not been particularly interested in the effects of comorbidity (which is often considered almost a nuisance variable) and so have not included the appropriate control groups (or even covariates) to be able to draw relevant conclusions. To study this issue carefully requires at least three groups—one with the anxiety disorder of interest but not a depressive disorder, one with comorbid disorders, and one with a depressive disorder alone—plus, ideally, healthy controls.

One example serves to illustrate this issue. As already noted, anxiety, but not depression, is usually associated with an attentional bias that occurs only at an early stage of processing (e.g., when stimuli are presented for only 30–500 msec). Depression, in contrast, is associated with an attentional bias toward negative information only when the stimuli are presented for a longer duration of 1000 msec or more, reflecting biased elaborative processing of negative information. For example, Mogg and Bradley (2005) reviewed evidence that individuals with GAD (but not depression) show an attentional bias for threatening information when stimuli are presented for very brief periods of time (30–500 msec). However, individuals with either depression alone or with *comorbid* GAD and depression do not show this attentional bias for negative information unless the stimuli are presented for more than 1000 msec and unless the material is self-relevant. One possible explanation for why this may occur is that individuals with depression (with or without comorbid GAD) may tend to show a depression-related motivational deficit that may occur because goal-engagement mechanisms are less readily activated during depression (see Mogg & Bradley, 2005). Thus the presence of depression seems to mask the bias that would otherwise be seen with GAD. Finally, research in this area is further complicated by the fact that cognitive biases differ somewhat across the different anxiety disorders. Unfortunately, this means that any simple conclusions about findings on the effects of comorbidity on cognitive biases much beyond those discussed here are simply not possible.

Examples from Neuroendocrine Research

Neuroendocrine research on the emotional disorders has focused on the primary hormonal output of the hypothalamic–pituitary–adrenal (HPA) axis: cortisol. The HPA axis and cortisol facilitate physiological adaptation to environmental demands, including stress, with actions such as increasing glucose availability in order to permit maintenance of homeostasis (see Fries, Dettenborn, & Kirschbaum, 2009). Although HPA dysregulation has been a long-standing focus of depression research, less attention has been given to this construct in research on anxiety disorders, despite the fact that activation of anxiety responses is known to trigger increases in cortisol release. Because HPA research in anxiety disorders lags behind parallel work in depression, conclusions that can be drawn at this time about common and specific factors are at best suggestive.

Two primary types of studies have examined HPA functioning in emotional disorders. First, studies of lab-induced acute stress have evaluated how cortisol levels change in response to a brief stressor. Many of these studies have used the Trier Social Stress Test (TSST; e.g., Kirschbaum, Pirke, & Hellhammer, 2008) or similar protocols designed to briefly induce stress in a laboratory setting using a speaking task and a mental arithmetic task performed for a panel of two aloof judges. One meta-analysis indicated that individuals with current depression show *attenuated* cortisol responses to the TSST and other similar protocols relative to healthy controls (Burke, Davis, Otte, & Mohr, 2005). Furthermore, one study using the TSST to examine individuals with pure social phobia, comorbid social phobia and depression, and healthy controls demonstrated that individuals with pure social phobia had the predicted exaggerated cortisol response to threat relative to controls on the TSST. However, this elevated response pattern was attenuated by comorbid depression, despite similar patterns of self-reported elevated anxious responding in the pure and comorbid groups relative to controls (Yoon & Joormann, 2012). This pattern of findings suggests that many individuals with depression experience a failure of neuroendocrine support for behavioral activation in response to threats to the self, whereas individuals with at least one pure anxiety disorder demonstrated the predicted exaggerated response to threat.

Second, naturalistic research has examined evidence for dysregulation of the diurnal rhythm of cortisol in anxiety and depression. One aspect of the diurnal rhythm that has received particular attention is the cortisol awakening response (CAR), the large increase in cortisol levels over already elevated waking cortisol levels that peaks 30–40 minutes after waking (Pruessner et al., 1997). Elevations in the CAR *prospectively* predicted both first onsets and recurrences of depression (Vrshek-Schallhorn et al., 2013). However, several cross-sectional studies have also shown that the CAR is *reduced* in current depression (e.g., Stetler & Miller, 2005). By contrast, cross-sectional data have suggested that the CAR, or morning cortisol, is *elevated* in individuals with current anxiety disorders or elevated anxiety. More specifically, in a study of more than 1,400 people, those with current anxiety disorders showed significantly greater CAR values than their remitted and never-disordered counterparts, an effect that may have been driven by cases of panic disorder (Vreeburg et al., 2010). New evidence from the Youth Emotion Project has also suggested that, even controlling for both past and future depression, higher levels of the CAR prospectively predicted first onsets of social phobia (Adam et al., 2014). Results concerning the relation of the CAR to other anxiety disorders were inconclusive, possibly due to inadequate power to detect effects.

One interpretation of this pattern of results is that heightened TSST reactivity and CAR levels capture a propensity to greater physiological reactivity among individuals at risk for depression. However, through allostatic wear-and-tear processes, currently depressed individuals seem to display evidence of a "collapse" in neuroendocrine activity, both in reactivity to lab-induced stress and in the CAR. Tentatively, therefore, it appears that heightened reactivity may be associated with anxiety, both cross-sectionally and prospectively; however, additional research is needed to confirm this conclusion.

Examples from Psychophysiological Research

Psychophysiological research provides several examples of common and specific features of depressive and anxiety disorders. For example, in an approach–withdrawal conceptualization of frontal asymmetry in brain activation, greater relative left than right frontal lobe activity (measured using electroencephalography [EEG]) is associated with behavioral approach states such as positive affect and anger. In contrast, reduced relative left frontal activity is associated with behavioral withdrawal states, including depression (for a review, see Coan & Allen, 2004). Such reduced resting state activation on the left side relative to the right side has been shown to prospectively predict first onsets of depression and also to be associated with a negative cognitive style (Nusslock et al., 2011). Interestingly, in another study, reduced relative left frontal activation during a reward anticipation task was specific to individuals with depression (irrespective of comorbid panic disorder) compared with individuals with pure panic disorder and with healthy controls (Shankman et al., 2013).

Others have emphasized the heterogeneous effects on regional brain activation associated with two types of anxiety symptoms: anxious anticipation, which occurs in GAD, and anxious physiological arousal, which occurs in panic disorder (Engels et al., 2007). Such groupings appear to be consistent with factor analytic evidence for anxious–misery and fear disorder distinctions in the anxiety disorders. During negative word trials on an Emotional Stroop Task, brain activation patterns differed between groups high on one or the other of these two types of symptoms. Those with high levels of anxious apprehension showed greater left hemisphere activation in several regions, and those with high levels of anxious arousal showed greater right hemisphere activation in one region. Importantly, the extent of each type of comorbid anxiety influenced lateralization of activity in depression as well. The characteristic pattern of reduced relative left activation (i.e., rightward lateralization) was present in individuals with depression during performance of an Emotional Stroop Task only in the context of high anxious arousal and low apprehension

(Engels et al., 2010). Such findings again illustrate the importance of accounting for comorbid anxiety when assessing the pathophysiology of depression.

In addition, one risk factor predicting anxiety disorders but not depression in the Youth Emotion Project was demonstrated using a fear-potentiation startle protocol in which participants were told they could receive an aversive stimulus to their arm during "danger" windows but not during "safe" windows. One such aversive stimulus occurred midway through the protocol. Greater magnitude startle responses during safe windows, after (but not before) the aversive stimulus occurred, significantly predicted risk for first onsets of anxiety disorders but not of depressive episodes (Craske et al., 2012). This finding is consistent with the notion that excessive threat anticipation is related to risk for anxiety disorders, but not depression. In addition to this prospective work, similar relations are evident cross-sectionally. For example, individuals with current panic disorder (irrespective of comorbid MDD) demonstrated heightened threat anticipation in a startle protocol compared with those with pure MDD and healthy controls (Shankman et al., 2013).

IMPLICATIONS

In conclusion, although the tripartite model in its earliest conceptualization continues to be refined, evidence from a range of research methodologies supports several of its key features. First, evidence that general distress (cf. neuroticism) is a common feature, and even a prospective predictor, of the array of emotional disorders comes from behavioral genetic and personality research. Behavioral genetic research indicates not only that comorbidity is in large part due to genetic (rather than environmental) factors but also that a substantial portion (one-third to one-half) of this common genetic variance is shared with neuroticism.

Second, multiple lines of research, including personality and psychophysiology studies, provide evidence of deficits in positive emotionality and related constructs in depression, but not in most anxiety disorders (however, we noted evidence of reduced positive emotionality in social phobia). The apparent collapse that occurs in the CAR during depression bears conceptual similarities to deficits in positive emotion and may signify a loss of physiological support for behavioral activation in depression. Third, there is evidence from psychophysiological research, neuroendocrine research, and information-processing research that anxiety disorders are characterized by greater reactivity and/or sensitivity to threatening stimuli, if not persistently elevated physiological arousal. These elevations in reactivity or sensitivity appear to be specific to the anxiety disorders and not depression, although more research is clearly needed to say this conclusively.

FUTURE DIRECTIONS FOR RESEARCH

The importance of identifying common and specific correlates and risk factors has gained substantial support in recent years and will shift the conceptualization of psychopathology and comorbidity from individual disorders to underlying dimensions. The Research Domain Criteria (RDoC) are a recent initiative of the National Institute of Mental Health (NIMH) aimed at creating a research classification system for psychopathology based on common and specific correlates and risk factors identified by neuroscience, genetics, and cognitive science. This initiative was motivated by the relative inability of dichotomous diagnostic systems to identify the common underlying causes of superficially distinct but ultimately related symptom presentations. As has been noted, this shortcoming leads to inefficiency and ineffectiveness of treatment efforts (Insel et al., 2010). An internal NIMH RDoC working group established a hierarchical scheme with proposed dimensions for study, nested within five broader domains—negative and positive valence systems, cognitive systems, systems for social processes, and arousal systems (Cuthbert & Insel, 2013). In addition to ultimately creating an evidence-based nosology, the RDoC initiative is poised to characterize common and specific features and hopefully also risk factors for the emotional disorders.

As this initiative progresses, what can researchers do to better delineate common and specific correlates and risk factors for depressive and anxious disorders? First, we must study multiple currently defined disorders (or their dimensions) simultaneously. For far too long, too many studies have compared individuals with a single, pure disorder with healthy controls. Although it would generally be unfeasible and cost-prohibitive for most investigators to study *all* depressive and anxiety disorders at once, even studying two carefully selected disorders or dimensions would represent an advance over the majority of research conducted to date. Ideally, studies would contrast individuals with pure disorders to those with comorbid conditions and to healthy controls. Particularly useful combinations of disorders may include depression, plus either GAD or PTSD (disorders loading on the anxious–misery subfactor of the internalizing dimension), plus either panic disorder or social phobia (disorders loading on the fear dimension). A problem we have noted in several areas is that research on the anxiety disorders lags somewhat behind that for depression. This is particularly true for neuroendocrine research and studies of environmental risk factors. Examining multiple disorders simultaneously will help to ameliorate this problem.

Second, in order to gain a better understanding of etiology and to develop effective preventive intervention efforts, we must recognize that the cross-sectional correlates of psychopathology may differ from prospective predictors because pathology may induce changes. Such differences between cross-sectional and prospective findings are particularly apparent in the neuroendocrine literature on depression. Finally, an important challenge to the field is to relate findings from disparate research methodologies to generate a cohesive biopsychosocial model of the emotional disorders that is valid across both neurobiological and psychological levels of analysis.

REFERENCES

Adam, E. K., Vrshek-Schallhorn, S., Kendall, A., Mineka, S. Zinbarg, R. E., & Craske, M. (2014). Prospective associations between the Cortisol Awakening Response and first onsets of anxiety disorders over a six-year follow-up—2013 Curt Richter Award Winner. *Psychoneuroendocrinology, 44*, 47–59.

Akiskal, H. S. (1990). Toward a clinical understanding of the relationship of anxiety and depressive disorders. In J. D. Maser & C. R. Cloninger (Eds.), *Comorbidity of mood and anxiety disorders* (pp. 597–607). Washington: American Psychiatric Press.

Alloy, L. B., Abramson, L. Y., Whitehouse, W. G., Hogan, M. E., Panzarella, C., & Rose, D. T. (2006). Prospective incidence of first onsets and recurrences of depression in individuals at high and low cognitive risk for depression. *Journal of Abnormal Psychology, 115*(1), 145–156.

Alloy, L. B., Kelly, K. A., Mineka, S., & Clements, C. M. (1990). Comorbidity of anxiety and depressive disorders: A helplessness–hopelessness perspective. In J. D. Maser & C. R.

Cloninger (Eds.), *Comorbidity of mood and anxiety disorders* (pp. 499–543). Washington, DC: American Psychiatric Association.

Andrews, G., Slade, T., & Issakidis, C. (2002). Deconstructing current comorbidity: Data from the Australian National Survey of Mental Health and Well-Being. *British Journal of Psychiatry, 181*(4), 306–314.

Bienvenu, O. J., Brown, C., Samuels, J. F., Liang, K.-Y., Costa, P. T., Eaton, W. W., et al. (2001). Normal personality traits and comorbidity among phobic, panic and major depressive disorders. *Psychiatry Research, 102*(1), 73–85.

Brown, T., Campbell, L., Lehman, C., Grisham, J., & Mancill, R. (2001). Current and lifetime comorbidity of the DSM-IV anxiety and mood disorders in a large clinical sample. *Journal of Abnormal Psychology, 110*(4), 585–599.

Brown, T., Chorpita, B., & Barlow, D. (1998). Structural relationships among dimensions of the DSM-IV anxiety and mood disorders and dimensions of negative affect, positive affect, and autonomic arousal. *Journal of Abnormal Psychology, 107*, 179–192.

Burke, H. M., Davis, M. C., Otte, C., & Mohr, D. C. (2005). Depression and cortisol responses to psychological stress: A meta-analysis. *Psychoneuroendocrinology, 30*(9), 846–856.

Byers, A. L., Yaffe, K., Covinsky, K. E., Friedman, M. B., & Bruce, M. L. (2010). High occurrence of mood and anxiety disorders among older adults: The National Comorbidity Survey Replication. *Archives of General Psychiatry, 67*(5), 489–496.

Caspi, A., Sugden, K., Moffitt, T. E., Taylor, A., Craig, I. W., Harrington, H., et al. (2003). Influence of life stress on depression: Moderation by a polymorphism in the 5-HTT gene. *Science, 301*, 386–389.

Chorpita, B., Albano, A., & Barlow, D. (1998). The structure of negative emotions in a clinical sample of children and adolescents. *Journal of Abnormal Psychology, 107*(1), 74–85.

Clark, L. (1989). The anxiety and depressive disorders: Descriptive psychopathology and differential diagnosis. In P. Kendall & D. Watson (Eds.), *Anxiety and depression: Distinctive and overlapping features* (pp. 83–129). San Diego, CA: Academic Press.

Clark, L., & Watson, D. (1991). Tripartite model of anxiety and depression: Psychometric evidence and taxonomic implications. *Journal of Abnormal Psychology, 100*(3), 316–336.

Coan, J. A., & Allen, J. J. (2004). Frontal EEG asymmetry as a moderator and mediator of emotion. *Biological Psychology, 67*(1), 7–49.

Craske, M. G., Wolitzky-Taylor, K. B., Mineka, S., Zinbarg, R., Waters, A. M., Vrshek-Schallhorn, S., et al. (2012). Elevated responding to safe conditions as a specific risk factor for anxiety versus depressive disorders: Evidence from a longitudinal investigation. *Journal of Abnormal Psychology, 121*(2), 315–324.

Cuijpers, P., van Straten, A., & Donker, M. (2005). Personality traits of patients with mood and anxiety disorders. *Psychiatry Research, 133*(2), 229–237.

Curry, J., Rohde, P., Simons, A., Silva, S., Vitiello, B., Kratochvil, C., et al. (2006). Predictors and moderators of acute outcome in the Treatment for Adolescents with Depression Study (TADS). *Journal of the American Academy of Child and Adolescent Psychiatry, 45*(12), 1427–1439.

Cuthbert, B. N., & Insel, T. R. (2013). Toward the future of psychiatric diagnosis: The seven pillars of RDoC. *BMC Medicine, 11*(1), 126.

de Graaf, R., Bijl, R., Ravelli, A., Smit, F., & Vollebergh, W. (2002). Predictors of first incidence of DSM-III-R psychiatric disorders in the general population: Findings from the Netherlands Mental Health Survey and Incidence Study. *Acta Psychiatrica Scandinavica, 106*(4), 303–313.

Engels, A., Heller, W., Mohanty, A., Herrington, J., Banich, M., Webb, A., et al. (2007). Specificity of regional brain activity in anxiety types during emotion processing. *Psychophysiology, 44*(3), 352–363.

Engels, A., Heller, W., Spielberg, J. M., Warren, S. L., Sutton, B. P., Banich, M. T., et al. (2010). Co-occurring anxiety influences patterns of brain activity in depression. *Cognitive, Affective, and Behavioral Neuroscience, 10*(1), 141–156.

Finlay-Jones, R., & Brown, G. W. (1981). Types of stressful life event and the onset of anxiety and depressive disorders. *Psychological Medicine, 11*(4), 803–815.

Fries, E., Dettenborn, L., & Kirschbaum, C. (2009). The cortisol awakening response (CAR): Facts and future directions. *International Journal of Psychophysiology, 72*(1), 67–73.

Green, J. G., McLaughlin, K. A., Berglund, P. A., Gruber, M. J., Sampson, N. A., Zaslavsky, A. M., et al. (2010). Childhood adversities and adult psychiatric disorders in the national comorbidity survey replication: I. Associations with first onset of DSM-IV disorders. *Archives of General Psychiatry, 67*(2), 113–123.

Griffith, J. W., Zinbarg, R. E., Craske, M. G., Mineka, S., Rose, R. D., Waters, A. M., et al. (2010). Neuroticism as a common dimension in the internalizing disorders. *Psychological Medicine, 40*(7), 1125–1136.

Heim, C., & Nemeroff, C. B. (2001). The role of childhood trauma in the neurobiology of mood and anxiety disorders: Preclinical and clinical studies. *Biological Psychiatry, 49*(12), 1023–1039.

Hettema, J., Neale, M., & Kendler, K. (2001). A review and meta-analysis of the genetic epidemiology of anxiety disorders. *American Journal of Psychiatry, 158*(10), 1568–1578.

Hettema, J., Neale, M., Myers, J., Prescott, C., & Kendler, K. (2006). A population-based twin study of the relationship between neuroticism and internalizing disorders. *American Journal of Psychiatry, 163*(5), 857–864.

Insel, T. R., Cuthbert, B. N., Garvey, M. A., Heinssen, R. K., Pine, D. S., Quinn, K. J., et al. (2010). Research domain criteria (RDoC): Toward a new classification framework for research on mental disorders. *American Journal of Psychiatry, 167*(7), 748–751.

Karg, K., Burmeister, M., Shedden, K., & Sen, S. (2011). The serotonin transporter promoter variant (*5-HTTLPR*), stress, and depression meta-analysis revisited: Evidence of genetic moderation. *Archives of General Psychiatry, 68*(5), 444–454.

Kendler, K., Hettema, J. M., Butera, F., Gardner, C. O., & Prescott, C. A. (2003). Life event dimensions of loss, humiliation, entrapment, and danger in the prediction of onsets of major depression and generalized anxiety. *Archives of General Psychiatry, 60*(8), 789–796.

Kendler, K., Prescott, C., Myers, J., & Neale, M. (2003). The structure of genetic and environmental risk factors for common psychiatric and substance use disorders in men and women. *Archives of General Psychiatry, 60*(9), 929–937.

Kendler, K., Walters, E., Neale, M., Kessler, R., Heath, A., & Eaves, L. (1995). The structure of the genetic and environmental risk factors for six major psychiatric disorders in women: Phobia, generalized anxiety disorder, panic disorder, bulimia, major depression, and alcoholism. *Archives of General Psychiatry, 52*(5), 374–383.

Kessler, R., Avenevoli, S., & Merikangas, K. (2001). Mood disorders in children and adolescents: An epidemiologic perspective. *Biological Psychiatry, 49*(12), 1002–1014.

Kessler, R., Berglund, P., Demler, O., Jin, R., Merikangas, K., & Walters, E. (2005). Lifetime prevalence and age-of-onset distributions of DSM-IV disorders in the National Comorbidity Survey Replication. *Archives of General Psychiatry, 62*(6), 593–603.

Kessler, R., Chiu, W. T., Demler, O., & Walters, E. E. (2005). Prevalence, severity, and comorbidity of 12-month DSM-IV disorders in the National Comorbidity Survey Replication. *Archives of General Psychiatry, 62*(6), 617–627.

Kessler, R., Nelson, C. B., McGonagle, K. A., & Liu, J. (1996). Comorbidity of DSM-III-R major depressive disorder in the general population: Results from the U.S. National Comorbidity Survey. *British Journal of Psychiatry, 168*(Suppl. 30), 17–30.

Khan, A. A., Jacobson, K. C., Gardner, C. O., Prescott, C. A., & Kendler, K. S. (2005). Personality and comorbidity of common psychiatric disorders. *British Journal of Psychiatry, 186*(3), 190–196.

Kirschbaum, C., Pirke, K.-M., & Hellhammer, D. H. (2008). The "Trier Social Stress Test": A tool for investigating psychobiological stress responses in a laboratory setting. *Neuropsychobiology, 28*(1–2), 76–81.

Krueger, R. (1999a). Personality traits in late adolescence predict mental disorders in early adulthood: A prospective–epidemiological study. *Journal of Personality, 67*(1), 39–65.

Krueger, R. (1999b). The structure of common mental disorders. *Archives of General Psychiatry, 56*, 921–926.

Krueger, R., Caspi, A., Moffitt, T., & Silva, P. (1998). The structure and stability of common mental disorders (DSM-III-R): A longitudinal–epidemiological study. *Journal of Abnormal Psychology, 107*, 216–227.

Krueger, R., Caspi, A., Moffitt, T., Silva, P., & McGee, R. (1996). Personality traits are differentially linked to mental disorders: A multitrait–multidiagnosis study of an adolescent birth cohort. *Journal of Abnormal Psychology, 105*, 299–312.

Krueger, R., McGue, M., & Iacono, W. (2001). The higher-order structure of common DSM mental disorders: Internalization, externalization, and their connections to personality. *Personality and Individual Differences, 30*(7), 1245–1259.

Levitan, R. D., Rector, N. A., Sheldon, T., & Goering, P. (2003). Childhood adversities associated with major depression and/or anxiety disorders in a community sample of Ontario: Issues of co-morbidity and specificity. *Depression and Anxiety, 17*(1), 34–42.

MacLeod, C., & Mathews, A. (2012). Cognitive bias modification approaches to anxiety. *Annual Review of Clinical Psychology, 8*, 189–217.

Mathews, A., & MacLeod, C. (2005). Cognitive vulnerability to emotional disorders. *Annual Review of Clinical Psychology, 1*, 167–195.

Mehta, D., & Binder, E. B. (2012). Gene × environment vulnerability factors for PTSD: The HPA axis. *Neuropharmacology, 62*(2), 654–662.

Merikangas, K., Akiskal, H. S., Angst, J., Greenberg, P. E., Hirschfeld, R., Petukhova, M., et al. (2007). Lifetime and 12-month prevalence of bipolar spectrum disorder in the National Comorbidity Survey replication. *Archives of General Psychiatry, 64*(5), 543–552.

Merikangas, K., He, J.-P., Burstein, M., Swanson, S. A., Avenevoli, S., Cui, L., et al. (2010). Lifetime prevalence of mental disorders in U.S. adolescents: Results from the National Comorbidity Survey Replication—Adolescent Supplement (NCS-A). *Journal of the American Academy of Child and Adolescent Psychiatry, 49*(10), 980–989.

Middeldorp, C., Cath, D., Van Dyck, R., & Boomsma, D. (2005). The co-morbidity of anxiety and depression in the perspective of genetic epidemiology: A review of twin and family studies. *Psychological Medicine, 35*(5), 611–624.

Mineka, S., Anand, D., & Sumner, J. A. (2014). Important issues in understanding comorbidity between generalized anxiety disorder and major depressive disorder. In C. S. Richards & M. W. O'Hara (Eds.), *Oxford handbook of depression and comorbidity* (pp. 129–147). New York: Oxford University Press.

Mineka, S., Watson, D., & Clark, L. (1998). Comorbidity of anxiety and unipolar mood disorders. *Annual Review of Psychology, 49*, 377–412.

Mogg, K., & Bradley, B. P. (2005). Attentional bias in generalized anxiety disorder versus depressive disorder. *Cognitive Therapy and Research, 29*(1), 29–45.

Monroe, S. (1990). Psychosocial factors in anxiety and depression. In J. D. Maser & C. R. Cloninger (Eds.), *Comorbidity of mood and anxiety disorders* (pp. 463–497). Washington, DC: American Psychiatric Press.

Monroe, S., & Harkness, K. (2005). Life stress, the "kindling" hypothesis, and the recurrence of depression: Considerations from a life-stress perspective. *Psychological Review, 112*(2), 417–444.

Monroe, S. M., Slavich, G. M., & Georgiades, K. (2009). The social environment and life stress in depression. In I. H. Gotlib & C. L. Hammen (Eds.), *Handbook of depression* (2nd ed., pp. 340–360). New York: Guilford Press.

Nusslock, R., Shackman, A. J., Harmon-Jones, E., Alloy, L. B., Coan, J. A., & Abramson, L. Y. (2011). Cognitive vulnerability and frontal brain asymmetry: Common predictors of first prospective depressive episode. *Journal of Abnormal Psychology, 120*(2), 497–503.

Provencher, M. D., Guimond, A.-J., & Hawke, L. D. (2012). Comorbid anxiety in bipolar spectrum disorders: A neglected research and treatment issue? *Journal of Affective Disorders, 137*(1), 161–164.

Pruessner, J., Wolf, O., Hellhammer, D., Buske-Kirschbaum, A., Von Auer, K., Jobst, S., et al. (1997). Free cortisol levels after awakening: A reliable biological marker for the assessment of adrenocortical activity. *Life Sciences, 61,* 2539–2549.

Robins, L., Locke, B., & Regier, D. (1991). An overview of psychiatric disorders in America. In L. Robins & D. Regier (Eds.), *Psychiatric disorders in America: The Epidemiological Catchment Area study* (pp. 328–366). New York: Free Press.

Roness, A., Mykletun, A., & Dahl, A. (2005). Help-seeking behaviour in patients with anxiety disorder and depression. *Acta Psychiatrica Scandinavica, 111*(1), 51–58.

Sareen, J., Cox, B., Afifi, T., de Graaf, R., Asmundson, G., ten Have, M., et al. (2005). Anxiety disorders and risk for suicidal ideation and suicide attempts: A population-based longitudinal study of adults. *Archives of General Psychiatry, 62*(11), 1249–1257.

Sen, S., Burmeister, M., & Ghosh, D. (2004). Meta-analysis of the association between a serotonin transporter promoter polymorphism (*5-HTTLPR*) and anxiety-related personality traits. *American Journal of Medical Genetics: Part B. Neuropsychiatric Genetics, 127*(1), 85–89.

Shankman, S. A., Nelson, B. D., Sarapas, C., Robison-Andrew, E. J., Campbell, M. L., Altman, S. E., et al. (2013). A psychophysiological investigation of threat and reward sensitivity in individuals with panic disorder and/or major depressive disorder. *Journal of Abnormal Psychology, 122*(2), 322–338.

Slade, T., & Watson, D. (2006). The structure of common DSM-IV and ICD-10 mental disorders in the Australian general population. *Psychological Medicine, 36*(11), 1593–1600.

Starr, L. R., & Davila, J. (2012). Temporal patterns of anxious and depressed mood in generalized anxiety disorder: A daily diary study. *Behaviour Research and Therapy, 50*(2), 131–141.

Stein, M. B., Schork, N. J., & Gelernter, J. (2007). Gene-by-environment (serotonin transporter and childhood maltreatment) interaction for anxiety sensitivity, an intermediate phenotype for anxiety disorders. *Neuropsychopharmacology, 33*(2), 312–319.

Stetler, C., & Miller, G. E. (2005). Blunted cortisol response to awakening in mild to moderate depression: Regulatory influences of sleep patterns and social contacts. *Journal of Abnormal Psychology, 114*(4), 697–705.

Sullivan, P., Neale, M., & Kendler, K. (2000). Genetic epidemiology of major depression: Review and meta-analysis. *American Journal of Psychiatry, 157*(10), 1552–1562.

Üstün, T., Ayuso-Mateos, J., Chatterji, S., Mathers, C., & Murray, C. (2004). Global burden of depressive disorders in the year 2000. *British Journal of Psychiatry, 184*(5), 386.

Vreeburg, S., Zitman, F., van Pelt, J., DeRijk, R., Verhagen, J., van Dyck, R., et al. (2010). Salivary cortisol levels in persons with and without different anxiety disorders. *Psychosomatic Medicine, 72*(4), 340–347.

Vrshek-Schallhorn, S., Doane, L. D., Mineka, S., Zinbarg, R., Craske, M., & Adam, E. K. (2013). The cortisol awakening response predicts major depression: Predictive stability over a four-year follow-up and effect of depression history. *Psychological Medicine, 43*(3), 483–493.

Watson, D. (2009). Differentiating the mood and anxiety disorders: A quadripartite model. *Annual Review of Clinical Psychology, 5,* 221–247.

Watson, D., Clark, L., Weber, K., Smith Assenheimer, J., Strauss, M. E., & McCormick, R. A. (1995). Testing a tripartite model: II. Exploring the symptom structure of anxiety and depression in student, adult, and patient samples. *Journal of Abnormal Psychology, 104,* 15–25.

Watson, D., Gamez, W., & Simms, L. J. (2005). Basic dimensions of temperament and their relation to anxiety and depression: A symptom-based perspective. *Journal of Research in Personality, 39*(1), 46–66.

Watson, D., Weber, K., Assenheimer, J., Clark, L., Strauss, M., & McCormick, R. (1995). Testing a tripartite model: I. Evaluating the convergent and discriminant validity of anxiety and depression symptom scales. *Journal of Abnormal Psychology, 104*(1), 3–14.

Weinstock, L. M., & Whisman, M. A. (2006). Neuroticism as a common feature of the depressive and anxiety disorders: A test of the revised integrative hierarchical model in a national sample. *Journal of Abnormal Psychology, 115*(1), 68–74.

Yoon, K. L., & Joormann, J. (2012). Stress reactivity in social anxiety disorder with and without comorbid depression. *Journal of Abnormal Psychology, 121*(1), 250–255.

Zinbarg, R., Mineka, S., Craske, M., Griffith, J., Sutton, J., Rose, R., et al. (2010). The Northwestern–UCLA Youth Emotion Project: Associations of cognitive vulnerabilities, neuroticism and gender with past diagnoses of emotional disorders in adolescents. *Behaviour Research and Therapy, 48*(5), 347–358.

Zinbarg, R., Mineka, S., Craske, M., Vrshek-Schallhorn, S., Griffith, J., Wolitzky-Taylor, K., et al. (2014). *Testing a hierarchical model of neuroticism and its facets: II. Prospective associations with onsets of anxiety disorders and unipolar mood disorders over three years in adolescents*. Manuscript submitted for publication.

CHAPTER 6

Emotional Functioning in Depression

JONATHAN ROTTENBERG *and* LAUREN M. BYLSMA

Emotions are quick-moving reactions that occur when an individual processes a meaningful stimulus, and these reactions involve loosely coordinated changes in subjective feelings, behavior, and physiology (Ekman, 1992; Keltner & Gross, 1999). Typically, emotional reactions promote dynamic adjustment to the threats and opportunities posed by a changing environment. Because of the central role of emotion in adaptation, emotion is recognized as a major domain of functioning, alongside cognition, social relations, and biological functioning. In fact, emotional disturbance, in one form or another, has long been recognized as central to many forms of psychopathology (American Psychiatric Association, 2013; Kring & Bachorowski, 1999). Increasingly, scientific work on the role of emotions in psychopathology has been facilitated by *affective science*, an often explicitly translational enterprise that seeks to bridge "basic" research on normative emotion functioning with "applied" research on clinical disorders (Kring & Sloan, 2009; Rottenberg & Johnson, 2007). To this end, the study of psychopathology has been enriched by the improvement in techniques for studying emotion, including better means of assessing emotion inside and outside the laboratory, and controlled procedures for reliably eliciting emotion in a laboratory setting.

Major depressive disorder (MDD) provides a great opportunity for affective science, in part because, at the broadest level, affective disturbance is at the core of the disorder. More specifically, a durable disturbance of mood is a key feature of a major depressive episode that is central to its diagnosis (American Psychiatric Association, 2013). Moods, in contrast to emotions, have been defined as diffuse, slow-moving feeling states that are weakly tied to specific stimuli in the environment (e.g., Watson, 2000). Diagnostic criteria for depression involve symptoms that implicate broad deficiencies in both positive affect (i.e., anhedonia) and excesses in negative affect (e.g., sadness, guilt). Consistent with these diagnostic criteria, people who are depressed reliably report low levels of positive affect and elevated negative affect across a variety of questionnaire and interview measures (e.g., Clark, Watson, & Mineka, 1994).

If MDD is quintessentially a disorder of mood, one key question is how this pervasive mood disturbance influences ongoing emotional reactivity (i.e., a positive or negative emotional response to a stimulus in the environment). Indeed, studying emotional reactivity in MDD forces us to reflect upon the relation between moods and emotions (Rottenberg & Gross, 2003), a fundamental but understudied issue. Although moods and emotions are distinguishable, these constructs are generally assumed to be interconnected, with moods altering the probability of having specific emotions (e.g., Rosenberg, 1998). A historical assumption in the field has been that moods will facilitate emotional reactions when the mood and emotion match in valence (Rosenberg, 1998). Thus, for people with MDD, the most intuitive predictions are that their pervasive negative moods will potentiate negative emotional reactions (negative potentiation) and that their notable absence of positive moods will attenuate positive emotional reactions (positive attenuation). In this chapter, we show that significant portions of the data do not match these expectations. Our view of emotional functioning in MDD, referred to as emotion-context insensitivity (ECI), is intended as a fuller account of what we know. In this chapter, we outline both the strengths and limitations of ECI and its implications for our understanding of depression and the mood–emotion relation more broadly.

The overall goal of this chapter is to synthesize what we have learned about the ways that MDD affects reactivity to emotion-generative stimuli. Although we focus on emotional reactivity, where possible we consider related subdomains of emotional functioning, such as emotion knowledge, meta-emotion, emotion perception, and the regulation of emotional responses. In addition to reviewing how emotional reactivity is altered during episodes of depression, we consider how changes in emotional reactivity might be related to different phases of depression, including MDD onset and the subsequent course of the disorder.

Our approach uses a multisystem, multicontext examination of emotional reactivity in depression. Emotions invariably involve multiple response systems and cannot be reduced to a single response. Indeed, one challenge in studying emotion is that it is common for response systems to dissociate (e.g., when attacked, a person reports anger but displays no facial behavior indicative of anger; Mauss, Levenson, McCarter, Wilhelm, & Gross, 2005). This review focuses largely on data from three systems that have historically been important to the study of emotion: emotional experience, emotional behavior, and autonomic physiology (heart rate, electrodermal activity; Lang, Greenwald, Bradley, & Hamm, 1993). We do not detail the growing body of work on neural aspects of emotion in depression, in part because of space considerations, and in part because this topic is reviewed elsewhere in this *Handbook* (see Pizzagalli & Treadway, Chapter 11, this volume).

We examine multiple assessment contexts because we believe a full description of depression-related changes in emotion requires assessing emotional functioning from a variety of angles. Specifically, we focus on experimental and naturalistic assessments, which can be seen as different yet highly complementary approaches. Experimental laboratory studies have the ability to achieve high internal validity through standardized stimulus presentation, control over the laboratory environment, and the relative ease of measuring emotion in a laboratory setting. However, the generalizability, or external validity, of laboratory findings to emotional functioning in everyday life is questionable. Naturalistic studies, by definition, have robust generalizability to everyday life and ecological validity, but they can be criticized as lacking in internal validity due to the typically uncontrolled nature of the stimuli and contexts in the natural environment.

As we show, putting together what we know from laboratory and naturalistic studies of emotion in people with depression reveals some convergences across assessments but also a number of conflicting, seemingly paradoxical findings. Rather than discounting these discrepancies, we try to synthesize them. Indeed, we argue that an accurate picture of how MDD affects emotional reactivity requires an integration of what we know from the laboratory and from real life. This integration includes interpretation of puzzling findings, acknowledgement of loose ends, and directions for future research to arrive at a fuller picture of emotional functioning in depression. In this context, our attempt at synthesis sets this review apart from prior efforts, which have generally focused on either laboratory *or* naturalistic findings (e.g., Bylsma, Morris, & Rottenberg, 2008; aan het Rot, Hogenelst, & Schoevers, 2012; Ebner-Priemer, & Trull, 2009).

EXPERIMENTAL LABORATORY STUDIES OF EMOTIONAL REACTIVITY IN DEPRESSION: SUPPORT FOR THE ECI VIEW

As a point of departure for our review of laboratory findings, we refer to our 2008 meta-analysis, currently the only quantitative review of emotional reactivity in MDD (Bylsma et al., 2008). We tested the extent to which data from laboratory studies supported three major views of emotional reactivity in depression: (1) negative potentiation, which predicts enhanced reactivity specific to negative stimuli and is consistent with cognitive perspectives that see preferential processing of negative material as central to depression (Beck, Rush, Shaw, & Emery, 1979; Scher, Ingram, & Segal, 2005); (2) positive attenuation, which predicts reduced reactivity specific to positive stimuli and is consistent with several psychobiological perspectives that see impaired hedonic functioning as central to depression (Depue & Iacono, 1989); and (3) ECI (Rottenberg, Gross, & Gotlib, 2005), which predicts reduced reactivity to positive *and* negative stimuli and is consistent with evolutionary perspectives that see environmental disengagement as central to depression (e.g., Nesse, 2000). We included data from laboratory studies that enrolled people diagnosed with MDD and healthy controls, that had one or more emotionally valenced conditions (and a neutral baseline comparison), and that reported data from one or more of three major emotion response systems: the self-report of emotional experience, behavior (primarily facial expressions), and autonomic physiology.

Omnibus analyses of 19 laboratory studies found that persons with MDD were characterized by reduced emotional reactivity to both positively and negatively valenced stimuli relative to healthy persons, with the reduction larger for positive stimuli ($d = -0.53$) than for negative stimuli ($d = -0.25$). Results were comparable when the three major emotion response systems (i.e., self-reported experience, expressive behavior, and peripheral physiology) were analyzed individually (Bylsma et al., 2008). The reductions in positive and negative emotional reactivity in MDD were robust in several respects. Both effects were highly statistically reliable, with file-drawer analyses indicating that the major results would hold even in the face of dozens of unpublished null findings. Finally, the reductions in reactivity appeared to generalize across different systems of emotional response and were not restricted to a single response system.

It is noteworthy that we found reliable reductions in positive emotional reactivity, indicating support for the positive attenuation view. At the same time, the ECI view uniquely predicts reduced reactivity to positive *and* negative emotional stimuli—so the ECI view was therefore the most parsimonious overall fit to laboratory results (at least as of 2008). Our interim conclusion was that accumulating evidence from laboratory studies indicated that MDD involves reduced emotional reactivity independent of valence. Contrary to intuitive predictions about how negative moods might influence reactivity to novel negative stimuli in the environment (negative potentiation), these findings indicated that clinically depressed moods actually *impede* reactivity to novel negative stimuli. That is, depressed persons exhibit a pattern of stereotyped and inflexible response, responding similarly to different kinds of valenced stimuli that are presented in a standardized laboratory context.

Led by these and other data, we have elaborated on ECI in MDD (e.g Rottenberg et al., 2005; Rottenberg & Vaughan, 2007), with both its implications for our understanding of depression and the nature of the mood–emotion relation. Why might severe mood disturbance inhibit reactivity to ongoing emotional elicitors in the environment? Briefly, the core idea draws on evolutionary accounts that describe depression as a defensive motivational state that fosters environmental disengagement (Nesse, 2000). According to this view, mood is linked to and provides support for motivated action. Severe depressive mood states evolved as internal signals to bias organisms against action in adverse situations in which continued activity might potentially be dangerous or wasteful (e.g., famine). In these situations, ongoing emotional reactivity is reduced as a part of a more general braking of purposive motivated behavior.

Although the term ECI is our coinage, other researchers have developed similar constructs to describe convergent phenomena. For example, Kuppens and colleagues have recently described the construct of emotional inertia (Kuppens, Allen, & Sheeber, 2010). Inertia is conceptualized in terms of affect persistence, which might jointly reflect decreased reactivity to ongoing emotional elicitors and poorer regulation (reduced ability to alter an affective response over time). This research group has operationalized emotional inertia via computing the autocorrelation of responses, where a high autocorrelation indicates that an emotional state is resistant to change. Empirical data from at least one laboratory study support the idea of increased emotional inertia in depression: Adolescents with depression exhibited higher levels of behavioral inertia during a laboratory interaction with their parents (pattern observed for happiness, anger, and dysphoria; see Kuppens et al., 2010, Study 2). Initial work on the proximal mechanisms for inertia (which may overlap with the mechanisms implicated in ECI) links emotional inertia to rumination (Nolen-Hoeksema, 2000), a perseverative inflexible cognitive style that has been associated with the maintenance of depression symptoms over time (Koval, Kuppens, Allen, & Sheeber, 2012).

Psychological (in)flexibility is another related construct that is relevant to ECI. Psychological flexibility, which has bases in personality, biology, and learning, is considered to be an important aspect of psychological health that facilitates the flexible, context-appropriate management of emotional impulses (Kashdan & Rottenberg, 2010). Emotional flexibility has been associated with trait resilience (Waugh, Thompson, & Gotlib, 2011), and several forms of psychopathology have been characterized by inflexibility (Gloster, Klotsche, Chaker, Hummel, & Hoyer, 2011). Moreover, some psychotherapy techniques are conceptualized as improving psychological flexibility. For example, acceptance and commitment therapy (ACT) targets habitual experiential avoidance by the use of mindfulness and cognitive defusion strategies to allow individuals to experience both positive and negative emotions more flexibly (e.g., Hayes, Strosahl, & Wilson, 2003).

This theme of undue persistence is also commensurate with research on the time course of emotional responses in depression (affective chronometry; Davidson, 1998). Here investigators have devoted explicit attention to the prolonged duration of emotional response in MDD (as opposed to its magnitude). There is evidence that MDD may indeed delay or impair physiological recovery after imposition of a psychological stressor (e.g., Salomon, Clift, Karlsdottir, & Rottenberg, 2009). Using pupil dilation as an index of attention to emotionally laden stimuli, individuals with MDD exhibit more sustained pupil dilations even after the stimuli are no longer present (Siegle, Granholm, Ingram, & Matt, 2001). Similar findings of sustained activation poststimulus have been obtained in the amygdala, an important brain structure in emotional responding (Siegle, Steinhauer, Thase, Stenger, & Carter, 2002). So although people with depression may exhibit less vigorous initial reactivity to negative stimuli or stressors, their negative affective responses last longer, contributing to a persistent negative mood state.

Corollaries and Implications of the ECI View

Taken together, the evidence for ECI and for related constructs such as inertia and psychological flexibility, along with evidence of prolonged reactions and poor recovery to negative stimuli, suggests an overall picture of persons with depression as having sluggish, inflexible reactions to emotion-generative stimuli presented in laboratory contexts. This view has several implications for emotional functioning in depression, some of which have been tested empirically.

One corollary concerns the relation to impairment: If ECI represents a core deficit in depression, it should be related to other depression-related impairments and should predict a worse course of disorder. Consistent with this formulation, a lack of sadness reactivity has been associated with lower global assessment of functioning scores (Rottenberg, Kasch, Gross, & Gotlib, 2002). While it must be granted that only a modest number of studies have examined emotional reactivity as a predictor of depression course, the ECI pattern has been shown to predict a worse course of depression among those who already have depression (see Morris, Bylsma, & Rottenberg, 2009, for a review). For example, lower levels of heart rate reactivity and reduced behavioral reactivity to positive emotion elicitors are related to poorer course of MDD (see Fraguas et al., 2007; Rottenberg et al., 2002). There is also evidence that diminished cardiovascular reactivity to negative elicitors or situations is associated with a worse course of disorder (Rottenberg et al., 2005). In related work, Coifman and Bonanno (2009, 2010) have developed the construct of "emotion-context sensitivity," which is the flip side of ECI. In a series of studies, flexible and situationally appropriate changes in emotion have been associated with resilience, including a resistance to depression following bereavement (Coifman & Bonanno, 2009, 2010). Studies examining the relation of emotional reactivity to first onset of MDD are even less common, but at least one result is consistent with the corollary that ECI would be harmful: Higher levels of emotional inertia in a laboratory task predicted onset of MDD among adolescents who had never had depression (Kuppens et al., 2012). Overall, initial evidence suggests that diminished reactivity in laboratory contexts is associated with depression-related impairment and poorer course of the disorder.

Emotional Functioning and Comorbidity

We know relatively little about the diagnostic specificity of emotional functioning in studies of MDD. The issue is challenging: Most samples of people with diagnosed MDD are not diagnostically "pure," and comorbidity with other disorders is the rule (i.e., anxiety disorders; Sartorius, Üstün, Lecrubier, & Wittchen, 1996), both in research studies and in the real world. In particular, MDD is highly comorbid with anxiety disorders (36% of those with MDD in the preceding year also had at least one anxiety disorder diagnosis; Hasin, Goodwin, Stinson, & Grant, 2005). It is therefore challenging to obtain a sample of "pure" MDD, and it is questionable whether such a sample would truly be representative of MDD. For the typical study that lacks a psychiatric control group, it is difficult to know the extent to which ECI, or any other pattern of emotional reactivity, is specific to depression or might interact with comorbid disorders.

One intriguing strategy to isolate the effects of MDD actually harnesses comorbidity rather than trying to eliminate it. Recent studies have examined whether depression affects the reactivity characteristics of other disorders and, if so, whether ECI is still observed when depression is comorbid with another disorder. We tested this idea with the emotion-modulated startle paradigm. It has long been known that, for healthy individuals, the defensive startle response is more vigorous in the presence of an aversive stimulus than in the presence of innocuous or positive stimuli (i.e., the emotion-modulated startle), and blunted emotion-modulated startle is one of the most reliable manifestations of ECI in MDD (Allen, Trinder, & Brennan, 1999; Dichter & Tomarken, 2008; Dichter, Tomarken, Shelton, & Sutton, 2004). Using the emotion-modulated startle paradigm, we contrasted emotional reactivity in persons with anxiety who either did or did not also have a current comorbid diagnosis of MDD. We found that, unlike anxiety alone, which did not blunt startle modulation, anxiety accompanied by depression was indeed associated with ECI (Clift, Morris, Rottenberg, & Kovacs, 2010; but see Shankman et al., 2013). Interestingly, Yoon and Joormann (2012) recently found a similar pattern in social anxiety disorder, in which blunted cortisol responses to an emotional stressor were detected only in people who had social anxiety that was comorbid with depression (but not social anxiety alone). These initial results suggest that depression can alter the emotional characteristics of other mental disorders in a manner consistent with ECI. It will also be important for future research to examine whether other forms of psychopathology may also independently contribute to ECI or whether ECI is specific to depression.

Key Unresolved Issues in Laboratory Studies

What Is the Relation between Depression Severity and Emotional Reactivity?

In this chapter we have focused on emotional reactivity in people who meet full syndrome criteria for MDD. One important unresolved issue concerns the relation between emotional reactivity and depression across the continuum of depression severity and the possibility of a nonlinear association. Specifically, low levels of depressive symptoms may be associated with negative potentiation, and ECI may be observed at high levels of depression severity. Interestingly, support for the negative potentiation hypothesis—when it is supported—comes in nondiagnosed samples of persons with dysphoria (e.g., Golin, Hartman, Klatt, Munz, & Wolfgang, 1977; Lewinsohn, Lobitz, & Wilson, 1973). However, other researchers have found the ECI pattern in nondiagnosed dysphoric samples (Moran, Mehta, & Kring, 2012; Schwerdtfeger, & Rosenkaimer, 2011). This issue remains open. To reach firmer conclusions, additional work is needed with much larger samples that test reactivity across the full range of depression severity.

Do Emotional Deficits Such as ECI Normalize upon Remission?

There are relatively few data that speak to whether emotional functioning normalizes upon remission from MDD. Relatively few laboratory studies of emotional reactivity focus on remitted depression. Inconsistent with ECI, Sigmon and Nelson-Gray (1992) found that individuals who were formerly and currently depressed more closely resembled each other, were both different from controls, and both exhibited potentiated electrodermal responding to negative stimuli. Consistent with the possibility that ECI is trait-like, however, Iacono and colleagues (1984) found that participants with current and formerly depression exhibited similarly attenuated electrodermal responding across both emotional and nonemotional stimuli relative to control participants. Also consistent with ECI being trait-like for positive stimuli, McCabe, Cowen, and Harmer (2009) found that unmedicated individuals who had recovered from MDD exhibited reduced neural responses to rewarding stimuli. Moreover, in a treatment study, Dichter and colleagues (2004) found that prior to beginning antidepressant treatment, emotion-startle modulation in individuals with depression was attenuated relative to control participants and remained attenuated even after symptomatic improvement.

Further muddling the picture, several studies that used stricter criteria for defining remitted depression (e.g., excluding individuals with current subthreshold symptoms) found essentially normal reactivity in persons with remitted depression. For example, Rottenberg and colleagues (2005) examined emotional reactivity to normative and idiographic films in individuals with current and remitted depression and observed that individuals with current depression reported less sadness reactivity and less happiness experience across all conditions relative to both controls and persons with remitted depression (who did not differ from one another). These results suggest mood-state-dependent changes in emotional reactivity that are most pronounced in self-reports of emotion experience. A similar mood-state-dependent pattern was found in autonomic physiology in three cross-sectional studies: diminished cardiovascular reactivity to stress was evident in people with current depression but *not* in those with former depression, who did not differ from healthy controls (Bylsma, Salomon, Taylor-Clift, Morris, & Rottenberg, 2014; Rottenberg Clift, Bolden, & Salomon 2007; Salomon, Bylsma, White, Panaite, & Rottenberg, 2013).

Given the conflicting findings, data are currently inconclusive concerning whether the changes in emotional reactivity observed in MDD are transient or trait-like. It is important to point out that depression has multiple phases (e.g., prodromal, residual) that change as symptoms wax and wane. At present, we know by far the most about emotional reactivity during the acute phase of depression. Depression is also episodic, and we know relatively little about how reactivity might change over episodes; it is possible that individuals may become less reactive only over repeated episodes or after a longer duration within episode (Forbes, Miller, Cohn, Fox, & Kovacs, 2005). Importantly, there may even be anomalies in emotional reactivity prior to the lifetime episode. Although a detailed review is beyond our scope, a number of studies of high-risk youth (due to having a parent with a history of depression) have started to shed light on abnormalities in emotional reactivity (Gotlib et al., 2010; see Gotlib & Colich, Chapter 13, this volume). For example, in a study utilizing event-related potentials, Kujawa, Hajcak, Torpey, Kim, and Klein (2012) found that children at high risk for depression exhibited a reduced electrocortical reactivity to emotional faces compared with their peers (as indexed by the late positive potential, a component that has been associated with emotional responding).

A mature view must accommodate the possibility that each phase of MDD is associated with distinct, systematic changes in emotional reactivity. Even if further data show that persons who formerly had depression do not markedly differ from those who never had depression in their emotional reactivity, it would be unwise to conclude that there is a broader based normalization in emotional functioning upon recovery from depression.

Early data elsewhere suggest that other aspects of emotional functioning remain problematic upon remission. For example, there is evidence that people with histories of depression report continuing problems in emotion regulation and tend to endorse strategies that clinicians and researchers regard as less healthy (e.g., D'Avanzato, Joormann, Siemer, & Gotlib, 2013; Kovacs, Rottenberg, & George, 2009). Relatedly, people who formerly had depression continue to endorse themselves as being high in the personality trait neuroticism, which is associated with reactivity to and difficulties in coping with life stressors, a process that may contribute to depressive relapse (Monroe & Harkness, 2005; see Monroe et al., Chapter 16, this volume).

Interim Conclusions

A preponderance of the evidence from a maturing body of laboratory designs supports ECI. Yet, despite advances in affective science and a rich vein of empirical work, much remains to be uncovered about emotional functioning in depression. Several key questions have not been definitively addressed, including the nature of the relation of emotional reactivity to diagnostic specificity, depression severity, or stability across different phases of depression. Moreover, important issues about emotional functioning in depression cannot easily be addressed in the laboratory. For example, it is difficult for laboratory assessments to address more complex patterning of emotional reactivity over time. There are limits to how many laboratory assessments of emotion are possible. That is, both the duration and frequency of assessments, as well as the number of emotion elicitors, are naturally constrained. There are also limits to the kinds of elicitations that can be used with people with depression. For example, many situations that drive reactivity in the real world, such as interpersonal rejection or feedback that one is a failure, are difficult to utilize in the laboratory in individuals with depression for ethical reasons. Finally, it is uncertain how reactivity in laboratory contexts generalizes to reactivity in real-world contexts, part of a historical tension between internal and external validity (Anderson & Bushman, 1997). Laboratory studies are not well suited to uncovering how emotional reactivity plays out in everyday life, yet understanding how individuals with depression function emotionally in their daily lives is of critical clinical significance. For all of these reasons, we believe that naturalistic studies, as a complement to laboratory assessments, are necessary to generate a complete picture of emotional functioning in MDD.

NATURALISTIC STUDIES OF EMOTION IN DEPRESSION

Ecological momentary assessment (EMA) approaches have been available for decades but have only more recently been applied to the study of psychopathology (e.g., Myin-Germeys et al., 2009; Trull & Ebner-Priemer, 2009; Wenze & Miller, 2010). EMA methods began as more simplistic daily diary formats that typically involved completing an end-of-day report for multiple days and have since evolved toward more sophisticated sampling throughout the day using computerized devices. Although relatively few studies have collected sophisticated sampling data on emotional functioning of people with clinical depression in everyday life settings, these methods have great potential for furthering our understanding of emotional functioning in this condition.

First, examining emotional reactivity in naturalistic settings arguably provides a more ecologically valid estimate of an individual's emotional functioning than does a laboratory study. Second, EMA permits multipoint assessments of emotional functioning, which have the potential to be more reliable than single-point assessments. Third, these assessments can be conducted in real time and, consequently, are less prone than single-point retrospective assessment to memory failure or memory bias (a particular concern with samples of depressed people; see Trull & Ebner-Priemer, 2009, for a review). Fourth, dense and repeated sampling of daily life allows the researcher to capture dynamic patterns of reactivity to the environment (Csikszentmihalyi & Larson, 1987), such as diurnal rhythms or patterns of response to particular environmental aspects (contextual features). The ability to study patterning is especially powerful when used with more sophisticated statistical methodologies (e.g., multilevel modeling) that are well suited for repeated assessments where multiple data points are nested within individuals over a number of days (e.g., Nezlek, 2012). Here we highlight how and why EMA can complement laboratory assessments. We also recognize challenges for integration that emerge from the initial EMA studies of samples of individuals with depression. We consider convergent results before turning to EMA findings that do not match the ECI view of depression as a condition of sluggish, unchanging, chronically high negative affect (NA) and chronically low positive affect (PA).

Converging Findings

It is reassuring that some findings converge across these very different assessments of emotional functioning. First, at least one study found reduced emotional reactivity to everyday life stressors in MDD (Peeters, Nicolson, Berkhof, Delespaul, & deVries, 2003) consistent with the unique prediction of ECI and prior laboratory results. Second, EMA studies found that relatively less reactivity to everyday negative events (Peeters, Berkhof, Rottenberg, & Nicolson, 2010) and reduced positive affect variability (Bylsma & Rottenberg, 2009) both predicted a worse course of MDD. Third, and also akin to laboratory results, two studies have found that emotional inertia outside of the lab was associated with depressive symptoms (Koval et al., 2012; Kuppens et al., 2010). However, no differences in emotional inertia were found between controls without depression and participants with diagnosed MDD (Thompson et al., 2012). Finally, it was recently reported that individuals with MDD had less differentiated reports of negative emotion than healthy controls without depression (Demiralp et al., 2012). This lack of emotion differentiation also reflects a stereotyped and inflexible pattern of response in that people with depression tend to report negative emotions as a response set—when they report one negative emotion, they tend to report other negative emotions at the same time.

Discrepant Findings

Increased Affective Instability

One set of puzzling EMA results that are in tension with laboratory findings relates to affective instability (e.g., Jahng, Wood, & Trull, 2008), which reflects mood variability over time not necessarily tied to specific triggers. If affect that is sluggish and slow to change characterizes depression, we would expect to see persons with depression exhibit reduced affective instability in everyday life, for both positive and negative emotions. The dense sampling strategies afforded by EMA are clearly well suited to assessing affective instability. Consistent with the need for multipoint EMA designs with dense assessments, results from single-point retrospective, "trait" assessments, or daily assessments with few time points have generated conflicting results (decreased variability: Cowdry, Gardner,

O'Leary, Leibenluft, & Rubinow, 1991; Golier, Yehuda, Schmeidler, & Siever, 2001; increased variability: Thompson, Berenbaum, & Bredemeier, 2011).

Both EMA studies that examined affective instability with dense sampling in diagnosed MDD cases found remarkably consistent results, with increased affective instability in persons with depression relative to healthy controls. In both cases, the finding was specific to negative affect and was not observed for positive affect (Peeters, Berkhof, Delespaul, Rottenberg, & Nicolson, 2006; Thompson et al., 2012). Importantly, Thompson and colleagues (2012) reported analyses that showed that the negative affect instability of persons with depression was not a function of other differences in emotional functioning. Specifically, it could not be accounted for by differences in negative affect reactivity nor by the reported intensity or frequency of positive or negative events.

Mood Brightening in Depression?

Basic research clearly establishes that even relatively minor pleasant and unpleasant daily life events, as defined by participants' own appraisals, are reliably associated with short-term emotional reactions (e.g., Gable, Reis & Elliot, 2000). EMA designs are well suited to examining whether MDD affects emotional reactivity to such daily life events. Here, we see a second set of nonconvergent EMA results regarding the reactivity of persons with depression to daily positive events.

Peeters, Nicolson, Berkhof, Delespaul and deVries (2003) found that, when responding to positive events, individuals with MDD reported greater reductions in negative affect and larger increases in positive affect relative to controls. To reiterate, ECI would predict reduced reactivity to both event types in MDD. In fact, no major theories (that we are aware of) would predict enhanced reactivity to pleasant events. Yet this effect increasingly appears credible: the Peeters and colleagues study was followed by two more recent additional investigations that found that the affective responses of persons with depression to daily positive events were enhanced. Bylsma, Taylor-Clift, and Rottenberg (2011) also reported greater decreases in negative affect to positive events for individuals diagnosed with MDD relative to controls. Similarly, Thompson and colleagues (2012) reported the mood-brightening finding, again, with greater decreases in negative affect to positive events for participants diagnosed with MDD. Finally, a few studies detected elements of the mood-brightening effect at lower levels of depression severity. We found the mood-brightening effect among individuals with minor depression (Bylsma et al., 2011), and a similar effect was reported in college students with high levels of depressive symptomatology (Gable & Nezlek, 1998; Nezlek & Gable, 2001).

Interpretations

Although these EMA results are puzzling when placed alongside laboratory results, there is no cause for great concern. First, the number of EMA studies remains small, and further data could substantially alter the picture. Second, tensions between laboratory and real-life data are common and are certainly not unique to depression. Indeed, discrepancies have been noted in schizophrenia, in which people with schizophrenia experienced demonstrated blunted emotional responses in laboratory assessments but also reported more intense and variable negative emotions in daily life (Myin-Germeys, Delespaul, & deVries, 2000). Nevertheless, the early EMA results for depression are consistent enough that interpretative efforts are warranted, and we believe several interpretations are viable.

One way to understand the instability finding is to consider the possibility that specific events in everyday life may alter the emotional dynamics of persons with depression more dramatically than those of persons without depression. Consistent with this possibility, Koval and Kuppens (2012) found that relative to participants low in depressive symptoms, those high in depressive symptoms were generally higher in emotional inertia and had more sudden decreases in inertia when anticipating a socially stressful event. These data raise the possibility that people with depression may appear more unstable in EMA because they are more vulnerable to the ebb and flow of cognitive events that arise from unpredictable daily life triggers (e.g., fear of social evaluation). Indeed, other data suggest that people with depression are more sensitive than people without depression to their own appraisals. Myin-Germeys and colleagues (2003) found that there was a stronger relation in people with depression than in controls between appraisals of stressfulness and reports of negative affect (i.e., negative affect intensified more with appraised stressfulness).

Another explanation of affective instability may stem from abnormalities in endogenous, biologically based rhythms. For example, depression has well-known links to circadian abnormalities, reflected in abnormal rhythms of sleep and the stress hormone cortisol, both of which have been linked to emotion (see Thase, Hahn, & Berton, Chapter 10, this volume). Consistent with an endogenous effect, Peeters and colleagues (2006) found abnormal diurnal mood patterns in negative affect among people with depression, who evidenced an inverted-U pattern, with mood worsening and then improving across the course of a day. Critically, *laboratory designs examine emotional responses seconds to minutes poststimulus, which is much too short a time scale to capture daily rhythms.* In contrast, naturalistic studies typically involve a longer time lag (often about 90 minutes) between assessments and are able to cover most waking hours of the day. Thus laboratory studies and EMA studies are examining instability on very different time scales; presumably, only instability at typical EMA time scales would be sensitive to disturbances in biorhythms.

We believe similar types of interpretations are viable for the puzzling mood-brightening data obtained with EMA designs. One interpretation concerns dynamic shifts in emotion regulation strategies. In an intriguing study designed to understand mood brightening, Takano, Sakamoto, and Tanno (2013) found that with participants who were high in depression symptoms the likelihood was greater that specific pleasant activities would temporarily interrupt their ruminative thinking. In turn, reductions in ruminative thinking were related to greater reductions in negative affect during these pleasant activities. Based on these results, it is plausible that fluctuations in everyday rumination among people with depression form a cognitive basis for the mood-brightening effect.

Another possible interpretation of the mood-brightening effect involves appraisal in depression as a cognitive influence on reactivity. Generally, appraisal theories of emotion posit that strength of an emotional reaction is related to how a stimulus is evaluated (e.g., Scherer, Shorr, & Johnstone, 2001), a premise that is also consistent with the tenets of cognitive therapy (see Hollon & Dimidjian, Chapter 27, this volume*)*. Importantly, in EMA designs people with depression appraise fewer events as pleasant, *consistently reporting fewer positive events than do persons without depression* (Bylsma et al., 2011; Peeters et al., 2003). This finding might reflect fewer positive events in reality and/or, just as plausibly, appraisal differences, such as that people with depression have more stringent standards for what is considered a pleasant event or tend to appraise a positive event, such as an intended compliment, as neutral or even negative (see Bylsma et al., 2011). Critically, unlike laboratory designs, in which pleasant events are usually predefined by the experimenter, pleasant events in EMA designs have no objective standard or definition and are necessarily dependent on participants' own appraisals. Thus we speculate that it is likely that people with depression are unreactive to many objectively pleasant everyday life events that are not appraised as pleasant in EMA designs and hence not picked up in EMA findings. If this were true, it would clearly reduce the discrepancy with the consistent blunting of hedonic responses found in laboratory designs. However, by extension, what the mood-brightening effect *also* tells us is that *if* a positive event does get through the cognitive filter of a person with depression and is appraised as pleasant, such people exhibit surprisingly robust reactivity to such events. That said, it should be clarified that the mood-brightening effect is a relative effect, not an absolute effect, as the negative affect values of persons with depression may remain higher than those of controls after positive events, as was observed by Bylsma and colleagues (2011). Nevertheless, the mood-brightening effect still may have clinical and therapeutic implications. It suggests that people with depression may have hidden reserves of reactivity, especially if a cognitively based therapy can shape the person's typical environmental appraisals.

TOWARD SYNTHESIS: A THEORY OF PUNCTUATED ECI?

Staying close to the data, many of the tensions between laboratory and EMA data may reveal differences between what these assessments are measuring rather than truly discrepant results. In fact, a closer view suggests that EMA results are helpful in clarifying the meaning of ECI in the laboratory and pointing to a larger synthesis of emotional functioning in depression.

First, although a wide range of emotion-eliciting procedures are utilized in the laboratory, with few exceptions, the stimuli used in laboratory settings, such as emotional pictures or films, are normative—that is, well known to elicit emotion in healthy participants. *What the laboratory data may tell us is that depression involves reduced flexibility and diminished reactivity specific to normative stimuli.* Thus ECI doesn't necessarily mean or imply that people with depression are always and everywhere unreactive, just that generic emotion-generative stimuli do not drive strong responses. In principle, laboratory designs could employ idiographic stimuli that are tailored to differ for each participant, but in practice it is challenging to use idiographic stimuli in the laboratory to elicit emotional reactivity in MDD, and such studies have been rare. One study using idiographic stimuli (i.e., participants describing an emotional memory on film) found that individuals with depression exhibited greater dysphoria in response to idiographic versus normative laboratory stimuli (Rottenberg et al., 2005). Another investigation found that a specific negative idiographic stimulus—critical letters from mothers—aroused negative affect more strongly in people who self-reported a depression diagnosis (Cuellar & Johnson, 2009). Thus early work suggests that integrating idiographic stimuli into laboratory designs will be important to understanding emotional functioning in MDD.

A second clarification returns to the briefer time frame of laboratory studies, which typically examine emotional responses in a temporal window at the level of seconds to minutes poststimulus (unlike naturalistic studies, in which observations are more widely spaced). At the shorter time scale of the laboratory, it appears that people with depression exhibit less dynamic change. This time scale is important because we usually conceive of emotions as short-term changes that last for seconds or minutes. If ECI applies at the shorter time scales (seconds or minutes) typically associated with emotion, we might ask whether the instability in EMA approaches should be understood in terms of a different affect-related construct, such as mood, that is associated with a longer time frame. Clearly, it is possible that the instability observed in the densely sampled EMA designs has a number of distinct sources. Although this depressive instability may appear random to a neutral observer, we think it likely has systemic sources of instability that include endogenous biorhythms, shifts in appraisal, and changes in other emotion regulation strategies, such as rumination.

Taken together, the two literatures suggest the possibility of a larger synthesis of emotional functioning in depression. Rather than depression involving only a single dysfunction, we should expect that multiple deficits apply to this condition, just as we see in other mature domains of investigation, such as cognition, where multiple deficits apply (e.g., biases in attention versus memory; see Joormann & Arditte, Chapter 14, this volume). As more data are reported, we suspect that the ECI model will need to be modified and refined, perhaps to a sort of punctuated ECI, in which ECI is observed in many, but not all, short-term contexts and other problems in emotional functioning are observed at longer time scales, likely reflecting other underlying mechanisms. Such a conclusion would be in keeping with a growing trend in work on emotion functioning toward contextually specific explanations (e.g., Aldao, 2013).

CONCLUSIONS AND FUTURE DIRECTIONS

In this chapter, we have begun to synthesize what laboratory assessment and naturalistic assessments of emotion teach us about emotional functioning in depression. In addition to research examining unresolved issues, such as the impact of comorbidity and symptom severity on emotional reactivity and how reactivity changes over different phases of depression, we prioritize three directions for future research to help us bridge the laboratory and the field and arrive at a more complete picture of emotional functioning in MDD.

One way to resolve tensions between laboratory and EMA data will be to examine their correspondence in designs in which both kinds of assessments are completed in the same sample of participants. Pioneer studies have demonstrated expected correspondences. For example, Silk and colleagues (2007) demonstrated in children with MDD that pupillary reactivity to emotional information in the laboratory is associated with higher levels of negative affect in the natural environment. In a similar vein, a study that assessed hedonic functioning using a functional magnetic resonance imaging (fMRI) guessing task and a cell phone EMA protocol found that relative to control adolescents, adolescents with MDD had altered processing in brain regions relevant to reward and that brain responses to monetary reward in adolescents with depression corresponded to their real-world positive affect (Forbes et al., 2009). The logical next step would be to conduct focal studies of phenomena such as mood brightening using multimodal assessments.

Another critical direction that will help us triangulate our findings on emotional functioning in MDD is to find ways to blend the two kinds of assessments to achieve "the best of both worlds" and to make the assessments more easily compared. For instance, it may be possible to introduce a greater degree of control within ambulatory assessments. Participants could be instructed through a mobile device to expose themselves to controlled emotion-eliciting situations (e.g., standardized stimuli or regulation instructions). Embedding controlled stimuli into EMA designs may be a way to "calibrate" emotion reactivity across assessment platforms (for a longer discussion, see Bylsma & Rottenberg, 2011). Similarly, although it is not possible to measure as many emotion response systems in EMA designs as it is in laboratory studies, some response systems, such as autonomic reactivity, can be added to EMA (i.e., ambulatory psychophysiology) to make daily life assessments more comparable to those in the laboratory and to aid in the overall interpretation of the data. One illustration of this point comes from Peeters, Nicolson, and Berkhof (2003), who examined cortisol response to daily events and demonstrated that individuals with MDD experienced more blunted increases in cortisol following negative events relative to healthy individuals. This finding was particularly apparent in individuals with depression who also had family histories of mood disorders, and the effects of negative events on cortisol appeared to be mediated by changes in mood.

Finally, a third future direction involves the explicit study of emotion regulation in an effort to integrate the role of emotion regulation in emotional reactivity across the different kinds of assessments. Not only is emotion regulation important in its own right, but discrepancies between lab and life emotion regulation may be important in explaining tension in emotional reactivity findings between laboratory and EMA data. For example, it is possible that individuals with and without depression use different emotion regulation strategies across assessment contexts. Moreover, some types of emotional regulation processes, such as situation selection or seeking out social support (e.g., Gross, 2008), are typically unavailable in the laboratory but may be frequently utilized in naturalistic settings. Similar context-specific processes may unfold with other coping strategies, such as reappraisal or rumination. The extent to which healthy persons and persons with depression differ in their regulatory tendencies in specific contexts (which is not currently known) could lead to discrepancies across EMA and laboratory findings. Some studies have begun to examine emotion regulation processes in daily life (e.g., Nezlek & Kuppens, 2008; Silk, Steinberg, & Morris, 2003). Clearly, there is a critical need for studies of emotion regulation processes using EMA designs in samples of individuals with clinical depression, as well as for studies that show the implications of laboratory emotion regulation for real-world affective functioning.

Ultimately, if we are able to take advantage of the complementary strengths of laboratory and daily life designs, we will achieve a more comprehensive picture of emotional functioning in depression. Effectively combining laboratory and EMA methods may help reveal how specific deficits observed in the laboratory manifest in the context of daily life, a finding that would be of critical importance for both clinical assessment and intervention efforts. The longer-term goals of affective science are not only to develop a full inventory of the problems in emotional functioning and the fundamental mechanisms underlying these problems, but also to use this information to develop more effective treatments for depression. In fact, based on the rapid rate of progress in this field, we are hopeful that it will be possible to develop treatments that explicitly target specific deficits in emotional reactivity and emotion regulation processes in MDD. Ultimately, we hope that an emotion-based therapy based on laboratory and daily life findings could be added to the armamentarium of psychosocial treatments for MDD.

REFERENCES

aan het Rot, M., Hogenelst, K., & Schoevers, R. A. (2012). Mood disorders in everyday life: A systematic review of experience sampling and ecological momentary assessment studies, *Clinical Psychology Review, 32,* 510–523.

Aldao, A. (2013). The future of emotion regulation research: Capturing context. *Perspectives on Psychological Science, 8,* 155–172.

Allen, N. B., Trinder, J., & Brennan, C. (1999). Affective startle modulation in clinical depression: Preliminary findings. *Biological Psychiatry, 46*(4), 542–550.

American Psychiatric Association. (2013). *Diagnostic and statistical manual of mental disorders* (5th ed.). Arlington, VA: American Psychiatric Publishing.

Anderson, C. A., & Bushman, B. J. (1997). External validity of "trivial" experiments: The case of laboratory aggression. *Review of General Psychology, 1*, 19–41.

Beck, A. T., Rush, J., Shaw, B. F., & Emery, G. (1979). *Cognitive therapy of depression.* New York: Guilford Press.

Bylsma, L. M., Morris, B. H., & Rottenberg, J. (2008). A meta-analysis of emotional reactivity in major depressive disorder. *Clinical Psychology Review, 28*(4), 676–691.

Bylsma, L. M. & Rottenberg, J. (2009, September). *High positive affective variability in Everyday life predicts depression remission.* Poster presented at the annual meeting of the Society for Research in Psychopathology, Minneapolis, MN.

Bylsma, L. M., & Rottenberg, J. (2011). Uncovering the dynamics of emotion regulation and dysfunction in daily life with ecological momentary assessment. In I. Nyklicek, A. J. J. M. Vingerhoets, & M. Zeelenberg (Eds.), *Emotion regulation and well-being: Part 3* (pp. 225–244). New York: Springer.

Bylsma, L. M., Salomon, K., Taylor-Clift, A., Morris, B. H., & Rottenberg, J. (2014). Respiratory sinus arrhythmia reactivity in current and remitted major depressive disorder. *Psychosomatic Medicine, 76*, 66–73.

Bylsma, L. M., Taylor-Clift, A., & Rottenberg, J. (2011). Emotional reactivity to daily events in major and minor depression. *Journal of Abnormal Psychology, 120*, 155.

Clark, L. A., Watson, D., & Mineka, S. (1994). Temperament, personality, and the mood and anxiety disorders. *Journal of Abnormal Psychology, 103*(1), 103–116.

Clift, A., Morris, B. H., Rottenberg, J., & Kovacs, M. (2010). Emotion-modulated startle in anxiety disorders is blunted by comorbid depressive episodes. *Psychological Medicine, 16*, 1–11.

Coifman, K. G., & Bonanno, G. A. (2009). Emotion context sensitivity in adaptation and recovery. In A. M. Kring & D. M. Sloan (Eds.), *Emotion regulation and psychopathology: A transdiagnostic approach to etiology and treatment* (pp. 157–173). New York: Guilford Press

Coifman, K. G., & Bonanno, G. A. (2010). When distress does not become depression: Emotion context sensitivity and adjustment to bereavement. *Journal of Abnormal Psychology, 119*(3), 479–490.

Cowdry, R. W., Gardner, D. L., O'Leary, K. M., Leibenluft, E., & Rubinow, D. R. (1991). Mood variability: A study of four groups. *American Journal of Psychiatry, 148*, 1505–1511.

Cuellar, A. K., & Johnson, S. L. (2009). Depressive symptoms and affective reactivity to maternal praise and criticism. *Journal of Social and Clinical Psychology, 28*, 1173–1194.

Csikszentmihalyi, M., & Larson, R. (1987). Validity and reliability of the experience-sampling method. *Journal of Nervous and Mental Disease, 175*, 526–536.

Davidson, R. J. (1989). Affective style and affective disorders: Perspectives from affective neuroscience. *Cognition and Emotion, 12*, 307–330.

D'Avanzato, C., Joormann, J., Siemer, M., & Gotlib, I. H. (2013). Emotion regulation in depression and anxiety: Examining diagnostic specificity and stability of strategy use. *Cognitive Therapy and Research, 37*, 968–980.

Demiralp, E., Thompson, R. J., Mata, J., Jaeggi, S. M., Buschkuehl, M., Barrett, L. F., et al. (2012). Feeling blue or turquoise? Emotional differentiation in major depressive disorder. *Psychological Science, 23*, 1410–1416.

Depue, R. A., & Iacono, W. G. (1989). Neurobehavioral aspects of affective disorders. *Annual Review of Psychology, 40*, 457?492.

Dichter, G. S., & Tomarken, A. J. (2008). The chronometry of affective startle modulation in unipolar depression. *Journal of Abnormal Psychology, 117*, 1–15.

Dichter, G. S., Tomarken, A. J., Shelton, R. C., & Sutton, S. K. (2004). Early and late-onset startle modulation in unipolar depression. *Psychophysiology, 41*, 433–440.

Ekman, P. (1992). An argument for basic emotions. *Cognition and Emotion, 6*, 169–200.

Ebner-Priemer, U. W., & Trull, T. J. (2009). Ecological momentary assessment of mood disorders and mood dysregulation. *Psychological Assessment, 21*(4), 463–475.

Forbes, E. E., Hariri, A. R., Martin, S. L., Silk J. S., Moyles D. L., & Fisher P. M., et al. (2009). Altered striatal activation predicting real-world positive affect in adolescent major depressive disorder. *American Journal of Psychiatry, 166,* 164–173.

Forbes, E. E., Miller, A., Cohn, J. F., Fox, N. A., & Kovacs, M. (2005). Affect-modulated startle in adults with childhood-onset depression: Relations to bipolar course and number of lifetime depressive episodes. *Psychiatry Research, 134,* 11–25.

Fraguas, R., Jr., Marci, C., Fava, M., Iosifescu, D. V., Bankier, B., Loh, R.,et al. (2007). Autonomic reactivity to induced emotion as potential predictor of response to antidepressant treatment. *Psychiatry Research, 151,* 169–172.

Gable, S. L., & Nezlek, J. B. (1998). Level and instability of day-to-day psychological well-being and risk for depression. *Journal of Personality and Social Psychology, 74,* 129–138.

Gable, S. L., Reis, H. T., & Elliot, A. J. (2000). Behavioral activation and inhibition in everyday life. *Journal of Personality and Social Psychology, 78*(6), 1135–1149.

Gloster, A. T., Klotsche, J., Chaker, S., Hummel, K. V., & Hoyer, J. (2011). Assessing psychological flexibility: What does it add above and beyond existing constructs? *Psychological Assessment, 23,* 970–982.

Golier, J. A., Yehuda, R., Schmeidler, J., & Siever, L. J. (2001). Variability and severity of depression and anxiety in post traumatic stress disorder and major depressive disorder. *Depression and Anxiety, 13*(2), 97–100.

Golin, S., Hartman, S. A., Klatt, E. N., Munz, K., & Wolfgang, G. L. (1977). Effects of self-esteem manipulation on arousal and reactions to sad models in depressed and nondepressed college students. *Journal of Abnormal Psychology, 86*(4), 435–439.

Gotlib, I. H., Hamilton, J. P., Cooney, R. E., Singh, M. K., Henry, M. L., & Joormann, J. (2010). Neural processing of reward and loss in girls at risk for major depression. *Archives of General Psychiatry, 67,* 380.

Gross, J. J. (2008). Emotion regulation. In M. Lewis, J. M. Haviland-Jones, & L. F. Barrett (Eds.), *Handbook of emotions* (3rd ed., pp. 497–512). New York: Guilford Press.

Hasin, D. S., Goodwin, R. D., Stinson, F. S., & Grant, B. F. (2005). Epidemiology of major depressive disorder: results from the National Epidemiologic Survey on Alcoholism and Related Conditions. *Archives of General Psychiatry, 62,* 1097–1106.

Hayes, S. C., Strosahl, K. D., & Wilson, K. G. (2003). *Acceptance and commitment therapy: An experiential approach to behavior change.* New York: Guilford Press.

Iacono, W. G., Peloquin, L. J., Lykken, D. T., Haroian, K. P., Valentine, R. H., & Tuason, V. B. (1984). Electrodermal activity in euthymic patients with affective disorders: One-year retest stability and the effects of stimulus intensity and significance. *Journal of Abnormal Psychology, 93,* 304–311.

Jahng, S., Wood, P. K., & Trull, T. J. (2008). Analysis of affective instability in ecological momentary assessment: Indices using successive difference and group comparison via multilevel modeling. *Psychological Methods, 13,* 354.

Kashdan, T. B., & Rottenberg, J. (2010). Psychological flexibility as a fundamental aspect of health. *Clinical Psychology Review, 30,* 865–878.

Keltner, D., & Gross, J. J. (1999). Functional accounts of emotions. *Cognition and Emotion, 13,* 467–480.

Kovacs, M., Rottenberg, J., & George, C. (2009). Maladaptive mood repair responses distinguish young adults with early onset depressive disorders and predict future depressive outcomes. *Psychological Medicine, 39,* 1841–1854.

Koval, P., & Kuppens, P. (2012). Changing emotion dynamics: Individual differences in the effect of anticipatory social stress on emotional inertia. *Emotion, 12*(2), 256–267.

Koval, P., Kuppens, P., Allen, N. B., & Sheeber, L. B. (2012). Getting stuck in depression: The roles of rumination and emotional inertia. *Cognition and Emotion, 26,* 1412–1427.

Kring, A. M., & Bachorowski, J. A. (1999). Emotions and psychopathology. *Cognition and Emotion, 13*(5), 575–599.

Kring, A. M., & Sloan, D. M. (Eds.). (2009). *Emotion regulation and psychopathology: A transdiagnostic approach to etiology and treatment.* New York: Guilford Press.

Kujawa, A., Hajcak, G., Torpey, D., Kim, J., & Klein, D. N. (2012). Electrocortical reactivity to emotional faces in young children and associations with maternal and paternal depression. *Journal of Child Psychology and Psychiatry, 53*(2), 207–215.

Kuppens, P., Allen, N. B., & Sheeber, L. B. (2010). Emotional inertia and psychological maladjustment. *Psychological Science, 21*, 984–991.

Kuppens, P., Sheeber, L. B., Yap, M. B. H., Whittle, S., Simmons, J. G., & Allen, N. B. (2012). Emotional inertia prospectively predicts the onset of depressive disorder in adolescence. *Emotion, 12*, 283–289.

Lang, P. J., Greenwald, M. K., Bradley, M. M., & Hamm, A. O. (1993). Looking at pictures: Affective, facial, visceral, and behavioral reactions. *Psychophysiology, 30*, 261–273.

Lewinsohn, P. M., Lobitz, W. C., & Wilson, S. (1973). "Sensitivity" of depressed individuals to aversive stimuli. *Journal of Abnormal Psychology, 81*, 259–263.

Mauss, I. B., Levenson, R. W., McCarter, L., Wilhelm, F. H., & Gross, J. J. (2005). The tie that binds? Coherence among emotion experience, behavior, and autonomic physiology. *Emotion, 5*, 175–190.

McCabe, C., Cowen, P. J., & Harmer, C. J. (2009). Neural representation of reward in recovered depressed patients. *Psychopharmacology, 205*(4), 667–677.

Monroe, S. M., & Harkness, K. L. (2005). Life stress, the" kindling" hypothesis, and the recurrence of depression: Considerations from a life stress perspective. *Psychological Review, 112*, 417–444.

Moran, E. K., Mehta, N., & Kring, A. M. (2012). Emotional responding in depression: Distinctions in the time course of emotion. *Cognition and Emotion, 26*(7), 1153–1175.

Morris, B. H., Bylsma, L. M., & Rottenberg, J. (2009). Does emotion predict the course of major depressive disorder?: A review of prospective studies. *British Journal of Clinical Psychology, 48*, 255–273.

Myin-Germeys, I., Delespaul, P. A. E. G., & deVries, M. W. (2000). Schizophrenia patients are more emotionally active than is assumed based on their behavior. *Schizophrenia Bulletin, 26*, 847–853.

Myin-Germeys, I., Oorschot, M., Collip, D., Lataster, J., Delespaul, P., & van Os, J. (2009). Experience sampling research in psychopathology: Opening the black box of daily life. *Psychological Medicine, 39*(9), 1533–1547.

Myin-Germeys, I., Peeters, F., Havermans, R., Nicolson, N. A., deVries, M. W., Delespaul, P., et al. (2003). Emotional reactivity to daily life stress in psychosis and affective disorder: An experience sampling study. *Acta Psychiatrica Scandinavica, 107*, 124–131.

Nesse, R. M. (2000). Is depression an adaptation? *Archives of General Psychiatry, 57*, 14.

Nezlek, J. B. (2012). Multilevel modeling for psychologists. In H. Cooper (Ed.), *APA handbook of research methods in psychology: Vol. 3. Data analysis and research publication* (pp. 219–241). Washington, DC: American Psychological Association.

Nezlek, J. B., & Gable, S. L. (2001). Depression as a moderator of relationships between positive daily events and day-to-day psychological adjustment. *Personality and Social Psychology Bulletin, 27*, 1692–1704.

Nezlek, J. B., & Kuppens, P. (2008). Regulating positive and negative emotions in daily life. *Journal of Personality, 76*, 561–580.

Nolen-Hoeksema, S. (2000). The role of rumination in depressive disorders and mixed anxiety/depressive symptoms. *Journal of Abnormal Psychology, 109*, 504–511.

Peeters, F., Berkhof, J., Delespaul, P., Rottenberg, J., & Nicolson, N. A. (2006). Diurnal mood variation in major depressive disorder. *Emotion, 6*, 383–391.

Peeters, F., Berkhof, J., Rottenberg, J., & Nicolson, N. A. (2010). Ambulatory emotional reactivity to negative daily life events predicts remission from major depressive disorder. *Behaviour Research and Therapy, 48*, 754–760.

Peeters, F., Nicolson, N. A., & Berkhof, J. (2003). Cortisol responses to daily events in major depressive disorder. *Psychosomatic Medicine, 65*(5), 836–841.

Peeters, F., Nicolson, N. A., Berkhof, J., Delespaul, P., & deVries, M. (2003). Effects of daily events on mood states in major depressive disorder. *Journal of Abnormal Psychology, 112*, 203–211.

Rosenberg, E. L. (1998). Levels of analysis and the organization of affect. *Review of General Psychology, 2*(3), 247–270.

Rottenberg, J., Clift, A., Bolden, S., & Salomon, K. (2007). *RSA fluctuation in major depressive disorder. Psychophysiology, 44*, 450–458.

Rottenberg, J., & Gross, J. J. (2003). When emotion goes wrong: Realizing the promise of affective science. *Clinical Psychology: Science and Practice, 10*, 227–232.

Rottenberg, J., Gross, J. J., & Gotlib, I. H. (2005). Emotion context insensitivity in major depressive disorder. *Journal of Abnormal Psychology, 114*(4), 627–639.

Rottenberg, J., & Johnson, S. L. (Eds.). (2007). *Emotion and psychopathology: Bridging affective and clinical science*. Washington, DC: APA Books.

Rottenberg, J., Kasch, K. L., Gross, J. J., & Gotlib, I. H. (2002). Sadness and amusement reactivity differentially predict concurrent and prospective functioning in major depressive disorder. *Emotion, 2*, 135–146.

Rottenberg, J., & Vaughan, C. (2007). Emotion expression in depression: Emerging evidence for emotion context-insensitivity. In A. Vingerhoets, I. Nyklí?ek, & J. Denollet (Eds.), *Emotion regulation: Conceptual and clinical issues* (pp. 125–139). New York: Springer.

Salomon, K., Bylsma, L. M., White, K. E., Panaite, V., & Rottenberg, J. (2013). Is blunted cardiovascular reactivity in depression mood-state dependent?: A comparison of major depressive disorder remitted depression and healthy controls. *International Journal of Psychophysiology, 90*(1), 50–57.

Salomon, K., Clift, A., Karlsdottir, M., & Rottenberg, J. (2009). Major depressive disorder is associated with attenuated cardiovascular reactivity and impaired recovery among those free of cardiovascular disease. *Health Psychology, 28*, 157–165.

Sartorius, N., Üstün, T. B., Lecrubier, Y., & Wittchen, H. U. (1996). Depression comorbid with anxiety: Results from the WHO study on psychological disorders in primary health care. *British Journal of Psychiatry, 168*, 38–43.

Scher, C. D., Ingram, R. F., & Segal, Z. V. (2005). Cognitive reactivity and vulnerability: Empirical evaluation of construct activation and cognitive diatheses in unipolar depression. *Clinical Psychology Review, 25*, 487?510.

Scherer, K. R., Shorr, A., & Johnstone, T. (Eds.). (2001). *Appraisal processes in emotion: Theory, methods, research*. Cary, NC: Oxford University Press.

Schwerdtfeger, A., & Rosenkaimer, A. K. (2011). Depressive symptoms and attenuated physiological reactivity to laboratory stressors. *Biological Psychology, 87*(3), 430–438.

Shankman, S. A., Nelson, B. D., Sarapas, C., Robison-Andrew, E. J., Campbell, M. L., Altman, S. E., et al. (2013). A psychophysiological investigation of threat and reward sensitivity in individuals with panic disorder and/or major depressive disorder. *Journal of Abnormal Psychology, 122*(2), 322–338.

Sigmon, S. T., & Nelson-Gray, R. O. (1992). Sensitivity to aversive events in depression: Antecedent, concomitant, or consequent? *Journal of Psychopathology and Behavioral Assessment, 14*, 225–246.

Siegle, G. J., Granholm, E., Ingram, R. E., & Matt, G. E. (2001). Pupillary and reaction time measures of sustained processing of negative information in depression. *Biological Psychiatry, 49*, 624–636.

Siegle, G. J., Steinhauer, S. R., Thase, M. E., Stenger, V. A., & Carter, C. S. (2002). Can't shake that feeling: Event-related fMRI assessment of sustained amygdala activity in response to emotional information in depressed individuals. *Biological Psychiatry, 51*(9), 693–707.

Silk, J. S., Dahl, R. E., Ryan, N. D., Forbes, E. E., Axelson, D. A., Birmaher, B., et al. (2007). Pupillary reactivity to emotional information in child and adolescent depression: Links to clinical and ecological measures. *American Journal of Psychiatry, 164*, 1873.

Silk, J. S., Steinberg, L., & Morris, A. S. (2003). Adolescents' emotion regulation in daily life: Links to depressive symptoms and problem behavior. *Child Development, 74*(6), 1869–1880.

Takano, K., Sakamoto, S., & Tanno, Y. (2013). Ruminative self-focus in daily life: Associations with daily activities and depressive symptoms. *Emotion, 13*(4), 657–667.

Thompson, R. J., Berenbaum, H., & Bredemeier, K. (2011). Cross-sectional and longitudinal relations between affective instability and depression. *Journal of Affective Disorders, 130*, 53–59.

Thompson, R. J., Mata, J., Jaeggi, S. M., Buschkuehl, M., Jonides, J., & Gotlib, I. H. (2012). The everyday emotional experience of adults with major depressive disorder: Examining emotional instability, inertia, and reactivity. *Journal of Abnormal Psychology, 121*(4), 819–829.

Trull, T. J., & Ebner-Priemer, U. W. (2009). Using experience sampling methods/ecological momentary assessment (ESM/EMA) in clinical assessment and clinical research: Introduction to the special section. *Psychological Assessment, 21*, 457–462.

Watson, D. (2000). *Mood and temperament.* New York: Guilford Press.

Waugh, C. E., Thompson, R. J., & Gotlib, I. H. (2011). Flexible emotional responsiveness in trait resilience. *Emotion, 11*, 1059–1067.

Wenze, S. J., & Miller, I. W. (2010). Use of ecological momentary assessment in mood disorders research. *Clinical Psychology Review, 30*, 794–804.

Yoon, K. L., & Joormann, J. (2012). Stress reactivity in social anxiety disorder with and without comorbid depression. *Journal of Abnormal Psychology, 121*, 250–255.

CHAPTER 7

Depression and Medical Illness

KENNETH E. FREEDLAND *and* ROBERT M. CARNEY

This chapter examines the relationship between depression and medical illness and the assessment and treatment of depression in medical patients.

RELATIONSHIPS BETWEEN DEPRESSION AND MEDICAL ILLNESS

Comorbidity and Multimorbidity

Depression co-occurs with a variety of medical conditions at rates that exceed chance. This fact raises many questions about the relationship between illness and depression. For example, does depression increase the risk of developing particular medical conditions, and if so, does it have a causal, etiological role? And when depression co-occurs with a particular condition, does it increase the risk of further medical morbidity and mortality? If so, how does it do this?

Much of the research on depression and medical illness consists of efforts to explain the comorbidity between depression and particular medical conditions. However, this kind of research has to take other comorbidities into account. Depression often co-occurs with other psychiatric conditions, and many patients have multiple medical conditions.

Medical comorbidities are usually taken into account in research on depression in specific medical conditions such as coronary heart disease (CHD), but they are not necessarily regarded as especially interesting or informative cofactors. This helps to keep the focus of the study on the relationship of primary interest, but it is also myopic in that it ignores the milieu in which this relationship is imbedded. Research on multimorbidity, that is, the coexistence of multiple chronic diseases, is an alternative to the traditional, narrow focus on isolated comorbidities. Definitions and measures of multimorbidity differ across studies (Diederichs, Berger, & Bartels, 2011), and further methodological work is needed. Nevertheless, multimorbidity research has already yielded new insights into depression in medically ill patients. For example, there is a "dose–response" relationship between multimorbidity and distress (Fortin et al., 2006), suggesting that isolated coprevalence rates (e.g., of depression with CHD) may underestimate the role of depression in medically complex subgroups.

Medical Illness as a Predictor of Depression

Chronic illness is a risk factor for major depression. However, chronic medical conditions seldom emerge until middle or old age, whereas the lifetime incidence of major depression increases sharply at puberty and gradually thereafter. The lifetime onset of major depression typically precedes the onset of chronic medical illnesses that are prevalent among adults, often by several decades. Nevertheless, chronic medical illness tends to be depressogenic.

In the Health and Retirement Study (Polsky et al., 2005), depression was no more common in participants with heart disease or diabetes (6%) than in healthy participants, and it was even less common in those with hypertension (4%) or arthritis (4%). In contrast, it affected 9%, 13%, and 13% of participants after the onset of stroke, pulmonary disease, or cancer, respectively. The risk of depression was elevated shortly after the diagnosis of cancer or lung disease, but it subsequently decreased. The risk of depression was fairly low in the first 2 years after the diagnosis of arthritis or heart disease, but it subsequently increased. This study shows that there is no simple answer to the question of whether newly diagnosed medical conditions increase the risk for depression. It depends on the medical condition, when it was diagnosed, and the burdens it imposes on the patient.

In the Alameda County study, poor health was one of the strongest predictors of depression (Roberts, Kaplan, Shema, & Strawbridge, 1997). In the Canadian National Population Health Survey (NPHS), respondents with chronic medical conditions had twice the risk of developing major depression. Painful conditions were some of the strongest predictors (Patten, 2001; Patten et al., 2005). In the Medical Outcomes Study (MOS), poor physical health predicted subsequent depression and vice versa (Hays, Marshall, Wang, & Sherbourne, 1994).

A quantitative review of 20 prospective studies found that neither medical illness nor poor health status was an *independent* risk factor for depression but that bereavement, sleep disturbances, disability, prior depression, and female gender were (Cole & Dendukuri, 2003). These findings, and those of the NPHS, suggest that pain and disability may be stronger risk factors for depression than is medical illness per se.

There is ample evidence from cross-sectional studies that depression is more prevalent among medically ill than physically healthy individuals. A Canadian study found that the prevalence of major depression was higher in chronically ill than in healthy respondents. This pattern held after adjustment for age, sex, social support, and stressful life events (Gagnon & Patten, 2002).

In the Canadian Community Health Survey (CCHS), chronic fatigue syndrome (CFS) and fibromyalgia were the conditions most strongly associated with major depression. Weaker associations were found for diabetes, heart disease, gastrointestinal disorders, and other conditions that tend to be less painful or fatiguing than CFS or fibromyalgia (Patten et al., 2005). This again suggests that depression is more strongly associated with pain, disability, and other burdens of illness than with medical illness per se.

Medical Illness as a Cause of Depression

Certain medical illnesses, such as hypothyroidism (Gold, Pottash, & Extein, 1981), Parkinson's disease (Cummings, 1992), and Huntington's disease (De Marchi & Mennella, 2000) do not merely predict depression; they can actually cause it. Most other chronic medical conditions have not been proven to cause depression through any known physiological pathway, despite the fact that depression is coprevalent with them. Nevertheless, because depression is a common problem in medically ill patients, it is often taken for granted that the depression is *caused* by medical illness. This is an example of the logical fallacy *post hoc, ergo propter hoc*. In reality, many patients who are depressed after the onset of medical illness were depressed before the onset; many have histories of depression that began decades before the onset of illness; and many other patients remain free of depression after becoming ill.

Depression as a Predictor of Incident Medical Illnesses

Multiple studies have shown that depression in healthy cohorts predicts medical illness later in life. The Western Electric Study (Persky, Kempthorne-Rawson, & Shekelle, 1987) and the Stirling County Study (Murphy et al., 1992) were among the first. In the Framingham Heart Study, depression did not predict cardiac events, but it did predict all-cause mortality (Wulsin et al., 2005). In a subsequent Framingham report, depression increased risk of stroke fourfold in those who were under age 65 at entry (Salaycik et al., 2007). In the Healthy Women Study, depression predicted incident metabolic syndrome (Raikkonen, Matthews, & Kuller, 2007).

Depression as a Risk Factor for Morbidity and Mortality in Medically Ill Patients

Numerous studies have shown that depression predicts further morbidity and mortality in patients with established heart disease, cancer, or other major illnesses. However, there is considerable uncertainty as to whether it is a causal risk factor in any of them. Formidable hurdles confront researchers who study this question (Freedland & Carney, 2013). Rigorous studies adjust for multiple confounders, but one can never be sure that every potential confounder has been addressed. For example, subclinical risk factors (e.g., undiagnosed diabetes) are easily missed. Many studies are limited to small samples; this constrains the number of confounders that can be evaluated without overfitting statistical models (Babyak, 2004). Paradoxically, it is more difficult to obtain gold standard medical measures in large studies than in small ones. Consequently, both large and small observational studies are vulnerable to questions about residual confounding, but for different reasons.

Randomized controlled trials (RCTs) are the crucibles of risk factor research. If treatment of a risk marker improves disease outcomes, its status may be elevated to that of a modifiable, causal risk factor. However, there are more ways for trials to fail than to succeed. For example, the Enhancing Recovery in Coronary Heart Disease (ENRICHD) trial tested the hypothesis that treating depression and low social support after an acute myocardial infarction (MI) reduces the risk of recurrent MI and death. The intervention had no effect on medical outcomes, but it also had only modest effects on depression and social support (Berkman et al., 2003). Thus ENRICHD did not provide a very strong test of the hypothesis.

Biobehavioral Mechanisms Linking Depression to Medical Illness

Depression increases the risk of morbidity and mortality in medically ill patients, but how it does so is unclear. Candidate biobehavioral mechanisms are factors that are affected by depression and that contribute to the progression of disease. Some are candidates in multiple diseases (Mykletun et al., 2007); others are disease-specific. For example, pro-coagulant factors might help to explain why depression predicts major adverse cardiovascular events (Serebruany et al., 2003), but not why it predicts mortality in women with AIDS (Cook et al., 2004).

Genetic and pathophysiological correlates of depression, such as autonomic dysregulation and inflammation, dominate the search for mechanisms (e.g., McCaffery et al., 2006). Behavioral correlates of depression, such as nonadherence to medical treatment regimens (DiMatteo, Lepper, & Croghan, 2000) and physical inactivity (Win et al., 2011), have also been studied. Mechanistic research has been summarized in a number of review articles (e.g., Gans, 2006; Skala, Freedland, & Carney, 2006; Spiegel & Giese-Davis, 2003).

ASSESSMENT OF DEPRESSION IN MEDICALLY ILL PATIENTS

Diagnosis of Depressive Disorders

DSM-5 (American Psychiatric Association, 2013) draws a clear distinction between forms of depression that are *direct pathophysiological consequences* of medical conditions such as hypothyroidism and ones that have a different relationship with medical illness. CHD, for example, is not known to cause depression through a direct pathophysiological pathway. In DSM-5, stressful illnesses such as CHD can promote or maintain depression without directly causing it. Thus, if depression follows an acute MI, it is an episode of "major depressive disorder," but if it is caused by hypothyroidism, it is classified as a "depressive disorder due to another medical condition, with major depressive-like episode."

DSM-5 notes that there are no perfect techniques for determining whether the relationship between a mood disturbance and a general medical condition is truly etiological. Factors to consider include (1) biological plausibility; (2) published evidence; (3) a consistent temporal relationship between the mood disturbance and the medical condition in terms of onset, worsening, improvement, and/or remission; and (4) an atypical presentation, such as depression in a patient with no history of depression and no recent exposure to any depressogenic stressors.

The DSM-5 criteria for depressive disorders include somatic symptoms that can be hard to interpret in medical patients. It is difficult to prove that a symptom such as fatigue is entirely due to direct pathophysiological effects of a medical illness and not at all due to depression. Such symptoms are nonspecific, that is, they can be simultaneously produced by two or more disorders, such as by depression and CHD. DSM-5 leaves room for clinical judgment as to whether to count nonspecific somatic symptoms such as fatigue or insomnia toward the diagnosis of depression in a medically ill patient. Several diagnostic schemes, ranging from highly exclusive (always exclude somatic symptoms) to highly inclusive (always include them), have been evaluated. There is a twofold difference between these extremes in the prevalence of major depression in medically ill older adults. The exclusive approach captures the most severe and persistent cases, but the inclusive approach is the most sensitive and reliable one, and it is a strong predictor of persistent depression (Koenig, George, Peterson, & Pieper, 1997).

This suggests that it is usually best to give the benefit of the doubt to the psychiatric disorder; that is, when in doubt, count somatic symptoms toward the diagnosis of depression, and do not exclude them except when they are clearly and entirely due to direct pathophysiological effects of medical illness. Rapid weight gain due to edema in heart failure is a rare example of an unquestionably excludable feature. In this situation, it is clearly not a sign of depression.

Measurement of Depression Symptoms

Research on depression in medically ill patients is often based on questionnaires that were originally developed for medically well individuals. The Beck Depression Inventories (BDI and BDI-II; Beck, Steer, & Brown, 1996; Beck, Ward, Mendelson, Mock, & Erbaugh, 1961) and the Center for Epidemiologic Studies Depression Scale (CES-D; Radloff, 1977) have been used in many studies. The Patient Health Questionnaire depression scale (PHQ-9; Spitzer, Kroenke, & Williams, 1999) was originally developed for primary care. Because of its brevity, ease of use, and diagnostic utility, it is very widely used in research on depression in medically ill patient populations. Among measures that were developed for research on medically ill patients, only the Hospital Anxiety and Depression Scale (HADS; Zigmond & Snaith, 1983) is widely used. It omits all of the somatic symptoms of depression, in line with the exclusive strategy.

The most controversial issue concerning depression questionnaires is whether they should be used for routine screening in medical care settings. For example, the American Heart Association recommends routine depression screening for patients with CHD (Lichtman et al., 2008), but this recommendation has been sharply criticized because routine screening has not been shown to improve clinical outcomes (Thombs et al., 2013). Consequently, this has become an active area of investigation (e.g., Rollman et al., 2012; Smolderen et al., 2011).

The performance of depression questionnaires in various medical patient populations has been evaluated in several disease-specific reviews and meta-analyses. These include reports focusing on diabetes (Roy, Lloyd, Pouwer, Holt, & Sartorius, 2012), heart disease (Thombs et al., 2007), cancer (Meijer, Roseman, et al., 2011), and others.

Depression as a Patient-Reported Outcome

The multiplicity of self-report outcome measures has made it difficult to compare or to meta-analyze studies of depression in medically ill patients. The Patient Reported Outcomes Measurement Information System (PROMIS) provides state-of-the-art measures of patient-reported outcomes, including depression (Pilkonis et al., 2011). Research on the validity, clinical utility, and prognostic value of the PROMIS depression scale in medically ill patients has just begun. It would be premature to rely solely on the PROMIS scale, but it should be included whenever possible, along with well-established measures such as the BDI-II or the PHQ-9, in future studies of comorbid depression in medical illness.

TREATMENT OF DEPRESSION IN MEDICAL PATIENTS

Randomized Controlled Trials

Medically ill patients have been excluded from most depression treatment trials. Safety concerns have made this necessary in some trials, but in others, a more salient concern has been that medically ill patients may be less responsive to treatment than healthier patients (Iosifescu et al., 2003). Because many patients with depression are also medically ill, this strategy has created an unrealistic picture of the safety and effectiveness of antidepressants.

However, medical illness exclusion criteria have been relaxed in a number of recent trials, such as in the Sequenced Treatment Alternatives to Relieve Depression (STAR*D) trial. The STAR*D investigators have not yet compared depression outcomes between participants with or without medical comorbidities, but they have compared the 22% of participants who would have been eligible for more restrictive Phase III efficacy trials and the 78% who would ordinarily be excluded from such trials due to medical comorbidities or for other reasons. The former subgroup tolerated citalopram better and had higher response (52% vs. 39%) and remission (34% vs. 25%) rates (Wisniewski et al., 2009).

Numerous trials have tested therapies that were originally developed for depressed but otherwise medically well patients, rather than ones designed de novo for medical patients. However, adaptations are necessary in some cases to meet the safety or accessibility needs of medical patients. For example, excessive behavioral activation can trigger serious adverse events in patients with certain medical conditions. In such cases, activation plans have to be carefully modified to ensure that they are safe (Skala, Freedland, & Carney, 2005).

Clinical Issues

More depression care is provided by primary care physicians than by mental health specialists (Mojtabai & Olfson, 2008). Medical comorbidities influence primary care for depression. For example, patients with medical comorbidities are more likely to be identified as depressed than are medically well patients. Paradoxically, patients with medical comorbidities are no more likely to receive adequate depression treatment or to be satisfied with their depression care than are healthier patients (Teh, Reynolds, & Cleary, 2008).

Because depression increases the risks of morbidity and mortality in a variety of medical illnesses, one might expect medically ill patients to be treated more aggressively for depression than healthier patients. However, in a study of primary care patients, 21% had a medical comorbidity and 6% had multimorbidity. Those with multimorbidity were *less* likely than other patients to receive an antidepressant (Gill, Klinkman, & Chen, 2010).

Safety issues constrain antidepressant options for some medical patients. For example, selective serotonin reuptake inhibitors (SSRIs) are generally safe for patients with CHD (Roose & Miyazaki, 2005), but they can interact with drugs that are metabolized by the same cytochrome P450 liver enzymes (Nemeroff, Preskorn, & Devane, 2007). Other factors, such as costs and regimen complexity, can also prevent medical patients from receiving adequate depression care (Mojtabai & Olfson, 2003).

Evidence-based psychotherapy should be considered, especially in primary care settings offering integrated behavioral services (Brawer, Martielli, Pye, Manwaring, & Tierney, 2010). There is evidence that cognitive-behavioral therapy (CBT; Wiles et al., 2013) and problem-solving therapy (PST; Unutzer et al., 2002) are effective in primary care for depression.

Psychosocial specialty services for patients with particular medical conditions have been established at many hospitals and clinics. For example, specialists in psychosocial oncology help cancer patients with depression and related problems (Hamilton, Jackson, Abbott, Zullig, & Provenzale, 2011; Preyde, Chevalier, Hatton-Bauer, & Barksey, 2010).

In-depth knowledge of the medical condition and its behavioral and psychosocial concomitants and advanced clinical training and experience can equip behavioral specialists to handle cases that might be too difficult or complex for generalists (Skala et al., 2005).

DEPRESSION IN RELATION TO SPECIFIC MEDICAL CONDITIONS

Obesity

Numerous studies over the past decade have examined associations between obesity and depression. A recent meta-analysis of 15 longitudinal studies ($n = 58,745$) found that obesity and overweight increase the risk of subsequent onset of depressive disorders and that depression increases the risk of developing obesity later in life (Luppino et al., 2010). Little is known about biobehavioral mechanisms that might explain these associations, although a recent study found that depression in women is associated with poorer diet quality (Appelhans et al., 2012).

A meta-analysis of 31 trials ($n = 7,937$) found that weight loss interventions reduce depressive symptoms as a secondary benefit. Lifestyle modification programs have larger effects on depression than dietary counseling or pharmacotherapy (Fabricatore et al., 2011). Weight loss following gastric-restrictive surgery is also associated with substantial decreases in depression in severely obese patients (Dixon, Dixon, & O'Brien, 2003). There is little evidence that antidepressant therapy reduces obesity as a collateral benefit. To the contrary, it is often associated with modest weight gain (Patten, Williams, Lavorato, Khaled, & Bulloch, 2011).

Metabolic Syndrome

Numerous studies over the past decade have identified a bidirectional relationship between depression and metabolic syndrome (MetS). In a recent meta-analysis of 29 cross-sectional studies ($n = 155,333$), 11 studies reported on depression as the outcome variable (odds ratio [OR] = 1.27), and 12 reported on MetS as the outcome (OR = 1.34). Out of 11 prospective studies, 9 studies ($n = 26,936$) reported on depression as the outcome (OR = 1.49), and 4 studies ($n = 3,834$) reported on MetS as the outcome (OR = 1.52). These findings show that depression increases the risk for MetS and vice versa (Pan et al., 2012).

Diabetes Mellitus

Recent meta-analyses confirm that there is a bidirectional relationship between depression and diabetes mellitus (DM), although depression seems to be a stronger predictor of DM than DM is of depression. In a meta-analysis of 11 prospective studies ($n = 172,521$), DM increased the relative risk of depression by 1.24 (Nouwen et al., 2010). A subsequent meta-analysis found that the risk of depression was elevated in individuals with diagnosed DM but not in those with undiagnosed DM or prediabetes (Nouwen et al., 2011). This suggests that the psychosocial impact of DM fosters depression but that glycemic dysregulation is not directly depressogenic.

Depression predicts adverse medical outcomes in DM. In a meta-analysis of 47 studies, depression was associated with nonadherence to diabetes treatment regimens, with an overall effect size $r = 0.21$ (Gonzalez et al., 2008). Depression in DM is also associated with poor glycemic control (Lustman, Anderson, et al., 2000), diabetic complications (de Groot, Anderson, Freedland, Clouse, & Lustman, 2001), CHD (Clouse et al., 2003), and dementia (Katon et al., 2012).

Early trials showed that depression can be treated in patients with DM with antidepressant medications (Lustman, Freedland, Griffith, & Clouse, 2000; Lustman et al., 2006) or CBT (Lustman, Griffith, Freedland, Kissel, & Clouse, 1998) and that treatment has additional benefits (e.g., better glycemic control). A recent trial tested systematic care management aimed at depression, hemoglobin A1c, systolic blood pressure, and low-density lipoprotein cholesterol levels in adults with depression and diabetes or CHD, who were recruited from primary care clinics. Compared with usual care controls, patients in the intervention arm had a mean of 114 additional depression-free days, an estimated 0.34 additional quality-adjusted life years, and lower costs for outpatient care (Katon et al., 2010).

Kidney Disease

Until recently, there was little interest in depression in chronic kidney disease (CKD) or in end-stage renal disease (ESRD), but research has grown rapidly in this area over the past few years. Major depression is prevalent in CKD; it affects about 40% of patients in stages 3–4 CKD (Hedayati, Minhajuddin, Toto, Morris, & Rush, 2009). A recent study of 598,153 veterans with CKD (stages 1–5) showed that depression decreases survival (hazard ratio [HR] = 1.55; Balogun et al., 2012). Depression is also prevalent in patients with ESRD on renal dialysis, and it predicts adverse outcomes. It is also associated with poor adherence to medications and dietary restrictions (Rosenthal, Ver Halen, & Cukor, 2012) and with worse survival rates (van Dijk et al., 2012).

Unfortunately, many patients with ESRD are unable to tolerate antidepressant medications, and research on treatment for depression in ESRD is at an early stage. One of the largest efforts is the ongoing Chronic Kidney Disease Antidepressant Sertraline Trial (CAST), which will randomize 200 patients with depression in stages 3–5 CKD to sertraline or placebo (Jain et al., 2013).

Sleep Apnea

Obstructive sleep apnea–hypopnea syndrome (OSAHS) is prevalent among obese individuals and older men, and it is a risk factor for mortality and a variety of other adverse health outcomes (e.g., Loke, Brown, Kwok, Niruban, & Myint, 2012). Major depression is present in about 1 out of 5 patients with OSAHS (Sharafkhaneh, Giray, Richardson, Young, & Hirshkowitz, 2005) and is associated with longer apneic episodes (Carney et al., 2006), worse fatigue, and poor subjective sleep quality (Bardwell, Ancoli-Israel, & Dimsdale, 2007; Wells, Day, Carney, Freedland, & Duntley, 2004). In a study of patients with a recent acute MI, those who had both depression and OSAHS were at higher risk of recurrent MI and mortality compared with patients with either condition alone or with neither condition (Hayano et al., 2012).

There is also emerging evidence that OSAHS can complicate the treatment of depression. Patients with depression and OSAHS tend to be less responsive to antidepressant therapy (Roest et al., 2012) and to CBT (Freedland et al., 2012) than similar patients with depression without OSAHS.

Coronary Heart Disease

There has been more research on depression in CHD than in any other chronic illness. Much of this work has focused on patients with a recent acute coronary syndrome (ACS), which includes acute MI and unstable angina. In a recent scientific statement, a review panel recommended that the American Heart Association should elevate depression to the status of a risk factor for adverse medical outcomes in patients with ACS (Lichtman et al., in press). A meta-analysis of 29 studies (n = 16,889) found that post-MI depression increases the risk of all-cause mortality (OR = 2.25), cardiac mortality (OR = 2.71), and composite outcomes of nonfatal and fatal cardiac events (OR = 1.59; Meijer, Conradi, et al., 2011).

A more recent meta-analysis of 22 prospective studies focused on the timing of depression in relation to cardiac death. Nine studies investigated premorbid depression in CHD-free cohorts, and 13 studies of patients with established CHD examined new-onset depression in comparison with past or recurrent depression. The risk ratios (RR) were 0.76 for past history of depression only, 1.79 for premorbid depression onset, 2.11 for postmorbid or new depression onset, and 1.59 for recurrent depression. Thus depression increases the risk of adverse outcomes regardless of whether it precedes or follows the onset of CHD, but a past history of depression without any current depression is not hazardous in CHD (Leung et al., 2012).

There is strong evidence that depression can be treated safely in patients with CHD with antidepressants such as sertraline (Glassman et al., 2002) or citalopram (Lespérance et al., 2007) or with evidence-based psychotherapies such as CBT (Freedland et al., 2009) or problem-solving therapy (PST; Davidson et al., 2010). The efficacy data are less consistent. Some of the smaller trials have yielded clinically significant effects on depression (e.g., Davidson et al., 2010; Freedland et al., 2009), but larger multicenter studies have produced modest effects. In ENRICHD, depression was treated with CBT and sertraline when indicated; Hamilton depression (HAMD) scores improved but only modestly (Berkman et al., 2003). In the Sertraline Antidepressant Heart Attack Randomized Trial (SADHART), there was no difference in HAMD scores between the sertraline and placebo arms in the primary analysis, although sertraline was superior to placebo by several points in a secondary analysis of the subgroup with the most severe depression (Glassman et al., 2002). Secondary analyses of data from these and other trials suggest that treatment of post-MI depression may improve survival (e.g., Carney et al., 2004), but none of the preplanned, primary analyses have provided any evidence for this effect (e.g., Berkman et al., 2003). A recent meta-analysis supports these conclusions (Baumeister, Hutter, & Bengel, 2011).

Collaborative care interventions offer a promising strategy for cost-effective treatment of depression in cardiac patients. In the Bypassing the Blues trial, patients who had recently undergone coronary artery bypass graft (CABG) surgery were randomly assigned to usual care or to a telephone-delivered, nurse-directed collaborative care intervention. HAMD scores were lower, and measures of functioning and health-related quality of life were significantly higher, in the intervention than in the usual care arm on follow-up assessments (Rollman et al., 2009).

Heart Failure

Heart failure (HF) is a debilitating condition with a poor prognosis. Its prevalence is expected to increase 25% by 2030, and its cost will increase by $70 billion per year (Go et al., 2013). Rehospitalizations account for much of the cost of HF care, and there is evidence that depression is a risk factor for HF rehospitalization (Albert et al., 2009). Depression is also a risk factor for HF mortality (Albert et al., 2009); this is not due to worse HF in patients with depression or to adverse effects of antidepressants (Gottlieb et al., 2009). Biobehavioral mechanisms that have been implicated in these associations include inadequate HF self-care, physical inactivity, inflammation, and others (Johansson et al., 2011; Zuluaga et al., 2010).

There have been few RCTs of treatments for depression in patients with HF, and the results so far have not been very encouraging. In SADHART–Chronic Heart Failure (CHF), patients were randomized to 12 weeks of sertraline or placebo. Sertraline was safe for HF patients, but it had no advantage over placebo for depression or cardiovascular outcomes (O'Connor et al., 2010). In the HF-ACTION trial, patients with HF were randomly assigned to either an aerobic exercise intervention or usual care. Between-group differences in BDI-II scores averaged less than 1 point at 3 and 12 months. In the primary outcome analysis, exercise training did not result in significant improvements in all-cause mortality or hospitalization, although some of the secondary analyses were promising (Blumenthal et al., 2012; O'Connor et al., 2009). Recent trials suggest that CBT and mindfulness yield modest improvements in depression, but that it may be possible to achieve larger gains by combining CBT with exercise (Dekker, Moser, Peden, & Lennie, 2012; Gary, Dunbar, Higgins, Musselman, & Smith, 2010; Sullivan et al., 2009).

Cerebrovascular Accident

Major depression affects approximately one out of every five stroke patients (Robinson, 2003). Depression is more likely to follow strokes in certain locations in the brain (Lassalle-Lagadec et al., 2012), and genetic factors such as serotonin transporter gene polymorphisms influence the risk of poststroke depression (Kohen et al., 2008). Depression also increases the risk of incident stroke (Glymour, Maselko, Gilman, Patton, & Avendano, 2010). A meta-analysis of 28 prospective studies (n = 317,540) showed that depression predicts both total stroke (HR = 1.45) and fatal stroke (HR = 1.55; Pan, Sun, Okereke, Rexrode, & Hu, 2011).

The depression treatment literature in stroke patients is small but encouraging. RCTs have confirmed that antidepressants and problem-solving therapy can prevent poststroke depression (Robinson et al., 2008) and that antidepressants can improve poststroke depression and functional outcomes (Narushima, Paradiso, Moser, Jorge, & Robinson, 2007).

Cancer

The current weight of evidence suggests that depression does not increase the risks of incident cancer, tumor progression, or metastasis. However, a recent meta-analysis of 25 studies showed that depression does predict cancer mortality (RR = 1.25) and that a diagnosis of major or minor depression confers an even higher risk (RR = 1.39), even after adjustment for clinical prognostic factors (Satin, Linden, & Phillips, 2009).

Recent studies have helped to allay concerns that antidepressant medications might increase the risks of colorectal, prostatic, breast, lung, or other forms of cancer (Cronin-Fenton et al., 2011; Haukka et al., 2010). Other studies show that widely used antidepressants can be prescribed for patients with diagnosed cancer without increasing the risks of recurrence or mortality, although tricyclic antidepressants may pose a risk in patients with colorectal cancer (Chubak et al., 2008; Walker, Grainge, Bates, & Card, 2012). Another exception to this favorable trend is that antidepressants such as paroxetine that strongly inhibit CYP2D6 can reduce the effectiveness of tamoxifen for breast cancer and thereby increase the risk of breast cancer mortality (Kelly et al., 2010). This possibility has led to a decline in prescriptions for strong CYP2D6 inhibitors among breast cancer patients and to interest in safer alternatives (Dusetzina, Alexander, Freedman, Huskamp, & Keating, 2013). Nevertheless, recent trials suggest that carefully selected antidepressants may help to improve depression and quality of life in patients with breast cancer (e.g., Park, Lee, Kim, Bae, & Hahm, 2012).

Psychotherapy may be a relatively safe option for cancer patients with depression. A recent meta-analysis of six psychotherapy RCTs found that psychotherapy was superior to control conditions for depression. CBT is more effective than problem-solving therapy for these patients, and it seems to be about as effective as antidepressant therapy (Hart et al., 2012).

HIV/AIDS

Depression is associated with HIV risk behaviors such as needle sharing and unprotected sex (Hutton, Lyketsos, Zenilman, Thompson, & Erbelding, 2004; Stein, Solomon, Herman, Anderson, & Miller, 2003). It also decreases the chances that an HIV-infected patient will initiate highly active antiretroviral therapy (HAART; Tegger et al., 2008), and it increases the risk of mortality (Leserman et al., 2007). Bipolar, but not unipolar, depression increases the risk of all-cause mortality among HIV-infected veterans (Nurutdinova et al., 2012).

Antidepressant therapy increases adherence to HAART among patients with depression (Cruess et al., 2012). It also decreases the desire for hastened death in patients with advanced AIDS (Breitbart et al., 2010). Little is known about whether antidepressants or psychotherapy for depression can improve survival in AIDS.

FUTURE DIRECTIONS

Several themes pervade the preceding sections. Depression is prevalent in all of the major chronic illnesses, and even more prevalent among patients with multimorbidity or with conditions that are painful or debilitating. Depression is a risk factor for the development (or early development) of certain medical conditions such as CHD, but not for others, such as various types of cancer. There is much more evidence that depression is a prognostic risk factor in various medical illnesses, and the evidence is particularly strong in relation to mortality. Considerable progress has been made in identifying biobehavioral mechanisms that may explain these effects, yet the causal status of depression as a risk factor for adverse medical outcomes remains as elusive as ever. Finally, efforts to identify safe, efficacious, and cost-effective treatments for depression in medically ill patients have produced inconsistent results. Pharmacological and psychotherapeutic interventions successfully relieve depression in many cases, but they fail to help many other patients. Treatment-resistant depression may be an especially risky subtype for medically ill patients, and, unfortunately, it is the one which (by definition) we know the least about how to treat.

Systematic treatment development research and rigorously designed and conducted RCTs are the best ways to make progress in this area over the next decade. It is sometimes assumed that clinical trials should be postponed until a complete mechanistic understanding of the target problem has been achieved. However, many mechanistically informed treatments do not work as expected.

Cardiologists learned this lesson the hard way from the unanticipated, lethal effects of anti-arrhythmic drugs in the Cardiac Arrhythmia Suppression Trial (Echt et al., 1991) and from many other disappointing trials. They have also learned that efficacious treatments can be developed without the benefit of a complete mechanistic understanding of the target problem or of the pathways through which the intervention affects the problem (DeMets & Califf, 2002). Such experiences show those of us who specialize in treating depression in medically ill patients that clinical trials should not be postponed until all of the key mechanistic questions have been definitively answered. Instead, clinical and mechanistic research should proceed in tandem, and each kind of research should be designed, whenever possible, to help to inform the other.

Another perennial issue is whether it is better to focus on primary, secondary, or tertiary prevention of depression. Most studies have focused on patients who are already medically ill, already depressed, and already at risk for further morbidity and mortality. There should be continued efforts in the coming decade to improve the state of the art of depression care for these patients. However, the lifetime onset of depression often precedes the onset of chronic medical illnesses by decades. Furthermore, depression in childhood, adolescence, and young adulthood may contribute to behavioral risk factors for chronic illness, such as smoking (Chaiton, Cohen, O'Loughlin, & Rehm, 2009; Rottenberg et al., 2014). Treatment of depression in young individuals may help to prevent recurrent depression and premature development of chronic medical illnesses.

In short, much has been learned over the past decade about the role and treatment of depression in a variety of medical illnesses. However, much more work remains to be done in this area. Both mechanistic and treatment research will remain important priorities.

REFERENCES

Albert, N. M., Fonarow, G. C., Abraham, W. T., Gheorghiade, M., Greenberg, B. H., Nunez, E. et al. (2009). Depression and clinical outcomes in heart failure: An OPTIMIZE-HF analysis. *American Journal of Medicine, 122,* 366–373.

American Psychiatric Association. (2013). *Diagnostic and statistical manual of mental disorders.* (5th ed.). Arlington, VA: Author.

Appelhans, B. M., Whited, M. C., Schneider, K. L., Ma, Y., Oleski, J. L., Merriam, P. A., et al. (2012). Depression severity, diet quality, and physical activity in women with obesity and depression. *Journal of the Academy of Nutrition and Dietetics, 112,* 693–698.

Babyak, M. A. (2004). What you see may not be what you get: A brief, nontechnical introduction to overfitting in regression-type models. *Psychosomatic Medicine, 66,* 411–421.

Balogun, R. A., Abdel-Rahman, E. M., Balogun, S. A., Lott, E. H., Lu, J. L., Malakauskas, S. M., et al. (2012). Association of depression and antidepressant use with mortality in a large cohort of patients with nondialysis-dependent CKD. *Clinical Journal of the American Society of Nephrology, 7,* 1793–1800.

Bardwell, W. A., Ancoli-Israel, S., & Dimsdale, J. E. (2007). Comparison of the effects of depressive symptoms and apnea severity on fatigue in patients with obstructive sleep apnea: A replication study. *Journal of Affective Disorders, 97,* 181–186.

Baumeister, H., Hutter, N., & Bengel, J. (2011). Psychological and pharmacological interventions for depression in patients with coronary artery disease. *Cochrane Database of Systematic Reviews,* Article No. CD008012, DOI: 10.1002/14651858.CD008012.pub3/abstract.

Beck, A. T., Steer, R. A., & Brown, G. K. (1996). *Manual for the Beck Depression Inventory—II.* San Antonio, TX: Psychological Corporation.

Beck, A. T., Ward, C. H., Mendelson, M., Mock, J. E., & Erbaugh, J. K. (1961). An inventory for measuring depression. *Archives of General Psychiatry, 4,* 561–571.

Berkman, L. F., Blumenthal, J., Burg, M., Carney, R. M., Catellier, D., Cowan, M. J., et al. (2003). Effects of treating depression and low perceived social support on clinical events after myocardial infarction: The Enhancing Recovery in Coronary Heart Disease Patients (ENRICHD) Randomized Trial.*Journal of the American Medical Association, 289,* 3106–3116.

Blumenthal, J. A., Babyak, M. A., O'Connor, C., Keteyian, S., Landzberg, J., Howlett, J., et al. (2012). Effects of exercise training on depressive symptoms in patients with chronic heart failure: The HF-ACTION randomized trial. *Journal of the American Medical Association,, 308,* 465–474.

Brawer, P. A., Martielli, R., Pye, P. L., Manwaring, J., & Tierney, A. (2010). St. Louis Initiative for Integrated Care Excellence (SLI(2)CE): Integrated-collaborative care on a large scale model. *Families, Systems, and Health, 28,* 175–187.

Breitbart, W., Rosenfeld, B., Gibson, C., Kramer, M., Li, Y., Tomarken, A., et al. (2010). Impact of treatment for depression on desire for hastened death in patients with advanced AIDS. *Psychosomatics, 51,* 98–105.

Carney, R. M., Blumenthal, J. A., Freedland, K. E., Youngblood, M., Veith, R. C., Burg, M. M., et al. (2004). Depression and late mortality after myocardial infarction in the Enhancing Recovery in Coronary Heart Disease (ENRICHD) study. *Psychosomatic Medicine, 66,* 466–474.

Carney, R. M., Howells, W. B., Freedland, K. E., Duntley, S. P., Stein, P. K., Rich, M. W., et al. (2006). Depression and obstructive sleep apnea in patients with coronary heart disease. *Psychosomatic Medicine, 68,* 443–448.

Chaiton, M. O., Cohen, J. E., O'Loughlin, J., & Rehm, J. (2009). A systematic review of longitudinal studies on the association between depression and smoking in adolescents. *BMC Public Health, 9,* 356.

Chubak, J., Buist, D. S., Boudreau, D. M., Rossing, M. A., Lumley, T., & Weiss, N. S. (2008). Breast cancer recurrence risk in relation to antidepressant use after diagnosis. *Breast Cancer Research and Treatment, 112,* 123–132.

Clouse, R. E., Lustman, P. J., Freedland, K. E., Griffith, L. S., McGill, J. B., & Carney, R. M. (2003). Depression and coronary heart disease in women with diabetes. *Psychosomatic Medicine, 65,* 376–383.

Cole, M. G., & Dendukuri, N. (2003). Risk factors for depression among elderly community subjects: A systematic review and meta-analysis. *American Journal of Psychiatry, 160,* 1147–1156.

Cook, J. A., Grey, D., Burke, J., Cohen, M. H., Gurtman, A. C., Richardson, J. L. et al. (2004). Depressive symptoms and AIDS-related mortality among a multisite cohort of HIV-positive women. *American Journal of Public Health, 94,* 1133–1140.

Cronin-Fenton, D. P., Riis, A. H., Lash, T. L., Dalton, S. O., Friis, S., Robertson, D., et al. (2011). Antidepressant use and colorectal cancer risk: A Danish population-based case-control study. *British Journal of Cancer, 104,* 188–192.

Cruess, D. G., Kalichman, S. C., Amaral, C., Swetzes, C., Cherry, C., & Kalichman, M. O. (2012). Benefits of adherence to psychotropic medications on depressive symptoms and antiretroviral medication adherence among men and women living with HIV/AIDS. *Annals of Behavioral Medicine, 43,* 189–197.

Cummings, J. L. (1992). Depression and Parkinson's disease: A review. *American Journal of Psychiatry, 149,* 443–454.

Davidson, K. W., Rieckmann, N., Clemow, L., Schwartz, J. E., Shimbo, D., Medina, V. et al. (2010). Enhanced depression care for patients with acute coronary syndrome and persistent depressive symptoms: Coronary psychosocial evaluation studies randomized controlled trial. *Archives of Internal Medicine, 170,* 600–608.

de Groot, M., Anderson, R., Freedland, K. E., Clouse, R. E., & Lustman, P. J. (2001). Association of depression and diabetes complications: A meta-analysis. *Psychosomatic Medicine, 63*, 619–630.

De Marchi, N., & Mennella, R. (2000). Huntington's disease and its association with psychopathology. *Harvard Review of Psychiatry, 7*, 278–289.

Dekker, R. L., Moser, D. K., Peden, A. R., & Lennie, T. A. (2012). Cognitive therapy improves three-month outcomes in hospitalized patients with heart failure. *Journal of Cardiac Failure, 18*, 10–20.

DeMets, D. L., & Califf, R. M. (2002). Lessons learned from recent cardiovascular clinical trials: Part I. *Circulation, 106*, 746–751.

Diederichs, C., Berger, K., & Bartels, D. B. (2011). The measurement of multiple chronic diseases: A systematic review on existing multimorbidity indices. *Journals of.Gerontology. Series A, Biological Sciences and Medical Sciences, 66*, 301–311.

DiMatteo, M. R., Lepper, H. S., & Croghan, T. W. (2000). Depression is a risk factor for noncompliance with medical treatment: Meta-analysis of the effects of anxiety and depression on patient adherence. *Archives of Internal Medicine, 160*, 2101–2107.

Dixon, J. B., Dixon, M. E., & O'Brien, P. E. (2003). Depression in association with severe obesity: Changes with weight loss. *Archives of Internal Medicine, 163*, 2058–2065.

Dusetzina, S. B., Alexander, G. C., Freedman, R. A., Huskamp, H. A., & Keating, N. L. (2013). Trends in co-prescribing of antidepressants and tamoxifen among women with breast cancer, 2004–2010. *Breast Cancer Research and Treatment, 137*, 285–296.

Echt, D. S., Liebson, P. R., Mitchell, L. B., Peters, R. W., Obias-Manno, D., Barker, A. H., et al. (1991). Mortality and morbidity in patients receiving encainide, flecainide, or placebo" The Cardiac Arrhythmia Suppression Trial. *New England Journal of Medicine, 324*, 781–788.

Fabricatore, A. N., Wadden, T. A., Higginbotham, A. J., Faulconbridge, L. F., Nguyen, A. M., Heymsfield, S. B., et al. (2011). Intentional weight loss and changes in symptoms of depression: A systematic review and meta-analysis. *International Journal of Obesity (London), 35*, 1363–1376.

Fortin, M., Bravo, G., Hudon, C., Lapointe, L., Dubois, M. F., & Almirall, J. (2006). Psychological distress and multimorbidity in primary care. *Annals of Family Medicine, 4*, 417–422.

Freedland, K. E., & Carney, R. M. (2013). Depression as a risk factor for adverse outcomes in coronary heart disease. *BMC Medicine, 11*, 131.

Freedland, K. E., Carney, R. M., Hayano, J., Steinmeyer, B. C., Reese, R. L., & Roest, A. M. (2012). Effect of obstructive sleep apnea on response to cognitive behavior therapy for depression after an acute myocardial infarction. *Journal of Psychosomatic Research, 72*, 276–281.

Freedland, K. E., Skala, J. A., Carney, R. M., Rubin, E. H., Lustman, P. J., Davila-Roman, V. G., et al. (2009). Treatment of depression after coronary artery bypass surgery: A randomized controlled trial. *Archives of General Psychiatry, 66*, 387–396.

Gagnon, L. M., & Patten, S. B. (2002). Major depression and its association with long-term medical conditions. *Canadian Journal of Psychiatry, 47*, 149–152.

Gans, R. O. (2006). The metabolic syndrome, depression, and cardiovascular disease: Interrelated conditions that share pathophysiologic mechanisms. *Medical Clinics of North America, 90*, 573–591.

Gary, R. A., Dunbar, S. B., Higgins, M. K., Musselman, D. L., & Smith, A. L. (2010). Combined exercise and cognitive behavioral therapy improves outcomes in patients with heart failure. *Journal of Psychosomatic Research, 69*, 119–131.

Gill, J. M., Klinkman, M. S., & Chen, Y. X. (2010). Antidepressant medication use for primary care patients with and without medical comorbidities: A national electronic health record (EHR) network study. *Journal of the American Board of Family Medicine, 23*, 499–508.

Glassman, A. H., O'Connor, C. M., Califf, R. M., Swedberg, K., Schwartz, P., Bigger, J. T., Jr., et al. (2002). Sertraline treatment of major depression in patients with acute MI or unstable angina. *Journal of the American Medical Association, 288*, 701–709.

Glymour, M. M., Maselko, J., Gilman, S. E., Patton, K. K., & Avendano, M. (2010). Depressive symptoms predict incident stroke independently of memory impairments. *Neurology, 75,* 2063–2070.

Go, A. S., Mozaffarian, D., Roger, V. L., Benjamin, E. J., Berry, J. D., Borden, W. B. et al. (2013). Executive summary: Heart disease and stroke statistics—2013 update: A report from the American Heart Association. *Circulation, 127,* 143–152.

Gold, M. S., Pottash, A. L., & Extein, I. (1981). Hypothyroidism and depression: Evidence from complete thyroid function evaluation. *Journal of the American Medical Association, 245,* 1919–1922.

Gonzalez, J. S., Peyrot, M., McCarl, L. A., Collins, E. M., Serpa, L., Mimiaga, M. J., et al. (2008). Depression and diabetes treatment nonadherence: A meta-analysis. *Diabetes Care, 31,* 2398–2403.

Gottlieb, S. S., Kop, W. J., Ellis, S. J., Binkley, P., Howlett, J., O'Connor, C., et al. (2009). Relation of depression to severity of illness in heart failure (from Heart Failure and a Controlled Trial Investigating Outcomes of Exercise Training [HF-ACTION]). *American Journal of Cardiology, 103,* 1285–1289.

Hamilton, N. S., Jackson, G. L., Abbott, D. H., Zullig, L. L., & Provenzale, D. (2011). Use of psychosocial support services among male Veterans Affairs colorectal cancer patients. *Journal of Psychosocial Oncology, 29,* 242–253.

Hart, S. L., Hoyt, M. A., Diefenbach, M., Anderson, D. R., Kilbourn, K. M., Craft, L. L., et al. (2012). Meta-analysis of efficacy of interventions for elevated depressive symptoms in adults diagnosed with cancer. *Journal of the National Cancer Institute, 104,* 990–1004.

Haukka, J., Sankila, R., Klaukka, T., Lonnqvist, J., Niskanen, L., Tanskanen, A., et al. (2010). Incidence of cancer and antidepressant medication: Record linkage study. *International Journal of Cancer, 126,* 285–296.

Hayano, J., Carney, R. M., Watanabe, E., Kawai, K., Kodama, I., Stein, P. K., et al. (2012). Interactive associations of depression and sleep apnea with adverse clinical outcomes after acute myocardial infarction. *Psychosomatic Medicine, 74,* 832–839.

Hays, R. D., Marshall, G. N., Wang, E. Y., & Sherbourne, C. D. (1994). Four-year cross-lagged associations between physical and mental health in the Medical Outcomes Study. *Journal of Consulting and Clinical Psychology, 62,* 441–449.

Hedayati, S. S., Minhajuddin, A. T., Toto, R. D., Morris, D. W., & Rush, A. J. (2009). Prevalence of major depressive episode in CKD. *American Journal of Kidney Diseases, 54,* 424–432.

Hutton, H. E., Lyketsos, C. G., Zenilman, J. M., Thompson, R. E., & Erbelding, E. J. (2004). Depression and HIV risk behaviors among patients in a sexually transmitted disease clinic. *American Journal of Psychiatry, 161,* 912–914.

Iosifescu, D. V., Nierenberg, A. A., Alpert, J. E., Smith, M., Bitran, S., Dording, C., et al. (2003). The impact of medical comorbidity on acute treatment in major depressive disorder. *American Journal of Psychiatry, 160,* 2122–2127.

Jain, N., Trivedi, M. H., Rush, A. J., Carmody, T., Kurian, B., Toto, R. D., et al. (2013). Rationale and design of the Chronic Kidney Disease Antidepressant Sertraline Trial (CAST). *Contemporary Clinical Trials, 34,* 136–144.

Johansson, P., Lesman-Leegte, I., Svensson, E., Voors, A., van Veldhuisen, D. J., & Jaarsma, T. (2011). Depressive symptoms and inflammation in patients hospitalized for heart failure. *American Heart Journal, 161,* 1053–1059.

Katon, W., Lyles, C. R., Parker, M. M., Karter, A. J., Huang, E. S., & Whitmer, R. A. (2012). Association of depression with increased risk of dementia in patients with type 2 diabetes: The Diabetes and Aging Study. *Archives of General Psychiatry, 69,* 410–417.

Katon, W. J., Lin, E. H., Von Korff, M., Ciechanowski, P., Ludman, E. J., Young, B., et al. (2010). Collaborative care for patients with depression and chronic illnesses. *New England Journal of Medicine, 363,* 2611–2620.

Kelly, C. M., Juurlink, D. N., Gomes, T., Duong-Hua, M., Pritchard, K. I., Austin, P. C., et al.

(2010). Selective serotonin reuptake inhibitors and breast cancer mortality in women receiving tamoxifen: A population-based cohort study. *British Medical Journal, 340,* c693.

Koenig, H. G., George, L. K., Peterson, B. L., & Pieper, C. F. (1997). Depression in medically ill hospitalized older adults: Prevalence, characteristics, and course of symptoms according to six diagnostic schemes. *American Journal of Psychiatry, 154,* 1376–1383.

Kohen, R., Cain, K. C., Mitchell, P. H., Becker, K., Buzaitis, A., Millard, S. P., et al. (2008). Association of serotonin transporter gene polymorphisms with poststroke depression. *Archives of General Psychiatry, 65,* 1296–1302.

Lassalle-Lagadec, S., Sibon, I., Dilharreguy, B., Renou, P., Fleury, O., & Allard, M. (2012). Subacute default mode network dysfunction in the prediction of post-stroke depression severity. *Radiology, 264,* 218–224.

Leserman, J., Pence, B. W., Whetten, K., Mugavero, M. J., Thielman, N. M., Swartz, M. S., et al. (2007). Relation of lifetime trauma and depressive symptoms to mortality in HIV. *American Journal of Psychiatry, 164,* 1707–1713.

Lespérance, F., Frasure-Smith, N., Koszycki, D., Laliberte, M. A., van Zyl, L. T., Baker, B., et al. (2007). Effects of citalopram and interpersonal psychotherapy on depression in patients with coronary artery disease: The Canadian Cardiac Randomized Evaluation of Antidepressant and Psychotherapy Efficacy (CREATE) trial. *Journal of the American Medical Association, 297,* 367–379.

Leung, Y. W., Flora, D. B., Gravely, S., Irvine, J., Carney, R. M., & Grace, S. L. (2012). The impact of premorbid and postmorbid depression onset on mortality and cardiac morbidity among patients with coronary heart disease: Meta-analysis. *Psychosomatic Medicine, 74,* 786–801.

Lichtman, J. H., Bigger, J. T., Jr., Blumenthal, J. A., Frasure-Smith, N., Kaufmann, P. G., Lesperance, F., et al. (2008). Depression and coronary heart disease: Recommendations for screening, referral, and treatment: A science advisory from the American Heart Association Prevention Committee of the Council on Cardiovascular Nursing, Council on Clinical Cardiology, Council on Epidemiology and Prevention, and Interdisciplinary Council on Quality of Care and Outcomes Research: Endorsed by the American Psychiatric Association. *Circulation, 118,* 1768–1775.

Lichtman, J. H., Froelicher, E. S., Blumenthal, J. A., Carney, R. M., Doering, L. V., Frasure-Smith, N., et al. (in press). Depression as a risk factor for poor prognosis among patients with acute coronary syndrome: Systematic review and recommendations: A scientific statement from the American Heart Association. *Circulation.*

Loke, Y. K., Brown, J. W., Kwok, C. S., Niruban, A., & Myint, P. K. (2012). Association of obstructive sleep apnea with risk of serious cardiovascular events: A systematic review and meta-analysis. *Circulation. Cardiovascular Quality and Outcomes., 5,* 720–728.

Luppino, F. S., de Wit, L. M., Bouvy, P. F., Stijnen, T., Cuijpers, P., Penninx, B. W., et al. (2010). Overweight, obesity, and depression: A systematic review and meta-analysis of longitudinal studies. *Archives of General Psychiatry, 67,* 220–229.

Lustman, P. J., Anderson, R. J., Freedland, K. E., de Groot, M., Carney, R. M., & Clouse, R. E. (2000). Depression and poor glycemic control: A meta-analytic review of the literature. *Diabetes Care, 23,* 934–942.

Lustman, P. J., Clouse, R. E., Nix, B. D., Freedland, K. E., Rubin, E. H., McGill, J. B., et al. (2006). Sertraline for prevention of depression recurrence in diabetes mellitus: A randomized, double-blind, placebo-controlled trial. *Archives of General Psychiatry, 63,* 521–529.

Lustman, P. J., Freedland, K. E., Griffith, L. S., & Clouse, R. E. (2000). Fluoxetine for depression in diabetes: A randomized double-blind placebo-controlled trial. *Diabetes Care, 23,* 618–623.

Lustman, P. J., Griffith, L. S., Freedland, K. E., Kissel, S. S., & Clouse, R. E. (1998). Cognitive behavior therapy for depression in type 2 diabetes mellitus: A randomized, controlled trial. *Annals of Internal Medicine, 129,* 613–621.

McCaffery, J. M., Frasure-Smith, N., Dube, M. P., Theroux, P., Rouleau, G. A., Duan, Q., et al.

(2006). Common genetic vulnerability to depressive symptoms and coronary artery disease: A review and development of candidate genes related to inflammation and serotonin. *Psychosomatic Medicine, 68*, 187–200.

Meijer, A., Conradi, H. J., Bos, E. H., Thombs, B. D., van Melle, J. P., & de Jonge, P. (2011). Prognostic association of depression following myocardial infarction with mortality and cardiovascular events: A meta-analysis of 25 years of research. *General Hospital Psychiatry, 33*, 203–216.

Meijer, A., Roseman, M., Milette, K., Coyne, J. C., Stefanek, M. E., Ziegelstein, R. C., et al. (2011). Depression screening and patient outcomes in cancer: a systematic review. *PLoS One, 6*, e27181.

Mojtabai, R., & Olfson, M. (2003). Medication costs, adherence, and health outcomes among Medicare beneficiaries. *Health Affairs (Millwood), 22*, 220–229.

Mojtabai, R., & Olfson, M. (2008). National patterns in antidepressant treatment by psychiatrists and general medical providers: Results from the National Comorbidity Survey replication. *Journal of Clinical Psychiatry, 69*, 1064–1074.

Murphy, J. M., Monson, R. R., Olivier, D. C., Zahner, G. E., Sobol, A. M., & Leighton, A. H. (1992). Relations over time between psychiatric and somatic disorders: The Stirling County Study. *American Journal of Epidemiology, 136*, 95–105.

Mykletun, A., Bjerkeset, O., Dewey, M., Prince, M., Overland, S., & Stewart, R. (2007). Anxiety, depression, and cause-specific mortality: The HUNT study. *Psychosomatic Medicine, 69*, 323–331.

Narushima, K., Paradiso, S., Moser, D. J., Jorge, R., & Robinson, R. G. (2007). Effect of antidepressant therapy on executive function after stroke. *British Journal of Psychiatry, 190*, 260–265.

Nemeroff, C. B., Preskorn, S. H., & Devane, C. L. (2007). Antidepressant drug–drug interactions: Clinical relevance and risk management. *CNS Spectrums, 12*, 1–13.

Nouwen, A., Nefs, G., Caramlau, I., Connock, M., Winkley, K., Lloyd, C. E., et al. (2011). Prevalence of depression in individuals with impaired glucose metabolism or undiagnosed diabetes: A systematic review and meta-analysis of the European Depression in Diabetes (EDID) Research Consortium. *Diabetes Care, 34*, 752–762.

Nouwen, A., Winkley, K., Twisk, J., Lloyd, C. E., Peyrot, M., Ismail, K., et al. (2010). Type 2 diabetes mellitus as a risk factor for the onset of depression: A systematic review and meta-analysis. *Diabetologia, 53*, 2480–2486.

Nurutdinova, D., Chrusciel, T., Zeringue, A., Scherrer, J. F., Al-Aly, Z., McDonald, J. R., et al. (2012). Mental health disorders and the risk of AIDS-defining illness and death in HIV-infected veterans. *AIDS, 26*, 229–234.

O'Connor, C. M., Jiang, W., Kuchibhatla, M., Silva, S. G., Cuffe, M. S., Callwood, D. D., et al. (2010). Safety and efficacy of sertraline for depression in patients with heart failure: Results of the SADHART-CHF (Sertraline Against Depression and Heart Disease in Chronic Heart Failure) trial. *Journal of the American College of Cardiology, 56*, 692–699.

O'Connor, C. M., Whellan, D. J., Lee, K. L., Keteyian, S. J., Cooper, L. S., Ellis, S. J., et al. (2009). Efficacy and safety of exercise training in patients with chronic heart failure: HF-ACTION randomized controlled trial. *Journal of the American Medical Association, 301*, 1439–1450.

Pan, A., Keum, N., Okereke, O. I., Sun, Q., Kivimaki, M., Rubin, R. R., et al. (2012). Bidirectional association between depression and metabolic syndrome: A systematic review and meta-analysis of epidemiological studies. *Diabetes Care, 35*, 1171–1180.

Pan, A., Sun, Q., Okereke, O. I., Rexrode, K. M., & Hu, F. B. (2011). Depression and risk of stroke morbidity and mortality: A meta-analysis and systematic review. *Journal of the American Medical Association, 306*, 1241–1249.

Park, H. Y., Lee, B. J., Kim, J. H., Bae, J. N., & Hahm, B. J. (2012). Rapid improvement of depression and quality of life with escitalopram treatment in outpatients with breast cancer: A 12-week, open-label prospective trial. *Progress in Neuro-Psychopharmacology and Biological Psychiatry, 36*, 318–323.

Patten, S. B. (2001). Long-term medical conditions and major depression in a Canadian population study at waves 1 and 2. *Journal of Affective Disorders, 63,* 35–41.

Patten, S. B., Beck, C. A., Kassam, A., Williams, J. V., Barbui, C., & Metz, L. M. (2005). Long-term medical conditions and major depression: Strength of association for specific conditions in the general population. *Canadian Journal of Psychiatry, 50,* 195–202.

Patten, S. B., Williams, J. V., Lavorato, D. H., Khaled, S., & Bulloch, A. G. (2011). Weight gain in relation to major depression and antidepressant medication use. *Journal of Affective Disorders, 134,* 288–293.

Persky, V. W., Kempthorne-Rawson, J., & Shekelle, R. B. (1987). Personality and risk of cancer: 20-year follow-up of the Western Electric Study. *Psychosomatic Medicine, 49,* 435–449.

Pilkonis, P. A., Choi, S. W., Reise, S. P., Stover, A. M., Riley, W. T., & Cella, D. (2011). Item banks for measuring emotional distress from the Patient-Reported Outcomes Measurement Information System (PROMIS(R)): Depression, anxiety, and anger. *Assessment, 18,* 263–283.

Polsky, D., Doshi, J. A., Marcus, S., Oslin, D., Rothbard, A., Thomas, N., et al. (2005). Long-term risk for depressive symptoms after a medical diagnosis. *Archives of Internal Medicine, 165,* 1260–1266.

Preyde, M., Chevalier, P., Hatton-Bauer, J., & Barksey, M. (2010). Exploratory survey of patients' needs and perceptions of psychosocial oncology. *Journal of Psychosocial Oncology, 28,* 320–333.

Radloff, L. S. (1977). The CES-D scale: A self-report depression scale for research in the general population. *Applied Psychological Measurement, 1,* 385–401.

Raikkonen, K., Matthews, K. A., & Kuller, L. H. (2007). Depressive symptoms and stressful life events predict metabolic syndrome among middle-aged women: A comparison of World Health Organization, Adult Treatment Panel III, and International Diabetes Foundation definitions. *Diabetes Care, 30,* 872–877.

Roberts, R. E., Kaplan, G. A., Shema, S. J., & Strawbridge, W. J. (1997). Prevalence and correlates of depression in an aging cohort: The Alameda County Study. *Journals of Gerontology. Series B, Psychological Sciences and Social Sciences, 52,* S252–S258.

Robinson, R. G. (2003). Poststroke depression: Prevalence, diagnosis, treatment, and disease progression. *Biological Psychiatry, 54,* 376–387.

Robinson, R. G., Jorge, R. E., Moser, D. J., Acion, L., Solodkin, A., Small, S. L., et al. (2008). Escitalopram and problem-solving therapy for prevention of poststroke depression: A randomized controlled trial. *Journal of the American Medical Association, 299,* 2391–2400.

Roest, A. M., Carney, R. M., Stein, P. K., Freedland, K. E., Meyer, H., Steinmeyer, B. C., et al. (2012). Obstructive sleep apnea/hypopnea syndrome and poor response to sertraline in patients with coronary heart disease. *Journal of Clinical Psychiatry, 73,* 31–36.

Rollman, B. L., Belnap, B. H., LeMenager, M. S., Mazumdar, S., Houck, P. R., Counihan, P. J., et al. (2009). Telephone-delivered collaborative care for treating post-CABG depression: A randomized controlled trial. *Journal of the American Medical Association, 302,* 2095–2103.

Rollman, B. L., Herbeck, B. B., Mazumdar, S., Houck, P. R., He, F., Alvarez, R. J., et al. (2012). A positive 2-item Patient Health Questionnaire depression screen among hospitalized heart failure patients is associated with elevated 12-month mortality. *Journal of Cardiac Failure, 18,* 238–245.

Roose, S. P., & Miyazaki, M. (2005). Pharmacologic treatment of depression in patients with heart disease. *Psychosomatic Medicine, 67*(Suppl. 1), S54–S57.

Rosenthal, A. D., Ver Halen, N., & Cukor, D. (2012). Depression and nonadherence predict mortality in hemodialysis treated end-stage renal disease patients. *Hemodialysis International, 16,* 387–393.

Rottenberg, J., Yaroslavsky, I., Carney, R. M., Freedland, K. E., George, C. J., Baji, I., et al. (2014). The association between major depressive disorder in childhood and risk factors for cardiovascular disease in adolescence. *Psychosomatic Medicine, 76,* 122–127.

Roy, T., Lloyd, C. E., Pouwer, F., Holt, R. I., & Sartorius, N. (2012). Screening tools used for measuring depression among people with Type 1 and Type 2 diabetes: A systematic review. *Diabetic Medicine, 29*, 164–175.

Salaycik, K. J., Kelly-Hayes, M., Beiser, A., Nguyen, A. H., Brady, S. M., Kase, C. S., et al. (2007). Depressive symptoms and risk of stroke: The Framingham Study. *Stroke, 38*, 16–21.

Satin, J. R., Linden, W., & Phillips, M. J. (2009). Depression as a predictor of disease progression and mortality in cancer patients: A meta-analysis. *Cancer, 115*, 5349–5361.

Serebruany, V. L., Glassman, A. H., Malinin, A. I., Nemeroff, C. B., Musselman, D. L., van Zyl, L. T., et al. (2003). Platelet/endothelial biomarkers in depressed patients treated with the selective serotonin reuptake inhibitor sertraline after acute coronary events: The Sertraline Antidepressant Heart Attack Randomized Trial (SADHART) Platelet Substudy. *Circulation, 108*, 939–944.

Sharafkhaneh, A., Giray, N., Richardson, P., Young, T., & Hirshkowitz, M. (2005). Association of psychiatric disorders and sleep apnea in a large cohort. *Sleep, 28*, 1405–1411.

Skala, J. A., Freedland, K. E., & Carney, R. M. (2005). *Heart disease.* Toronto, Ontario, Canada: Hogrefe & Huber.

Skala, J. A., Freedland, K. E., & Carney, R. M. (2006). Coronary heart disease and depression: A review of recent mechanistic research. *Canadian Journal of Psychiatry, 51*, 738–745.

Smolderen, K. G., Buchanan, D. M., Amin, A. A., Gosch, K., Nugent, K., Riggs, L., et al. (2011). Real-world lessons from the implementation of a depression screening protocol in acute myocardial infarction patients: Implications for the American Heart Association depression screening advisory. *Circulation. Cardiovascular Quality and Outcomes, 4*, 283–292.

Spiegel, D., & Giese-Davis, J. (2003). Depression and cancer: Mechanisms and disease progression. *Biological Psychiatry, 54*, 269–282.

Spitzer, R. L., Kroenke, K., & Williams, J. B. (1999). Validation and utility of a self-report version of PRIME-MD: The PHQ primary care study. Primary Care Evaluation of Mental Disorders. Patient Health Questionnaire. *Journal of the American Medical Association, 282*, 1737–1744.

Stein, M. D., Solomon, D. A., Herman, D. S., Anderson, B. J., & Miller, I. (2003). Depression severity and drug injection HIV risk behaviors. *American Journal of Psychiatry, 160*, 1659–1662.

Sullivan, M. J., Wood, L., Terry, J., Brantley, J., Charles, A., McGee, V., et al. (2009). The Support, Education, and Research in Chronic Heart Failure Study (SEARCH): A mindfulness-based psychoeducational intervention improves depression and clinical symptoms in patients with chronic heart failure. *American Heart Journal, 157*, 84–90.

Tegger, M. K., Crane, H. M., Tapia, K. A., Uldall, K. K., Holte, S. E., & Kitahata, M. M. (2008). The effect of mental illness, substance use, and treatment for depression on the initiation of highly active antiretroviral therapy among HIV-infected individuals. *AIDS Patient Care and STDs, 22*, 233–243.

Teh, C. F., Reynolds, C. F., & Cleary, P. D. (2008). Quality of depression care for people with coincident chronic medical conditions. *General Hospital Psychiatry, 30*, 528–535.

Thombs, B. D., Magyar-Russell, G., Bass, E. B., Stewart, K. J., Tsilidis, K. K., Bush, D. E., et al. (2007). Performance characteristics of depression screening instruments in survivors of acute myocardial infarction: Review of the evidence. *Psychosomatics, 48*, 185–194.

Thombs, B. D., Roseman, M., Coyne, J. C., de Jonge, P., Delisle, V. C., Arthurs, E., et al. (2013). Does evidence support the American Heart Association's recommendation to screen patients for depression in cardiovascular care?: An updated systematic review. *PLoS One, 8*, e52654.

Unutzer, J., Katon, W., Callahan, C. M., Williams, J. W., Jr., Hunkeler, E., Harpole, L., et al. (2002). Collaborative care management of late-life depression in the primary care setting: A randomized controlled trial. *Journal of the American Medical Association, 288*, 2836–2845.

van Dijk, S., van den Beukel, T. O., Dekker, F. W., le Cessie, S., Kaptein, A. A., Honig, A. et al. (2012). Short-term versus long-term effects of depressive symptoms on mortality in patients on dialysis. *Psychosomatic Medicine, 74*, 854–860.

Walker, A. J., Grainge, M., Bates, T. E., & Card, T. R. (2012). Survival of glioma and colorectal cancer patients using tricyclic antidepressants post-diagnosis. *Cancer Causes and Control, 23,* 1959–1964.

Wells, R. D., Day, R. C., Carney, R. M., Freedland, K. E., & Duntley, S. P. (2004). Depression predicts self-reported sleep quality in patients with obstructive sleep apnea. *Psychosomatic Medicine, 66,* 692–697.

Wiles, N., Thomas, L., Abel, A., Ridgway, N., Turner, N., Campbell, J., et al. (2013). Cognitive behavioural therapy as an adjunct to pharmacotherapy for primary care based patients with treatment resistant depression: Results of the CoBalT randomised controlled trial. *Lancet, 381,* 375–384.

Win, S., Parakh, K., Eze-Nliam, C. M., Gottdiener, J. S., Kop, W. J., & Ziegelstein, R. C. (2011). Depressive symptoms, physical inactivity and risk of cardiovascular mortality in older adults: The Cardiovascular Health Study. *Heart, 97,* 500–505.

Wisniewski, S. R., Rush, A. J., Nierenberg, A. A., Gaynes, B. N., Warden, D., Luther, J. F., et al. (2009). Can phase III trial results of antidepressant medications be generalized to clinical practice?: A STAR*D report. *American Journal of Psychiatry, 166,* 599–607.

Wulsin, L. R., Evans, J. C., Vasan, R. S., Murabito, J. M., Kelly-Hayes, M., & Benjamin, E. J. (2005). Depressive symptoms, coronary heart disease, and overall mortality in the Framingham Heart Study. *Psychosomatic Medicine, 67,* 697–702.

Zigmond, A. S., & Snaith, R. P. (1983). The Hospital Anxiety and Depression Scale. *Acta Psychiatrica Scandinavica, 67,* 361–370.

Zuluaga, M. C., Guallar-Castillon, P., Rodriguez-Pascual, C., Conde-Herrera, M., Conthe, P., & Rodriguez-Artalejo, F. (2010). Mechanisms of the association between depressive symptoms and long-term mortality in heart failure. *American Heart Journal, 159,* 231–237.

CHAPTER 8

Features and Course of Bipolar Disorder

ERIC YOUNGSTROM *and* GUILLERMO PEREZ ALGORTA

An adolescent is hospitalized for mania, recovers, and never has another clinically significant mood disturbance. Another person has a manic episode around the same age, and then spends decades battling recurrent, paralyzing depressions and alcoholism. Do they have the same illness? Current classification is based on symptoms, regardless of underlying etiology, and definitions use a polythetic approach, in which two people could meet criteria for the "same" disorder with nonoverlapping sets of symptoms. This creates tremendous heterogeneity within what nominally are cases of the same disorder. Within-disorder heterogeneity reaches its zenith in bipolar disorder (BD), a label encompassing a wide array of clinical presentations and equally complex variations of longitudinal course.

This chapter reviews BD's definition, highlighting the potential impact of changes DSM-5 introduced, then lists associated features, including BD's symptoms, comorbidity, and correlated aspects of functioning. We describe its course, defining key issues such as the distinction between rapid relapse versus mood instability. Measurement issues have slowed progress toward an integrated developmental understanding of BD; we outline them and then delineate three models of longitudinal course, concluding with recommendations for methods likely to accelerate the consolidation of constructs and models of BD.

FEATURES OF BD

The defining features of BD are manic and hypomanic symptoms and episodes. There are a wide variety of associated features, including depressive symptoms, as well as changes in cognition, sleep, and behavioral activity levels. Several different conceptual frameworks have been superimposed on the range of clinical phenomena associated with BD, reviewed later. None to date completely covers the complex range of presentations, nor has any succeeded in demonstrating sharp boundaries with similar conditions.

Mood Symptoms and Episodes

Mania

The diagnosis of BD-I hinges on the presence of a manic episode. Although it previously was called "manic–depressive" illness, DSM-5 (American Psychiatric Association, 2013) and the *International Classification of Diseases* (ICD-10; World Health Organization, 1992) do not require a history of depression. A sizable minority of people experience only mania or hypomania without any depressive episodes (see Johnson, Cuellar, & Peckham, Chapter 17, this volume; Merikangas et al., 2012). The current definition of mania emphasizes an episode in which functioning clearly differs from what is typical for the person, consistent with Kraepelin's (1921) use of episodic presentation to distinguish manic–depression from dementia praecox (schizophrenia). Mania's key feature is a disturbance of mood or energy/activity level, lasting much of the day most days of the week, for at least a week. If the severity warrants psychiatric hospitalization, then the week-duration requirement is waived. DSM-5 specifies that the mood change be *unusually elated or irritable mood that lasts an abnormally long time, and unusual and long-lasting increases in energy and activity, especially focused on a project or goal.* Activity and energy may be easier for people to recognize in themselves than shifts in mood, and the recollection may be less influenced by social desirability, mood congruent recall effects, or cultural factors (Angst et al., 2010). However, the DSM's using *and* instead of *or* makes the definition more narrow, requiring the presence of *both* mood and energy/activity change. This will likely decrease the definition's sensitivity to cases with BD.

Seven additional symptoms also indicate manic episodes: a grandiose sense of self, needing markedly less sleep than usual, getting more talkative and difficult to interrupt, having ideas that seem accelerated or to fly from one topic to another, physical agitation or periods of heightened energy, or taking risks because of the potential excitement or fun with apparent disregard of the possible negative consequences. (DSM-5 criteria omit the statement that these risky activities are often pleasurable.) None is necessary or sufficient for diagnosis of a manic episode. Other symptoms may be associated with mania, although not considered formal diagnostic features of it, such as increased vividness of sensory perception, heightened creativity, impulsivity, and sensation seeking. The symptoms canonized as part of the diagnostic criteria are not a comprehensive description of the manic picture, nor are they limited to features that are specific to the syndrome, adding ambiguity to differential diagnosis.

Hypomania

Hypomanic episodes are manic episodes but with less intensity and with a lower minimum duration. DSM-5 continues to require a 4-day minimum duration for an index episode of hypomania, despite epidemiological and clinical data that people frequently experience 2–3 day hypomanic periods that are still associated with impairment (Angst et al., 2010; Axelson et al., 2006; Youngstrom, Birmaher, & Findling, 2008).

Depression

Depressive episodes and symptoms are often an associated feature of BD. The diagnostic nosology is confusing because patients need never have had a major depressive episode to be diagnosed with BD-I, but BD-II requires lifetime history of at least one major depressive and least one hypomanic episode. Depressive episodes preclude the diagnosis of cyclothymic disorder in DSM-5 (American Psychiatric Association, 2013, p. 139; Criterion C), and they are excluded from most forms of other specified bipolar and related disorders (previously termed "bipolar disorder not otherwise specified" in DSM-IV [American Psychiatric Association, 1994] and most of the extant research). Thus depressive episodes are required, optional, or exclusionary, depending on the specific BD in the current DSM system.

Does the depressed phase of a bipolar illness differ in important respects from unipolar depression? Recurrent depressions, earlier age of onset of depression, acute onset, atypical features—such as hypersomnia and increased appetite, along with interpersonal rejection sensitivity—psychotic features, and poor response to antidepressants all may be associated with bipolar depression (Goodwin & Jamison, 2007). These findings are inconsistent and likely to represent small or medium effect sizes aggregated across studies.

Mixed Mood

DSM-IV (American Psychiatric Association, 1994) defined a mixed episode as meeting full criteria for mania, with at least five of nine symptoms of major depression also occurring much of the day, most days of the week, during the same episode. DSM-5 (American Psychiatric Association, 2013) dropped "mixed" as a separate episode and added a specifier "with mixed features" that could be coded on top of a hypomanic or depressive, as well as a manic, episode. Mixed presentations subsume many clinical pictures, including dysphoric mania and agitated depressions, as well as periods of intense mood lability that oscillate frequently (Kraepelin, 1921; Youngstrom, 2009). Mixed mood may be more common in younger people (Algorta et al., 2011; Birmaher et al., 2006; Kraepelin, 1921), perhaps reflecting immaturity of the emotion regulation centers in the brain (Strakowski et al., 2012).

MOOD CATEGORIES VERSUS CONTINUA

The DSM approach assesses lifetime history of mood episodes and then assembles these into categorical diagnoses. Each is treated as a distinct category; however, their descriptions imply differences in degree of symptom intensity and duration. Studies formally testing whether mood symptoms behave in a more categorical or dimensional manner tend to find more evidence for a dimensional model for both depression (Haslam, Holland, & Kuppens, 2012) and mania (Prisciandaro & Roberts, 2011)—consistent with mood disorders being polygenic (Kelsoe, 2003) and having multiple environmental risk factors (Tsuchiya, Byrne, & Mortensen, 2003). Categorical models arguably have pragmatic advantages in terms of treatment selection, billing, and reimbursement (Helzer, Kraemer, & Krueger, 2006); but models ought to aim for fidelity to the construct under study (Borsboom, 2006).

Dimensional models imply the existence of missing categories in the current classification system, such as mild or moderate depression, falling along the continuum between major depression and mild distress. There are similar gaps in the categorical labels for mixed presentations. Angst (2007) proposed a notation system that concisely summarized the history of most severe mood states for an individual patient, using M = mania, D = major depression, m = hypomania, and d = minor depression; minor depression is not well captured in the DSM system. DSM-5 addressed some prior omissions by changing "mixed features" to a specifier that can be coded on top of mania, hypomania, or major depression, persistent depressive disorder, or mood due to other medical conditions—but not the "other specified bipolar and related disorder" (OS-BRD) definitions. The specifier approach is a partial solution, accommodating the previously problematic cases of mixed hypomania or mixed features on predominantly depressive presentations; but the exclusion of OS-BRD omits what may be the most prevalent form of presentation in both epidemiological (Van Meter, Moreira, & Youngstrom, 2011) and clinical samples (Merikangas & Pato, 2009). Hypomanic–manic and depressive symptoms usually have positive skew or zero inflated distributions, whereas most cases have low scores, and the number with moderate elevations far outnumber those with extreme scores. Figure 8.1 illustrates how the dimensional and categorical approaches label the space of potential mood presentations.

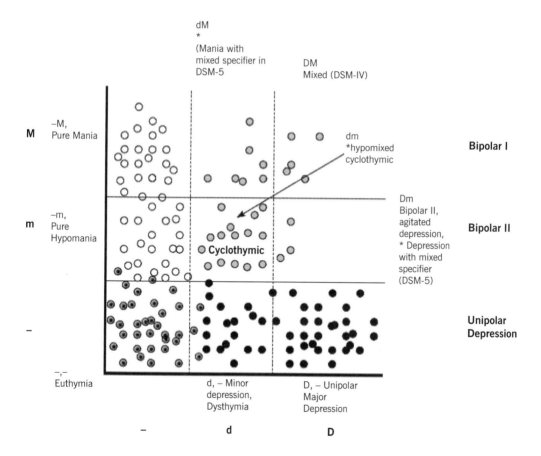

FIGURE 8.1. Mapping a two-dimensional model of mood symptoms onto diagnostic categories for mood episodes and disorders, as well as Angst's taxonomy. *Note.* In Angst's (2007) taxonomy, M, mania; m, hypomania; D, major depression; d, minor depression or dysthymia. This schematic omits issues of duration, which are important both for assigning DSM diagnoses and predicting longitudinal course.

Dimensional Models of BD

What are the major dimensions underlying BD? The simplest model would be that depression and mania are opposite extremes of a single dimension of mood dysfunction. Data strongly refute this, though. Whereas happy and sad emotions might be nearly opposite emotional states, they are almost independent at the trait level. Similarly, the correlation between lifetime depressive symptoms and hypomanic–manic symptoms is low, pulled down by the large number of people experiencing depression without any corresponding history of mood elevation.

Factor analyses of mood symptoms yield mixed results. There are more studies of depression, and they often use larger item pools, increasing the power to detect an underlying dimension. For example, the Young Mania Rating Scale cannot test whether elated mood and irritability represent separate factors contributing to mania because it contains only one elation item and two referring to irritability and aggressive behavior. In contrast, most measures of depression have 17 or more items, potentially allowing identification of four or more robust underlying factors. Analyses of depression tend to find multiple underlying factors, consistent with the methodological advantage of having a larger pool of indicators. Unfortunately, structures rarely replicate across studies. Many studies use an item pool from DSM criteria or the content of established measures. Thus most studies are more accurately described as checking the factor structure of DSM criteria or of a particular instrument rather than the structure of mania or depression per se. This is not an academic distinction: If relevant clinical phenomena are omitted from the diagnostic criteria or the published version of the measure, or if the item pool does not include enough indicators of an underlying factor, then the narrow set of items cannot recover the structure of the broader construct. Analyses with larger item sets have identified additional dimensions underlying both depression and mania, including irritability, psychomotor activation or retardation, and cognitive dysfunction (see Goodwin & Jamison, 2007, Tables 2-9 and 2-10, for summary).

Theories try to impose organization on the riot of disparate findings, and the obstinate data push back. The two-dimensional model of positive affect (PA) and negative affect (NA) got more elaborate as data accumulated about the structure underlying depression and anxiety (Tellegen, Watson, & Clark, 1999). The tripartite model added physiological hyperarousal and summarized the latent structure underlying depression and anxiety based on levels of the three dimensions. Extending the tripartite model to BD, pure mania could be conceptualized as elevated PA and mixed mood states as either simultaneous activation of PA and NA or rapid oscillation between the two. There are few direct empirical tests of this model yet, but anger and irritability pose a major conceptual issue. In two-dimensional models of affect, anger coincides with fear at the nexus of strong negative valence and high activation/arousal. Anger does not follow fear onto the physiological hyperarousal dimension, but it also loads highly on measures of both mania and depression. Physiological studies place anger on an approach dimension, which also saturates a variety of positive emotions (Harmon-Jones & Allen, 1998). Three-dimensional models of affect typically include dominance as a third factor that differentiates anger (high dominance) from fear (low dominance). Dominance is also likely to contribute to the grandiosity, assertiveness, and goal pursuit aspects of mania, as well as irritability and anger when goal pursuit is interrupted (Johnson, Leedom, & Muhtadie, 2012; Youngstrom & Izard, 2008). Measures such as the Positive and Negative Affect Schedule (PANAS) may not adequately tap the dominance construct because they were optimized for assessment of the other two dimensions (Watson & Clark, 1994).

The behavioral inhibition system and behavioral activation system (BIS/BAS) model is another major theoretical model. BIS aligns roughly with NA, or with trait neuroticism and emotional instability in major personality models. By extrapolation, we would expect BIS to positively correlate with depression and anxiety, as well as the depressed or anxious component of mixed mood presentations. BAS is more congruent with the mania dimension. High BAS activation is accruing support as a correlate of mania, and low BAS could conform with the low PA portion of the tripartite model of depression. The BAS model also accounts better for anger and irritability as approach-oriented phenomena. Together, BIS and BAS tell a compelling story about depression, anxiety, and mania, and they offer possible conceptual advantages in linking to neuropsychological and animal models, as well as accommodating irritability and aggression in mania. BAS dysregulation models test whether mania and hypomania can be modeled as disruption of BAS activation thresholds or regulation. Correlations between extant BAS measures and manic symptoms are in the moderate range, indicating that much variance in mania is linked to other factors.

The National Institute of Mental Health (NIMH) Research Domain Criteria (RDoC) offer another dimensional heuristic that may help perceive unifying patterns that cut across diagnoses and levels of analysis (Sanislow et al., 2010). The hope is that a fundamental set of core dimensions can integrate genetic, cellular, circuit, system, behavioral, and interpersonal levels of analysis and delineate processes contributing to multiple forms of psychopathology. RDoC has organized a matrix of several different constructs, including positive valence, negative valence, social dominance, and cognitive functioning (e.g., Robinson et al., 2006; Walshaw, Alloy, & Sabb, 2010), that assimilate many of the constructs relevant to BD.

BD may fundamentally be characterized by instability and change. Rather than residing at a particular set of coordinates in a multivariate map, BD may be a peripatetic condition most notable for its wanderings, sometimes into zones of reckless impulsivity, and other times into overcautious withdrawal; venturing into gregariousness, gambling, and lust, then retreating into tension and torpor. Kraepelin (1921, Figure 20) described manic–depression in terms of oscillations among three major symptom clusters: the intellective (cognitive), volitional (somatic and energy), and emotional. The operational definition of BD may be the high variance on key dimensions—both within a group of cases and also within the same person's life tracked over time—not extremity of mean scores. Examples of larger standard deviations in measures of mood and energy in bipolar groups dot the literature (Lovejoy & Steuerwald, 1995), suggesting that investment in this research definition will be profitable (cf. Trull & Ebner-Priemer, 2013).

Episodic versus Chronic Distinction

Longitudinal course of illness was one of the primary differences between manic–depression and dementia praecox, according to Kraepelin (1921) and contemporaries. Episodic course, with periods of mood disturbance interrupting good functioning, typified manic–depression, whereas a more insidious onset, chronic impairment, and progressively worsening course were more indicative of dementia praecox. Modern conceptualizations of BD also tend to emphasize episodic presentation and change in functioning as ways of differentiating mood disorder from other neurodevelopmental conditions that may have a more chronic presentation (American Psychiatric Association, 2013; Ghaemi et al., 2008). More episodic presentation may predict better response to lithium treatment

(Alda, Grof, Rouleau, Turecki, & Young, 2005). What might seem to be the same symptom based on a snapshot of behavior can have different meaning when viewed unfolding over time. Chronic difficulty concentrating suggests an attention-deficit/hyperactivity disorder (ADHD), whereas episodes would suggest hypomania; continual worry suggests generalized anxiety disorder, whereas distinct patches might indicate mood disorder (American Psychiatric Association, 2013; Youngstrom, Birmaher, & Findling, 2008). Irritable mood has provoked heated debate about pediatric presentations and the boundaries of BD. A narrow definition of pediatric BD tightens the DSM definition by requiring elated mood or grandiosity for diagnosis, whereas the intermediate DSM definition would permit primarily irritable mood with clear change in functioning and supporting manic symptoms. A broad phenotype of pediatric BD would accept primarily irritable mood and an insidious onset or nonepisodic presentation. DSM-5 authors, concerned about the overdiagnosis of pediatric BD, added disruptive mood dysregulation disorder (DMDD), modifying prior research operational definitions. Available evidence suggests that DMDD has different family history, imaging responses, and treatment response than pediatric BD (Leibenluft, 2011; Youngstrom, 2009).

Several findings have blunted episode's sharp edge as a tool for carving BD away from other disorders. Clinical samples have high rates of relapse, often accompanied by partial remission, and high levels of symptomatology between episodes, eroding confidence in the Kraepelinian vision of episodes having clear offset. Schizoaffective disorder challenges the idea that schizophrenia and BD are distinct, suggesting that they may all be on a continuum instead. Genetic and imaging studies find much overlap, blurring boundaries between underlying mechanisms. Frequent comorbidity between BD and anxiety disorders, ADHD, and other conditions that have more chronic presentations grind against efforts to dissect distinct causes. Comorbidity also creates a background camouflage of symptoms against which it is hard to discern the movements of mood disorder.

Affective temperament and cyclothymic disorder further corrode the distinction about episode and clear onset of illness. Multiple questionnaire and interview studies report evidence of affective temperaments, interpreted as biological dispositions toward depression, anxiety, irritability, and hypomania or mania. To an extent, these studies relabel aspects of what others have construed as personality or basic motivational systems. These dimensions show concurrent criterion validity with diagnoses of mood disorder, and they also prospectively predict the onset of new mood episodes. The theoretical problem comes from their chronicity—temperament is by definition a cross-situational individual difference. Cyclothymia is essentially "chronic instability" that lacks clear episodes of mania or major depression, or else the diagnosis would change to a different mood disorder; so there is no episodic touchstone to help guide recognition. It is hard to tease apart the fibers of cyclothymia from other chronic conditions, such as ADHD or anxiety; and if chronic mood instability can grow seamlessly into a full mania or depression, then insidious onset blurs the episodic boundary. More work needs to clarify (1) how affective temperaments overlap with other temperament and personality constructs (cf. Shiner, 1998), (2) whether there are clusters within affective temperaments or whether we should treat them strictly as dimensions, and (3) whether temperament and cyclothymia are best considered diatheses for other mood disorders, general pathology risk factors, prodromes, early stages of illness, or pathological entities (Parker, McCraw, & Fletcher, 2012).

Despite obdurate counterexamples, the chronic-versus-episodic distinction retains considerable heuristic value. In clinical work, asking about episodicity solicits both confirming and disconfirming evidence for a mood diagnosis, and it also informs case conceptualization. Chronic irritability shows differences in course, family history, and neurocognitive performance when compared with episodic irritability in BD.

COMORBIDITIES AND ASSOCIATED FEATURES

Patterns of psychiatric comorbidity look similar among cases with BD drawn from clinical (Goodwin & Jamison, 2007) or epidemiological (Merikangas & Pato, 2009) settings. Comorbidity is also similar between pediatric and adult samples (Youngstrom, Birmaher, & Findling, 2008). BD is one of the most highly comorbid mental illnesses: More than 95% of adults meeting criteria for BD-I or II and more than 75% of those with bipolar spectrum disorders meet criteria for at least one other major mental health diagnosis (Merikangas et al., 2011). Rates are equally high in pediatric clinical samples (Kowatch, Youngstrom, Danielyan, & Findling, 2005). High comorbidity rates suggest a process driving the association, which could be either "artifactual" or "true" comorbidity (Caron & Rutter, 1991). True comorbidity could be the product of shared causal mechanisms—one of the main theses of the RDoC initiative. Developmental sequencing, or heterotypical continuity—such as occurs when a condition presents first as anxiety, then later as depression, and yet later as mania—is another example of true comorbidity.

Organizing the patterns along the lines of major dimensions, BD shows high rates of comorbidity with other disorders involving high NA, including depressive disorders, anxiety disorders, posttraumatic stress disorder, and eating disorders. It also shows high comorbidity with other disorders characterized by marked impulsivity, poor sensitivity to cues of threat, and high reward salience, including ADHD, conduct disorder and antisocial personality disorder, gambling, and substance misuse. BD also shows elevated rates with other psychotic disorders. Differences in rates of comorbidity across samples are principally due to main effects of age and referral pattern, not to a significant interaction between age and BD. For example, younger samples tend to have higher rates of comorbid ADHD in direct proportion to the base rate of ADHD at that age range (Galanter & Leibenluft, 2008). Plausibly, some of the lifetime comorbidity is due to heterotypical continuity as well. Generalized anxiety disorder often precedes major depression developmentally, and other studies find that depression is followed by hypomania or mania in a quarter to a third of cases (Angst et al., 2011; Angst, Gamma, Sellaro, Lavori, & Zhang, 2003; Fiedorowicz et al., 2011).

Personality and Temperament

In addition to the associations with PA, NA, BIS/BAS, and the affective temperament models noted previously, research has documented differences in major personality dimensions associated with BD during periods of euthymia, as well as in the midst of mood episodes. Major findings include low agreeableness (i.e., more hostility), decreased extraversion, increased openness to new experiences, and low conscientiousness but high levels of trait neuroticism or emotional instability (Bagby et al., 1996; Barnett et al., 2011), as well as high trait sensation seeking and impulsivity, measured by performance tests as well as self-report measures (Swann, Dougherty, Pazzaglia, Pham, & Moeller, 2004) . Neuroticism and high trait NA are overlapping if not identical constructs, and low agreeableness dovetails with clinical observations of irritability. Low conscientiousness may interfere with treatment more than any other trait, as the disorganization and chaos of the patient's life lead to forgotten medication doses or missed appointments (Barnett et al., 2011).

Somatic and Medical Correlates

BD is associated with tremendous impairment and premature morbidity, not only because of days lost to mood episodes or increased risk of suicide but also because of much higher rates of cancer, heart disease, and other forms of chronic illness (Gore et al., 2011; Lopez, Mathers, Ezzati, Jamison, & Murray, 2006). Some of the physiological effects could be the product of allostatic load, metabolic effects of medications, or the harmful correlates of poverty and social isolation. But emerging evidence also suggests a direct pathway between metabolic syndrome, inflammatory response, and increased mood and psychotic symptoms (Goldstein, Kemp, Soczynska, & McIntyre, 2009). Trials of anti-inflammatory agents have provided promising initial results (Berk et al., 2008), spurring a rush of interest in exploring metabolic pathways as mechanisms of risk, as well as potential avenues for intervention. Regardless of the ultimate outcome of these trials, it will be helpful to explore conceptualizing BD as a systemic illness involving the whole body and perhaps the extended microbiome, not just the brain.

COURSE OF BD

Duration of Episode

Duration of episode helps separate pathological mood from more typical responses to events (American Psychiatric Association, 2013). Establishing a set threshold can help improve reliability of diagnostic decisions. Duration also has prognostic value: Longer durations augur less crisp response to acute treatment, higher risk of residual symptoms, and greater chance of a subsequent episode also having a long duration (Klein, 2008). Unfortunately, duration has been damnably hard to measure precisely. Prospective efforts have been cumbersome even when people are feeling well, let alone when mood swings to extremes; and retrospection is a hazy lens that is easily retinted by current mood. Insight into one's own hypomania is a tenuous thing at any time (Pini, Dell'Osso, & Amador, 2001), but memory fails faster for past hypomania than for depression or manias that led to incontrovertible events such as hospitalizations or arrests. The lack of strong measurement data means that thresholds rest on clay foundations rather than bedrock.

DSM-Specified Threshold Durations

DSM-5 retained the threshold durations used in DSM-IV. Major depressive episodes need to last a minimum of 2 weeks. The bar for mania still is set at 1 week, with the symptoms present "much of the day, most days," unless they are severe enough to trigger hospitalization. The index episode of hypomania requires 4 consecutive days of mood and energy disturbance, "much of the day, most days." Pervasive depressive episodes (previously called dysthymia) and cyclothymia require durations of 24 months with no more than 2 months symptom free, or at least a year in youths. All of these thresholds represent committee consensus rather than unambiguous boundaries emerging from data. These also are minimal thresholds to establish the presence of an episode that would change diagnosis, not a "typical" length of episode.

Hypomania, cyclothymia, and dysthymia are intrinsically ambiguous. Symptoms cannot be too intense, or they would move into territory claimed by major depression or mania. Cyclothymia's long duration shades imperceptibly into the realm of temperament or chronic conditions. Conversely, hypomania's brevity combined with the stricture that it be a change in functioning—but not too big—make it prone to overdiagnosis or letting instances escape. The preponderance of data indicate that the modal hypomania lasts 2 days, not 4, in youth (Youngstrom, Birmaher, & Findling, 2008), in adult epidemiological samples (Merikangas & Pato, 2009), and in longitudinal follow-up (Angst et al., 2003). Retaining the 4-day threshold improves specificity, avoiding pseudo-bipolar false alarms; but many 2- and 2-day hypomanias are linked with substantial impairment (Axelson et al., 2011; Van Meter, Youngstrom, Youngstrom, Feeny, & Findling, 2011). Keeping the hypomania threshold at 4 consecutive days shifts cases that would otherwise meet criteria for BD-II into the OS-BRD category, adding both to its high prevalence and associated burden.

Definitions of Offset: Treatment Response and Remission

We also need clear terms with precise meaning to describe the ends of episodes. A recent task force of the International Society for Bipolar Disorders published consensus operational definitions for nine terms: *response, remission, recovery, relapse, recurrence, subsyndromal states, predominant polarity, switch,* and *functional outcome* (Tohen et al., 2009). Greater consistency using these terms would help integrate research findings.

Confusion around the term *rapid cycling* provides a cautionary tale. *Rapid cycling* originally referred to rapid recurrence of episodes, entailing at least four distinct mood episodes in the course of a year, demarcated by periods of remission or definite change in predominant polarity (Dunner, Patrick, & Fieve, 1977). Although DSM formally incorporated this definition, usage in clinical practice and many research studies focused more on apparent polarity change than on distinct episodes separated by periods of remission. "Ultradian" cycling (Geller, Tillman, & Bolhofner, 2007)—experiencing highs and lows in the same day—could also be conceptualized as mood lability or instability (MacKinnon & Pies, 2006). Calling it "cycling" blurred the distinction about number of episodes, which has substantial prognostic value with regard to course and treatment response (Youngstrom, Birmaher, & Findling, 2008).

MEASUREMENT ISSUES

Measurement of psychiatric diagnoses and mental health constructs is still imprecise. Many of the standard obstacles are yet more pernicious in the instance of BD.

Reliability Travails

Reliability, or the reproducibility of a diagnosis or score, establishes the upper bound for the validity of any decision or inference based on the variable. Interrater reliability for psychiatric diagnosis fares poorly, with one meta-analysis finding an average κ of .3 when comparing clinical diagnoses with semistructured interviews with the same people, and the κ dropped below .10 when focusing on bipolar diagnoses (Rettew, Lynch, Achenbach, Dumenci, & Ivanova, 2009). When two clinicians use their typical approaches to independently diagnose the same patient, agreement is often even lower (Garb, 1998). The reliability in the DSM-5 field trials ranged from • = .56 for BD-I down to .28 for major depression and .25 for disruptive mood dysregulation disorder (Regier et al., 2013).

Why would the assessment of BDs be worse than for other conditions? Many factors add to the task diagnosticians confront. If the condition is episodic, then the hallmark features will not always be present, and what the clinician observes today may be quite different from the behaviors manifesting 2 weeks ago. Training is inconsistent about the degree and methods used to probe past hypomanic or manic episodes, a procedure that would reveal that the current depression is actually a bipolar illness. Clinicians watching the same video disagree about how manic the patient is, with the country in which they practice explaining a large portion of the variance (Mackin, Targum, Kalali, Rom, & Young, 2006). Clinicians reading the same vignette show literally 100% range of opinion about the probability that the case has a bipolar diagnosis (Jenkins, Youngstrom, Washburn, & Youngstrom, 2011), and favored diagnoses varied significantly according to where the person worked (Dubicka, Carlson, Vail, & Harrington, 2008).

Referral biases and poor insight further obscure the trail of hidden hypomanias. People with hypomania are unlikely to see it as a problem, and the behaviors are not so extreme as to compel intervention by others. There is a powerful distinction between subjective and interpersonal perceptions of manic behaviors, blending the actor–observer bias (Jones & Nisbett, 1971) with differences in the degree of mania required for recognition of the same symptom in oneself versus another (Freeman, Youngstrom, Freeman, Youngstrom, & Findling, 2011). Agreement between parent and youth or adult and partner about manic symptoms typically falls in the low to moderate range (r of .2 to .3; Youngstrom et al., 2004), clinically underwhelming but significant and in line with typical benchmarks for cross-informant ratings of emotional and behavioral problems (Achenbach, McConaughy, & Howell, 1987). Patients are more motivated to seek help when depressed, and they are unlikely to mention past hypomania in their description of the presenting problem. The cognitive heuristics we evolved to deal with complex information quickly can lead us astray in clinical interviews (Garb, 1998): Confirmation bias chases down evidence supporting an initial hypothesis of depression—or antisocial behavior, or schizophrenia, if the presenting problem includes aggression or psychosis. We discount disconfirming evidence, and unstructured interviews do not organize systematic consideration of alternate explanations (Croskerry, 2003). Considering the combined effect of these factors, it is no longer surprising that bipolar is frequently a contentious diagnosis.

Validity Issues

The validity of a diagnosis, or the score on the same rating scale, also will change as a function of the type of informant. The issue is most salient in the assessment of children and adolescents. Young children will not be able to read checklists, and they do not have the same meta-cognitive skills and psychological mindedness that adolescents or adults would. Teachers frequently provide ratings of youth behavior, and they observe the youth in a different social context and with different expectations and standards for comparison than parents would. When any two of these three major sources of information share less than 10% of the variance in their perceptions in common, it calls into question the validity of the diagnosis. What does it mean if a parent insists that the youth was flagrantly manic but the youth and teacher report only modest concerns (Carlson & Youngstrom, 2011)? Mania seems as though it should pervade across situations, obvious to all interested observers.

Across all measures and samples examined to date, the parent report has significantly higher validity coefficients than adolescent self-report or teacher report (Hazell, Carr, Lewin, & Sly, 2003; Youngstrom, Joseph, & Greene, 2008). Yet agreement between parent, teacher, and youth about mood symptoms is significantly better than typical agreement between these dyads about other problems (Youngstrom, Meyers, Youngstrom, Calabrese, & Findling, 2006b). The seeming paradox comes from the effect sizes involved: Typical cross-informant agreement is only modest. It is significantly less modest in cases with BD, though still far short of what would be decisive from the standpoint of making or refuting high-stakes clinical decisions. All perspectives may have a role. Parent report is more sensitive to acute pharmacological treatment effects (e.g., Youngstrom et al., 2013) and relates to imaging and genetic findings; but teacher and youth reports also show distinct behavioral genetic correlates (Bartels et al., 2003), and self-report is a crucial to treatment engagement. The high validity of collateral report about hypomanic symptoms, repeatedly evident in youth data, exposes a major opportunity for research in adults.

Charting Course

Accurate identification of BD hinges on detection of multiple episodes, placing great weight on longitudinal assessment, rather than thorough cross-sectional analysis of the presenting problem. Checklists and interviews are heavily influenced by current mood state, making them less sensitive or even biased in their representation of past events. There are three main designs for charting the course of illness.

Adult retrospective studies begin by evaluating current status and then asking the person to retrospectively describe what he or she remembers about his or her past mood and energy. This is the weakest design from a research perspective and the most vulnerable to forgetting and other reporting biases. It also is the most commonly used format in clinical practice, abetting the almost criminally low reliability of bipolar diagnoses. The validity of information gathered via retrospective methods is improved by using more structured methods, such as semistructured diagnostic interviews and checklists. More ambitious approaches include retrospective life charting methods, using significant events as anchors to orient week-by-week ratings of past functioning (Denicoff et al., 1997). Because retrospective designs are the least expensive, they are the most commonly used. Their shortcomings pervade the extant literature about BD. When these designs indicate that the first episode of bipolar illness is often depression, the caveat is that the methods are especially weak at recording prior hypomania and even moderate mania due to the combined effects of retrospection and lack of insight compromising self-report.

Prospective studies in adulthood also start with careful evaluating of present functioning and then regularly follow up with repeated assessments of mood and energy. The crudest version is the "How have things been going?" query at each treatment session. Upgrades could include using brief checklists or semistructured interviews at each contact, in the same manner as longitudinal research would do at each wave. More intensive approaches include prospective mood charting methods—acquiring daily instead of weekly ratings, actimetry, and using software to monitor light exposure or online activity, among other behavioral traces. The major advantage of these methods is greater sensitivity to mild and moderate fluctuations that might be discounted in retrospective reports. Concerns about antidepressant coincident mania have been inflated by this improved vigilance: The clinician and patient often don't ask and don't tell about prior hypomanias, but then do thorough education about and evaluation of potential subsequent hypomania. The improved assessment leads to better sensitivity, but blinded studies typically find that the rate of treatment-emergent affective switches are not significantly different in the antidepressant versus placebo arms (Joseph, Youngstrom, & Soares, 2009; Licht, Gijsman, Nolen, & Angst, 2008).

The most expensive research design is the prospective study beginning in childhood, particularly if it is enrolling youth in the general population or in enriched, at-risk samples. These designs combine the expense of interviewing multiple informants, often assessing a large number of cases that may never develop BD, with all the usual costs attached to prospective longitudinal work. Due to the costs, these are rare (see Youngstrom & Algorta, 2014, for a review). These generally use similar methods to the adult studies, with the added wrinkle of including caregiver interviews and reports. The lack of self-report rating scales prior to age 11 and the discontinuation of parent reports after age 18 in most studies confounds changes in source with changes due to development. It will be vital to address the confound in future work, perhaps by augmenting with actimetry and other performance measures, as well as adding collateral informants, given that parent and adolescent reports show large differences in sensitivity to hypomanic symptoms. Peer reports could offer a developmentally appropriate collateral perspective in adolescence and young adulthood. Prospective studies starting in childhood have played a valuable role in demonstrating developmental continuity between bipolar presentations in youth and adolescence or early adulthood (Axelson et al., 2011; Geller, Tillman, Bolhofner, & Zimerman, 2008).

These methods are crucial for charting the course of illness, and the most valuable information comes from designs that complement clinical practice by following people even when they do not come to the clinic. Clinical samples face "Berkson's bias" (1946): Those seeking services are not a random sample of all that have the condition, thus confounding associated features and comorbidity estimates. Milder cases are systematically underrepresented. Clinical samples also have the problem of differential attrition. Those who recover do not spontaneously return to a clinic, and they are more likely to withdraw from research; the resulting bias overestimates risk of recurrence and severity of illness course. The field needs a combination of designs that mirror clinical practice, augmented with longitudinal epidemiological studies that inform about community rates of recovery.

THREE LONGITUDINAL COURSE MODELS

Despite more than a century of clinical observation, there is no conclusive support for a single model of the longitudinal course of BD. The measurement issues discussed herein increase the uncertainty. It is likely that all three models are accurate for subsets of cases meeting current criteria for BD, reflecting the heterogeneity of etiology and trajectory in a group in which membership is defined by symptom criteria and imperfect measurement. We cannot yet gauge the relative frequency of each of these models, nor can we yet tell which pathway an individual person might follow. Keeping these models clearly in mind will help refine both research and case formulation.

Progressive Deterioration Model

The dominant narrative is that BD follows a recurrent course with progressive deterioration. In clinical samples, each mood episode appears to increase the odds that there will be another in the future, as well as greater treatment resistance (Scott et al., 2006). The recurrence crescendo could support synaptic kindling (Post, Weiss, & Leverich, 1994), or increased allostatic load as people accumulate more stressors, trauma, and toxin exposure, or pharmacotoxicity due to long-term effects of well-intentioned interventions (Reichart & Nolen, 2004). The bulk of evidence for progressive deterioration has been based on clinical samples, in which selective attrition will exaggerate the degree of persistence and progression. Clinical samples also have a "chicken and egg" problem: Drugs also change the nervous system. How much blame to assign BD versus psychotropic side effects—or to indirect effects via more substance use and trauma exposure—is not yet clear. Proponents of prevention and targeted intervention tend to invoke the progressive deterioration model (Miklowitz & Chang, 2008).

Diathesis–Stress and Reactivity Models

A second model focuses on mood episodes as a reaction to environmental triggers, which could include interpersonal stressors, dietary factors, disruption of circadian rhythms, or other factors. This set of models could subsume the diathesis–stress model, in which genetic or other early biological factors convey a propensity for mood dysregulation but which requires an outside factor to trigger it (Zuckerman, 1999). The diathesis–stress/reactivity model accommodates the data showing high but imperfect concordance for BD in monozygotic twins (Smoller & Finn, 2003), along with the large number of replicated but nonspecific environmental risk factors (Tsuchiya et al., 2003). In theory, diathesis–stress models could support both pharmacological interventions—ostensibly targeting the diathesis—and psychosocial interventions—moderating the environmental factors—potentially also thus changing gene activation. Those preferring the progressive deterioration model point out that subsequent episodes may require fewer environmental precipitants to produce a recurrence; but again, differential attrition in most samples makes it uncertain whether this is an artifact of who keeps returning to the clinic.

Developmentally Limited Model

The most provocative model posits that there might be a group that has mood episodes in youth, then outgrows them and has no recurrences in later life. The developmentally limited model inverts the conventional wisdom about BD, which has framed it as an illness of early adulthood, with less certainty about whether it manifests at younger ages. Evidence for a developmentally limited subtype comes from reanalysis of the follow-up data from two large epidemiological samples, finding that the rate of mania dropped from 6% in the 18- to 24-year-old cohort to 3% when they were followed up at ages 25–29 (Cicero, Epler, & Sher, 2009). Even allowing for differential attrition, many cases may remit and the individuals function well afterward, staying out of view of those working in clinical settings (Cicero et al., 2009).

A developmentally limited form of BD fits with general trends in neurocognitive development, including normative patterns of myelination in the dorsolateral and orbitofrontal cortices and other regions involved in emotion regulation (Gogtay et al., 2007) and changes in socioemotional recognition and interpersonal relations (McClure-Tone, 2009). For a subset of cases, BD could be reframed as a "developmental delay" in emotion regulation, and intervention could be geared to providing temporary scaffolding until adequate maturation occurred. Developmentally limited course holds far greater hope for affected individuals, which sadly means that there are risks to misclassifying people as being on this trajectory when in fact they are still prone to relapse. Ironically, the subgroup that might provide the most information about resilience and recovery is also the group most likely to be systematically missing from clinical data.

CONCLUSIONS AND FUTURE DIRECTIONS

As this chapter makes clear, the elements contributing to BD are not qualitatively different from those involved in normal development. Instead, what constitutes a bipolar "disorder" is a difference in degree of extremity or instability, or situational appropriateness, in emotion regulation and expression, or in sleep pattern or cognition. Greater priority should be given to dimensional approaches to understanding the underpinnings and outgrowths of BD. The complexity of dimensional approaches will be more than offset by their greater fidelity to the phenomena. DSM-5 encouraged dimensional ratings, but it retained a categorical classification system that is largely at odds with the empirical investigations of the boundaries of conditions (Haslam et al., 2012).

More could be done to use dimensional approaches in research and also in clinical applications. Some examples of things that would yield immediate benefits include using continuous scores from rating scales and checklists rather than dichotomizing them. Most popular rating scales, such as the General Behavior Inventory or the Mood Disorder Questionnaire, have algorithms for determining a "screen positive" or "caseness." However, the behavior of these algorithms necessarily changes as a function of the base rate of BD and other conditions in the sample (Kraemer, 1992). Using an algorithm that was optimal in one setting will be less accurate when applied in situations in which the true rate of BD is different (Miller, Johnson, Kwapil, & Carver, 2011; Youngstrom, Meyers, Youngstrom, Calabrese, & Findling, 2006a), and dichotomizing things that have continuous underlying distributions always reduces statistical power and precision of estimation (Cohen, 1983). Other approaches to measuring key dimensions of BD could include using area under the curve as a measure of mood dysregulation and summarizing a long series of daily reports using life-charting methods. Dimensional approaches offer an opportunity to better investigate liminal areas that are not well represented in the current nosology, such as minor depression, mixed hypomania, or short-duration cyclothymia.

The continuity between pathological states and normal functioning makes it vital to investigate the role of temperament and personality. "Affective temperament" models need to be integrated with prevailing models of adult personality, such as the Big Five, as well as linked developmentally to normative temperament models. Shiner (1998) has done outstanding work synthesizing these models, and the RDoC initiative may help spur further reorganization and integration. There are more measures and names for constructs than there are underlying dimensions, and identification of a parsimonious set of dimensions that can be studied developmentally would accelerate progress.

Does temperament represent a diathesis, a prodrome, or an early stage of illness? We do not yet know. Cyclothymia is a case in point: It is conceptualized as either a temperamental style or a long-duration categorical disorder, yet neither model has been rigorously tested. Diathesis and prodrome models are not mutually exclusive, but they make distinct predictions. In diathesis–stress models a stressor is necessary for illness, whereas a prodrome could progress to illness even absent a stressor. Mood episodes can generate new stressors, underscoring the importance of prospective investigation to disentangle associations with ambiguous directionality in cross-sectional data (Hammen, 1992).

Technology is creating new methods for tracking mood and energy in real time. Online mood-charting tools and smart phone applications make it more convenient. The sensors built into smart phones can turn the device into an actimeter, measure light exposure, or track behavioral "scrapings," such as online social media postings, using changes in frequency or content to mark mood shifts (Trull & Ebner-Priemer, 2013). These reduce burden, perhaps requiring no more effort than simply continuing to use the smart phone as normal. Yet these techniques increase generalizability, bypassing major hurdles that block assessments relying on interviews or self-report, such as the lack of insight or social desirability biases. The next decade promises fundamental change in our understanding of BD as we harness new technologies and statistical methods to advance our dimensional approaches to understanding its core processes and their development over a lifetime.

REFERENCES

Achenbach, T. M., McConaughy, S. H., & Howell, C. T. (1987). Child/adolescent behavioral and emotional problems: Implication of cross-informant correlations for situational specificity. *Psychological Bulletin, 101*, 213–232.

Alda, M., Grof, P., Rouleau, G. A., Turecki, G., & Young, L. T. (2005). Investigating responders to lithium prophylaxis as a strategy for mapping susceptibility genes for bipolar disorder. *Progress in Neuro-psychopharmacology and Biological Psychiatry, 29*, 1038–1045.

Algorta, G. P., Youngstrom, E. A., Frazier, T. W., Freeman, A. J., Youngstrom, J. K., & Findling, R. L. (2011). Suicidality in pediatric bipolar disorder: Predictor or outcome of family processes and mixed mood presentation? *Bipolar Disorders, 13*, 76–86.

American Psychiatric Association. (1994). *Diagnostic and statistical manual of mental disorders* (4th ed.). Washington, DC: Author.

American Psychiatric Association. (2013). *Diagnostic and statistical manual of mental disorders* (5th ed.). Arlington, VA: Author.

Angst, J. (2007). The bipolar spectrum. *British Journal of Psychiatry, 190*, 189–191.

Angst, J., Azorin, J. M., Bowden, C. L., Perugi, G., Vieta, E., Gamma, A., et al. (2011). Prevalence and characteristics of undiagnosed bipolar disorders in patients with a major depressive episode: The BRIDGE study. *Archives of General Psychiatry, 68*, 791–798.

Angst, J., Gamma, A., Sellaro, R., Lavori, P. W., & Zhang, H. (2003). Recurrence of bipolar disorders and major depression: A life-long perspective. *European Archives of Psychiatry and Clinical Neuroscience, 253*, 236–240.

Angst, J., Meyer, T. D., Adolfsson, R., Skeppar, P., Carta, M., Benazzi, F., et al. (2010). Hypomania: A transcultural perspective. *World Psychiatry, 9*, 41–49.

Axelson, D. A., Birmaher, B., Strober, M., Gill, M. K., Valeri, S., Chiappetta, L., et al. (2006). Phenomenology of children and adolescents with bipolar spectrum disorders. *Archives of General Psychiatry, 63*, 1139–1148.

Axelson, D. A., Birmaher, B., Strober, M. A., Goldstein, B. I., Ha, W., Gill, M. K., et al. (2011). Course of subthreshold bipolar disorder in youth: Diagnostic progression from bipolar disorder not otherwise specified. *Journal of the American Academy of Child and Adolescent Psychiatry, 50*, 1001–1016.e3.

Bagby, R. M., Young, L. T., Schuller, D. R., Bindseil, K. D., Cooke, R. G., Dickens, S. E., et al. (1996). Bipolar disorder, unipolar depression and the Five-Factor Model of personality. *Journal of Affective Disorders, 41*, 25–32.

Barnett, J. H., Huang, J., Perlis, R. H., Young, M. M., Rosenbaum, J. F., Nierenberg, A. A., et al. (2011). Personality and bipolar disorder: Dissecting state and trait associations between mood and personality. *Psychological Medicine, 41*, 1593–1604.

Bartels, M., Hudziak, J. J., van den Oord, E. J. C. G., van Beijsterveldt, C. E. M., Rietveld, M. J. H., & Boomsma, D. I. (2003). Co-occurrence of aggressive behavior and rule-breaking behavior at age 12: Multi-rater analyses. *Behavior Genetics, 33*, 607–621.

Berk, M., Copolov, D. L., Dean, O., Lu, K., Jeavons, S., Schapkaitz, I., et al. (2008). N-acetyl cysteine for depressive symptoms in bipolar disorder—a double-blind randomized placebo-controlled trial. *Biological Psychiatry, 64*, 468–475.

Berkson, J. (1946). Limitations of the application of fourfold tables to hospital data. *Biometrics Bulletin, 2*, 47–53.

Birmaher, B., Axelson, D., Strober, M., Gill, M. K., Valeri, S., Chiappetta, L., et al. (2006). Clinical course of children and adolescents with bipolar spectrum disorders. *Archives of General Psychiatry, 63*, 175–183.

Borsboom, D. (2006). The attack of the psychometricians. *Psychometrika, 71*, 425–440.

Carlson, G. A., & Youngstrom, E. A. (2011). Two opinions about one child: What's the clinician to do? *Journal of Child and Adolescent Psychopharmacology, 21*, 385–387.

Caron, C., & Rutter, M. (1991). Comorbidity in child psychopathology: Concepts, issues and research strategies. *Journal of Child Psychology and Psychiatry, 32*, 1063–1080.

Cicero, D. C., Epler, A. J., & Sher, K. J. (2009). Are there developmentally limited forms of bipolar disorder? *Journal of Abnormal Psychology, 118*, 431–447.

Cohen, J. (1983). The cost of dichotomization. *Applied Psychological Measurement, 7*, 249–253.

Croskerry, P. (2003). The importance of cognitive errors in diagnosis and strategies to minimize them. *Academic Medicine, 78*, 775–780.

Denicoff, K. D., Smith-Jackson, E. E., Disney, E. R., Suddath, R. L., Leverich, G. S., & Post, R. M. (1997). Preliminary evidence of the reliability and validity of the prospective life-chart methodology (LCM-p). *Journal of Psychiatric Research, 31*, 593–603.

Dubicka, B., Carlson, G. A., Vail, A., & Harrington, R. (2008). Prepubertal mania: Diagnostic differences between U.S. and U.K. clinicians. *European Child and Adolescent Psychiatry, 17*, 153–161.

Dunner, D. L., Patrick, V., & Fieve, R. R. (1977). Rapid cycling manic depressive patients. *Comprehensive Psychiatry, 18*, 561–566.

Fiedorowicz, J. G., Endicott, J., Leon, A. C., Solomon, D. A., Keller, M. B., & Coryell, W. H. (2011). Subthreshold hypomanic symptoms in progression from unipolar major depression to bipolar disorder. *American Journal of Psychiatry, 168*, 40–48.

Freeman, A. J., Youngstrom, E. A., Freeman, M. J., Youngstrom, J. K., & Findling, R. L. (2011). Is caregiver–adolescent disagreement due to differences in thresholds for reporting manic symptoms? *Journal of Child and Adolescent Psychopharmacology, 21*, 425–432.

Galanter, C. A., & Leibenluft, E. (2008). Frontiers between attention deficit hyperactivity disorder and bipolar disorder. *Child and Adolescent Psychiatric Clinics of North America, 17*, 325–346.

Garb, H. N. (1998). *Studying the clinician: Judgment research and psychological assessment.* Washington, DC: American Psychological Association.

Geller, B., Tillman, R., & Bolhofner, K. (2007). Proposed definitions of bipolar I disorder episodes and daily rapid cycling phenomena in preschoolers, school-aged children, adolescents, and adults. *Journal of Child and Adolescent Psychopharmacology, 17*, 217–222.

Geller, B., Tillman, R., Bolhofner, K., & Zimerman, B. (2008). Child bipolar I disorder: Prospective continuity with adult bipolar I disorder; characteristics of second and third episodes; predictors of 8-year outcome. *Archives of General Psychiatry, 65*, 1125–1133.

Ghaemi, S. N., Bauer, M., Cassidy, F., Malhi, G. S., Mitchell, P., Phelps, J., et al. (2008). Diagnostic guidelines for bipolar disorder: a summary of the International Society for Bipolar Disorders Diagnostic Guidelines Task Force Report. *Bipolar Disorders, 10*, 117–128.

Gogtay, N., Ordonez, A., Herman, D. H., Hayashi, K. M., Greenstein, D., Vaituzis, C., et al. (2007). Dynamic mapping of cortical development before and after the onset of pediatric bipolar illness. *Journal of Child Psychology and Psychiatry, 48*, 852–862.

Goldstein, B. I., Kemp, D. E., Soczynska, J. K., & McIntyre, R. S. (2009). Inflammation and the phenomenology, pathophysiology, comorbidity, and treatment of bipolar disorder: A systematic review of the literature. *Journal of Clinical Psychiatry, 70*, 1078–1090.

Goodwin, F. K., & Jamison, K. R. (2007). *Manic-depressive illness* (2nd ed.). New York: Oxford University Press.

Gore, F. M., Bloem, P. J., Patton, G. C., Ferguson, J., Joseph, V., Coffey, C., et al. (2011). Global burden of disease in young people aged 10–24 years: A systematic analysis. *Lancet, 377*, 2093–2102.

Hammen, C. (1992). Cognitive, life stress, and interpersonal approaches to a developmental psychopathology model of depression. *Development and Psychopathology, 4*, 189–206.

Harmon-Jones, E., & Allen, J. J. B. (1998). Anger and frontal brain activity: EEG asymmetry consistent with approach motivation despite negative affective valence. *Journal of Personality and Social Psychology, 74*, 1310–1316.

Haslam, N., Holland, E., & Kuppens, P. (2012). Categories versus dimensions in personality and psychopathology: A quantitative review of taxometric research. *Psychological Medicine, 42*, 903–920.

Hazell, P. L., Carr, V., Lewin, T. J., & Sly, K. (2003). Manic symptoms in young males with ADHD predict functioning but not diagnosis after 6 years. *Journal of the American Academy of Child and Adolescent Psychiatry, 42*, 552–560.

Helzer, J. E., Kraemer, H. C., & Krueger, R. F. (2006). The feasibility and need for dimensional psychiatric diagnoses. *Psychological Medicine, 36*, 1671–1680.

Jenkins, M. M., Youngstrom, E. A., Washburn, J. J., & Youngstrom, J. K. (2011). Evidence-based strategies improve assessment of pediatric bipolar disorder by community practitioners. *Professional Psychology: Research and Practice, 42*, 121–129.

Johnson, S. L., Leedom, L. J., & Muhtadie, L. (2012). The dominance behavioral system and psychopathology: Evidence from self-report, observational, and biological studies. *Psychological Bulletin, 138*, 692–743.

Jones, E. E., & Nisbett, R. E. (1971). *The actor and the observer: Divergent perceptions of the causes of behavior.* New York: General Learning Press.

Joseph, M., Youngstrom, E. A., & Soares, J. C. (2009). Antidepressant-coincident mania in children and adolescents treated with selective serotonin reuptake inhibitors. *Future Neurology, 4*, 87–102.

Kelsoe, J. R. (2003). Arguments for the genetic basis of the bipolar spectrum. *Journal of Affective Disorders, 73*, 183–197.

Klein, D. N. (2008). Classification of depressive disorders in the DSM-V: Proposal for a two-dimension system. *Journal of Abnormal Psychology, 117*, 552–560.

Kowatch, R. A., Youngstrom, E. A., Danielyan, A., & Findling, R. L. (2005). Review and meta-analysis of the phenomenology and clinical characteristics of mania in children and adolescents. *Bipolar Disorders, 7*, 483–496.

Kraemer, H. C. (1992). *Evaluating medical tests: Objective and quantitative guidelines.* Newbury Park, CA: Sage.

Kraepelin, E. (1921). *Manic-depressive insanity and paranoia.* Edinburgh, UK: Livingstone.

Leibenluft, E. (2011). Severe mood dysregulation, irritability, and the diagnostic boundaries of bipolar disorder in youths. *American Journal of Psychiatry, 168*, 129–142.

Licht, R. W., Gijsman, H., Nolen, W. A., & Angst, J. (2008). Are antidepressants safe in the treatment of bipolar depression? A critical evaluation of their potential risk to induce switch into mania or cycle acceleration. *Acta Psychiatrica Scandinavica, 118*, 337–346.

Lopez, A. D., Mathers, C. D., Ezzati, M., Jamison, D. T., & Murray, C. J. (2006). Global and regional burden of disease and risk factors, 2001: Systematic analysis of population health data. *Lancet, 367*, 1747–1757.

Lovejoy, M. C., & Steuerwald, B. L. (1995). Subsyndromal unipolar and bipolar disorders: Comparisons on positive and negative affect. *Journal of Abnormal Psychology, 104*, 381–384.

Mackin, P., Targum, S. D., Kalali, A., Rom, D., & Young, A. H. (2006). Culture and assessment of manic symptoms. *British Journal of Psychiatry, 189*, 379–380.

MacKinnon, D. F., & Pies, R. (2006). Affective instability as rapid cycling: Theoretical and clinical implications for borderline personality and bipolar spectrum disorders. *Bipolar Disorders, 8*, 1–14.

McClure-Tone, E. B. (2009). Socioemotional functioning in bipolar disorder versus typical development: Behavioral and neural differences. *Clinical Psychology: Science and Practice, 16*, 98–113.

Merikangas, K. R., Cui, L., Kattan, G., Carlson, G. A., Youngstrom, E. A., & Angst, J. (2012). Mania with and without depression in a community sample of U.S. adolescents. *Archives of General Psychiatry, 69*, 943–951.

Merikangas, K. R., Jin, R., He, J.-P., Kessler, R. C., Lee, S., Sampson, N. A., et al. (2011). Prevalence and correlates of bipolar spectrum disorder in the World Mental Health Survey Initiative. *Archives of General Psychiatry, 68*, 241–251.

Merikangas, K. R., & Pato, M. (2009). Recent developments in the epidemiology of bipolar disorder in adults and children: Magnitude, correlates, and future directions. *Clinical Psychology: Science and Practice, 16*, 121–133.

Miklowitz, D. J., & Chang, K. D. (2008). Prevention of bipolar disorder in at-risk children: Theoretical assumptions and empirical foundations. *Development and Psychopathology, 20*, 881–897.

Miller, C. J., Johnson, S. L., Kwapil, T. R., & Carver, C. S. (2011). Three studies on self-report scales to detect bipolar disorder. *Journal of Affective Disorders, 128*, 199–210.

Parker, G., McCraw, S., & Fletcher, K. (2012). Cyclothymia. *Depression and Anxiety, 29*(6), 487–494.

Pini, S., Dell'Osso, L., & Amador, X. F. (2001). Insight into illness in schizophrenia, schizoaffective disorder, and mood disorders with psychotic features. *American Journal of Psychiatry, 158*, 122–125.

Post, R. M., Weiss, S. R. B., & Leverich, G. S. (1994). Recurrent affective disorder: Roots in developmental neurobiology and illness progression based on changes in gene expression. *Development and Psychopathology, 6*, 781–813.

Prisciandaro, J. J., & Roberts, J. E. (2011). Evidence for the continuous latent structure of mania in the Epidemiologic Catchment Area from multiple latent structure and construct validation methodologies. *Psychological Medicine, 41*, 575–588.

Regier, D. A., Narrow, W. E., Clarke, D. E., Kraemer, H. C., Kuramoto, S. J., Kuhl, E. A., et al. (2013). DSM-5 field trials in the United States and Canada: Pt. II. Test–retest reliability of selected categorical diagnoses. *American Journal of Psychiatry, 170*(1), 59–70.

Reichart, C. G., & Nolen, W. A. (2004). Earlier onset of bipolar disorder in children by antidepressants or stimulants? An hypothesis. *Journal of Affective Disorders, 78*, 81–84.

Rettew, D. C., Lynch, A. D., Achenbach, T. M., Dumenci, L., & Ivanova, M. Y. (2009). Meta-analyses of agreement between diagnoses made from clinical evaluations and standardized diagnostic interviews. *International Journal of Methods in Psychiatric Research, 18*, 169–184.

Robinson, L. J., Thompson, J. M., Gallagher, P., Goswami, U., Young, A. H., Ferrier, I. N., & Moore, P. B. (2006). A meta-analysis of cognitive deficits in euthymic patients with bipolar disorder. *Journal of Affective Disorders, 93*, 105–115.

Sanislow, C. A., Pine, D. S., Quinn, K. J., Kozak, M. J., Garvey, M. A., Heinssen, R. K., et al. (2010). Developing constructs for psychopathology research: Research domain criteria. *Journal of Abnormal Psychology, 119*, 631–639.

Scott, J., Paykel, E., Morriss, R., Bentall, R., Kinderman, P., Johnson, T., et al. (2006). Cognitive-behavioural therapy for severe and recurrent bipolar disorders: Randomised controlled trial. *British Journal of Psychiatry, 188*, 313–320.

Shiner, R. L. (1998). How shall we speak of children's personalities in middle childhood? A preliminary taxonomy. *Psychological Bulletin, 124*, 308–332.

Smoller, J. W., & Finn, C. T. (2003). Family, twin, and adoption studies of bipolar disorder. *American Journal of Medical Genetics: Part C. Seminars in Medical Genetics, 123C*(1), 48–58.

Strakowski, S. M., Adler, C. M., Almeida, J., Altshuler, L. L., Blumberg, H. P., Chang, K. D., et al. (2012). The functional neuroanatomy of bipolar disorder: A consensus model. *Bipolar Disorders, 14*, 313–325.

Swann, A. C., Dougherty, D. M., Pazzaglia, P. J., Pham, M., & Moeller, F. G. (2004). Impulsivity: A link between bipolar disorder and substance abuse. *Bipolar Disorders, 6*, 204–212.

Tellegen, A., Watson, D., & Clark, L. A. (1999). On the dimensional and hierarchical structure of affect. *Psychological Science, 10*, 297–303.

Tohen, M., Frank, E., Bowden, C. L., Colom, F., Ghaemi, S. N., Yatham, L. N., et al. (2009). The International Society for Bipolar Disorders (ISBD) Task Force report on the nomenclature of course and outcome in bipolar disorders. *Bipolar Disorders, 11*(5), 453–473.

Trull, T. J., & Ebner-Priemer, U. (2013). Ambulatory assessment. *Annual Review of Clinical Psychology, 9*, 151–176.

Tsuchiya, K. J., Byrne, M., & Mortensen, P. B. (2003). Risk factors in relation to an emergence of bipolar disorder: A systematic review. *Bipolar Disorders, 5*, 231–242.

Van Meter, A., Moreira, A. L., & Youngstrom, E. A. (2011). Meta-analysis of epidemiological studies of pediatric bipolar disorder. *Journal of Clinical Psychiatry, 72*, 1250–1256.

Van Meter, A., Youngstrom, E. A., Youngstrom, J. K., Feeny, N. C., & Findling, R. L. (2011). Examining the validity of cyclothymic disorder in a youth sample. *Journal of Affective Disorders, 132*, 55–63.

Walshaw, P. D., Alloy, L. B., & Sabb, F. W. (2010). Executive function in pediatric bipolar disorder and attention-deficit hyperactivity disorder: In search of distinct phenotypic profiles. *Neuropsychology Review, 20*, 103–120.

Watson, D., & Clark, L. A. (1994). *The PANAS-X: Manual for the Positive and Negative Affect Schedule—Expanded Form*. Cedar Rapids: University of Iowa.

World Health Organization. (1992). *The ICD-10 Classification of Mental and Behavioural Disorders: Clinical Descriptions and Diagnostic Guidelines*. London: World Health Organization.

Youngstrom, E., Zhao, J., Mankoski, R., Forbes, R. A., Marcus, R. M., Carson, W., et al. (2013). Clinical significance of treatment effects with aripiprazole versus placebo in a study of manic or mixed episodes associated with pediatric bipolar I disorder. *Journal of Child and Adolescent Psychopharmacology, 23*, 72–79.

Youngstrom, E. A. (2009). Definitional issues in bipolar disorder across the life cycle. *Clinical Psychology: Science and Practice, 16*, 140–160.

Youngstrom, E. A., Birmaher, B., & Findling, R. L. (2008). Pediatric bipolar disorder: Validity, phenomenology, and recommendations for diagnosis. *Bipolar Disorders, 10*, 194–214.

Youngstrom, E. A., Findling, R. L., Calabrese, J. R., Gracious, B. L., Demeter, C., DelPorto Bedoya, D., et al. (2004). Comparing the diagnostic accuracy of six potential screening instruments for bipolar disorder in youths aged 5 to 17 years. *Journal of the American Academy of Child and Adolescent Psychiatry, 43*, 847–858.

Youngstrom, E. A., & Izard, C. E. (2008). Functions of emotions and emotion-related dysfunction. In A. J. Elliot (Ed.), *Handbook of approach and avoidance motivation* (pp. 367–384). New York: Psychology Press.

Youngstrom, E. A., Joseph, M. F., & Greene, J. (2008). Comparing the psychometric properties of multiple teacher report instruments as predictors of bipolar disorder in children and adolescents. *Journal of Clinical Psychology, 64*, 382–401.

Youngstrom, E. A., Meyers, O. I., Youngstrom, J. K., Calabrese, J. R., & Findling, R. L. (2006a). Comparing the effects of sampling designs on the diagnostic accuracy of eight promising screening algorithms for pediatric bipolar disorder. *Biological Psychiatry, 60*, 1013–1019.

Youngstrom, E. A., Meyers, O. I., Youngstrom, J. K., Calabrese, J. R., & Findling, R. L. (2006b). Diagnostic and measurement issues in the assessment of pediatric bipolar disorder: Implications for understanding mood disorder across the life cycle. *Development and Psychopathology, 18*, 989–1021.

Youngstrom, E. A., & Algorta, G. P. (2014). Pediatric bipolar disorder. In E. J. Mash & R. A. Barkley (Eds.), *Child psychopathology* (3rd ed.). New York: Guilford Press.

Zuckerman, M. (1999). *Vulnerability to psychopathology: A biosocial model*. Washington, DC: American Psychological Association.

PART II

VULNERABILITY, RISK, AND MODELS OF DEPRESSION

Many approaches have been taken by theorists in attempts to identify factors involved in the etiology and maintenance of depression. Whereas some of these approaches involve an examination of genetic factors and biological functioning, other approaches focus on personal characteristics of individuals who statistically are vulnerable to depressive episodes and on aspects of the social environments that are posited to increase risk for depression. The nine chapters in this section describe approaches and models developed to explain vulnerability and risk for depressive disorders. Lau, Lester, Hodgson, and Eley (Chapter 9) describe the genetic foundations of depression and discuss studies that have examined specific genes involved in the heritability of this disorder. Continuing with a focus on biological factors in depression, Thase, Hahn, and Berton (Chapter 10) and Pizzagalli and Treadway (Chapter 11) describe biological aspects of depressive disorders. Whereas Thase et al. focus on the role of neurotransmitters in the onset and maintenance of depression, Pizzagalli and Treadway describe neuroanatomical structures and the neural circuits that are increasingly being implicated in this disorder. Goodman and Lusby (Chapter 12) also discuss biological aspects of vulnerability to depression but broaden the focus to include psychosocial factors early in life that appear to increase risk for depression. Gotlib and Colich (Chapter 13) review the growing literature that documents the adverse effects of parental depression on children's functioning, focusing on methodological issues in this research and on mechanisms and mediators of the effects of parental depression on the functioning of their offspring. Joormann and Arditte (Chapter 14) describe the growing body of research examining cognitive models of depression and of risk for this disorder and present findings of recent studies using paradigms adapted from experimental cognitive psychology to assess biases in information processing in depression. Hammen and Shih (Chapter 15) describe aspects of the interpersonal context of depression, presenting research documenting the interpersonal consequences of depression, as well as interpersonal risk factors for this disorder and the possible origins of these vulnerabilities. Monroe, Slavich, and Georgiades (Chapter 16) complement this chapter by adopting a diathesis–stress perspective in examining the social environments of individuals with depression. Finally, Johnson, Cuellar, and Peckham (Chapter 17) discuss biological, social, and psychosocial risk factors and predictors of bipolar disorder.

CHAPTER 9

The Genetics of Mood Disorders

JENNIFER Y. F. LAU, KATHRYN J. LESTER, KAREN HODGSON,
and THALIA C. ELEY

Major depressive disorder (MDD) is remarkably common, disabling, and costly (see Kessler et al., Chapter 1, this volume). Why some individuals develop these debilitating conditions while others remain relatively unscathed by affective symptoms—and why some people get better and others relapse—are questions that have attracted much interest from clinical scientists. In this chapter we focus on how genetic differences can explain individual differences in the risk for depression and can also predict treatment outcomes. We also consider how genetic liability and resilience are expressed through interplay with the environment and with intermediate neural circuits involved in information processing.

THE CASE FOR A GENETIC BASIS OF DEPRESSION: QUANTITATIVE GENETIC STUDIES

Early support for the heritability of depression came from quantitative genetic studies. These studies investigate genetic contributions to behavior by assessing resemblance among different pairs of genetically related individuals. Genetic influences are inferred if the similarity on depression measures across individuals increases as a function of shared genes. For example, finding that first-degree relatives (who share on average 50% of their genes) are more similar than second-degree relatives (who share on average 25% of their genes) in the propensity to experience depression in family studies or that identical twin pairs (who share 100% of their genes) are more concordant for depressive disorder than nonidentical twins (who share on average 50% of their genes) in twin studies indicates genetic influence. In family studies, rates of MDD in first-degree relatives of individuals with depression are elevated compared with those of relatives of healthy controls (see Shih, Belmonte, & Zandi, 2004, for a review), with odds ratios (ORs) of 1.70 to 3.98 (Rice, Harold, & Thapar, 2002; Sullivan, Neale, & Kendler, 2000). Interestingly, the upper end of this range (a nearly fourfold increase in risk for depression) was found for top-down studies only (Rice et al., 2002); that is, those that examined disorder rates in the offspring of parents with depression (rather than in the family members of offspring with depression). The greater transmission of depression from parents to offspring raises questions about whether factors other than genes may also be inherited, such as the rearing environment. This possibility highlights a limitation of family studies: They cannot easily distinguish shared genetic from shared environmental explanations for familiality.

Twin studies partition these confounding influences by comparing the similarity between identical (monozygotic, MZ) and nonidentical (dizygotic, DZ) twins. As MZ twins are genetically more alike than DZ twins but are assumed to share their family or common environment to the same degree, any greater behavioral resemblance among MZ twins is attributed to genetic factors. Any resemblance in MZ twins not due to genetic effects is accounted for by the shared (common) environment, whereas differences between MZ twins are attributed to nonshared (individual specific) environmental contributions. Twin studies suggest that 30–40% of the variance in adult MDD is due to genetics (Shih et al., 2004, Sullivan et al., 2000), with the remaining variance due to the nonshared environment.

Adoption studies draw upon the differential relationships among adoptive family members, biological (birth) family members, and nonadoptive biological (control) family members. Put simply, adoption designs compare behavioral similarity among "environmental" relatives, "genetic" relatives, and "environmental plus genetic" relatives. A handful of adoption studies have explored the genetics of depression (Shih et al., 2004), but only one has reported convincing genetic effects (Wender et al., 1986). However, a more recent study suggests that genetic liabilities may only be expressed in the presence of certain rearing environments (Natsuaki et al., 2010)—a gene–environment interaction, discussed later.

Family, twin, and adoption studies are not without their limitations (see Plomin, DeFries, Knopnik, & Neiderhiser, 2013, for discussion). For example, differences in how the intrauterine environment is experienced by different types of twins and how this might inflate MZ similarity over DZ twins have not gone unnoticed. Nor has the confound that biological mothers pass on certain prenatal environments to their offspring that adopted mothers do not—which could also contribute as a nongenetic factor to similarity among the former dyads but not among the latter. Because there is increasing recognition that prenatal factors can influence early-emerging behavioral and emotional difficulties, newer designs that capitalize on parent–child dyads from assisted conception procedures such as *in vitro* fertilization (IVF) may further dissociate these various sources of influence. For example, one could compare similarity between children and parents conceived through various different IVF methods: homologous (genetically related to both parents), sperm donation (genetically related to mother only), egg donation (genetically related to father only), or embryo donation (genetically related to neither parent; Rice et al., 2009).

Quantitative designs have allowed other questions to be asked concerning the nature of genetic risks on depression. Studies investigating gender differences have reported similar patterns of genetic influence in males and females (Sullivan et al., 2000). Data on age trends suggest that across key developmental transitions such as adolescence—a period associated with heightened vulnerability for the emergence of mood symptoms—new genetic factors come online to influence continuity of symptoms (Kendler, Gardner, & Lichtenstein, 2008; Lau & Eley, 2006). Simple cross-sectional comparisons of heritability estimates suggest a similar magnitude of genetic effects across clinical and community twin samples (Glowinski, Madden, Bucholz, Lynskey, & Heath, 2003). In contrast, however, studies using recurrence of depressive episodes as an index of severity yield higher MDD rates in relatives of probands with recurrent MDD compared with those with single episodes (Sullivan et al., 2000). Finally, data suggest that whereas strong genetic links characterize depression, generalized anxiety, and bipolar affective disorder, genetic ties between depression and other types of anxiety, such as specific phobias and panic disorder, are more tenuous (Kendler, Prescott, Myers, & Neale, 2003; McGuffin et al., 2003).

PROGRESS IN FINDING SPECIFIC GENES FOR DEPRESSION: MOLECULAR GENETIC STUDIES

Liability for depression is likely to arise from the effects of multiple susceptibility genes, each of a small effect that is neither necessary nor sufficient for disease development. Three main strategies have been used to detect these "quantitative trait loci" (QTLs): linkage, candidate–gene association approaches, and genomewide association studies (GWAS). All three compare genetic markers—stretches of DNA that vary between members of a population—either between affected and unaffected family members or between cases and controls. Of note, the different versions of genetic markers are called alleles. Individuals can be homozygous (two copies of the same allele) or heterozygous (different alleles) at a particular locus.

In linkage studies, coinheritance of genetic markers with a disease (or high levels of a phenotypic trait) is investigated in families. A genetic marker is linked to a disease if it is more prevalent among affected than among unaffected family members. However, linkage could occur to markers that are not the susceptibility gene but are located within close proximity. As the probability of recombination decreases for alleles that are positioned closer (i.e., having a lesser chance of crossover of alleles in neighboring loci during meiosis), such alleles will often be coinherited. Thus demonstrating an excess of marker sharing among affected family members within the same broad region of the chromosome helps narrow down the search for the susceptibility genes to a particular region. Linkage methods often rely on systematic investigation of a large number of markers uniformly distributed throughout the entire genome and can be very powerful in detecting disease-associated variants across large genomic distances. However, these methods are better suited to diseases resulting from a small number of genetic variants, each of large effect, in which the presence or absence of a single variant is likely to drive the presence or absence of disease for an individual within a high-risk family.

Although three main genomic regions have been implicated at chromosomes 3p25–26, 12q22–24 and 15q25–26 across genomewide linkage studies, these have not been replicated robustly. This may be due to different analysis methodology and use of different phenotypic definitions of depression. A key issue is lack of statistical power in many studies used to detect signals. It has been estimated that around 1,000 affected sibling pairs are required to detect a single locus that causes a 25–30% MDD risk increase for siblings (Hauser, Boehnke, Guo, & Risch, 1996). Only two studies have come close to this sample size. In the initial report from GenRED, a genomewide significant association with the 15q25–26 region was found in their sample of 297 families with recurrent early-onset MDD (Holmans et al., 2004). However, when an additional 359 families were recruited in wave 2, this signal was attenuated (Holmans et al., 2007). The region was investigated in further detail in a companion article, and with fine mapping (where 88 single-nucleotide polymorphisms [SNPs] within the region were genotyped), the signal became highly significant at a genomewide level (Levinson et al., 2007). The authors proposed that this area contained either one single locus that increases sibling MDD risk by around 20% or multiple loci of smaller effect. In the first report of the Depression Network (DeNT) sample of 417 families, suggestive signals were also observed in the same 15q region, along with signals at 1p, 12q, and 13q locations (McGuffin et al., 2005). However, as seen in the GenRED study, in a final report from the DeNT sample (combining wave 1 and wave 2 data, to give a total of 839 families), these regions showed no strong evidence of linkage (Breen et al., 2011). Nevertheless, when the analysis was restricted to patients with more severe forms of recurrent MDD, a genomewide significant association in the 3p25-26 region was observed and subsequently replicated in a closely overlapping location in an independent sample (Pergadia et al., 2011).

Association studies also aim to identify genetic markers but at more precise locations. Association studies document relations between allelic markers and susceptibility to a disorder in unrelated individuals. In some studies, frequencies of genetic markers are compared in affected individuals (cases) and unaffected individuals (controls), whereas in others, phenotypic behaviors are compared across individuals with different genotypes. As these studies involve simple group comparisons, care is needed to match groups in terms of potential confounders. One of these is population stratification, in which other sources of genetic variability, such as ethnicity, may spuriously account for group differences in terms of allelic frequencies. To minimize these confounds, studies have focused on one ethnic group and/or controlled for variation relating to ancestry in analyses (Price et al., 2006).

Association studies often focus on candidate genes where prior knowledge targets allelic markers thought to influence variation in a relevant neurobiological system. But the literature on significant gene associations with depression is extremely inconsistent. One reason for this is that effect sizes in MDD are anticipated to be small. As such, much larger samples of cases and controls are required to achieve adequate statistical power. Many studies undertaking candidate gene research have been grossly underpowered. This issue has been addressed by the use of meta-analyses, in which the data from a number of different studies are pulled together. These show that the literature is focused on a small number of "favorite" candidate genes, with only 6% of genes being considered in three or more independent studies (López-León et al., 2007), and, of those for which sufficient replication attempts were available (20 genes), only a quarter were significantly associated with MDD. These were *APOE, GNB3, MTHFR, SLC6A3,* and *SLC6A4*. Another problem that could be affecting low replication rates is publication bias, through which positive associations are more likely to be published than null results, with smaller studies being particularly vulnerable (Bosker et al., 2011). Finally, our ability to select appropriate candidate genes is also constrained by a lack of understanding of the pathological processes involved in depression.

The complementary strengths offered by linkage and association, notably the systematic yet hypothesis-free nature of linkage studies, combined with better localization of DNA polymorphisms in candidate-gene association studies, have given rise to GWAS. GWAS have been made possible by microarray technology, by which genotyping is performed at 500,000 to upward of 1 million SNPs, capturing the majority of common genetic variation. Yet performing over 500,000 tests of association confers a massive multiple-hypothesis testing burden. To protect against Type I errors, it is necessary to impose a stringent significance threshold so that conventionally $p < 5 \times 10^{-8}$ is considered a statistically significant result (Dudbridge & Gusnanto, 2008), whereas a threshold of $p < 5 \times 10^{-6}$ indicates a "suggestive" hit. These thresholds consider not only the number of SNPs tested but also the local correlation (linkage disequilibrium) that is seen between SNPs. These stringent thresholds of genomewide significance and the small genetic effect sizes predicted mean that power to detect association is a critical issue in GWAS. Thus collection of very large cohorts is imperative and has led to formation of large consortia.

The largest MDD GWAS to date was completed by the Psychiatric GWAS Consortium (PGC). Data collated from nine GWAS included 9,240 cases and 9,519 controls (MDD Working Group of the PGC, 2013) in a discovery phase. The top hits were then evaluated in a replication phase drawing from seven independent samples (including 6,783 cases). No genetic variants have yet reached genomewide significance. Despite this, there is evidence that the genetic information captured in GWAS does play an important role in liability to MDD (Lubke et al., 2012). In a study estimating the proportion of phenotypic variance that can be explained by the SNPs genotyped on a GWAS microarray chip, genomewide SNP data explained 28–32% of the variance in MDD liability, comparing favorably with estimates from twin studies.

UNDERSTANDING GENE ACTION: GENE–ENVIRONMENT INTERPLAY

The study of gene–environment interplay has informed questions about genetic risk mechanisms by examining how genetic factors influence exposure to the environment (gene–environment correlation [rGE]), how genetic factors influence responsivity to the environment (gene–environment interaction [G × E]), and how environmental factors can induce chemical changes that influence expression of genes on behavioral outcomes (epigenetics).

Gene–Environment Correlation

Correlations between genes and the environment arise when the number of individuals carrying a particular genotype (genotypic frequencies) is not randomly distributed across levels of environmental risk (e.g., parents' educational background) but rather occur more frequently within a certain environmental stratum (e.g., low parental education). Conceptually, rGE occurs when genetic factors influence exposure to an environmental condition. This effect can arise through three processes (Scarr & McCartney, 1983). Passive rGE comes about when the effects of parental genotype are related to the family environments children are exposed to. For example, children of gifted musicians both inherit genes that influence musical talent and experience early exposure to music in childhood. Evocative rGE occurs when individuals elicit reactions from others consistent with their genetic propensities. Thus the same offspring of gifted musicians who perform well in music classes may be more likely to draw the attention of their music teachers at school. Finally, active rGE occurs when individuals select, create, and modify their environmental experiences based on genetic dispositions. Thus offspring of gifted musicians may be more likely to seek out activities that nurture developing musical abilities, such as participation in an orchestra.

Quantitative genetic designs have yielded genetic effects on many environmental measures, including life events (Kendler & Karkowski-Shuman, 1997); family relationships (Jacobson & Rowe, 1999); parenting and parent–child interactions assessed by questionnaires (Lau, Rijsdijk, & Eley, 2006) and observation (O'Connor, Hetherington, Reiss, & Plomin, 1995); across mothers (Neiderhiser et al., 2004) and fathers (Neiderhiser,

Reiss, Lichtenstein, Spotts, & Ganiban, 2007); marital quality (Spotts et al., 2004) and divorce (O'Connor, Caspi, DeFries, & Plomin, 2000); social support (Agrawal, Jacobson, Prescott, & Kendler, 2002) and peer relationships (Iervolino et al., 2002); and job-related stress (Middeldorp, Cath, & Boomsma, 2006). In many of these studies, genetic risks on environmental measures also overlap with those for depressive symptoms. A few studies have begun to search for genes for some of these environmental measures. Burt (2008) measured popularity among peers and showed that men carrying at least one copy of the G allele located in the serotonin transporter receptor 2A (5-HT2A) gene received higher sociometric ratings from their peers than did men carrying two copies of the A allele. These findings, although intriguing, suffer from the same criticisms as those of candidate-gene studies of behavior but could benefit from better measures of the phenotype under study (i.e., the environment) to minimize problems of nonreplication.

Gene–Environment Interactions

Interactions arise when the effects of one variable on an outcome measure vary at different levels of another variable. G × E interactions occur when genetic factors influence responsivity to the environment or when environmental factors "trigger" or "inhibit" genetic diatheses.

Early support for G × E relied on quantitative genetic designs, comparing responses to naturally occurring environmental events across family members who were at high genetic risk with those who were defined as low in genetic risk. High genetic risk can be inferred from the genetic relationship with individuals with depression, whereas low genetic risk can be inferred from the genetic relationship to psychiatrically healthy (or low-depression-scoring) individuals. In twin studies, DZ twins who have a cotwin with depression are defined as having a lower genetic risk than MZ twins whose cotwins have MDD. These studies are generally consistent in finding that genetic risk predicts the likelihood of developing or reporting depressive symptoms only following acute life events (Kendler et al., 1995) or chronic stressors (Eley et al., 2004). That is, the effects of these stressors on subsequent depressive symptoms are greatest among those defined as at high genetic risk. Other studies have examined the degree to which estimated heritability for depression changes across levels of an environmental factor. Most data suggest that genetic effects increase with higher levels of stress, including negative life events (Lau & Eley, 2008b), family conflict (Rice, Harold, Shelton, & Thapar, 2006), negative parenting (Lau & Eley, 2008b), and, in adult women, the absence of a marriage-like relationship (Heath, Eaves, & Martin, 1998). Presumably in these studies, social stressors may trigger latent genetic risks.

A groundbreaking study investigated interactions between a specific genetic polymorphism found in the serotonin transporter gene (5-HTTLPR) and stressful life events on depression (Caspi et al., 2003). The effects of stressful life events on depression symptoms were significantly stronger among individuals carrying one or two copies of the short form of the allele. The short allele also enhanced the longitudinal effects of childhood maltreatment on adult depression symptoms, showing that the moderation effects apply to distal stressors, too. Results of this study have inspired a new wave of investigations focusing on this candidate gene and its interaction with social stressors. However, these effects have been controversial, with some meta-analyses painting a rather pessimistic picture of nonreplications (Chipman et al., 2007; Munafo, Durrant, Lewis, & Flint, 2009; Risch et al., 2009) and attributing previously reported positive results to little more than chance findings. However, others, taking a less selective approach to the papers included, find support of the effect (Karg, Burmeister, Shedden, & Sen, 2011). Given the large sample sizes required for demonstrating main effects of genes on a phenotype, it is perhaps not surprising that finding interactions is even more challenging. One clear finding to emerge from the literature is that the effect may be sensitive to certain characteristics of the data, such as age and gender of the sample (Uher & McGuffin, 2008). Furthermore, it appears that studies that use highest quality measures of the environment are those that show the interaction. Overall, it appears likely that this is a genuine effect, but it is small and very sensitive to measurement issues.

A recent suggestion is that the same genetic polymorphisms that enhance risks for depressive symptoms under conditions of environmental risk also enhance resilience against symptoms when exposed to positive environments. This "differential susceptibility" framework has gained momentum following a review of prior G × E findings (van IJzendoorn, Belsky, & Bakermans-Kranenburg, 2012) and has led to the view that certain genes should be considered "plasticity" genes rather than "vulnerability" genes given that these appear to enhance susceptibility to the environment.

Epigenetics

Epigenetic processes modify the quantity, location, and timing of gene products (proteins) through chemically modulated "marks" on DNA transcriptional activity. These chemical changes likely involve cytosine methylation (where methyl groups are attached directly to cytosine bases in DNA) and histone modifications (where the histone proteins around which DNA is wrapped are methylated, phosphorylated or acetylated), both of which are associated with gene silencing and lowering of gene expression (see Mill & Petronis, 2007, for further details). Because early environmental factors can trigger epigenetic processes (along with hormones and random cellular factors), there has been growing interest in how early adverse environments can modulate gene expression of key neurophysiological systems to shape emergent emotional behaviors and phenotypes such as depression (Meaney & Szyf, 2005).

The earliest set of studies showing that epigenetics can explain variation in depressive-like behaviors were based on an established observation, notably that normal variations in maternal care, such as degree of licking and grooming and arch-backed nursing in rats, influenced behavioral and physiological indices of stress reactivity in the pups (Meaney, 2001). A crucial discovery, however, was that these effects were found to be mediated through epigenetic processes (Fish et al., 2004) that resulted in sustained changes in hippocampal glucocorticoid receptor mRNA expression, enhanced glucocorticoid negative feedback sensitivity, and decreased hypothalamic CRH mRNA levels (Caldji, Diorio, & Meaney, 2000; Caldji, Francis, Sharma, Plotsky, & Meaney, 2000).

Other groups have also reported that other environmental factors can leave methyl marks on other genes. For example, brief separation of mouse pups from their mothers reduced methylation of an important regulatory region that affected expression of the arginine vasopressin gene (Murgatroyd & Spengler, 2011). Arginine vasopressin is a hormone thought to modulate social behavior. In other studies, abusive caregiving environments administered to rats resulted in persistent changes in the methylation of brain-derived neurotrophic factor (BDNF) DNA, which affected expression of this growth factor in the adult prefrontal cortex (Roth, Lubin, Funk, & Sweatt, 2009). Although human equivalents of these studies have been limited (due mainly to reliance on postmortem tissue upon which to study the role of epigenetic processes in human behavior), at least two studies have reported epigenetic differences in a neuron-specific glucocorticoid receptor (NR3C1) promoter in suicide victims with and without a history of childhood maltreatment and controls (Labonte et al., 2012; McGowan et al., 2009)—and others using methyl marks assayed from peripheral DNA have shown that childhood abuse is associated with increased methylation of the promoter region of the serotonin transporter gene (although these findings do not withstand correction for multiple comparisons; Beach, Brody, Todorov, Gunter, & Philibert, 2010, 2011; Vijayendran, Beach, Plume, Brody, & Philibert, 2012). Together, these studies provide a molecular "genomic imprinting" mechanism that complements long-standing associations between early environments such as parent–child relationships and developmental outcomes of maladaptive emotional behavior (Ainsworth, Boston, Bowlby, & Rosenbluth, 1956).

Understanding Gene Action: The Search for Biomarkers

Biomarkers (also known as endophenotypes) are vulnerability traits thought to be more proximal and therefore more directly influenced by the genes relevant to a behavioral disorder than are its signs and symptoms. The search for biomarkers has become important for molecular geneticists, as use of these in gene-finding studies rather than behavioral measures may increase statistical power for the detection of susceptibility genes in two ways. First, as biomarkers fall upstream to the products of gene expression but downstream from the clinical phenotype, these may reflect more simplistic genetic phenomena. Second, as numerous routes to the same behavioral phenotype are likely, identifying subsamples on the basis of biomarkers may create more homogenous samples for gene-finding studies.

One of the first reviews of biomarkers for MDD discussed possible neurobiological and psychological/cognitive factors as genetic mediators (Hasler, Drevets, Manji, & Charney, 2004). Although many of these were clearly associated with depression, the biggest problem lay in establishing whether these reflected genetic (or even familial) influences or whether they were driven by environmental exposure. Given this gap, there has been an expansion of work assessing linkages between gene variants and patterns of brain activation but also with cognitive measures of information processing. These studies make use of candidate-gene association approaches in tandem with imaging tools such as magnetic resonance imaging (MRI) and positron emission tomography (PET) scans, as well as experimental tasks of information processing.

The first wave of "imaging genetics" data reported an association between the serotonin transporter gene (5-HTTLPR) variants and amygdala activity assayed during the presentation of fearful and angry faces in a face-matching task (Hariri et al., 2002). Individuals with at least one copy of the short variant of the polymorphism showed greater activation in the right amygdala when viewing negative face emotions. Moreover, genotype differences on brain activity occurred without differences in task performance, implying that gene variants directly modulated brain function rather than by driving differences in behavior. There have been several attempts at replication, and conclusions drawn from meta-analyses of these gene–brain associations have been more positive than those drawn from gene–behavior and gene–environment behavior linkage data (Munafo, Brown, & Hariri, 2008). Nevertheless, uneasy tension exists over issues of sample size; whereas imaging studies typically involve 40–50 participants, far larger numbers are required for molecular genetic studies to address concerns over power. Given huge costs of imaging studies, this has not been easy to achieve. Regardless, a number of imaging phenotypes relevant to depression have been unveiled (Savitz & Drevets, 2009). These include: increased activity of the subgenual anterior cingulate cortex and reduced connectivity between this region and the amygdala; hippocampal volume loss and gray-matter volume loss in the anterior cingulate cortex; and, from PET scans, decreased *5-HT(1A)* binding potential in the raphe, medial temporal lobe, and medial prefrontal cortex and altered binding potential of the serotonin transporter.

Fewer psychological markers have been identified. Quantitative genetic studies have focused on personality traits, such as neuroticism and harm avoidance (Fanous, Gardner, Prescott, Cancro, & Kendler, 2002; Farmer et al., 2002) and on information-processing characteristics such as emotion recognition (Lau et al., 2009) and fear learning (Hettema, Annas, Neale, Kendler, & Fredrikson, 2003), attributional style (Lau & Eley, 2008a), and social cognition (Gregory et al., 2007). The paucity of research in this area is most likely due to increased measurement errors associated with experimental methods (Brown et al., 2014). These design-related artifacts may artificially change the magnitude of twin correlations, affecting the interpretability of results, particularly those of null heritability but large nonshared environmental effects (Lau et al., 2012). Efforts aimed at identifying cognitive phenotypes for genetic research have also started to employ molecular genetic methods. These studies report promising associations between variants of the serotonin transporter gene and attention-orienting biases for threat (Armbruster et al., 2009; Fox, Ridgewell, & Ashwin, 2009), but they require further replication.

GENETICS OF TREATMENT

Over 50% of patients with depression fail to respond adequately to the first antidepressant they are prescribed (Trivedi et al., 2006; see Gitlin, Chapter 26, this volume), and approximately 40% of people retain significant impairments following cognitive-behavioral therapy (CBT; DeRubeis et al., 2005; see Hollon & Dimidjian, Chapter 27, this volume). Yet there has been limited progress in identifying robust predictors of treatment response despite the potential for improved patient outcomes, substantial cost and time savings, and a shift toward individualized treatment approaches. A recent focus is investigating genetic factors as a potential source of individual differences in response to treatment for depression. It may be that the same genetic and environmental factors implicated in the origins of depression are also involved in differential responses to treatment (Uher, 2008). The interaction between genotype and response to antidepressants or psychological therapy represents a special case of G × E (Uher, 2011) and provides an elegant test of the vantage sensitivity concept, which refers specifically to the "bright side" of the differential susceptibility hypothesis that individuals will vary in the extent to which they gain benefit from positive environments (Pluess & Belsky, 2012).

A considerable body of research exists investigating genetic predictors of response to pharmacological treatments for mood disorders. Carriers of one or more copies of the high-expression L allele of the *5-HTTLPR* may be more likely to respond to selective serotonin reuptake inhibitors (SSRIs) but not tricyclic antidepressants (Kato & Serretti, 2010). However, this effect has failed to replicate in several large datasets, including the Sequenced Treatment Alternatives to Relieve Depression (STAR*D) study, and, overall, a meta-analysis reported a nonsignificant association (Taylor, Sen, & Bhagwagar, 2010). Significant associations with improved antidepressant response have also been reported with the TT genotype at rs1360780 in *FKBP5* (Binder et al., 2004); however, a meta-analysis reported overall negative results (Zou, Wang, et al., 2010). Similarly, the Met allele of *BDNF* and variation in *CRHR1* and *NR3C1*, genes encoding components of the hypothalamic–pituitary–adrenocortical (HPA) axis, have all been associated with a better response to antidepressant medication (Kato & Serretti, 2010; Licinio et al., 2004; Liu et al., 2007; Uher et al., 2009; Zou, Ye, et al., 2010). However, as with the *5-HTTLPR*, the strength of associations has been weak, and the replicability of candidate gene pharmacogenetic associations has been disappointing. Yet, despite this, GWAS are under way and have so far reported a small number of plausible but as yet unreplicated hits. Moreover, it is reassuring that recently developed analytical methods have estimated that common genetic polymorphisms on a GWAS microarray explain approximately 42% of the variance in antidepressant response (Tansey et al., 2013). As next-generation sequencing methods become increasingly affordable, higher density genotyping may also identify other rare genetic variants.

Only a few studies have investigated genetic predictors of individual differences in response to psychological treatments (Eley et al., 2012). "Therapygenetics" is very much in its infancy, and this is apparent in the small, highly heterogeneous and preliminary nature of the studies published thus far. The majority of research has investigated response to psychological treatments for anxiety disorders, with only a handful of studies investigating depressive disorders (for a review, see Lester & Eley, 2013). All studies have used a candidate gene approach focusing on variants within the serotonergic system with the *5-HTTLPR* being the most widely assessed polymorphism. The low-expression SS genotype of the *5-HTTLPR* was associated with a larger reduction in depression scores in response to a brief problem-solving intervention plus concurrent antidepressant regimen in a sample of clinically depressed older adults after ischemic stroke (Kohen et al., 2011). However, a second study failed to find any association with *5-HTTLPR* genotype and time to recurrence following a brief course of CBT in individuals with recurrent depression (Bockting, Mocking, Lok, Koeter, & Schene, 2012). The contradictory findings observed for the *5-HTTLPR* are also reflected in the anxiety literature, with one study reporting an association between SS genotype carriers and improved response to CBT for child anxiety disorders (Eley et al., 2012), a second study reporting an association between the SS genotype and fewer treatment gains in patients undergoing exposure-based CBT for PTSD (Bryant et al., 2010), and five studies reporting no significant association (Furmark et al., 2010; Hedman et al., 2012; Lonsdorf et al., 2010; Sakolsky et al., 2011; Wang et al., 2009). Small sample sizes, varying clinical phenotypes, and the role of medication may explain mixed results.

Significant associations with improved treatment response and greater likelihood of remission of depression have also been reported in carriers of one or more copies of the 12 repeat alleles of the *STin2* VNTR of the *5-HTT* gene (Kohen et al., 2011). This result is in contrast to those reported in some studies for response to SSRIs, which have found poorer remission rates for major depression in 12/12 genotype carriers (Mrazek et al., 2009). This suggests a potential interesting double dissociation between response to psychological and pharmacological treatment modalities. Likewise, carriers of the G allele at rs7997012 in the *HTR2A* gene had a significantly larger reduction in depression symptom scores to CBT for unipolar depression than AA homozygotes (Kotte, McQuaid, & Kelsoe, 2007). In contrast, AA homozygotes had a reduction in risk of nonresponse to SSRIs compared with GG homozygote carriers in the STAR*D sample (McMahon et al., 2006; Paddock et al., 2007). These early therapygenetics research findings require replication in adequately powered samples, but they serve to open up exciting avenues for future research in this field.

Concluding Remarks and Future Directions

Understanding the genetic basis of depression has never been more exciting. Here, we focus on three avenues in which research efforts could be directed. First, although there has been disappointment over identification of susceptibility genes, efforts are now being directed toward GWAS. By comparing what we know about the relative prevalence of schizophrenia and MDD, in order to replicate the success of GWAS in schizophrenia (in which a number of genomewide significant hits have been identified), it has been suggested that sample sizes in MDD will need to be much larger. This creates an impetus for mega-analytic attempts to pool data across multiple sites. To this end, search for biomarkers both at the neurobiological and psychological level may be important for identifying subtypes for genetic analysis, too.

Second, epigenetic research provides an appealing explanation for how the social environment can modulate gene expression on emotional functioning. For those studying depression, this opens up many interesting questions: Are there critical periods for environmentally induced changes in the epigenome? Can later adverse events have similar (long-term) impacts on gene expression? Can the effects of altered gene expression be reversed by protective environments, such as more social support, or even through therapies focusing on cognitive change? The ability to address these questions will depend on advances in laboratory techniques aimed at optimal measurements of human DNA methylation.

Third, the replicability of genetic effects for the treatment of depression has yet to be established, and existing findings are not sufficiently strong to suggest immediate translational applications into clinical practice. To achieve clinically meaningful prediction, future research efforts may need to integrate genetic information with neurophysiological, psychological, and behavioral measures to better understand the background on which treatments act and to elucidate mechanisms that mediate the effect of genetic variants on treatment response. This research may improve outcomes and enhance understanding of the pathophysiology of mood disorders.

REFERENCES

Agrawal, A., Jacobson, K. C., Prescott, C. A., & Kendler, K. S. (2002). A twin study of sex differences in social support. *Psychological Medicine, 32*(7), 1155–1164.

Ainsworth, M., Boston, M., Bowlby, J., & Rosenbluth, D. (1956). The effects of mother–child separation: A follow-up study. *British Journal of Medical Psychology, 29*(3–4), 211–247.

Armbruster, D., Moser, D. A., Strobel, A., Hensch, T., Kirschbaum, C., Lesch, K. P., et al. (2009). Serotonin transporter gene variation and stressful life events impact processing of fear and anxiety. *International Journal of Neuropsychopharmacology, 12*(3), 393–401.

Beach, S. R., Brody, G. H., Todorov, A. A., Gunter, T. D., & Philibert, R. A. (2010). Methylation at SLC6A4 is linked to family history of child abuse: An examination of the Iowa adoptee sample. *American Journal of Medical Genetics: Part B. Neuropsychiatric Genetics, 153B*(2), 710–713.

Beach, S. R., Brody, G. H., Todorov, A. A., Gunter, T. D., & Philibert, R. A. (2011). Methylation at *5HTT* mediates the impact of child sex abuse on women's antisocial behavior: An examination of the Iowa adoptee sample. *Psychosomatic Medicine, 73*(1), 83–87.

Binder, E. B., Salyakina, D., Lichtner, P., Wochnik, G. M., Ising, M., Putz, B., et al. (2004). Polymorphisms in FKBP5 are associated with increased recurrence of depressive episodes and rapid response to antidepressant treatment. *Nature Genetics, 36*, 1319–1325.

Bockting, C. L. H., Mocking, R. J., Lok, A., Koeter, M. W. J., & Schene, A. H. (2012). Therapy-genetics: The 5HTTLPR as a biomarker for response to psychological therapy? *Molecular Psychiatry, 18*(7), 744–745.

Bosker, F. J., Hartman, C. A., Nolte, I. M., Prins, B. P., Terpstra, P., Posthuma, D., et al. (2011). Poor replication of candidate genes for major depressive disorder using genome-wide association data. *Molecular Psychiatry, 16*(5), 516–532.

Breen, G., Webb, B. T., Butler, A. W., van den Oord, E. J., Tozzi, F., Craddock, N., et al. (2011). A genome-wide significant linkage for severe depression on chromosome 3: The Depression Network Study. *American Journal of Psychiatry, 168*(8), 840–847.

Brown, H., Eley, T. C., Broeren, S., MacLeod, C., Rinck, M., Hadwin, J., et al. (2014). Psychometric properties of reaction time-based experimental paradigms measuring anxiety-related information-processing biases in children. *Journal of Anxiety Disorders, 28*(1), 97–107.

Bryant, R. A., Felmingham, K. L., Falconer, E. M., Pe Benito, L., Dobson-Stone, C., Pierce, K. D., et al. (2010). Preliminary evidence of the short allele of the serotonin transporter gene predicting poor response to cognitive-behavior therapy in posttraumatic stress disorder. *Biological Psychiatry, 67*(12), 1217–1219.

Burt, S. A. (2008). Genes and popularity: Evidence of an evocative gene–environment correlation. *Psychological Science, 19*(2), 112–113.

Caldji, C., Diorio, J., & Meaney, M. J. (2000). Variations in maternal care in infancy regulate the development of stress reactivity. *Biological Psychiatry, 48*(12), 1164–1174.

Caldji, C., Francis, D., Sharma, S., Plotsky, P. M., & Meaney, M. J. (2000). The effects of early rearing environment on the development of GABAA and central benzodiazepine receptor levels and novelty-induced fearfulness in the rat. *Neuropsychopharmacology, 22*(3), 219–229.

Caspi, A., Sugden, K., Moffitt, T. E., Taylor, A., Craig, I. W., Harrington, H., et al. (2003). Influence of life stress on depression: Moderation by a polymorphism in the 5-HTT gene. *Science, 301*, 386–389.

Chipman, P., Jorm, A. F., Prior, M., Sanson, A., Smart, D., Tan, X., et al. (2007). No interaction between the serotonin transporter polymorphism (5-HTTLPR) and childhood adversity or recent stressful life events on symptoms of depression: Results from two community surveys. *American Journal of Medical Genetics: Part B. Neuropsychiatric Genetics, 144B*(4), 561–565.

DeRubeis, R. J., Hollon, S. D., Amsterdam, J. D., Shelton, R. C., Young, P. R., Salomon, R. M., et al. (2005). Cognitive therapy vs medications in the treatment of moderate to severe depression. *Archives of General Psychiatry, 62*(4), 409–416.

Dudbridge, F., & Gusnanto, A. (2008). Estimation of significance thresholds for genomewide association scans. *Genetic Epidemiology, 32*(3), 227–234.

Eley, T. C., Hudson, J. L., Creswell, C., Tropeano, M., Lester, K. J., Cooper, P., et al. (2012). Therapygenetics: The *5HTTLPR* and response to psychological therapy. *Molecular Psychiatry, 17*, 236–237.

Eley, T. C., Liang, H., Plomin, R., Sham, P., Sterne, A., Williamson, R., et al. (2004). Parental familial vulnerability, family environment, and their interactions as predictors of depressive symptoms in adolescents. *Journal of the American Academy of Child and Adolescent Psychiatry, 43*(3), 298–306.

Fanous, A., Gardner, C. O., Prescott, C. A., Cancro, R., & Kendler, K. S. (2002). Neuroticism, major depression and gender: A population-based twin study. *Psychological Medicine, 32*(4), 719–728.

Farmer, A., Redman, K., Harris, T., Mahmood, A., Sadler, S., Pickering, A., et al. (2002). Neuroticism, extraversion, life events and depression: The Cardiff Depression Study. *British Journal of Psychiatry, 181*, 118–122.

Fish, E. W., Shahrokh, D., Bagot, R., Caldji, C., Bredy, T., Szyf, M., et al. (2004). Epigenetic programming of stress responses through variations in maternal care. *Annals of the New York Academy of Sciences, 1036*, 167–180.

Fox, E., Ridgewell, A., & Ashwin, C. (2009). Looking on the bright side: Biased attention and the human serotonin transporter gene. *Proceedings. Biological Sciences, 276*, 1747–1751.

Furmark, T., Carlbring, P., Hammer, S., Wahlgren, I., Ekselius, L., Eriksson, E., et al. (2010). Effects of serotonin transporter and tryptophan hydroxylase-2 gene variation on the response to cognitive-behavior therapy in individuals with social anxiety disorder. *Biological Psychiatry, 67*(9, Suppl.), 114S.

Glowinski, A. L., Madden, P. A., Bucholz, K. K., Lynskey, M. T., & Heath, A. C. (2003). Genetic epidemiology of self-reported lifetime DSM-IV major depressive disorder in a population-based twin sample of female adolescents. *Journal of Child Psychology and Psychiatry, 44*(7), 988–996.

Gregory, A. M., Rijsdijk, F. V., Lau, J. Y., Napolitano, M., McGuffin, P., & Eley, T. C. (2007). Genetic and environmental influences on interpersonal cognitions and associations with depressive symptoms in 8-year-old twins. *Journal of Abnormal Psychology, 116*(4), 762–775.

Hariri, A. R., Mattay, V. S., Tessitore, A., Kolachana, B., Fera, F., Goldman, D., et al. (2002). Serotonin transporter genetic variation and the response of the human amygdala. *Science, 297*, 400–403.

Hasler, G., Drevets, W. C., Manji, H. K., & Charney, D. S. (2004). Discovering endophenotypes for major depression. *Neuropsychopharmacology, 29*(10), 1765–1781.

Hauser, E. R., Boehnke, M., Guo, S. W., & Risch, N. (1996). Affected-sib-pair interval mapping and exclusion for complex genetic traits: Sampling considerations. *Genetic Epidemiology, 13*(2), 117–137.

Heath, A. C., Eaves, L. J., & Martin, N. G. (1998). Interaction of marital status and genetic risk for symptoms of depression. *Twin Research, 1*(3), 119–122.

Hedman, E., Andersson, E., Ljótsson, B., Andersson, G., Schalling, M., Lindefors, N., et al. (2012). Clinical and genetic outcome determinants of Internet- and group-based cognitive-behavior therapy for social anxiety disorder. *Acta Psychiatrica Scandinavica, 126*(2), 126–136.

Hettema, J. M., Annas, P., Neale, M. C., Kendler, K. S., & Fredrikson, M. (2003). A twin study of the genetics of fear conditioning. *Archives of General Psychiatry, 60*(7), 702–708.

Holmans, P., Weissman, M. M., Zubenko, G. S., Scheftner, W. A., Crowe, R. R., Depaulo, J. R., Jr., et al. (2007). Genetics of recurrent early-onset major depression (GenRED): Final genome scan report. *American Journal of Psychiatry, 164*(2), 248–258.

Holmans, P., Zubenko, G. S., Crowe, R. R., DePaulo, J. R., Jr., Scheftner, W. A., Weissman, M. M., et al. (2004). Genomewide significant linkage to recurrent, early-onset major depressive disorder on chromosome 15q. *American Journal of Human Genetics, 74*(6), 1154–1167.

Iervolino, A. C., Pike, A., Manke, B., Reiss, D., Hetherington, E. M., & Plomin, R. (2002). Genetic and environmental influences in adolescent peer socialization: Evidence from two genetically sensitive designs. *Child Development, 73*(1), 162–174.

Jacobson, K. C., & Rowe, D. C. (1999). Genetic and environmental influences on the relationships between family connectedness, school connectedness, and adolescent depressed mood: Sex differences. *Developmental Psychology, 35*(4), 926–939.

Karg, K., Burmeister, M., Shedden, K., & Sen, S. (2011). The serotonin transporter promoter variant (5-HTTLPR), stress, and depression meta-analysis revisited: Evidence of genetic moderation. *Archives of General Psychiatry, 68*(5), 444–454.

Kato, M., & Serretti, A. (2010). Review and meta-analysis of antidepressant pharmacogenetic findings in major depressive disorder. *Molecular Psychiatry, 15*(5), 473–500.

Kendler, K. S., Gardner, C. O., & Lichtenstein, P. (2008). A developmental twin study of symptoms of anxiety and depression: Evidence for genetic innovation and attenuation. *Psychological Medicine, 38*(11), 1567–1575.

Kendler, K. S., & Karkowski-Shuman, L. (1997). Stressful life events and genetic liability to major depression: Genetic control of exposure to the environment? *Psychological Medicine, 27*(3), 539–547.

Kendler, K. S., Kessler, R. C., Walters, E. E., MacLean, C., Neale, M. C., Heath, A. C., et al.

(1995). Stressful life events, genetic liability, and onset of an episode of major depression in women. *American Journal of Psychiatry, 152*(6), 833–842.

Kendler, K. S., Prescott, C. A., Myers, J., & Neale, M. C. (2003). The structure of genetic and environmental risk factors for common psychiatric and substance use disorders in men and women. *Archives of General Psychiatry, 60*(9), 929–937.

Kohen, R., Cain, K. C., Buzaitis, A., Johnson, V., Becker, K. J., Teri, L., et al. (2011). Response to psychosocial treatment in poststroke depression is associated with serotonin transporter polymorphisms. *Stroke, 42*(7), 2068–2070.

Kotte, A., McQuaid, J. R., & Kelsoe, J. (2007, May). *HTR2A: Genotypic predictor of depression psychotherapy treatment outcome.* Paper presented at the 62nd annual scientific convention and meeting of the Society of Biological Psychiatry, San Diego, CA.

Labonte, B., Yerko, V., Gross, J., Mechawar, N., Meaney, M. J., Szyf, M., et al. (2012). Differential glucocorticoid receptor exon 1(B), 1(C), and 1(H) expression and methylation in suicide completers with a history of childhood abuse. *Biological Psychiatry, 72*(1), 41–48.

Lau, J. Y., Burt, M., Leibenluft, E., Pine, D. S., Rijsdijk, F., Shiffrin, N., et al. (2009). Individual differences in children's facial expression recognition ability: The role of nature and nurture. *Developmental Neuropsychology, 34*(1), 37–51.

Lau, J. Y., & Eley, T. C. (2006). Changes in genetic and environmental influences on depressive symptoms across adolescence: A twin and sibling study. *British Journal of Psychiatry, 189*, 422–427.

Lau, J. Y., & Eley, T. C. (2008a). Attributional style as a risk marker of genetic effects for adolescent depressive symptoms. *Journal of Abnormal Psychology, 117*(4), 849–859.

Lau, J. Y., & Eley, T. C. (2008b). Disentangling gene–environment correlations and interactions on adolescent depressive symptoms. *Journal of Child Psychology and Psychiatry, 49*(2), 142–150.

Lau, J. Y., Hilbert, K., Goodman, R., Gregory, A. M., Pine, D. S., Viding, E. M., et al. (2012). Investigating the genetic and environmental bases of biases in threat recognition and avoidance in children with anxiety problems. *Biology of Mood and Anxiety Disorders, 2*(1), 12.

Lau, J. Y., Rijsdijk, F., & Eley, T. C. (2006). I think, therefore I am: A twin study of attributional style in adolescents. *Journal of Child Psychology and Psychiatry, 47*(7), 696–703.

Lester, K. J., & Eley, T. C. (2013). Therapygenetics: Using genetic markers to predict response to psychological treatment for mood and anxiety disorders. *Biology of Mood and Anxiety Disorders, 3*(1), 4.

Levinson, D. F., Evgrafov, O. V., Knowles, J. A., Potash, J. B., Weissman, M. M., Scheftner, W. A., et al. (2007). Genetics of recurrent early-onset major depression (GenRED): Significant linkage on chromosome 15q25-q26 after fine mapping with single nucleotide polymorphism markers. *American Journal of Psychiatry, 164*(2), 259–264.

Licinio, J., O'Kirwan, F., Irizarry, K., Merriman, B., Thakur, S., Jepson, R., et al. (2004). Association of a corticotropin-releasing hormone receptor 1 haplotype and antidepressant treatment response in Mexican-Americans. *Molecular Psychiatry, 9*, 1075–1082.

Liu, Z., Zhu, F., Wang, G., Xiao, Z., Tang, J., Liu, W., et al. (2007). Association study of corticotropin-releasing hormone receptor 1 gene polymorphisms and antidepressant response in major depressive disorders. *Neuroscience Letters, 414*(2), 155–158.

Lonsdorf, T. B., Ruck, C., Bergstrom, J., Andersson, G., Ohman, A., Lindefors, N., et al. (2010). The COMTval158met polymorphism is associated with symptom relief during exposure-based cognitive-behavioral treatment in panic disorder. *BMC Psychiatry, 10*, 99.

López-León, S., Janssens, A. C., González-Zuloeta Ladd, A. M., Del-Favero, J., Claes, S. J., Oostra, B. A., et al. (2007). Meta-analyses of genetic studies on major depressive disorder. *Molecular Psychiatry, 13*(8), 772–785.

Lubke, G. H., Hottenga, J. J., Walters, R., Laurin, C., de Geus, E. J., Willemsen, G., et al. (2012). Estimating the genetic variance of major depressive disorder due to all single nucleotide polymorphisms. *Biological Psychiatry, 72*(8), 707–709.

Major Depressive Disorder Working Group of the Psychiatric GWAS Consortium. (2013). A mega-analysis of genome-wide association studies for major depressive disorder. *Molecular Psychiatry, 18*(4), 497–511.

McGowan, P. O., Sasaki, A., D'Alessio, A. C., Dymov, S., Labonte, B., Szyf, M., et al. (2009). Epigenetic regulation of the glucocorticoid receptor in human brain associates with childhood abuse. *Nature Neuroscience, 12*(3), 342–348.

McGuffin, P., Knight, J., Breen, G., Brewster, S., Boyd, P. R., Craddock, N., et al. (2005). Whole genome linkage scan of recurrent depressive disorder from the depression network study. *Human Molecular Genetics, 14*(22), 3337–3345.

McGuffin, P., Rijsdijk, F., Andrew, M., Sham, P., Katz, R., & Cardno, A. (2003). The heritability of bipolar affective disorder and the genetic relationship to unipolar depression. *Archives of General Psychiatry, 60*(5), 497–502.

McMahon, F. J., Buervenich, S., Charney, D., Lipsky, R., Rush, A. J., Wilson, A. F., et al. (2006). Variation in the gene encoding the serotonin 2A receptor is associated with outcome of antidepressant treatment. *American Journal of Human Genetics, 78*(5), 804–814.

Meaney, M. J. (2001). Maternal care, gene expression, and the transmission of individual differences in stress reactivity across generations. *Annual Review of Neuroscience, 24,* 1161–1192.

Meaney, M. J., & Szyf, M. (2005). Environmental programming of stress responses through DNA methylation: Life at the interface between a dynamic environment and a fixed genome. *Dialogues in Clinical Neuroscience, 7*(2), 103–123.

Middeldorp, C. M., Cath, D. C., & Boomsma, D. I. (2006). A twin-family study of the association between employment, burnout and anxious depression. *Journal of Affective Disorders, 90*(2–3), 163–169.

Mill, J., & Petronis, A. (2007). Molecular studies of major depressive disorder: The epigenetic perspective. *Molecular Psychiatry, 12*(9), 799–814.

Mrazek, D. A., Rush, A. J., Biernacka, J. M., O'Kane, D. J., Cunningham, J. M., Wieben, E. D., et al. (2009). SLC6A4 variation and citalopram response. *American Journal of Medical Genetics: Part B. Neuropsychiatric Genetics, 150B*(3), 341–351.

Munafo, M. R., Brown, S. M., & Hariri, A. R. (2008). Serotonin transporter (5-HTTLPR) genotype and amygdala activation: A meta-analysis. *Biological Psychiatry, 63*(9), 852–857.

Munafo, M. R., Durrant, C., Lewis, G., & Flint, J. (2009). Gene × environment interactions at the serotonin transporter locus. *Biological Psychiatry, 65*(3), 211–219.

Murgatroyd, C., & Spengler, D. (2011). Epigenetic programming of the HPA axis: Early life decides. *Stress: The International Journal on the Biology of Stress, 14*(6), 581–589.

Natsuaki, M. N., Ge, X., Leve, L. D., Neiderhiser, J. M., Shaw, D. S., Conger, R. D., et al. (2010). Genetic liability, environment, and the development of fussiness in toddlers: The roles of maternal depression and parental responsiveness. *Developmental Psychology, 46*(5), 1147–1158.

Neiderhiser, J. M., Reiss, D., Lichtenstein, P., Spotts, E. L., & Ganiban, J. (2007). Father–adolescent relationships and the role of genotype–environment correlation. *Journal of Family Psychology, 21*(4), 560–571.

Neiderhiser, J. M., Reiss, D., Pedersen, N. L., Lichtenstein, P., Spotts, E. L., Hansson, K., et al. (2004). Genetic and environmental influences on mothering of adolescents: A comparison of two samples. *Developmental Psychology, 40*(3), 335–351.

O'Connor, T. G., Caspi, A., DeFries, J. C., & Plomin, R. (2000). Are associations between parental divorce and children's adjustment genetically mediated?: An adoption study. *Developmental Psychology, 36*(4), 429–437.

O'Connor, T. G., Hetherington, E. M., Reiss, D., & Plomin, R. (1995). A twin-sibling study of observed parent–adolescent interactions. *Child Development, 66*(3), 812–829.

Paddock, S., Laje, G., Charney, D., Rush, J., Wilson, A. F., Sorant, A. J. M., et al. (2007). Association of GRIK4 with outcome of antidepressant treatment in the STAR*D cohort. *American Journal of Psychiatry, 164,* 1181–1188.

Pergadia, M. L., Glowinski, A. L., Wray, N. R., Agrawal, A., Saccone, S. F., Loukola, A., et al.(2011). A 3p26-3p25 genetic linkage finding for DSM-IV major depression in heavy smoking families. *American Journal of Psychiatry, 168*(8), 848–852.

Plomin, R., DeFries, J. C., Knopnik, V. S., & Neiderhiser, J. M. (2013). *Behavioral genetics* (5th ed.). New York: Worth Books.

Pluess, M., & Belsky, J. (2012). Vantage sensitivity: Individual differences in response to positive experiences. *Psychological Bulletin, 139*(4), 901–916.

Price, A. L., Patterson, N. J., Plenge, R. M., Weinblatt, M. E., Shadick, N. A., & Reich, D. (2006). Principal components analysis corrects for stratification in genome-wide association studies. *Nature Genetics, 38*(8), 904–909.

Rice, F., Harold, G. T., Boivin, J., Hay, D. F., van den Bree, M., & Thapar, A. (2009). Disentangling prenatal and inherited influences in humans with an experimental design. *Proceedings of the National Academy of Sciences of the USA, 106*(7), 2464–2467.

Rice, F., Harold, G. T., Shelton, K. H., & Thapar, A. (2006). Family conflict interacts with genetic liability in predicting childhood and adolescent depression. *Journal of the American Academy of Child and Adolescent Psychiatry, 45*(7), 841–848.

Rice, F., Harold, G. T., & Thapar, A. (2002). The genetic aetiology of childhood depression: A review. *Journal of Child Psychology and Psychiatry, 43*(1), 65–79.

Risch, N., Herrell, R., Lehner, T., Liang, K. Y., Eaves, L., Hoh, J., et al. (2009). Interaction between the serotonin transporter gene (5-HTTLPR), stressful life events, and risk of depression: A meta-analysis. *Journal of the American Medical Association, 301*(23), 2462–2471.

Roth, T. L., Lubin, F. D., Funk, A. J., & Sweatt, J. D. (2009). Lasting epigenetic influence of early-life adversity on the BDNF gene. *Biological Psychiatry, 65*(9), 760–769.

Sakolsky, D., Nurmi, E., Birmaher, B., March, J. S., Walkup, J., Piacentini, J., et al. (2011). *Serotonin transporter variation and treatment response in the Child/Adolescent Anxiety Multimodal Study (CAMS).* Paper presented at the annual meeting of the American Academy of Child and Adolescent Psychiatry, Toronto.

Savitz, J. B., & Drevets, W. C. (2009). Imaging phenotypes of major depressive disorder: Genetic correlates. *Neuroscience, 164*(1), 300–330.

Scarr, S., & McCartney, K. (1983). How people make their own environments: A theory of genotype greater than environment effects. *Child Development, 54*(2), 424–435.

Shih, R. A., Belmonte, P. L., & Zandi, P. P. (2004). A review of the evidence from family, twin and adoption studies for a genetic contribution to adult psychiatric disorders. *International Review of Psychiatry, 16*(4), 260–283.

Spotts, E. L., Neiderhiser, J. M., Towers, H., Hansson, K., Lichtenstein, P., Cederblad, M., et al. (2004). Genetic and environmental influences on marital relationships. *Journal of Family Psychology, 18*(1), 107–119.

Sullivan, P. F., Neale, M. C., & Kendler, K. S. (2000). Genetic epidemiology of major depression: Review and meta-analysis. *American Journal of Psychiatry, 157*(10), 1552–1562.

Tansey, K. E., Guipponi, M., Hu, X., Domenici, E., Lewis, G., Malafosse, A., et al. (2013). Contribution of common genetic variants to antidepressant response. *Biological Psychiatry, 73*(7), 679–682.

Taylor, M. J., Sen, S., & Bhagwagar, Z. (2010). Antidepressant response and the serotonin transporter gene-linked polymorphic region. *Biological Psychiatry, 68*(6), 536–543.

Trivedi, M. H., Rush, A. J., Wisniewski, S. R., Nierenberg, A. A., Warden, D., Ritz, L., et al. (2006). Evaluation of outcomes with citalopram for depression using measurement-based care in STAR*D: Implications for clinical practice. *American Journal of Psychiatry, 163*(1), 28–40.

Uher, R. (2008). The implications of gene–environment interactions in depression: Will cause inform cure? *Molecular Psychiatry, 13*(12), 1070–1078.

Uher, R. (2011). Genes, environment, and individual differences in responding to treatment for depression. *Harvard Review of Psychiatry, 19*(3), 109–124.

Uher, R., Huezo-Diaz, P., Perroud, N., Smith, R., Rietschel, M., Mors, O., et al. (2009). Genetic predictors of response to antidepressants in the GENDEP project. *Pharmacogenomics Journal, 9*(4), 225–233.

Uher, R., & McGuffin, P. (2008). The moderation by the serotonin transporter gene of environmental adversity in the aetiology of mental illness: Review and methodological analysis. *Molecular Psychiatry, 13*(2), 131–146.

van IJzendoorn, M. H., Belsky, J., & Bakermans-Kranenburg, M. J. (2012). Serotonin transporter genotype *5HTTLPR* as a marker of differential susceptibility?: A meta-analysis of child and adolescent gene-by-environment studies. *Translational Psychiatry, 2*, e147.

Vijayendran, M., Beach, S. R., Plume, J. M., Brody, G. H., & Philibert, R. A. (2012). Effects of genotype and child abuse on DNA methylation and gene expression at the serotonin transporter. *Frontiers in Psychiatry, 3*, 55.

Wang, Z., Harrer, J., Tuerk, P., Acierno, R., Hamner, M., Timmerman, M. A., et al. (2009, May). *5-HTTLPR influence PTSD treatment outcome.* Paper presented at the annual scientific convention and meeting of the Society of Biological Psychiatry, Vancouver, Canada.

Wender, P. H., Kety, S. S., Rosenthal, D., Schulsinger, F., Ortmann, J., & Lunde, I. (1986). Psychiatric disorders in the biological and adoptive families of adopted individuals with affective disorders. *Archives of General Psychiatry, 43*(10), 923–929.

Zou, Y.-F., Wang, F., Feng, X.-L., Li, W.-F., Tao, J.-H., Pan, F.-M., et al. (2010). Meta-analysis of FKBP5 gene polymorphisms association with treatment response in patients with mood disorders. *Neuroscience Letters, 484*(1), 56–61.

Zou, Y.-F., Ye, D.-Q., Feng, X.-L., Su, H., Pan, F.-M., & Liao, F.-F. (2010). Meta-analysis of BDNF Val66Met polymorphism association with treatment response in patients with major depressive disorder. *European Neuropsychopharmacology, 20*(8), 535–544.

CHAPTER 10

Neurobiological Aspects of Depression

MICHAEL E. THASE, CHANG-GYU HAHN, *and* OLIVIER BERTON

Since antiquity, there have been speculations about the biological basis of depression. It is only during the past 50 years, however, that the methodology has been available to study directly alterations in brain function associated with depression. What has emerged from this half-century of research has been an evolving process, answering some questions and opening new, more sophisticated lines of inquiry. One certainty is that the heterogeneous conditions now grouped together under the construct of "clinical depression" are biopsychosocial disorders, which have multifactorial causality.

The neurobiology of depression has been reviewed in the previous editions of this *Handbook*, and across the past decade various hypotheses have been advanced, tested, and either rejected or modified as knowledge about the function of the central nervous system (CNS) in health, disease, and various states of duress has grown. Significant advances have come from basic research on the intracellular processes that link transporters and receptors to the up- or down-regulation of gene activity, including transcription factors and neurotrophins. Notable recent advances in genetics (Lau et al., Chapter 9, this volume) and neuroimaging (Pizzagalli & Treadway, Chapter 11, this volume) are reviewed in more detail elsewhere in this volume. In this chapter, research using other neurobiological paradigms is reviewed, updating key developments since the last edition of this volume.

BACKGROUND

In the late 1950s, several converging lines of evidence pointed to the possibility that depression is caused by dysfunction of CNS systems subserved by the monoamine neurotransmitters, particularly the catecholamine norepinephrine (NE) and the indoleamine serotonin (also known as 5-hydroxytryptamine [5-HT]). Early studies indicated that these neurotransmitters were important regulators of bodily functions that are commonly disturbed in depression, including sleep, appetite, libido, and psychomotor tone;

by the mid-1960s, there was strong evidence that the tricyclic antidepressants (TCAs) and monoamine oxidase inhibitors (MAOIs) rapidly increased concentrations of NE and/ or 5-HT at neuronal synapses. Thus it was thought that depression was caused by deficits of 5-HT or NE activity and mania was caused by increased NE activity (Bunney & Davis, 1965; Glassman, 1969; Schildkraut, 1965). It was further suggested that a third monoamine, dopamine (DA), was involved in some symptoms of depression, including fatigue, anhedonia, and psychomotor retardation (Korf & van Praag, 1971). However, by the mid-1990s it was clear that such simplistic models were not supported by the evidence (see, e.g., Duman, Heninger, & Nestler, 1997; Ressler & Nemeroff, 1999; Schatzberg & Schildkraut, 1995).

Nevertheless, three findings from this first generation of research have ongoing relevance. First, although depression is not caused by deficits of NE or 5-HT, subgroups of patients with depression have low urinary levels of the NE metabolites (Ressler & Nemeroff, 1999; Schatzberg & Schildkraut, 1995) or low cerebrospinal fluid (CSF) levels of the serotonin metabolite 5-hydroxy-indoleacetic acid (5-HIAA; Maes & Meltzer, 1995). These findings are relevant because the former abnormality is associated with psychomotor retardation (Schatzberg & Schildkraut, 1995) and the latter is associated with increased risk of suicidal behaviors (Maes & Meltzer, 1995; Mann, Brent & Arango, 2001). Second, some depressed patients hypersecrete the glucocorticoid hormone cortisol, the primary effector of stress responses (Holsboer, 1995; Swaab et al., 2005); increased hypothalamic–pituitary–adrenal (HPA) axis activity also is revealed by challenge paradigms such as the dexamethasone suppression test (DST) and the combined dexamethasone (DEX)/corticotropin-releasing hormone (CRH) test (Holsboer, 2001). Hypercortisolism is linked to older age, recurrence risk, and increased syndromal symptom severity, including psychosis and suicidal ideation, as well as to a lower response to placebo and nonspecific therapeutic interventions. A third set of pivotal findings emanate from the transition of older paradigms to assess brain activity, such as polysomnography and evoked potentials, to newer neuroimaging strategies such as positron emission tomography (PET) and functional magnetic resonance imaging (fMRI). There is now good evidence that depression is linked to disturbances of several key neural circuits, including a medial prefrontal–limbic network that primarily subserves the regulation of emotional arousal and a reward network centered on the ventral striatum with orbitofrontal and medial prefrontal interconnections (Kupfer, Frank, & Phillips, 2012).

ABNORMALITIES OF MONOAMINERGIC SYSTEMS

Noradrenergic Systems

Almost all of the NE cell bodies in the brain are located in a single pontine nucleus, the locus ceruleus (LC). Noradrenergic neurons project from the LC to the thalamus, hypothalamus, limbic system, basal ganglia, and cerebral cortex, reflecting the role of NE in initiating and maintaining arousal in the brainstem, limbic system, and cerebral cortex (Kandel, Schwartz, & Jessell, 1991; Kingsley, 2000). Noradrenergic projections to the amygdala and hippocampus have been implicated in behavioral sensitization to stress, and stimulation of noradrenergic fibers in the medial forebrain bundle enhances attention and increases levels of appetitive behavior (Aston-Jones, Rajkowski, & Cohen, 1999).

Noradrenergic neurotransmission has a fundamental role in stress response. Perception of novel or threatening stimuli is relayed from the cerebral cortex to the LC via the thalamus and from the periphery via the nucleus prepositus hypoglossi, provoking an almost immediate increase in NE activity. Cognitive processes thus can amplify or dampen NE cellular responses to stress. In addition, activation from glutamatergic fibers projecting from the nucleus paragigantocellularis and release of CRH can "turn on" the LC (Nestler, Alreja, & Aghajanian, 1999).

The peripheral component of stress response is transmitted from the LC via the sympathoadrenal pathway to the endochromafin cells of the adrenal glands, which release NE into systemic circulation. The peripherally arousing effects of the sympathoadrenal response are largely mediated by cells expressing the α_1 and β type of NE receptors.

The activity of NE neurons is regulated by the autoinhibitory effects of α_2 receptors. Neuronal release of NE almost immediately begins to decrease the sensitivity of LC neurons to repeated firing. α_2 receptors also are located on serotoninergic cell bodies, and stimulation of these heteroceptors activates nearby (colocalized) inhibitory 5-HT neurons. A sustained increase in LC firing also causes the number of α_1 and β receptors to decrease, a process known as down-regulation. Together, these actions (i.e., α_2 autoinhibition, α_1 and β receptor down-regulation, and activation of adjacent inhibitory 5-HT neurons) constitute a homeostatic counterregulatory force that dampens responses to threat. If, however, the stress is sustained, intracellular stores of NE may become depleted, which can result in diminished inhibitory α_2 and 5-HT input to the LC, which in turn will dysregulate homeostasis of NE neurotransmission. Over time, the net effect is that ascending central NE neurotransmission will decrease (which is probably the cause of reduced urinary excretion of NE metabolites in depression), although the output of the adrenal medulla may remain high (which may explain the observation of high levels of NE and its metabolites in some patients with severe depression).

The consequences of sustained stress on NE systems in animals can result in a behavioral state known as learned helplessness (Maier & Seligman, 1976). Learned helplessness is not an exact analogue of human depression; cognitions about powerlessness or hopelessness distinguish depression from the behavioral states experienced by rodents and dogs in learned helplessness experiments (Gilbert, 1992). Nevertheless, the changes in NE activity observed in learned helplessness experiments do parallel those associated with other animal models of depression, such as social defeat, and are associated with increased glucocorticoid activity and alterations in gene transcription factors (Berton et al., 2007; Maier & Watkins, 2005).

Serotonin Systems

Most of the serotonin (5-HT) in the brain is synthesized in the dorsal raphé nuclei, which are located in the pons. These neurons project to the cerebral cortex, hypothalamus, thalamus, basal ganglia, septum, and hippocampus (Kandel et al., 1991; Kingsley, 2000). Serotonin pathways are largely colocalized with NE pathways and generally have tonic or inhibitory effects that counterbalance NE activity (Kingsley, 2000). Serotonin neurons projecting to the suprachiasmatic nucleus (SCN) of the anterior hypothalamus help to regulate circadian rhythms (e.g., sleep–wake cycles, body temperature, and HPA axis function; Duncan, 1996) and the 90-minute infraradian cycle of alternating periods of rapid eye movement (REM) and non-REM sleep (Duncan, 1996).

All 5-HT neurons express membrane-bound transporters (5-HTT), which permit the uptake of 5-HT from the synaptic cleft. The antidepressant activity of the selective serotonin reuptake inhibitors (SSRIs) and serotonin–norepinephrine reuptake inhibitors (SNRIs) is initiated by blocking this transporter. A functional polymorphism in the promoter region of the gene that codes for the 5-HTT has been associated with individual differences in response to stress (Caspi et al., 2003). Of the many types of serotonin receptors in the mammalian brain, $5\text{-}HT_{1A}$ and $5\text{-}HT_{2A}$ have the greatest relevance to the pathophysiology and treatment of depression (Mann et al., 2001).

An intact tonic level of 5-HT neurotransmission is necessary for affiliative behaviors and modulates the goal-directed motor and appetitive behaviors that are primarily mediated by NE and DA. The tonic level of 5-HT neurotransmission in primates is relatively stable and is partly under genetic control (Higley et al., 1996), with heritability at least partly determined by a polymorphism in the promoter region of the gene that codes for the 5-HTT. In rodents, social defeat reliably lowers basal 5-HT tone, and, similarly, primates with lower rankings on social dominance hierarchies have lower CSF 5-HIAA levels (Higley et al., 1996). In primates, animals manifesting at least one copy of the short (*s*) allele, which is less functional (i.e., less transporter is synthesized), show greater behavioral dysfunction and more exaggerated responses to stress than do animals who have two copies of the more common long (*l*) form of the allele (Shannon et al., 2005; see Lau et al., Chapter 9, this volume).

Humans show a similar *s* polymorphism of the 5-HTT, as well as a second, less functional variant of the *l* form. Studies of these polymorphisms have yielded evidence of gene–environment interactions. Specifically, the *s* allele of the serotonin transporter is associated with an increased risk of depression following exposure to stress (Caspi et al., 2003; see Lau et al., Chapter 9, this volume). Two functional correlates of such heightened vulnerability are increased limbic activation to threat (Hariri et al., 2002) and cortisol secretion to stress (Gotlib, Joormann, Minor, & Hallmayer, 2008). In addition, individuals carrying at least one *s* allele show greater vulnerability on cognitive measures such as neuroticism (Jacobs et al., 2006) and dysfunctional attitudes (Hayden et al., 2008), use more passive coping strategies (Wilhelm et al., 2007) and have greater negative recall bias (Hayden et al., 2013).

Evidence from studies using receptor imaging techniques suggests that dysfunction of $5\text{-}HT_{1A}$ receptors is clearly implicated in depression (Drevets et al., 2007). In the absence of a heritable risk factor, down-regulation of $5\text{-}HT_{1A}$ receptors is most likely a consequence of exposure to chronic stress (Embree et al., 2013).

The integrity of 5-HT neurotransmission can be transiently compromised by eliminating the essential amino acid precursor tryptophan from the food source. Complete disruption of 5-HT synthesis has little immediate impact on mood in studies of healthy individuals, but it does have an impact on some aspects of cognitive–affective processing (Robinson, Cools, & Sahakian, 2012). In clinical studies, a brief period of tryptophan depletion does not worsen untreated depression but reliably reverses antidepressant response overnight in about 50–60% of people treated with SSRI antidepressants (Delgado, 2004). Tryptophan depletion does not affect response to norepinephrine reuptake inhibitors (NRIs; Delgado, 2004), placebo (Delgado, 2004), repetitive transcranial magnetic stimulation (O'Reardon et al., 2006), and cognitive therapy (O'Reardon et al., 2004), underscoring the specificity of this mechanism.

Dopaminergic Systems in Depression

There are four principal DA pathways in the brain (Kandel, Schwartz, & Jessell, 1991; Kingsley, 2000). The tuberoinfundibular system projects from cell bodies in the hypothalamus to the pituitary and inhibits secretion of the hormone prolactin. The nigrostriatral system, which helps to regulate psychomotor activity, originates from cell bodies in the substantia nigra and projects to the basal ganglia. The mesolimbic pathway begins with cell bodies located in the ventral tegmentum and projects to the nucleus accumbens, amygdala, hippocampus, medial dorsal nucleus of the thalamus, and cingulate gyrus. The mesolimbic DA pathway modulates emotional expression and goal-directed or appetitive behavior. Down-regulation of this pathway invariably accompanies learned helplessness and social defeat; consequently, identifying individual differences in susceptibility has important implications for research on depression (Willner, Scheel-Krüger & Belzung, 2012). The mesocortical DA pathway, which projects from the ventral tegmentum orbitofrontal and prefrontal cerebral cortex, subserves motivation, initiation of goal-directed tasks, and "executive" cognitive processes. Decreased DA activity has obvious implications in the motoric, hedonic, and cognitive symptoms of depression (Willner et al., 2012). Of note, an allelic variation in the gene coding for the enzyme catechol-O-methyltransferase (COMT)—the Val(158)Met polymorphism—is associated with significant differences in affective processing and, as such, may indirectly contribute to the risk of depression (Antypa, Drago, & Serretti, 2013).

As with the other monoamines, chronic stress reduces DA levels and results in behavioral changes suggestive of depression (Willner et al., 2012). Chronic mild stress, for example, reduces the reinforcing effects of low concentrations of sucrose water.

Dopaminergic neurotransmission is partly dependent on the integrity of 5-HT systems (Willner et al., 2012), providing another example of how dysfunction in one system can provoke secondary changes in the others. Animal studies have shown that antidepressants of various classes can reverse or prevent the DA dysfunction caused by chronic stress (Willner et al., 2012).

Stress, Monoamines, and the HPA Axis

The foregoing discussion has emphasized the changes in monoamine function that are linked to depression, particularly in relation to the neurobiological consequences of sustained, unresolvable stress. Elevated HPA activity is the hallmark of mammalian stress responses, and the regulation of the axis is partly under the control of phasic NE (activating) and tonic 5-HT (inhibitory) neurotransmission. This axis has four levels of organization and modulation. In relevant areas of the cerebral cortex, the threat and contextual significance of the stressor are perceived, and the signal is relayed to the HPA. With respect to the role of the higher brain regions in HPA regulation, neurons containing the neuropeptides CRH and arginine vasopressin are diffusely located throughout the cerebral cortex, with particularly high concentrations within the thalamus, amygdala, and other components of the limbic system, and these regions "light up" immediately following exposure to stress (Bonfiglio et al., 2011; Swaab et al., 2005). Furthermore, CRH activation of the LC provokes NE stimulation of the thalamus, hypothalamus, and amygdala, creating a "reverberating circuit" or a positive feedback loop. Activating inputs from neurons are transmitted to the hypothalamus, where CRH also is released and travels systemically to the adjacent pituitary. Specialized cells in the anterior pituitary respond to CRH via release of adrenocorticotropic hormone (ACTH), which travels via the bloodstream to the cortex of the adrenal glands, where glucocorticoids are released and, if the stressor is sustained, synthesis is increased. The impact of CRH stimulation is increased by simultaneous release of arginine vasopressin, which is intensified during chronic stress (Bonfiglio et al., 2011; Swaab et al., 2005).

The cellular effects of glucocorticoids are triggered by intracellular glucocorticoid receptors (GR), which migrate between the cell membrane and cell nuclei, effecting changes in the activity of many genes. Once cortisol release is stimulated by ACTH, it is released into the circulation and exerts a large number of physiological actions on various end-organs, including anti-inflammatory effects on immune function and insulin-antagonist effects on glucose and lipid metabolism. Overall, these acute changes promote short-term survival in response to overwhelming or life-threatening circumstances. Such benefits are time-limited, however, and negative compensatory (allostatic) changes will begin to accumulate if cortisol levels remain elevated for prolonged periods (McEwen & Gianaros, 2011).

The HPA axis, like the NE and 5-HT components of stress response, is regulated by a redundant, multileveled system of inhibitory control. This type of negative feedback inhibition occurs at all levels of the axis, including the hippocampus, hypothalamus, pituitary, and adrenal cortex. As acute stresses pass or resolve, the elevated plasma cortisol levels of healthy humans will normalize within a matter of minutes or hours. Sustained hypercortisolism thus can result from increased CRH drive (from the hypothalamus or cerebral cortex), increased secretion of ACTH (secreted, e.g., by a pituitary tumor), unrestrained noradrenergic stimulation from the locus ceruleus, and/or the failure of one or more mechanisms of feedback inhibition (Swaab et al., 2005).

It has been known for several decades that sustained hypercortisolism can cause lasting damage to the integrity of HPA axis regulation (Bremner, 1999; Sapolsky, 1996). Exposure to various forms of stress early in life has been shown to compromise the regulation of HPA activity for a lifetime (Heim et al., 2009). In animal models of early trauma, even brief periods of maternal separation can result in long-standing changes in stress responses (Coplan et al., 2001, 2006). Stress in later life appears to accelerate the slow decline in the integrity of HPA axis regulation that normally accompanies aging.

Hypercortisolism suppresses neurogenesis by decreasing neuronal synthesis of BDNF (Anacker et al., 2013) and, consequently, is posited to play a role in the reductions in the volume of several areas of the cortex associated with depression. Importantly, treatments that reduce hypercortisolism have also been shown to at least partly reverse hippocampal volume reduction in other conditions, including posttraumatic stress disorder (Bremner, 1999), Cushing's disease (Starkman et al., 1999), and depression (Bellani, Dusi, Yeh, Soares, & Brambilla, 2011). In one study with a 3-year follow-up, patients who remitted showed significantly less cortical volume reduction than did those who had persistent depression (Frodl et al., 2008). However, given that reduced hippocampal volume has been documented in patients experiencing their first lifetime depressive episode (Frodl et al., 2002), this may also be a risk factor for chronic or persistent depression, as well as a consequence. Consistent with this view, primates with smaller hippocampal volumes have been found to have increased cortisol responses to experimentally induced stress (Lyons, Parker, Zeitzer, Buckmaster, & Schatzberg, 2007).

Dysregulation of HPA activity plays an important role in the pathophysiology of depression and, ultimately, may prove to be a target for novel therapeutics of severe depressive disorders (Holsboer & Ising, 2010). Nevertheless, like stress itself, hypercortisolism is not unique to depression and is evident in a significant minority of people suffering from acute schizophrenia, mania, posttraumatic stress disorder, and other distressing mental disorders. Abnormalities of HPA regulation also commonly occur in advanced Alzheimer's disease, presumably due to acceleration of hippocampal cell death (Swaab et al., 2005).

Antidepressants, Monoamine Receptors, and Intracellular Mechanisms

Although it was known by the mid-1960s that TCAs and MAOIs enhance NE and 5-HT neurotransmission, several puzzling discrepancies indicated that the mechanisms underlying antidepressant response were not due simply to monoamine agonist effects. For example, although increased NE or 5-HT levels were available in the synaptic cleft within hours of administration of NE or 5-HT reuptake inhibitors, antidepressant responses took weeks to emerge (Duman et al., 1997; Shelton, 2007). By contrast, some NE agonists, as exemplified by cocaine, were shown to have rapid mood-elevating properties but no sustained antidepressant effects. The MAOIs, which increase synaptic monoamine levels by inhibiting intracellular degradation of NE, 5-HT, and DA, similarly were associated with a time course of antidepressant effects that typically lagged at least several weeks behind the biochemical effects.   It is now clear that the synaptic effects of antidepressant medications only initiate a sequence or cascade of effects that culminate within the nuclei of serotoninergic and noradrenergic neurons, modulating the activity of specific genes (Duman, Heninger & Nestler, 1997; Shelton, 2007). Thus the interplay resulting from effects on monoamine reuptake transporters and changes in the "signal" of cellular electrical activity is transduced into a series of intracellular reactions of second and third messengers that activate or inhibit the activity of selected genes. The pathway of action of antidepressant medication initiates an effect at 5-HT or NE receptors, whether by diffusely increasing the availability of monoamines at the synapse (i.e., the MAOIs) or selectively by inhibiting monoamine reuptake or blocking postsynaptic receptors. Receptor binding activates membrane-bound g-proteins and enzymes such as phospholipase C (PLC), protein kinase C, and adenylate cyclase (AC) (Shelton, 2007). These enzymes catalyze the formation of second messengers, such as cyclic adenomonophosphate (cAMP) and diacylglycerol. The second messengers, in turn, activate protein kinases A and C (PKA and PKC, respectively), which phosphorylate the gene transcription factor CREB (cAMP response element binding protein). CREB appears to be the first common step shared by antidepressants that selectively modulate NE or 5-HT neurotransmission (Shelton, 2007).

Phosphorylated CREB regulates the activity of a number of genes related to stress responses, including the genes that code for CRH, GRs, brain-derived neurotropic factor (BDNF), and tropomyosin-related kinase B (TRKB), which is the intracellular receptor for BDNF (Duman et al., 2007; Shelton, 2007). As noted earlier, BDNF has received considerable attention over the past decade because it has been shown to reverse or inhibit stress-induced apoptosis, because it is necessary for neurogenesis, and because it plays a key role in neuroplasticity (Jiang & Salton, 2013; Pittenger & Duman, 2008). BDNF levels are significantly decreased by a variety of stressors and increased by a variety of antidepressant interventions (Pittenger & Duman, 2008). Importantly, whereas BDNF promotes stress resilience in brain regions such as the hippocampus, it reduces appetitive and exploratory behavior in mesolimbic regions and plays an important role in mediating behavioral responses to social defeat (Pittenger & Duman, 2008).

Levels of BDNF are reduced in the plasma of people with depression (Molendijk et al., in press). This abnormality appears to be reversed by antidepressant treatment and, as such, may be a state-dependent marker of depressive symptom severity (see, e.g., Sen, Duman, & Sanacora, 2008). Although it remains to be seen whether this is a direct correlate of antidepressant action or an epiphenomenon, interventions that target BDNF synthesis in the hippocampus nevertheless continue to be an important area of treatment development.

Glutamate, NMDA Receptors, and Ketamine

The excitatory amino acid glutamate is the most widely distributed neurotransmitter in the CNS (Kingsley, 2000) and, following the initial confirmation of the rapid antidepressant effects of the glutamatergic antagonist ketamine (Zarate et al., 2006), there has been intense interest in this ubiquitous excitatory neurotransmitter (see, e.g., Krystal, Sanacora, & Duman, 2013).

There are two types of glutamate receptors: the α-amino-3-hydroxy-5-methylisoxazole-4-propionic acid (AMPA) receptor and the N-methyl-D-aspartate (NMDA) receptor. AMPA receptors are ionotropic (i.e., cation channels) transmembrane receptors that mediate fast synaptic transmission in the brain. AMPA receptors (AMPAR), which are essential for development of long-term potentiation (LTP) of neurons, are composed of four types of subunits, designated as Glu_{R1}, Glu_{R2}, Glu_{R3}, and Glu_{R4}. Most AMPARs are either homo-tetramers (i.e., four units of Glu_{R1} or Glu_{R4}) or symmetric combinations of two units of Glu_{R2} and a second dimer consisting of Glu_{R1}, $Glu_{R3,}$ or Glu_{R4}; each subunit has a binding site for glutamate. The ion channel opens when at least two sites are occupied. Most AMPA receptors in the brain include Glu_{R2} subunits, which are impermeable to calcium and hence help to guard against neurotoxicity.

The NMDA receptor is an ionotropic receptor for glutamate (and, to a lesser extent, aspartate); activation of these receptors open nonselective ion channels that allow sodium and calcium influx and potassium efflux. It is the calcium influx that results in the critical role that NMDA receptors play in both synaptic plasticity and neurotoxicity. NMDA receptors consist of heterodimers formed by NR_1 and NR_2 subunits; there are multiple receptor isoforms, which are characterized by distinct patterns of distribution within the brain and unique functional properties. Each receptor has three regions, constituting the extracellular, membrane, and intracellular domains. The extracellular domain includes NR_1 subunits that bind to glycine and NR_2 subunits that bind to glutamate. The membrane domain includes the channel pores, which are highly permeable to calcium and are subject to a voltage-dependent magnesium block. The intracellular domain contains residues that are modifiable by protein kinases and protein phosphatases.

The potential relevance of drugs that block NMDA receptors is arguably the topic of the greatest research activity in antidepressant therapeutics (Krystal et al., 2013). Importantly, neurons and glial cells in the hippocampus and amygdala have high concentrations of NMDA receptors, and intracellular accumulation of glutamate can have neurotoxic effects (Sanacora & Banasr, 2013). Thus reductions in the number or function of glial cells that can occur as a consequence of chronic stress may have particularly detrimental effects with respect to neuronal exposure to glutamate (Sanacora & Banasr, 2013). With respect to the dramatic antidepressant effects of ketamine, it is proposed that the effect is mediated by activation of synaptic plasticity mechanisms (Kavalali & Monteggia, 2012), and ketamine infusion causes a rapid increase in plasma BDNF levels (Duncan, Selter, et al., 2013).

More research is needed to determine whether this remarkable effect can be safely harnessed for more routine clinical use: Ketamine has psychomimetic effects and abuse potential, and it is not yet know whether tolerance will develop to its therapeutic effects or whether repeated exposure will be associated with adverse consequences, such as neurotoxicity. However, the complexity of the NMDA receptor offers multiple potential targets for novel drugs and, because the psychotomimetic and antidepressant effects of ketamine infusion are uncorrelated, there is reason for optimism that safer compounds may be identified.

γ-Aminobutyric Acid

γ-aminobutyric acid (GABA) has inhibitory effects on NE and DA pathways. GABA receptors are densely localized in the thalamus and ascending mesocortical and mesolimbic systems (Kingsley, 2000; Paul, 1995). GABA is released in a calcium (Ca^{2+})–dependent fashion from interneurons in the cortex, brainstem, and spinal cord and dampens the activity of excitatory neural circuits. Through this mechanism, inhibitory GABA-ergic neurons help to mediate the expression of the behaviors associated with learned helplessness (Berton et al., 2007). There are two principal subtypes of GABA receptors, referred to as A and B (Paul, 1995). Benzodiazepines and barbiturates attach to $GABA_A$ receptors, which serve to "gate" the control of membrane chloride (Cl^-) ion channels. This results in localized hyperpolarization of neurons, which decreases their responsivity to excitatory neurotransmitters. $GABA_B$ receptors are indirectly coupled to membrane potassium (K^+) channels via a G-protein and have uncertain clinical relevance (Kingsley, 2000; Paul, 1995).

Chronic stress can reduce or deplete GABA levels in these regions of the brain, perhaps reflecting, yet again, an example of an excessive demand outstripping the capacity for synthesis (Weiss & Kilts, 1998). Although definitive evidence is lacking, there has been ongoing interest in the role of deficient GABA-ergic inhibition in depressive disorders (Croarkin, Levinson, & Daskalakis, 2011). Reduction of GABA levels in depression has been observed in plasma and CSF specimens (Petty, 1995), in postmortem tissues of suicide victims (Rajkowska, O'Dwyer, Teleki, Stockmeier, & Miguel-Hidalgo, 2007; Sequeria et al., 2007), and *in vivo* in studies using proton magnetic resonance spectroscopy (Hasler et al., 2007).

Acetylcholine

Neuron fibers containing acetylcholine (ACH) are distributed diffusely throughout the cerebral cortex and interact extensively with monoamine and glucocorticoid systems (Kingsley, 2000). At the most general level, ACH neurons have alerting or activating acute effects on brain systems, as reflected by increased release of ACTH and cortisol, increased nocturnal awakenings, and increased firing of LC neurons (Janowsky & Overstreet, 1995). The two principal subtypes of ACH receptors are called nicotinic and muscarinic receptors.

It has long been known that drugs that have agonist and antagonist effects on ACH have opposing effects on depressive symptoms (Janowsky & Overstreet, 1995). Behavioral changes following administration of an ACH agonist include lethargy, anergia, and psychomotor retardation in normal participants and, among patients, exacerbation of depression, as well as weak and transient antimanic effects (Janowsky & Overstreet, 1995).

There is evidence from studies of animals and humans that heightened muscarinic ACH receptor sensitivity can induce some of the neurobiological changes associated with depression (Janowsky & Overstreet, 1995). For example, a strain of mice bred to be supersensitive to cholinergic effects develops learned helplessness quickly when exposed to inescapable stress (Overstreet, 1993). Similarly, some remitted patients with recurrent mood disorders, as well as their never-ill first-degree relatives, manifest a trait-like supersensitivity to cholinergic agonists (Sitaram, Dubé, Keshavan, Davies, & Reynal, 1987). Elevated choline levels in depression likewise have been detected by *in vivo* studies utilizing magnetic resonance spectroscopy, particularly in basal ganglia regions (Yildiz-Yesiloglu & Ankerst, 2006). A specific gene accounting for such heightened activity has not yet been confirmed, although a polymorphism of the type 2 muscarinic receptor has been implicated. A state of cholinergic supersensitivity also can be induced by attenuating adrenergic activity (Schittecatte et al., 1992). Interest in the therapeutic potential of cholinergic antagonists has recently been reactivated by the work of Drevets, Zarate, and Furey (2013), who have found that intravenous scopolamine has robust and relatively sustained antidepressant effects.

Abnormalities of Other Hormonal Regulatory Systems

Thyroid Axis Dysregulation

Thyroid gland dysfunction has long known to be associated with an increased risk for depression (Fountoulakis et al., 2006), and there has been sustained interest in the relation of the brain's regulation of the thyroid axis to depressive disorders (Hage & Azar, 2012). In particular, studies have examined the role of the hypothalamic (thyrotropin-releasing hormone [TRH]) and pituitary (thyroid-stimulating hormone [TSH]) neuropeptides that drive the thyroid axis in relation to the pathophysiology of depression (Hage & Azar, 2012). It is important to note, however, that relatively few people who seek treatment for depression have frank hypothyroidism, and only a small percentage have subclinical hypothyroidism (Fountoulakis et al., 2006). Nevertheless, it is also true that normal thyroid function is essential for central control of energy metabolism (Hage & Azar, 2012) and neurogenesis (Montero-Pedrazuela et al., 2006), as well as a precondition for antidepressant response (Cole et al., 2002). Interestingly, the therapeutic potential of adjunctive therapy with l-triiodothyronine, which has been used in combination with antidepressants with mixed results, may be limited to those patients with depression who carry a less functional polymorphism of the gene for type 1 deiodinase, which is involved in the conversion of thyroid hormone in the brain (Cooper-Kazaz et al., 2009).

A significant minority of patients with depression with otherwise normal basal thyroid hormone levels—up to 40% in studies of inpatients with depression—manifest a blunted TSH response to a test dose of TRH (Hage & Azar, 2012). Given that this abnormality does not rapidly reverse with effective treatment and is predictive of increased risk of depressive relapse (Kirkegaard & Faber, 1998), it may be a potential trait marker for illness vulnerability. Within the context of normal basal levels of thyroid hormones, a blunted TSH response to TRH is indicative of down-regulation of thyrotropin responsiveness as a consequence of increased extra-hypothalamic "drive" on the thyroid axis (Hage & Azar, 2012). It is likely that this represents a nonspecific consequence of a chronic stress-related process.

Growth Hormone and Somatostatin

Growth hormone (GH) is secreted by cells in the anterior pituitary in response to the hypothalamic neuropeptide growth hormone–releasing factor (GHRF), as well as noradrenergic stimulation via α_2 receptors (Holsboer, 1995). GH secretion is principally inhibited by the neuropeptides somatostatin and CRH. Significant concentrations of somatostatin are found in the amygdala, hippocampus, nucleus accumbens, prefrontal cortex, and LC (Plotsky, Owens, & Nemeroff, 1995). GH secretion normally follows a 24-hour circadian rhythm, with highest levels between 2300 and 0200 hours (i.e., normally during the first 2–3 hours of sleep). The nocturnal rise in GH secretion thus coincides with the greatest amount of deep, slow-wave sleep (SWS; Steiger, 2007). The most consistent alteration of GH associated with depression is blunted release in response to a variety of agents with noradrenergic agonist effects, including antidepressants such as desipramine and the selective α_2 agonist clonidine (Holsboer, 1995). Blunted GH release has been documented in childhood-onset depression (Dahl et al., 2000) and appears to be both trait-like (Coplan et al., 2000) and most pronounced among people with depression with diminished SWS (Steiger, 2007).

Alterations of Sleep Neurophysiology

The neurochemical processes that mediate sleep are well characterized (Steiger, Dresler, Kluge, & Schüssler, 2013). The diurnal sleep–wake circadian rhythm is "paced" by the suprachiasmatic nucleus of the hypothalamus. The propensity to sleep is marked by a nocturnal rise in the pineal hormone melatonin, which coincides with low levels of ACTH and cortisol. Melatonin is released from the pineal gland following the onset of darkness in response to β-adrenergic stimulation. There is also a 90-minute infradian cycle oscillating between REM and non-REM sleep; this cycle is normally suppressed during wakefulness. The desynchronization of electroencephalographic (EEG) rhythms following sleep onset partly reflects decreased activity of the LC and increased inhibitory activity of GABA-ergic and 5-HT neurons; the latter effect appears to be mediated by 5-HT$_2$ receptors (Horne, 1992; Steiger et al., 2013). Beyond facilitating sleep onset, 5-HT neurons tonically inhibit the onset of REM sleep; this effect appears to be mediated by 5-HT$_{1A}$ receptors. Near the end of each 90-minute REM–non-REM cycle, 5-HT neurons cease firing, which "releases" the pontine cholinergic neurons that initiate rapid eye movements. The depth of sleep also is facilitated by certain neuropeptides, including growth hormone-releasing hormone, ghrelin, galanin, and neuropeptide Y, and disrupted by others, including CRH and somatostatin (Steiger et al., 2013).

A significant proportion of people with depression manifest reduced SWS and an early onset of the first period of REM (also referred to as reduced REM latency), although neither of these abnormalities is specific to depression (Thase, 2006). Reduced REM latency and decreased SWS are significantly correlated, in large part because 30–40 minutes of SWS during the first non-REM sleep period normally inhibits the onset of the first REM period. SWS propensity is partly under genetic control and, consistent with trait-like behavior, reduced SWS often persists following clinical recovery (Kupfer & Ehlers, 1989). Decreased SWS activity has been proposed to represent a marker of impaired neuroplasticity in depression (Duncan, Selter, et al., 2013). Although both of these changes in sleep electrophysiology are observed with aging, depression appears to accelerate this process by a decade or more (Thase, 2006).

Compared with age-matched healthy controls, people with depression also experience an increase in nocturnal awakenings and a decrease in total sleep time. Whereas reduced SWS appears to be state-independent with conventional antidepressant therapies, sleep continuity disturbances associated with depression are correlated with symptom severity. Unlike normal aging, depression is also associated with an increase in the frequency and amplitude of REM sleep (Thase, 2006). Such changes in the phasic activity of REM sleep, quantified as measures of REM intensity or density, are greatest during the first several REM periods. Increased "phasic" REM sleep typically co-occurs with other state-dependent biological abnormalities, including hypercortisolemia (Thase & Howland, 1995). Increased phasic REM sleep is more pronounced in recurrent depression compared with a single lifetime episode and is one component of a profile of sleep disturbances associated with poorer response to psychotherapy (Thase et al., 1998). Although linked to severity and at least partly reversible with effective treatment, increased indices of phasic REM sleep also appear to characterize people at high risk for depressive disorder (Modell, Ising, Holsboer, & Lauer, 2005).

Antidepressants have variable effects on measures of sleep efficiency, which are largely the result of sedative properties that are largely attributable to antihistaminic effects (Thase, 2006). Potent monoamine reuptake inhibitors that are not sedating tend to be relatively sleep-neutral, with some tendency toward a lighter level of sleep that is offset by improvements in subject complaints of insomnia (Thase, 2006). Drugs that block 5-HT$_{2C}$ receptors, including mirtazapine and agomelatine, may have an advantage over SSRIs and SNRIs in terms of improvements in sleep efficiency (Thase, 2006). Interestingly, a ketamine infusion has been shown to cause an increase in slow-wave activity (Duncan, Sarasso, et al., 2013), which is not typically observed during antidepressant therapy, further differentiating the effects of this drug from conventional antidepressants.

Most antidepressants, including the SSRIs, SNRIs, TCAs, and MAOIs, rapidly delay the onset of REM sleep and suppress phasic REM sleep (Thase, 2006). Pharmacological REM suppression is mediated by stimulation of 5-HT$_{1A}$ receptors, as well as by less well-characterized effects of NE neurotransmission. Although it was once thought that REM suppression might be a necessary action of antidepressant therapies, it is now clear that REM suppression is only weakly correlated with antidepressant efficacy, and several antidepressants have little to no effect on REM sleep (Thase, 2006). Effective treatment with psychotherapy also does not reliably change REM sleep parameters (Thase, Fasiczka, Berman, Simons, & Reynolds, 1998). Together, these findings indicate that REM suppression is neither a necessary nor a sufficient element of antidepressant therapy.

Depression and Circadian Rhythms

Sleep disturbances, increased cortisol secretion, blunted nocturnal growth-hormone secretion, and elevated nocturnal body temperature all reflect abnormalities of circadian biological rhythms, with severe depression possibly representing an abnormal phase advancement of circadian rhythms (Wirz-Justice, 2009). It was also noted that people with depression suffer from disruptions of the social zeitgebers (i.e., meal times, periods of companionship, and exercise) that help to entrain circadian rhythms (Ehlers, Frank, & Kupfer, 1988). Indeed, the alterations in circadian rhythms associated with depression are likely better viewed as a disorganization of functions than as a phase advance. Thus the state of dysphoric activation that characterized more severe depressions—whether mediated by increased levels of CRH and/or glutamatergic drive or decreased inhibitory neurotransmission from 5-HT or GABA pathways—may disrupt the more subtle regulation of circadian rhythms. There is, however, evidence of a circadian phase delay in the subset of patients who experience recurrent winter depression (Lewy et al., 2007) that is responsive to manipulations of the photoperiod via bright white morning light or dawn stimulation (Lewy et al., 2007; Wirz-Justice, 2009).

Immunological Disturbances

Depressive disorders are associated with several immunological abnormalities, including decreased lymphocyte proliferation in response to mitogens and other forms of impaired cellular immunity (Felger & Lotrich, 2013; Raison, Capuron, & Miller, 2006). These lymphocytes and macrophages produce proinflammatory peptides such as C-reactive protein (CRP) and cytokines such the interleukins (IL), which in turn interact with neuromodulators such as BDNF and CRH (Felger & Lotrich, 2013; Raison et al., 2006). In fact, patients with low pretreatment levels of BDNF are at greatest risk for development of depression during interferon therapy for hepatitis (Lotrich, Albusaysi, & Ferrell, 2013).

Although depression is not invariably associated with alterations in immune response, the number of studies reporting positive associations is too great to discount, and this relation is likely to contribute to the increased risk of inflammatory diseases, including arthritis, allergy, and atherosclerosis, associated with depression (Glassman & Miller, 2007). For this reason, a placebo-controlled study was undertaken evaluating the potential therapeutic value of tumor necrosis factor antagonist infliximab in 60 patients with treatment-resistant depression (Raison et al., 2013). Although the investigators observed no significant effect for infliximab infusions overall, there was a large effect favoring the active therapy group among the subset of 22 patients with elevated CRP levels. If replicated, this finding would suggest an alternate therapeutic pathway for the subset of treatment-resistant depressed patients with elevated inflammatory markers.

As noted earlier, studies of the behavioral and neurochemical effects associated with interferon treatment have provided a rich area for investigating relations between depression and immune function (see, e.g., Lotrich et al., 2013; Sarkar & Schaefer, in press). The risk of depression during interferon therapy has been linked to an allelic variation in several genes relevant to BDNF and serotoninergic neurotransmission (Lotrich et al., 2013). Furthermore, the risk of depression during interferon therapy is significantly reduced by pretreatment with antidepressants (Sarkar & Schaefer, in press).

Cerebral Metabolism and Blood Flow in Depressive Disorders

The activity of neuronal circuitry may be visualized in the living brain via PET or fMRI scans. In studies utilizing PET to measure cerebral glucose utilization (because glucose is the primary source of energy for neurons, it is an excellent marker of neuronal activity), experimentally provoked dysphoria has been shown to increase cerebral blood flow (CBF) to the thalamus, medial prefrontal cortex, and amygdala in healthy individuals (Mayberg, 2003), with deactivation of the dorsolateral prefrontal cortex (DLPC) observed in some studies (see Freed & Mann, 2007). The most widely replicated PET finding associated with clinical depression is reduced glucose utilization in the anterior cortical structures, including DLPC (Drevets, 2000; Mayberg, 2003). Reductions in DLPC activity have also been documented in studies using fMRI (Hamilton et al., 2012; Siegle, Thompson, Carter, Steinhauer, & Thase, 2007). Frontal hypometabolism has been shown to be reversible following switches from depression into mania in bipolar depression (Ketter et al., 1994), as well as in response to both psychotherapy and pharmacotherapy (Bellani et al., 2011; Siegle, Carter, & Thase, 2006).

In addition to a global reduction of anterior cerebral metabolism, increased glucose metabolism has been observed in several limbic regions, most prominently the amygdala and anterior cingulate (Drevets, 2000; Hamilton et al., 2012). The strongest evidence of limbic hypermetabolism is found in studies of patients with a family history of severe, recurrent depression, or hypercortisolemia (Drevets, 2000). Among this high-risk group, limbic hypermetabolism is suppressed by pharmacotherapy but re-emerges when patients are taken off medication (Bellani et al., 2011).

As noted earlier, amygdalar hypermetabolism appears to be the emotional "amplifier" that helps to distort the stress responses of vulnerable people. Abnormalities of prefrontal and limbic systems appear to be unrelated (i.e., having one does not increase the likelihood of manifesting the other), at least in patients with mild to moderate depression (Siegle et al., 2007) and thus may represent separate targets for therapy (Siegle et al., 2006, 2012). There is some evidence that cognitive-behavioral therapy and antidepressant medication result in different patterns of changes in cerebral blood flow, with psychotherapy showing a greater impact on anterior cortical structures and medication having a greater effect on subcortical structures, including the amygdala (Kennedy et al., 2007).

SUMMARY, SYNTHESIS, AND FUTURE DIRECTIONS

Major depressive disorder is a heterogeneous clinical entity and, not surprisingly, is associated with a wide range of neurobiological disturbances. The characteristics that have been shown to be at least partly state-dependent—including elevated peripheral levels of NE metabolites, increased phasic REM sleep, poor sleep maintenance, hypercortisolism, impaired cellular immunity, and decreased DLPC activity—tend to coaggregate among more severely symptomatic patients, particularly older patients who have experienced recurrent depressive episodes; this constellation partly maps on the classic clinical prototype of endogenous depression or melancholia.

The trait-like neurobiological characteristics of depression—including low 5-HIAA, decreased SWS, reduced REM latency, blunted nocturnal growth hormone response, and increased limbic response to stress—are associated with an early age of onset and greater heritability. In people manifesting these traits, symptom expression early in the course of the illness may be shaped by the developmental trajectory of functional inhibitory response systems (i.e., 5-HT and GABA), resulting in symptoms that are atypical of melancholia, such as overeating and oversleeping. Given that estrogen enhances these inhibitory responses, it is not surprising that reverse neurovegetative features are most common among premenopausal women with depression (see Hilt & Nolen-Hoeksema, Chapter 19, this volume).

Nevertheless, it is also true that responses to stress, aging, and neurobiological sequelae of recurrent depression are almost inextricably interwoven. During youth and young adult life, the onset of the first depressive episode usually is associated with significant stress, a relation that is strongest with individuals with a history of increased genetic risk (Caspi et al., 2003). This association tends to unravel in midlife for individuals with a history of recurrent depressive episodes (Kendler, Thornton, & Gardner, 2001), in concert with the increasing prevalence of state-dependent neurobiological abnormalities.

Although many aspects of the neurobiology of depression remain only partly understood, there has been tremendous progress since the previous edition of this *Handbook*. The major developments include further elucidation of the intracellular processes that are relevant to both the illness and treatment response. Using messenger RNA, it is now possible to determine which genes are turned on or turned off by particular stressors or interventions. To the extent that gene products can be measured reliably in plasma or CSF, or if gene products can be tagged with radionucleotides that permit visualization of gene activity in the living brain, these techniques are increasingly relevant in clinical research.

Following completion of the mapping of the human genome, it has become possible to study the relations among various polymorphisms for genes related to neurotransmission and risk of mood disorders, as illustrated by the explosion of research that followed recognition of the link between the *s* allele of the serotonin transporter and stress response (Caspi et al., 2003; Hariri et al., 2002). Research on epigenetic effects, particularly in relation to the lasting effects of early childhood trauma, holds similar promise for the next decade. Studies evaluating various resilience factors, both psychological and neurobiological, may hold comparable promise (Karatsoreos & McEwen, 2013; Southwick, Vythilingam & Charney, 2005). The next generation of studies not only will help to further clarify the complex biopsychosocial pathways of illness transmission but may also identify new mechanisms for treatments that have more enduring or truly curative effects.

REFERENCES

Anacker, C., Cattaneo, A., Luoni, A., Musaelyan, K., Zunszain, P. A., Milanesi, E., et al. (2013) Glucocorticoid-related molecular signaling pathways regulating hippocampal neurogenesis. *Neuropsychopharmacology, 38*, 872–883.

Antypa, N., Drago, A., & Serretti, A. (2013).The role of COMT gene variants in depression: Bridging neuropsychological, behavioral and clinical phenotypes. *Neuroscience and Biobehavioral Reviews, 37*, 1597–1610.

Aston-Jones, G., Rajkowski, J., & Cohen, J. (1999). Role of locus coeruleus in attention and behavioral flexibility. *Biological Psychiatry, 46*, 1309–1320.

Bellani, M., Dusi, N., Yeh, P. H., Soares, J. C., & Brambilla, P. (2011). The effects of antidepressants on human brain as detected by imaging studies: Focus on major depression. *Progress in Neuropsychopharmacology and Biological Psychiatry, 35*, 1544–1552.

Berton, O., Covington, H. E., III, Ebner, K., Tsankova, N. M., Carle, T. L., Ulery, P., et al. (2007). Induction of deltaFosB in the periaqueductal gray by stress promotes active coping responses. *Neuron, 55*, 289–300.

Bonfiglio, J. J., Inda, C., Refojo, D., Holsboer, F., Arzt, E., & Silberstein, S. (2011). The corticotropin-releasing hormone network and the hypothalamic–pituitary–adrenal axis: Molecular and cellular mechanisms involved. *Neuroendocrinology, 94*, 12–20.

Bremner, J. D. (1999). Does stress damage the brain? *Biological Psychiatry, 45*, 797–780

Bunney, W. E., Jr., & Davis, J. M. (1965). Norepinephrine and depressive reactions: A review. *Archives of General Psychiatry, 13*, 483–494.

Caspi, A., Sugden, K., Moffitt, T. E., Taylor, A., Craig, I. W., Harrington, H., et al. (2003). Influence of life stress on depression: Moderation by a polymorphism in the 5-HTT gene. *Science, 301*(5631), 386–389.

Cole, D. P., Thase, M. E., Mallinger, A. G., Soares, J. C., Luther, J. F., Kupfer, D. J., et al. (2002). Lower pretreatment thyroid function predicts a slower treatment response in bipolar depression. *American Journal of Psychiatry, 159*, 116–121.

Cooper-Kazaz, R., van der Deure, W. M., Medici, M., Visser, T. J., Alkelai, A., Glaser, B., et al. (2009). Preliminary evidence that a functional polymorphism in type 1 deiodinase is associated with enhanced potentiation of the antidepressant effect of sertraline by triiodothyronine. *Journal of Affective Disorders, 116*, 113–116

Coplan, J. D., Smith, E. L., Altemus, M., Mathew, S. J., Perera, T., Kral, J. G., et al. (2006). Maternal–infant response to variable foraging demand in nonhuman primates: Effects of timing of stressor on cerebrospinal fluid corticotropin-releasing factor and circulating glucocorticoid concentrations. *Annals of the New York Academy of Sciences, 1071*, 525–533.

Coplan, J. D., Smith, E. L. P., Altemus, M., Scharf, B. A., Owens, M. J., Nemeroff, C. B., et al. (2001). Variable foraging demand rearing: Sustained elevations in cisternal cerebrospinal fluid corticotropin-releasing factor concentrations in adult primates. *Biological Psychiatry, 50*, 200–204.

Coplan, J. D., Wolk, S. I., Goetz, R. R., Ryan, N. D., Dahl, R. E., Mann, J. J., et al. (2000). Nocturnal growth hormone secretion studies in adolescents with or without major depression reexamined: Integration of adult clinical follow-up data. *Biological Psychiatry, 47*, 594–604.

Croarkin, P. E., Levinson, A. J., & Daskalakis, Z. J. (2011). Evidence for GABAergic inhibitory deficits in major depressive disorder. *Neuroscience and Biobehavioral Reviews, 35*, 818–825.

Dahl, R. E., Birmaher, B., Williamson, D. E., Dorn, L., Perel, J., Kaufman, J., et al. (2000). Low growth hormone response to growth hormone-releasing hormone in child depression. *Biological Psychiatry, 48*, 981–988.

Delgado, P. L. (2004). How antidepressants help depression: Mechanisms of action and clinical response. *Journal of Clinical Psychiatry, 65*(Suppl. 4), 25–30.

Drevets, W. C. (2000). Functional anatomical abnormalities in limbic and prefrontal cortical structures in major depression. *Progress in Brain Research, 126,* 413–431.

Drevets, W. C., Thase, M. E., Moses-Kolko, E. L., Price, J., Frank, E., Kupfer, D. J., et al. (2007). Serotonin-1A receptor imaging in recurrent depression: Replication and literature review. *Nuclear Medicine and Biology, 34,* 865–877.

Drevets, W. C., Zarate, C. A., Jr., & Furey, M. L. (2013). Antidepressant effects of the muscarinic cholinergic receptor antagonist scopolamine: A review. *Biological Psychiatry, 73,* 1156–1163.

Duman, R. S., Heninger, G. R., & Nestler, E. J. (1997). A molecular and cellular theory of depression. *Archives of General Psychiatry, 54,* 597–606.

Duncan, W. C., Sarasso, S., Ferrarelli, F., Selter, J., Riedner, B. A., Hejazi, N. S., et al. (2013). Concomitant BDNF and sleep slow wave changes indicate ketamine-induced plasticity in major depressive disorder. *International Journal of Neuropsychopharmacology, 16,* 301–311.

Duncan, W. C., Jr. (1996). Circadian rhythms and the pharmacology of affective illness. *Pharmacology Therapy, 71,* 253–312.

Duncan, W. C., Jr., Selter, J., Brutsche, N., Sarasso, S., & Zarate, C. A., Jr. (2013). Baseline delta sleep ratio predicts acute ketamine mood response in major depressive disorder. *Journal of Affective Disorders, 145,* 115–119.

Ehlers, C. L., Frank, E., & Kupfer, D. J. (1988). Social zeitgebers and biological rhythms: A unified approach to understanding the etiology of depression. *Archives of General Psychiatry, 45,* 948–952.

Embree, M., Michopoulos, V., Votaw, J. R., Voll, R. J., Mun, J., Stehouwer, J. S., et al. (2013). The relation of developmental changes in brain serotonin transporter (5HTT) and 5HT1A receptor binding to emotional behavior in female rhesus monkeys: Effects of social status and 5HTT genotype. *Neuroscience, 228,* 83–100.

Felger, J. C., & Lotrich, F. E. (2013). Inflammatory cytokines in depression: Neurobiological mechanisms and therapeutic implications. *Neuroscience, 246,* 199–229.

Fountoulakis, K. N., Kantartzis, S., Siamouli, M., Panagiotidis, P., Kaprinis, S., Iacovides, A., et al. (2006). Peripheral thyroid dysfunction in depression. *World Journal of Biological Psychiatry, 7,* 131–137.

Freed, P. J., & Mann, J. J. (2007). Sadness and loss: Toward a neurobiopsychosocial model. *American Journal of Psychiatry, 164,* 28–34.

Frodl, T. S., Koutsouleris, N., Bottlender, R., Born, C., Jäger, M., Scupin, I., et al. (2008). Depression-related variation in brain morphology over 3 years: Effects of stress? *Archives of General Psychiatry, 65,* 1156–1165.

Frodl, T., Meisenzahl, E. M., Zetzsche, T., Born, C., Groll, C., Jäger, M., et al. (2002). Hippocampal changes in patients with a first episode of major depression. *American Journal of Psychiatry, 159,* 1112–1118.

Gilbert, P. (1992). *Depression: The evolution of powerlessness.* Hove, UK: Erlbaum.

Glassman, A. (1969). Indoleamines and affective disorders. *Psychosomatic Medicine, 31,* 107–114.

Glassman, A. H., & Miller, G. E. (2007). Where there is depression, there is inflammation . . . sometimes! *Biological Psychiatry, 62,* 280–281.

Gotlib, I. H., Joormann, J., Minor, K. L., & Hallmayer, J. (2008). HPA axis reactivity: A mechanism underlying the associations among *5-HTTLPR,* stress, and depression. *Biological Psychiatry, 63,* 847–851.

Hage, M. P., & Azar, S. T. (2012). The link between thyroid function and depression. *Journal of Thyroid Research, 2012,* 590648

Hamilton, J. P., Etkin, A., Furman, D. J., Lemus, M. G., Johnson, R. F., & Gotlib, I. H. (2012). Functional neuroimaging of major depressive disorder: A meta-analysis and new integration of base line activation and neural response data. *American Journal of Psychiatry, 169,* 693–703.

Hariri, A. R., Mattay, V. S., Tessitore, A., Kolachana, B., Fera, F., Goldman, D., et al. (2002).

Serotonin transporter genetic variation and the response of the human amygdala. *Science, 297,* 400–403.

Hasler, G., van der Veen, J. W., Tumonis, T., Meyers, N., Shen, J., & Drevets, W. C. (2007). Reduced prefrontal glutamate/glutamine and gamma-aminobutyric acid levels in major depression determined using proton magnetic resonance spectroscopy. *Archives of General Psychiatry, 64,* 193–200.

Hayden, E. P., Dougherty, L. R., Maloney, B., Olino, T. M., Sheikh, H., Durbin, C. E., (2008). Early-emerging cognitive vulnerability to depression and the serotonin transporter promoter region polymorphism. *Journal of Affective Disorders, 107,* 227–230.

Hayden, E. P., Olino, T. M., Bufferd, S. J., Miller, A., Dougherty, L. R., Sheikh, H. I., et al. (2013). The serotonin transporter linked polymorphic region and brain-derived neurotrophic factor valine to methionine at position 66 polymorphisms and maternal history of depression: Associations with cognitive vulnerability to depression in childhood. *Developmental Psychopathology, 25,* 587–98.

Heim, C., Bradley, B., Mletzko, T. C., Deveau, T. C., Musselman, D. L., Nemeroff, C. B., et al. (2009). Effect of childhood trauma on adult depression and neuroendocrine function: Sex-specific moderation by CRH receptor 1 gene. *Frontiers in Behavioral Neuroscience, 3,* 41.

Higley, J. D., Mehlman, P. T., Higley, S. B., Fernald, B., Vickers, J., Lindell, S. G., et al. (1996). Excessive mortality in young free-ranging male nonhuman primates with low cerebrospinal fluid 5-hydroxyindoleacetic acid concentrations. *Archives of General Psychiatry, 53,* 537–543.

Holsboer, F. (1995). Neuroendocrinology of mood disorders. In F. E. Bloom & D. J. Kupfer (Eds.), *Psychopharmacology: The fourth generation of progress* (pp. 957–969). New York: Raven Press.

Holsboer, F. (2001). Stress, hypercortisolism and corticosteroid receptors in depression: Implications for therapy. *Journal of Affective Disorders, 62,* 77–91.

Holsboer, F., & Ising, M. (2010). Stress hormone regulation: Biological role and translation into therapy. *Annual Review of Psychology, 61,* 81–109.

Horne, J. (1992). Human slow-wave sleep and the cerebral cortex. *Journal of Sleep Research, 1,* 122–124.

Jacobs, N., Kenis, G., Peeters, F., Derom, C., Vlietinck, R., & van Os, J. (2006). Stress-related negative affectivity and genetically altered serotonin transporter function: Evidence of synergism in shaping risk of depression. *Archives of General Psychiatry, 63,* 989–996.

Janowsky, D. S., & Overstreet, D. H. (1995). The role of acetylcholine mechanisms in mood disorders. In F. E. Bloom & D. J. Kupfer (Eds.), *Psychopharmacology: The fourth generation of progress* (pp. 945–956). New York: Raven Press.

Jiang, C., & Salton, S. R. (2013). The role of neurotrophins in major depressive disorder. *Translational Neuroscience, 4,* 46–58.

Kandel, E. R., Schwartz, J. H., & Jessell, T. M. (1991). *Principles of neural science* (3rd ed.). New York: Elsevier Press.

Karatsoreos, I. N., & McEwen, B. S. (2013). Annual Research Review: The neurobiology and physiology of resilience and adaptation across the life course. *Journal of Child Psychology and Psychiatry, 54,* 337–347.

Kavalali, E. T., & Monteggia, L. M. (2012). Synaptic mechanisms underlying rapid antidepressant action of ketamine. *American Journal of Psychiatry, 169,* 1150–1156.

Kendler, K. S., Thornton, L. M., & Gardner, C. O. (2001). Genetic risk, number of previous depressive episodes, and stressful life events in predicting onset of major depression. *American Journal of Psychiatry, 158,* 582–586.

Kennedy, S. H., Konarski, J. Z, Segal, Z. V., Lau, M. A., Bieling, P. J., McIntyre, R. S., et al. (2007). Differences in brain glucose metabolism between responders to CBT and venlafaxine in a 16-week randomized controlled trial. *American Journal of Psychiatry, 164,* 778–788.

Ketter, T. A., George, M. S., Ring, H. A., Pazzaglia, P., Marangell, L., Kimbrell, T. A., et al. (1994).

Primary mood disorders: Structural and resting functional studies. *Psychiatric Annals, 24,* 637–642.

Kingsley, R. E. (2000). *Concise text of neuroscience* (2nd ed.). Philadelphia: Lippincott Williams & Wilkins.

Kirkegaard, C., & Faber, J. (1998). The role of thyroid hormones in depression. *European Journal of Endocrinology, 138,* 1–9.

Korf, J., & van Praag, H. M. (1971). Retarded depressions and the dopamine metabolism. *Psychopharmacologia, 19,* 199–203.

Krystal, J. H., Sanacora, G., & Duman, R. S. (2013) Rapid-acting glutamatergic antidepressants: The path to ketamine and beyond. *Biological Psychiatry, 73,* 1133–1141.

Kupfer, D. J., & Ehlers, C. L. (1989). Two roads to rapid eye movement latency. *Archives of General Psychiatry, 46,* 945–948.

Kupfer, D. J., Frank, E., & Phillips, M. L. (2012). Major depressive disorder: New clinical, neurobiological, and treatment perspectives. *Lancet, 379,* 1045–1055.

Lewy, A. J., Rough, J. N., Songer, J. B., Mishra, N., Yuhas, K., & Emens, J. S. (2007). The phase shift hypothesis for the circadian component of winter depression. *Dialogues in Clinical Neuroscience, 9,* 291–300.

Lotrich, F. E., Albusaysi, S., & Ferrell, R. E. (2013). Brain-derived neurotrophic factor serum levels and genotype: Association with depression during interferon-α treatment. *Neuropsychopharmacology, 38,* 985–995.

Lyons, D. M., Parker, K. J., Zeitzer, J. M., Buckmaster, C. L., & Schatzberg, A. F. (2007). Preliminary evidence that hippocampal volumes in monkeys predict stress levels of adrenocorticotropic hormone. *Biological Psychiatry, 62,* 1171–1174.

Maes, M., & Meltzer, H. Y. (1995). The serotonin hypothesis of major depression. In F. E. Bloom & D. J. Kupfer (Eds.), *Psychopharmacology: The fourth generation of progress* (pp. 933–944). New York: Raven Press.

Maier, S. F., & Seligman, M. E. P. (1976). Learned helplessness: Theory and evidence. *Journal of Experimental Psychology, 105,* 3–46.

Maier, S. F., & Watkins, L. R. (2005). Stressor controllability and learned helplessness: The roles of the dorsal raphe nucleus, serotonin, and corticotropin-releasing factor. *Neuroscience and Biobehavioral Reviews, 29,* 829–841.

Mann, J. J., Brent, D. A., & Arango, V. (2001). The neurobiology and genetics of suicide and attempted suicide: A focus on the serotonergic system. *Neuropsychopharmacology, 24,* 467–477.

Mayberg, H. S. (2003). Positron emission tomography imaging in depression: A neural systems perspective. *Neuroimaging Clinics of North America, 13,* 805–815.

McEwen, B. S., & Gianaros, P. J. (2011). Stress- and allostasis-induced brain plasticity. *Annual Review of Medicine, 62,* 431–445.

Modell, S., Ising, M., Holsboer, F., & Lauer, C. J. (2005). The Munich vulnerability study on affective disorders: Premorbid polysomnographic profile of affected high-risk probands. *Biological Psychiatry, 58,* 694–699.

Molendijk, M. L., Spinhoven, P., Polak, M., Bus, B. A., Penninx, B. W., & Elzinga, B. M. (in press). Serum BDNF concentrations as peripheral manifestations of depression: Evidence from a systematic review and meta-analyses on 179 associations (N = 9484). *Molecular Psychiatry.*

Montero-Pedrazuela, A., Venero, C., Lavado-Autric, R., Fernández-Lamo, I., García-Verdugo, J. M., Bernal, J., et al. (2006). Modulation of adult hippocampal neurogenesis by thyroid hormones: Implications in depressive-like behavior. *Molecular Psychiatry, 11,* 361–371.

Nestler, E. J., Alreja, M., & Aghajanian, G. K. (1999). Molecular control of locus coeruleus neurotransmission. *Biological Psychiatry, 46,* 1131–1139.

O'Reardon, J. P., Chopra, M. P., Bergan, A., Gallop, R., DeRubeis, R. J., & Crits-Christoph, P. (2004). Response to tryptophan depletion in major depression treated with either cognitive therapy or selective serotonin reuptake inhibitor antidepressants. *Biological Psychiatry, 55,* 957–959.

O'Reardon, J. P., Cristancho, P., Pilania, P., Bapatla, K. B., Chuai, S., & Peshek, A. D. (2006). Patients with a major depressive episode responding to treatment with repetitive transcranial magnetic stimulation (rTMS) are resistant to the effects of rapid tryptophan depletion. *Depression and Anxiety, 24,* 537–544.

Overstreet, D. H. (1993). The Flinders sensitive line rats: A genetic animal model of depression. *Neuroscience and Biobehavioral Reviews, 17,* 51–68.

Paul, S. M. (1995). GABA and glycine. In F. E. Bloom & D. J. Kupfer (Eds.), *Psychopharmacology: The fourth generation of progress* (pp. 87–94). New York: Raven Press.

Petty, F. (1995). GABA and mood disorders: A brief review and hypothesis. *Journal of Affective Disorders, 34,* 275–281.

Pittenger, C., & Duman, R. S. (2008). Stress, depression, and neuroplasticity: A convergence of mechanisms. *Neuropsychopharmacology, 33,* 88–109.

Plotsky, P. M., Owens, M. J., &. Nemeroff, C. B. (1995). Neuropeptide alterations in mood disorders. In F. E. Bloom & D. J. Kupfer (Eds.), *Psychopharmacology: The fourth generation of progress* (pp. 971–981). New York: Raven Press.

Raison, C. L., Capuron, L., & Miller, A. H. (2006). Cytokines sing the blues: Inflammation and the pathogenesis of depression. *Trends in Immunology, 27,* 24–31.

Raison, C. L., Rutherford, R. E., Woolwine, B. J., Shuo, C., Schettler, P., Drake, D. F., et al. (2013). A randomized controlled trial of the tumor necrosis factor antagonist infliximab for treatment-resistant depression: The role of baseline inflammatory biomarkers. *Journal of the American Medical Association Psychiatry, 70,* 31–41.

Rajkowska, G., O'Dwyer, G., Teleki, Z., Stockmeier, C. A., & Miguel-Hidalgo, J. J. (2007). GABAergic neurons immunoreactive for calcium binding proteins are reduced in the prefrontal cortex in major depression. *Neuropsychopharmacology, 32,* 471–482.

Ressler, K. J., & Nemeroff, C. B. (1999). Role of norepinephrine in the pathophysiology and treatment of mood disorders. *Biological Psychiatry, 46,* 1219–1233.

Robinson, O. J., Cools, R., & Sahakian, B. J. (2012). Tryptophan depletion disinhibits punishment but not reward prediction: Implications for resilience. *Psychopharmacology, 219,* 599–605.

Sanacora, G., & Banasr, M. (2013). From pathophysiology to novel antidepressant drugs: Glial contributions to the pathology and treatment of mood disorders. *Biological Psychiatry, 73,* 1172–1179.

Sapolsky, R. M. (1996). Why stress is bad for your brain. *Science, 273,* 749–750.

Sarkar, S., & Schaefer, M. (in press). Antidepressant pretreatment for the prevention of interferon alfa-associated depression: A systematic review and meta-analysis. *Psychosomatics.*

Schatzberg, A. F., & Schildkraut, J. J. (1995). Recent studies on norepinephrine systems in mood disorders. In F. E. Bloom & D. J. Kupfer (Eds.), *Psychopharmacology: The fourth generation of progress* (pp. 911–920). New York: Raven Press.

Schildkraut, J. J. (1965). The catecholamine hypothesis of affective disorder: A review of supporting evidence. *American Journal of Psychiatry, 122,* 509–522.

Schittecatte, M., Charles, G., Machowski, R., Garcia-Valentin, J., Mendlewicz, J., & Wilmotte, J. (1992). Reduced clonidine rapid eye movement sleep suppression in patients with primary major affective illness. *Archives of General Psychiatry, 49,* 637–642.

Sen, S., Duman, R., & Sanacora, G. (2008). Serum brain-derived neurotrophic factor, depression, and antidepressant medications: Meta-analyses and implications. *Biological Psychiatry, 64,* 527–532.

Sequeira, A., Klempan, T., Canetti, L., ffrench-Mullen, J., Benkelfat, C., Rouleau, G. A., et al. (2007). Patterns of gene expression in the limbic system of suicides with and without major depression. *Molecular Psychiatry, 12,* 640–655.

Shannon, C., Schwandt, M. L., Champoux, M., Shoaf, S. E., Suomi, S. J., Linnoila, M., et al. (2005). Maternal absence and stability of individual differences in CSF *5-HIAA* concentrations in rhesus monkey infants. *American Journal of Psychiatry, 162,* 1658–1664.

Shelton, R. C. (2007).The molecular neurobiology of depression. *Psychiatric Clinics of North America, 30,* 1–11.

Siegle, G. J., Carter, C. S., & Thase, M. E. (2006). fMRI predicts recovery in cognitive behavior therapy for unipolar depression. *American Journal of Psychiatry, 163*, 735–735.

Siegle, G. J., Thompson, W., Carter, C. S., Steinhauer, S. R., & Thase, M. E. (2007). Increased amygdala and decreased dorsolateral prefrontal BOLD responses in unipolar depression: Related and independent features. *Biological Psychiatry, 61*, 198–209.

Siegle, G. J., Thompson, W. K., Collier, A., Berman, S. R., Feldmiller, J., Thase, M. E., et al. (2012). Toward clinically useful neuroimaging in depression treatment: Prognostic utility of subgenual cingulate activity for determining depression outcome in cognitive therapy across studies, scanners, and patient characteristics. *Archives of General Psychiatry, 69*, 913–924.

Sitaram, N., Dubé, S., Keshavan, M., Davies, M., & Reynal, P. (1987). The association of supersensitive cholinergic REM-induction and affective illness within pedigrees. *Biological Psychiatry, 21*, 487–497.

Southwick, S. M., Vythilingam, M., & Charney, D. S. (2005). The psychobiology of depression and resilience to stress: Implications for prevention and treatment. *Annual Review of Clinical Psychology, 1*, 255–291.

Starkman, M. N., Giordani, B., Gebarski, S. S., Berent, S., Schork, M. A., & Schteingart, D. E. (1999). Decrease in cortisol reverses human hippocampal atrophy following treatment of Cushing's disease. *Biological Psychiatry, 46*, 1595–1602.

Steiger, A. (2007). Neurochemical regulation of sleep. *Journal Psychiatric Research, 41*, 537–552.

Steiger, A., Dresler, M., Kluge, M., & Schüssler, P. (2013). Pathology of sleep, hormones and depression. *Pharmacopsychiatry, 46*(Suppl. 1), S30–35.

Swaab, D. F., Bao, A. M., & Lucassen, P. J. (2005). The stress system in the human brain in depression and neurodegeneration. *Ageing Research Reviews, 4*, 141–194.

Thase, M. E. (2006). Depression and sleep: Pathophysiology and treatment. *Dialogues in Clinical Neuroscience, 8*, 217–226.

Thase, M. E., Fasiczka, A. L., Berman, S. R., Simons, A. D., & Reynolds, C. F., III. (1998). Electroencephalographic sleep profiles before and after cognitive behavior therapy of depression. *Archives of General Psychiatry, 55*, 138–144.

Thase, M. E., & Howland, R. H. (1995). Biological processes in depression: An updated review and integration. In E. E. Beckham & W. R. Leber (Eds.), *Handbook of depression* (2nd ed., pp. 213–279). New York: Guilford Press.

Weiss, J. M., & Kilts, C. D. (1998). Animal models of depression and schizophrenia. In A. F. Schatzberg & C. B. Nemeroff (Eds.), *Textbook of psychopharmacology* (2nd ed., pp. 89–131). Washington, DC: American Psychiatric Press.

Wilhelm, K., Siegel, J. E., Finch, A. W., Hadzi-Pavlovic, D., Mitchell, P. B., Parker, G., et al. (2007). The long and the short of it: Associations between *5-HTT* genotypes and coping with stress. *Psychosomatic Medicine, 69*, 614–620.

Willner, P., Scheel-Krüger, J., & Belzung, C. (2012). The neurobiology of depression and antidepressant action. *Neuroscience and Biobehavioral Reviews, 37*(10), 2331–2371.

Wirz-Justice, A. (2009). From the basic neuroscience of circadian clock function to light therapy for depression: On the emergence of chronotherapeutics. *Journal of Affective Disorders, 116*, 159–160.

Yildiz-Yesiloglu, A., & Ankerst, D. P. (2006). Review of 1H magnetic resonance spectroscopy findings in major depressive disorder: A meta-analysis. *Psychiatry Research, 147*, 1–25.

Zarate, C. A., Jr., Singh, J. B., Carlson, P. J., Brutsche, N. E., Ameli, R., Luckenbaugh, D. A., et al. (2006). A randomized trial of an N-methyl-D-aspartate antagonist in treatment-resistant major depression. *Archives of General Psychiatry, 63*, 856–864.

CHAPTER 11

Neuroimaging Approaches to the Study of Major Depressive Disorder
From Regions to Circuits[1]

DIEGO A. PIZZAGALLI *and* MICHAEL T. TREADWAY

The neuroimaging literature of major depressive disorder (MDD) has exploded in recent years, with the current pace of research including over 250 new articles published each year, as estimated by PubMed. This substantial increase in neuroimaging research reflects great strides in identifying specific regions, neurotransmitter systems, and networks associated with depressive illness. Despite these discoveries, fundamental questions remain about the pathophysiology and etiology of MDD. More importantly, the neuroimaging literature has done little to directly influence clinical practice. Diagnosis of mental disorders such as MDD via objective measures has long been a goal for the fields of clinical psychology and psychiatry. Frustratingly little progress has been made on this front, however, and the "gold standard" of diagnostic validity and reliability remains expert consensus (Kapur, Phillips, & Insel, 2012).

It is against this backdrop that we present the current chapter. Given the rich literature of targeted reviews that are already available to the field, our primary goal is to provide a general survey of key findings from different neuroimaging approaches, including structural, functional and neurochemical imaging studies. Following this summary, we discuss some of the current conceptual obstacles to better understanding the etiopathophysiology of depression. We end the chapter by highlighting important directions for future studies.

---

[1] Portions of this chapter were previously published as a review article (see Treadway & Pizzagalli, in press).

Neuroimaging and the Pathophysiology of MDD

Structural Neuroimaging Studies

Adult mammalian brain systems are significantly more malleable than once believed. Indeed, at the microcircuit level, neurons are constantly altering their structure in terms of gene expression, process development, receptor density, and so on. Microbiological approaches to the study of neurons have revealed that a great proportion of these adaptations are activity-dependent, meaning that the changes are stimulated by input from other neurons. Importantly, these local activity-dependent alterations in individual neurons result in larger-scale changes in functional networks, receptor expression, and regional morphology that are detectable using *in vivo* neuroimaging methods. Examples of this include volumetric changes in brain regions associated with complex visual motion after people learn to juggle (Draganski et al., 2004), white-matter changes after adults acquire a second language (Schlegel, Rudelson, & Tse, 2012), and receptor expression changes as individuals train on a cognitive task (McNab et al., 2009). Given these readily observable changes in gross morphology associated with modest time involved in acquiring a new skill, it stands to reason that a shift as substantial as entering into a depressive episode is also associated with structural changes.

To date, a large number of studies of MDD have indeed highlighted structural alternations in multiple tissue classes. These findings have been summarized using meta-analytic approaches reporting on structural alterations observed using regions-of-interest (ROI) tracing-based methods (Kempton et al., 2011; Koolschijn, van Haren, Lensvelt-Mulders, Hulshoff Pol, & Kahn, 2009), voxel-based methods (VBM; Bora, Fornito, Pantelis, & Yucel, 2011), postmortem tissue analysis (Cotter, Mackay, Landau, Kerwin, & Everall, 2001), and diffusion tensor imaging of white-matter integrity (Liao et al., 2013). The most frequently replicated results using tracer-based methods include reduced hippocampal volume and enlarged ventricles. These results have largely been recapitulated by meta-analyses of voxel-based results, which tend to offer evidence for a more widely distributed network of structural alterations associated with MDD, including the anterior cingulate cortex (ACC), medial prefrontal cortex (mPFC), orbitofrontal cortex (OFC), dorsolateral prefrontal cortex (dlPFC), the striatum, and the amygdala.

In addition to these cross-sectional findings, a handful of studies have further identified evidence for structural fluctuations as a function of depressive state and treatment outcome. For some regions, including the hippocampus and medial prefrontal areas, several studies have suggested that volumetric differences do not emerge until after multiple episodes (McKinnon, Yucel, Nazarov, & MacQueen, 2009; Yucel et al., 2008). In contrast, the amygdala may become enlarged prior to a first depressive episode (van Eijndhoven et al., 2009). Finally, hippocampal volumes have been found to predict treatment outcome at both 1- and 3-year follow-ups (Frodl et al., 2004, 2008).

Convergent evidence of morphometrical alterations in MDD comes from preclinical work that has identified cellular and molecular mechanisms that link common risk factors for MDD—such as stress—to structural damage (McEwen, 2007; Sapolsky, 2000). Two of the most common regions identified by this work include the hippocampus and mPFC. These regions are well known to play a critical role in the regulation of stress hormones via direct and indirect projections to the hypothalamus and have been shown to be structurally vulnerable to glucocorticoid-mediated excitotoxicity. Given that elevated stress is a major precipitant of first-time depressive episodes (Hammen, 2005), the association between stress and regional microdamage is highly relevant. Similar morphometric changes in these regions have also been associated with high levels of trait negative affect in individuals without depression who have a genetic profile for developing MDD. This has been observed using both genomewide analysis (Holmes et al., 2012) and examinations of individuals without depression but with a family history of MDD (Amico et al., 2011; Saleh et al., 2012), consistent with the hypothesis that these structural decreases reflect an endophenotype marker (Hasler & Northoff, 2011).

Functional Neuroimaging Studies

The functional neuroimaging literature has grown substantially over the last two decades, with over 150 papers published each year since 2008. A wide variety of functional domains have been probed in depression, using a large number of tasks. Here, we focus on two general domains that have been most frequently examined in depression studies: (1) emotion processing and emotion regulation; and (2) reward processing. For a more comprehensive discussion of other aspects of the functional neuroimaging literature in MDD, we refer readers to the following excellent reviews and meta-analyses: Diener and colleagues (2012), Hamilton and colleagues (2012), and Pizzagalli (2011).

Functional Neuroimaging of Emotion Processing

Arguably the most common domain assessed by functional imaging studies of depression is responses to emotional stimuli. Examples include studies of responses to both explicit and implicit presentations of affect-laden stimuli (Fu et al., 2004; Siegle, Steinhauer, Thase, Stenger, & Carter, 2002; Victor, Furey, Fromm, Ohman, & Drevets, 2010), recruitment of cognitive control mechanisms required to gate out affective "distracters" during simple working memory and attention tasks (Mitterschiffthaler et al., 2008; Siegle, Thompson, Carter, Steinhauer, & Thase, 2007), and deliberate top-down control of affective responses to positive and negative stimuli (Beauregard, Paquette, & Levesque, 2006; Dillon & Pizzagalli, 2013; Erk et al., 2010; Johnstone, van Reekum, Urry, Kalin, & Davidson, 2007). The most replicated result observed during passive presentation of emotional stimuli is a heightened responsivity in limbic regions—especially the amygdala—to negatively valenced stimuli in individuals with depression. For tasks that require participants to efficiently "gate out" affective content in order to better attend to nonemotional aspects of a task or stimulus, elevated limbic activity is often accompanied by hypoactivation in prefrontal areas, including aspects of ventromedial PFC, ventrolateral prefrontal cortex (vlPFC), ACC, and dlPFC. It is noteworthy that these same regions frequently exhibit volumetric, volume density, and cortical thickness abnormalities in depression.

Although prefrontal hypoactivations are commonly interpreted as evidence of a top-down control "deficit," it is unclear whether they reflect a local deficit in network recruitment or simply a failure to engage in the task as effectively as controls. Interestingly, when task performance is matched across individuals with and without depression, there is evidence for hyperresponse in prefrontal areas (Matsuo et al., 2007; Wagner et al., 2006), possibly indicating cortical inefficiency. In addition, the specificity of alterations in amygdalar and prefrontal networks to depression is unclear. Specifically, similar patterns are frequently observed in studies of anxiety, and only a few direct comparison studies have been conducted to date (Beesdo et al., 2009; Etkin & Schatzberg, 2011). Future research is needed to further isolate the specific alterations in cortico-limbic responses to emotion in MDD and to determine the extent to which these effects are specific to a depressed mood or share a common mechanism associated with other forms of internalizing psychopathology.

In contrast to experimental paradigms that require either passive emotional processing or implicit emotion regulation in the form of attentional control, findings of studies of directed emotion regulation in MDD are highly variable. In healthy controls, down-regulation of negative emotion has been consistently associated with increased activation in mPFC and dlPFC areas and reduced activity in the amygdala (Ochsner et al., 2004). These observations, combined with observations of impaired functional coupling between mPFC and amygdala during passive viewing of affective stimuli (Matthews, Strigo, Simmons, Yang, & Paulus, 2008), led investigators to hypothesize that patients with depression would be less successful in reducing amygdala reactivity—and associated negative emotions—when explicitly regulating emotional responses to negative stimuli. Empirical support for this hypothesis, however, has been mixed. Only one study has reported that patients with depression experience more difficulty in decreasing sadness than do controls (Beauregard et al., 2006), whereas others have found no differences (Dillon & Pizzagalli, 2013; Erk et al., 2010; Johnstone et al., 2007). These studies have also generally failed to observe impaired cortico-amygdala interactions during explicit emotion regulation in MDD. Consequently, these data suggest that emotion regulation deficits in MDD do not reflect a true inability to regulate emotion when explicitly directed to do so.

Functional Neuroimaging of Reward Processing

Another primary area of functional neuroimaging research in MDD involves responses to rewarding stimuli. Although early functional magnetic resonance imaging (fMRI) (and nonimaging) studies frequently operationalized reward in terms of the passive viewing or consumption of positively valenced stimuli (e.g., Keedwell, Andrew, Williams, Brammer, & Phillips, 2005; Mitterschiffthaler et al., 2003; Surguladze et al., 2005), more recent work has increasingly emphasized constructs of reward anticipation (Dichter et al., 2009; Forbes et al., 2009; Gotlib et al., 2010; Pizzagalli et al., 2009), reinforcement learning (Kumar et al., 2008; Pizzagalli, Iosifescu, Hallett, Ratner, & Fava, 2008) and motivation (Clery-Melin et al., 2011; Sherdell, Waugh, & Gotlib, 2011; Treadway, Bossaller, Shelton, & Zald, 2012). This shift has been motivated largely by the enhanced understanding of functional segregation of dopaminergic cortico-striatal systems in reward processing, which have been found to underlie anticipation, learning, and salience of rewards, rather than affective responses to them (Berridge, 2007). Indeed, reward-related symptoms are especially amenable to a translational neuroscience approach, given how well characterized reward-related pathways are by both preclinical and human neuroeconomic studies (see Treadway & Zald, 2011, for a longer discussion). The most common observation from this body of work is hyporecruitment of striatal regions associated with reward salience, anticipation, and learning in MDD, possibly reflecting alterations in the availability of presynaptic pools in dopaminergic afferents to striatal subregions (Capuron et al., 2012; see also discussion of dopamine imaging studies later in the chapter). In addition, altered cross-talk between cortical and ventral striatal regions has been associated with rapid habituation to rewarding stimuli, also consistent with anhedonic presentation (Heller et al., 2009).

Taken together, this work highlights cortico-striatal pathways as critically involved in specific symptom domains of MDD. Of note, there is arguably greater consistency in studies of reward processing in MDD than of other cognitive processes or imaging modalities. This may reflect the facts that reward processing studies have focused on a more homogeneous symptom domain and that the neurobiology of normative functioning is better understood.

Neurochemical Imaging Studies

The hypothesis that specific neurotransmitter systems represent a core pathology of mood disorders is among the oldest in biological psychiatry (e.g., Schildkraut, 1965). For most of modern psychiatric history, this line of work has emphasized alterations in monoamines, given early observations that administration of various monoaminergic drugs could induce depressive symptoms. This approach to inferring pathophysiological mechanisms is substantially limited, however, given that the presence of drug effects that mimic a disorder does not necessarily implicate that system as a substrate of endogenous disease. Consequently, direct investigation of the role of monoamines and other neurochemicals in the pathophysiology of depression would have to wait until *in vivo* interrogation of these systems could be achieved.

Currently, the two most widely used approaches to human neurochemical imaging in psychiatric populations are positron emission tomography (PET) and magnetic resonance spectroscopy (MRS). A less commonly used technique is single-photon emission computed tomography (SPECT). Both PET and SPECT rely on the measurement of radioactive decay from an isotope that has been injected into the participant as the basis of targeting the spatial distribution of a particular receptor or protein. In contrast, MRS takes advantage of the different magnetic resonance signatures associated with distinct metabolites and is commonly used to assess the neurotransmitters glutamate (Glu) and γ-aminobutyric acid (GABA). Both of these methods have led to significant contributions to the study of pathophysiology in MDD. In this section, we review some of the primary neurotransmitter systems that have been investigated in MDD using these techniques and highlight some of the key findings to emerge regarding the molecular pathophysiology of the disorder.

Neurochemical Imaging of Serotonin Systems in MDD

Interest in serotonin (5-HT) has been central to depression research over the last three decades, owing primarily to reported success of antidepressant pharmacotherapies that selectively target the serotonergic system in both human and animal models. Evidence from preclinical studies further supports a role for serotonin in MDD symptoms, particularly those related to the processing of stress. Under normal conditions of wakefulness, serotonin neurons are tonically active (Jacobs & Fornal, 1999), and the distribution of serotonergic tone is relatively even across most brain regions (Daubert & Condron, 2010), which has been found to support normal network functioning for a variety of cognitive and goal-directed behaviors. In contrast, exposure to stress can produce a surge in 5-HT signaling, which has been found to disrupt the emotion-regulatory functions of cortico-amygdalar networks (Jasinska, Lowry, & Burmeister, 2012). Furthermore, evidence suggests that medial prefrontal projections to serotonin-releasing neurons in the dorsal raphe play a crucial role in determining adaptive versus nonadaptive responses to stress (Amat et al., 2005; Amat, Paul, Watkins, & Maier, 2008). Consequently, impaired serotonin signaling may be a substrate involved in stress vulnerability and a key risk factor in the development of MDD (Hammen, 2005; Kendler, Karkowski, & Prescott, 1999; Kessler, 1997).

For these reasons, serotonin is among the most widely imaged neurochemical systems in MDD, with more than 35 studies exploring group differences in the expression of serotonin receptor subtypes as well as the serotonin transporter (for recent reviews, see Savitz & Drevets, 2013; Smith & Jakobsen, 2013). To date, however, results have been mixed, with investigators frequently reporting higher or lower serotonin receptor or transporter expression in MDD participants than in controls (Savitz & Drevets, 2013). For example, of the 15 studies investigating expression of 5-HT$_{1A}$ receptor in patients with depression relative to healthy controls, nine reported decreased expression in MDD, four reported increased expression, and two observed no change. Similar discrepancies have been observed for other proteins involved in 5-HT signaling pathways, including the 5-HT$_{2A}$ receptor, 5-HT$_{1B}$ receptor, and the serotonin transporter.

It is important to note that most of these studies are relatively small in size (9–22 patients with MDD) and, therefore, underpowered to explore within-sample relations between serotonin function and specific symptom dimensions. This is a potentially critical limitation, as the substantial heterogeneity of MDD is likely to be associated with divergent effects on neurotransmitter systems. In addition, most of these studies have not investigated the function of serotonin signaling systems compared with baseline expression. Therefore, where there are group differences, it is difficult to know whether they should be interpreted as a primary deficit, a downstream consequence, a risk factor, or a compensatory mechanism. Consequently, although human neuroimaging data support the hypothesis that 5-HT systems are affected in MDD, future research is needed to identify the precise role of 5-HT in the pathophysiology of the disorder.

Neurochemical Imaging of Dopamine Systems in MDD

Another monoamine that has long been associated with MDD is dopamine (DA) (van Praag, Korf, & Schut, 1973; Willner, 1983). DA is well established as being necessary for motivation, reward-based learning, and goal-directed behavior (Berridge, 2007; Salamone & Correa, 2012; Schultz, 2007) and, therefore, is believed to be a substrate of reward-related symptoms such as anhedonia, fatigue, and anergia in psychiatric disorders (Barch & Dowd, 2010; Treadway & Zald, 2013). Unlike 5-HT, which is relatively uniform in its distribution across the brain, DA expression is densest in the striatum, a key structure involved in valuation, decision making, and action.

Neuroimaging evidence supporting the hypothesis that DA systems are altered in MDD has come primarily from PET and SPECT studies. This research has found that MDD is associated with changes in DA synthesis capacity as indexed by L-dopa uptake (Agren & Reibring, 1994), as well as changes in the regional distribution and availability of DA receptors and the DA transporter (DAT). As with the 5-HT studies summarized before, imaging studies of DA systems have produced conflicting results. In PET and SPECT studies of DAT, MDD has been associated with both lower (Meyer et al., 2001) and higher (Amsterdam & Newberg, 2007; Laasonen-Balk et al., 1999; Yang et al., 2008) binding potential in the striatum. Interestingly, however, all studies reporting DAT increases have used SPECT, which has much lower sensitivity than PET (Rahmim & Zaidi, 2008). Moreover, postmortem studies support the observation of reduced DAT expression (Klimek, Schenck, Han, Stockmeier, & Ordway, 2002).

Studies of DA receptor availability in MDD have also yielded mixed results. In some cases, increased striatal D2/D3 receptor binding has been shown to occur in heterogeneous samples of individuals with depression (D'Haenen & Bossuyt, 1994; Shah, Ogilvie,

Goodwin, & Ebmeier, 1997). This increase in D2/D3 receptor availability appears to contradict animal data in which antidepressant responses are associated with increased D2-like binding in the striatum (Gershon, Vishne, & Grunhaus, 2007). Other studies using medication-naïve or medication-free patients have failed to find group differences in striatal receptor binding (Hirvonen et al., 2008; Parsey et al., 2001), whereas one additional small study showed variable changes in D2-like binding following treatment with SSRIs, with patients who showed increased binding exhibiting more clinical improvement than those who did not (Klimke et al., 1999). With respect to the D1 receptor, fewer studies have examined this system given the lack of available ligands that reliably distinguish between D1 and serotonin 5-HT$_{2A}$ receptor, especially in extrastriatal areas where the receptor density of D1 and 5-HT$_{2A}$ is roughly equivalent. One study reported reduced D1 availability in left middle caudate (Cannon et al., 2009), but this finding has not yet been replicated. Taken together, these studies suggest a possible role of D2-like receptors in downstream effects of antidepressant treatment, although the precise nature of the effect and how alterations in D2-like receptor availability may be related to DA function are unclear.

As with other conflicting reports in neuroimaging studies of MDD, part of the discrepancy across studies likely reflects the heterogeneity of the disorder. Supporting this is the observation of slightly more consistent effects when MDD samples are selected on the basis of a particular symptom profile. For example, one study that restricted its MDD patient sample to individuals with anhedonic symptoms reported decreased DAT binding (Sarchiapone et al., 2006). In addition, assessments of L-dopa alterations in the striatum are present in individuals with depression with flat affect or psychomotor slowing but not in individuals without these symptoms who are not depressed (Bragulat et al., 2007; Martinot et al., 2001). Decreases in DA synthesis have also been observed in patients who develop depressive symptoms after undergoing interferon alpha therapy. This therapy stimulates inflammation-signaling cascades, which have been found to disrupt DA synthesis and may provide a link between elevated inflammation in MDD and specific symptoms related to perturbances of DA signaling, such as motivation and anhedonia (Capuron et al., 2012; Haroon, Raison, & Miller, 2011).

Taken together, these studies provide mixed evidence for general DA alterations in MDD, with additional evidence highlighting the importance of examining links between DA systems and specific symptoms in MDD, rather than in the disorder as a whole.

Neurochemical Imaging of Glutamatergic Systems in MDD

In recent years there has been substantial interest in the contribution of neurotransmitters other than monoamines to the pathophysiology of MDD, particularly the excitatory and inhibitory amino-acid transmitters of glutamate (Glu) and GABA, respectively. At an intuitive level, the hypothesis that these systems would be implicated in depression offers significant appeal. The innervation of Glu- and GABA-releasing neurons vastly outnumbers all other neurotransmitter systems in the brain, making these two neurochemicals responsible for the bulk of human information processing. Indeed, Glu and GABA signaling are heavily implicated in numerous processes relating to learning, cognition, memory, and decision making (Sanacora, Treccani, & Popoli, 2012). When considering the scope of this diverse functional anatomy, it is difficult to imagine that Glu and GABA would not be involved in at least a subset of symptoms that characterize MDD.

Evidence for alterations of Glu transmission in MDD have long been reported, but findings have been mixed, with decreases in Glu observed in CNS fluid (Altamura et al., 1993; Kim, Schmid-Burgk, Claus, & Kornhuber, 1982) and increases often found in postmortem tissue (Hashimoto, Sawa, & Iyo, 2007). These discrepancies may be due in part to the multiple roles that Glu plays in the brain (for a longer discussion, see Yuksel & Ongur, 2010). The use of *in vivo* imaging techniques such as MRS has provided more consistent evidence; a recent meta-analysis found that MDD was associated with a substantial decrease in Glu levels within mPFC/ACC (Luykx et al., 2011), though it should be noted that not all included studies were able to distinguish between Glu and glutamine, a common metabolite of astrocyte reuptake processes. Studies published after (or omitted from) this meta-analysis provided additional evidence of reduced Glu concentration in the mPFC of participants with MDD (Jarnum et al., 2011; Merkl et al., 2010; Portella et al., 2010), and similar alterations have also been detected in children with depressive symptoms (Kondo et al., 2011), as well as individuals with remitted MDD (Portella et al., 2010), raising the possibility that they constitute a trait-like vulnerability factor for MDD. Highlighting the clinical significance of these findings, among participants with MDD, increased pretreatment Glu levels predicted better ECT response (Merkl et al., 2010).

Treatment studies also implicate this neurotransmitter in MDD. The rapid-acting effects of ketamine (Berman et al., 2000; Zarate et al., 2006) have been localized to its actions on N-methyl-D-aspartate (NMDA) receptors, which are common postsynaptic targets of glutamate transmission (Duman & Aghajanian, 2012). Importantly, aberrations in Glu signaling and Glu neurotoxicity have been associated with mPFC volumetric reductions discussed earlier (Sanacora et al., 2012). Taken together, investigation of Glu dysfunction in MDD is relatively new, and questions remain regarding how alterations in Glu symptoms may result in specific symptoms. Nevertheless, given the near ubiquitous distribution of Glu signaling throughout the brain, it is likely that many of the alterations in neural circuit function observed using fMRI studies partially reflect Glu-related pathology.

Neurochemical Imaging of GABA in MDD

Investigators have documented alterations in GABA function in MDD (Hasler & Northoff, 2011; Luscher, Shen, & Sahir, 2010), including reports of reduced GABA levels in plasma and cerebrospinal fluid (Gerner & Hare, 1981; Petty & Schlesser, 1981; Petty & Sherman, 1981), as well as specific GABA reductions in mPFC in MDD (Gabbay et al., 2012; Hasler et al., 2007), as assessed with MRS. Moreover, GABA function in this region has been suggested to play a critical role in mediating negative feedback of HPA-axis activity (Radley, Gosselink, & Sawchenko, 2009; Radley & Sawchenko, 2011). Thus decreased GABA-ergic tone may foment excess glucocorticoid exposure in mPFC, as reviewed previously. The combination of increased glucocorticoid exposure and elevated GABA has been hypothesized to be a combination that may lead to increased excitotoxicity in these regions, thereby partially explaining the structural alterations in these areas summarized in the preceding section.

Integrative Summary of Neuroimaging Studies

In the preceding review of findings, two common themes emerge. The most promising result is that regardless of imaging modality, neuroimaging studies repeatedly isolate a similar network of regions in which MDD patients differ from controls. Indeed, the greatest success of neuroimaging studies in MDD has been the identification of core nodes involved in the expression of depressive symptoms. This discovery alone has been useful. In addition, neural responses in cortico-limbic circuits have been shown to discriminate between responders to different treatment modalities (McGrath et al., 2013; Pizzagalli, 2011) and have been the empirical foundation for new treatment techniques, such as deep-brain stimulation (Malone et al., 2009; Mayberg et al., 2005) and transcranial magnetic stimulation (Carpenter et al., 2012).

In spite of this progress, caveats remain. For example, while the same regions are often implicated, the direction of the effects is often contradictory (e.g., greater or lesser BOLD signal, depending on the task). Moreover, some of this consistency is undoubtedly due to confirmatory bias in ROI selection; that is, reports of group differences in a given region increase the probability that future studies will focus on the region, either with targeted measurement (e.g., volumetric tracing) or with more liberal statistical thresholds in voxel-based studies (e.g., small-volume correction). Even when group differences emerge, they are often present only at the level of group average, with comparable ranges for both groups. As a result, the field has been unable to identify and replicate neural signatures that may serve as useful biomarkers in the diagnosis of MDD or guide treatment selection.

FUTURE DIRECTIONS

Despite this progress toward localization of depressive symptomatology, neuroimaging research to date has failed to identify reliable etiopathophysiological mechanisms that can offer causal explanations of the disorder that lead to objective, biological-based diagnostic tests. Arguably, this null result has important implications both for our understanding of the biological basis of depression and for directions for future studies.

Testing Dimensional Models

A recurring theme that appears to motivate many neuroimaging studies of MDD and other psychiatric disorders is the desire to find a "final common pathway" for one or more aspects of the disease. The hope is that one might be able to identify a core pathology that—despite the possibility of diverse origins and heterogeneous symptom expression—is nevertheless both necessary and sufficient for the presence of the disorder. Examples of such primary pathologies include dopamine cell death in Parkinson's disease and possibly beta-amyloid accumulation in Alzheimer's disease. Given the increasing recognition that DSM-based diagnostic categories are unlikely to be sufficiently homogenous in terms of symptom presentation, etiology, and progression, the search for disorder-specific final common pathways has been widely criticized (Insel, 2009) with the argument that case-control studies that seek to identify the pathology of psychiatric symptoms will generally fail to observe true effects. This failure can result from case-control designs that emphasize mean group differences rather than dimensional predictors and that can inadvertently compare individuals who may or may not be far apart on a given trait (Plomin, Haworth, & Davis, 2009). Alternatively, and more endemic to psychopathology research, is a reliance on extreme-groups designs in which a target clinical phenotype is compared against so-called "super normal." Such studies often yield group differences, so it can be hard to know which end of the distribution accounts for these effects.

The need to eschew DSM-based study designs in favor of more dimensional approaches to psychiatric research is now relatively widely accepted and has received substantial institutional support from major funding agencies. For example, the Research Domain

Criteria (RDoC) initiative led by the National Institute of Mental Health (NIMH) is specifically oriented toward this goal (Insel et al., 2010; Sanislow et al., 2010). Nevertheless, progress on this front will require changes in expectations that journal reviewers and editors demand for clinical studies.

From Symptoms to Function

For the reasons highlighted herein, NIMH has increasingly emphasized the importance of moving away from DSM-based diagnostic categories in biomedical research on mental disorders. In its place has been the pursuit of symptom-level final common pathways. The underlying hypothesis is that the experience of a discrete symptom (e.g., anhedonia in MDD) may show greater clinical and biological homogeneity than depression as a whole. However, this formulation may be vulnerable to a similar problem; the expression of even a single psychiatric symptom often reflects the emergent properties of multiple large-scale neural networks interacting over time. At the biological level, functional vulnerabilities in these networks can result from a wide range of biological abnormalities such that common forms of network dysfunction may be unlikely to reduce to common molecular mechanisms (Villoslada, Steinman, & Baranzini, 2009). For example, the studies of familial forms of Parkinson's disease have identified six distinct genes involved in the death of dopamine neurons, which have very distinct functional targets. Consequently, it is only in certain combinations that particular allelic variants in these genes actual confer risk. Importantly, these interactive effects are revealed only through detailed pathway-level analysis.

Furthermore, it is not clear whether current operational definitions and assessments of given psychiatric symptoms are specific enough to reveal meaningful correlations with measures of biological processes (Kagan, 2007). Consider the case of anhedonia, which was once perceived as a unitary symptom construct. Anhedonia has gradually come to be recognized as involving multiple subcomponents, each of which involves distinct biological mechanisms (Barch & Dowd, 2010; Kring & Sloan, 2010; Pizzagalli, in press; Treadway & Zald, 2013). Additional challenges come from individual differences in language expression and introspective accuracy that may negatively affect assessment of nonbehavioral psychiatric symptoms. When studies use symptom inventories that ask participants to rate their affective experience "on average" over the course of a week or more, there is a critical assumption that variability in reporting accuracy is not too large to obscure any meaningful relation between reported severity level and the biological dimension of interest. However, this assumption has received little empirical investigation and may critically undermine many dimensional studies (Conner & Barrett, 2012).

Consider the Larger Context: Interactions between Biological and Contextual Risk Factors

Lastly, we encourage researchers to consider how the study of systems neuroscience at the individual level can be integrated into the broader context of etiological risk factors for MDD. Although MDD is generally conceptualized as a disease that affects individuals, there are many situational, cultural, and interpersonal factors that are not reducible to neurobiology (Kendler, 2008). Importantly, these aspects of disease risk are not adequately explained by simple diathesis–stress models, as they often involve recursive feedback loops that transcend levels of analysis. To illustrate this point, consider the role of neurotic personality traits in increasing the risk for depression. Diathesis–stress models posit that neurotic traits lead to depression through impoverished coping with life stressors, a model that can easily be studied at the level of systems and molecular neuroscience. Neurotic individuals may show both stronger affective responses to stress and difficulty exerting cognitive control over emotionally arousing stimuli. This in turn can result in prolonged exposure to the damaging effects of stress-related signaling cascades, further weakening structures involved in negative feedback regulation. Although this type of model has been highly productive for the field, individual reactions to stress cannot fully account for risk conferred by neurotic traits. In addition to their own reactivity to stress, individuals with neurotic traits are often experienced as difficult to be around, making them less desirable social companions. Consequently, psychologically healthy individuals may seek to minimize contact with individuals with neurotic traits, leaving them to experience more isolation and rejection than normally occurs (Kendler et al., 1999) or to seek out the company of those who are willing to engage in corumination, which may exacerbate the development of symptoms (Rose, Carlson, & Waller, 2007; Stone, Hankin, Gibb, & Abela, 2011). In other words, neuroticism increases risk for depression in part due to intraindividual factors but also through interactions with the environment (Kendler et al., 1999). Importantly, the effects of these interactions cannot always be reduced to the level of individual neurobiology.

Consequently, neuroimaging studies will need to do more than rely on experimental psychopathology approaches that seek to recapitulate symptom experiences in the scanner environment. Increasingly, efforts must be made to study psychopathology in real-world contexts, while using imaging as a means of understanding the basic cognitive architecture and individual parameters that guide such real-world behaviors. Progress to this end has already begun, with studies increasingly taking advantage of ecological moment assessment techniques to detect relations between neuroimaging variables and real-world affect (e.g., Forbes et al., 2009). However, we need to make further progress in this direction.

CONCLUSION

In sum, the neuroimaging literature of depression has grown tremendously over the last several decades. The primary fruit of these efforts has been to localize brain regions and structures that are most critical to the expression of depressive symptomatology while also increasing our knowledge of how these regions interact with particular neurotransmitter systems, neurochemicals, hormones, and other signaling proteins. Moreover, neuroimaging has yielded promising markers predicting treatment outcome (e.g., Pizzagalli, 2011) and, recently, treatment-specific markers (McGrath et al., 2013). Although these findings await replications, neuroimaging holds great promise for the development of "personalized treatments" in psychiatry. Critically, however, in order to move from questions of location to questions of circuit function, future research will need to incorporate dimensional, real-world assessments that are not constrained by clinician-derived diagnostic categories and symptom definitions.

REFERENCES

Agren, H., & Reibring, L. (1994). PET studies of presynaptic monoamine metabolism in depressed patients and healthy volunteers. *Pharmacopsychiatry, 27*(1), 2–6.

Altamura, C. A., Mauri, M. C., Ferrara, A., Moro, A. R., D'Andrea, G., & Zamberlan, F. (1993).

Plasma and platelet excitatory amino acids in psychiatric disorders. *American Journal of Psychiatry, 150*(11), 1731–1733.

Amat, J., Baratta, M. V., Paul, E., Bland, S. T., Watkins, L. R., & Maier, S. F. (2005). Medial prefrontal cortex determines how stressor controllability affects behavior and dorsal raphe nucleus. *Nature Neuroscience, 8*(3), 365–371.

Amat, J., Paul, E., Watkins, L. R., & Maier, S. F. (2008). Activation of the ventral medial prefrontal cortex during an uncontrollable stressor reproduces both the immediate and long-term protective effects of behavioral control. *Neuroscience, 154*(4), 1178–1186.

Amico, F., Meisenzahl, E., Koutsouleris, N., Reiser, M., Moller, H. J., & Frodl, T. (2011). Structural MRI correlates for vulnerability and resilience to major depressive disorder. *Journal of Psychiatry and Neuroscience, 36*(1), 15–22.

Amsterdam, J. D., & Newberg, A. B. (2007). A preliminary study of dopamine transporter binding in bipolar and unipolar depressed patients and healthy controls. *Neuropsychobiology, 55*(3–4), 167–170.

Barch, D. M., & Dowd, E. C. (2010). Goal representations and motivational drive in schizophrenia: The role of prefrontal–striatal interactions. *Schizophrenia Bulletin, 36*(5), 919–934.

Beauregard, M., Paquette, V., & Levesque, J. (2006). Dysfunction in the neural circuitry of emotional self-regulation in major depressive disorder. *NeuroReport, 17*(8), 843–846.

Beesdo, K., Lau, J. Y., Guyer, A. E., McClure-Tone, E. B., Monk, C. S., Nelson, E. E., et al. (2009). Common and distinct amygdala-function perturbations in depressed vs. anxious adolescents. *Archives of General Psychiatry, 66*(3), 275–285.

Berman, R. M., Cappiello, A., Anand, A., Oren, D. A., Heninger, G. R., Charney, D. S., et al. (2000). Antidepressant effects of ketamine in depressed patients. *Biological Psychiatry, 47*(4), 351–354.

Berridge, K. C. (2007). The debate over dopamine's role in reward: The case for incentive salience. *Psychopharmacology, 191*(3), 391–431.

Bora, E., Fornito, A., Pantelis, C., & Yucel, M. (2011). Gray matter abnormalities in major depressive disorder: A meta-analysis of voxel-based morphometry studies. *Journal of Affective Disorders, 138*(1–2), 9–18.

Bragulat, V., Paillere-Martinot, M. L., Artiges, E., Frouin, V., Poline, J. B., & Martinot, J. L. (2007). Dopaminergic function in depressed patients with affective flattening or with impulsivity: [18F]fluoro-L-dopa positron emission tomography study with voxel-based analysis. *Psychiatry Research, 154*(2), 115–124.

Cannon, D. M., Klaver, J. M., Peck, S. A., Rallis-Voak, D., Erickson, K., & Drevets, W. C. (2009). Dopamine type-1 receptor binding in major depressive disorder assessed using positron emission tomography and [11C]NNC-112. *Neuropsychopharmacology, 34*(5), 1277–1287.

Capuron, L., Pagnoni, G., Drake, D. F., Woolwine, B. J., Spivey, J. R., Crowe, R. J., et al. (2012). Dopaminergic mechanisms of reduced basal ganglia responses to hedonic reward during interferon alfa administration. *Archives of General Psychiatry, 69*(10), 1044–1053.

Carpenter, L. L., Janicak, P. G., Aaronson, S. T., Boyadjis, T., Brock, D. G., Cook, I. A., et al. (2012). Transcranial magnetic stimulation (TMS) for major depression: A multisite, naturalistic, observational study of acute treatment outcomes in clinical practice. *Depression and Anxiety, 29*(7), 587–596.

Clery-Melin, M. L., Schmidt, L., Lafargue, G., Baup, N., Fossati, P., & Pessiglione, M. (2011). Why don't you try harder?: An investigation of effort production in major depression. *PLoS One, 6*(8), e23178.

Conner, T. S., & Barrett, L. F. (2012). Trends in ambulatory self-report: The role of momentary experience in psychosomatic medicine. *Psychosomatic Medicine, 74*(4), 327–337.

Cotter, D., Mackay, D., Landau, S., Kerwin, R., & Everall, I. (2001). Reduced glial cell density and neuronal size in the anterior cingulate cortex in major depressive disorder. *Archives of General Psychiatry, 58*(6), 545–553.

Daubert, E. A., & Condron, B. G. (2010). Serotonin: A regulator of neuronal morphology and circuitry. *Trends in Neurosciences, 33*(9), 424–434.

D'Haenen, H. A., & Bossuyt, A. (1994). Dopamine D2 receptors in depression measured with single photon emission computed tomography. *Biological Psychiatry, 35*(2), 128–132.

Dichter, G. S., Felder, J. N., Petty, C., Bizzell, J., Ernst, M., & Smoski, M. J. (2009). The effects of psychotherapy on neural responses to rewards in major depression. *Biological Psychiatry, 66*(9), 886–897.

Diener, C., Kuehner, C., Brusniak, W., Ubl, B., Wessa, M., & Flor, H. (2012). A meta-analysis of neurofunctional imaging studies of emotion and cognition in major depression. *Neuroimage, 61*(3), 677–685.

Dillon, D. G., & Pizzagalli, D. A. (2013). Evidence of successful modulation of brain activation and subjective experience during reappraisal of negative emotion in unmedicated depression. *Psychiatry Research, 212*(2), 99–107.

Draganski, B., Gaser, C., Busch, V., Schuierer, G., Bogdahn, U., & May, A. (2004). Neuroplasticity: Changes in grey matter induced by training. *Nature, 427*, 311–312.

Duman, R. S., & Aghajanian, G. K. (2012). Synaptic dysfunction in depression: Potential therapeutic targets. *Science, 338*, 68–72.

Erk, S., Mikschl, A., Stier, S., Ciaramidaro, A., Gapp, V., Weber, B., et al. (2010). Acute and sustained effects of cognitive emotion regulation in major depression. *Journal of Neuroscience, 30*, 15726–15734.

Etkin, A., & Schatzberg, A. F. (2011). Common abnormalities and disorder-specific compensation during implicit regulation of emotional processing in generalized anxiety and major depressive disorders. *American Journal of Psychiatry, 168*(9), 968–978.

Forbes, E. E., Hariri, A. R., Martin, S. L., Silk, J. S., Moyles, D. L., Fisher, P. M., et al. (2009). Altered striatal activation predicting real-world positive affect in adolescent major depressive disorder. *American Journal of Psychiatry, 166*(1), 64–73.

Frodl, T., Jager, M., Smajstrlova, I., Born, C., Bottlender, R., Palladino, T., et al. (2008). Effect of hippocampal and amygdala volumes on clinical outcomes in major depression: A 3-year prospective magnetic resonance imaging study. *Journal of Psychiatry and Neuroscience, 33*(5), 423–430.

Frodl, T., Meisenzahl, E. M., Zetzsche, T., Hohne, T., Banac, S., Schorr, C., et al. (2004). Hippocampal and amygdala changes in patients with major depressive disorder and healthy controls during a 1-year follow-up. *Journal of Clinical Psychiatry, 65*(4), 492–499.

Fu, C. H., Williams, S. C., Cleare, A. J., Brammer, M. J., Walsh, N. D., Kim, J., et al. (2004). Attenuation of the neural response to sad faces in major depression by antidepressant treatment: A prospective, event-related functional magnetic resonance imaging study. *Archives of General Psychiatry, 61*(9), 877–889.

Gabbay, V., Mao, X., Klein, R. G., Ely, B. A., Babb, J. S., Panzer, A. M., et al. (2012). Anterior cingulate cortex gamma-aminobutyric acid in depressed adolescents: Relationship to anhedonia. *Archives of General Psychiatry, 69*(2), 139–149.

Gerner, R. H., & Hare, T. A. (1981). CSF GABA in normal subjects and patients with depression, schizophrenia, mania, and anorexia nervosa. *American Journal of Psychiatry, 138*(8), 1098–1101.

Gershon, A. A., Vishne, T., & Grunhaus, L. (2007). Dopamine D2-like receptors and the antidepressant response. *Biological Psychiatry, 61*(2), 145–153.

Gotlib, I. H., Hamilton, J. P., Cooney, R. E., Singh, M. K., Henry, M. L., & Joormann, J. (2010). Neural processing of reward and loss in girls at risk for major depression. *Archives of General Psychiatry, 67*(4), 380–387.

Hamilton, J. P., Etkin, A., Furman, D. J., Lemus, M. G., Johnson, R. F., & Gotlib, I. H. (2012). Functional neuroimaging of major depressive disorder: A meta-analysis and new integration of base line activation and neural response data. *American Journal of Psychiatry, 169*(7), 693–703.

Hammen, C. (2005). Stress and depression. *Annual Review of Clinical Psychology, 1*, 293–319.

Haroon, E., Raison, C. L., & Miller, A. H. (2011). Psychoneuroimmunology meets neuropsychopharmacology: Translational implications of the impact of inflammation on behavior. *Neuropsychopharmacology, 37*(1), 137–162.

Hashimoto, K., Sawa, A., & Iyo, M. (2007). Increased levels of glutamate in brains from patients with mood disorders. *Biological Psychiatry, 62*(11), 1310–1316.

Hasler, G., & Northoff, G. (2011). Discovering imaging endophenotypes for major depression. *Molecular Psychiatry, 16*(6), 604–619.

Hasler, G., van der Veen, J. W., Tumonis, T., Meyers, N., Shen, J., & Drevets, W. C. (2007). Reduced prefrontal glutamate/glutamine and gamma-aminobutyric acid levels in major depression determined using proton magnetic resonance spectroscopy. *Archives of General Psychiatry, 64*(2), 193–200.

Heller, A. S., Johnstone, T., Shackman, A. J., Light, S. N., Peterson, M. J., Kolden, G. G., et al. (2009). Reduced capacity to sustain positive emotion in major depression reflects diminished maintenance of fronto-striatal brain activation. *Proceedings of the National Academy of Sciences of the USA, 106*, 22445–22450.

Hirvonen, J., Karlsson, H., Kajander, J., Markkula, J., Rasi-Hakala, H., Nagren, K., et al. (2008). Striatal dopamine D2 receptors in medication-naive patients with major depressive disorder as assessed with [11C]raclopride PET. *Psychopharmacology, 197*(4), 581–590.

Holmes, A. J., Lee, P. H., Hollinshead, M. O., Bakst, L., Roffman, J. L., Smoller, J. W., et al. (2012). Individual differences in amygdala-medial prefrontal anatomy link negative affect, impaired social functioning, and polygenic depression risk. *Journal of Neuroscience, 32*, 18087–18100.

Insel, T., Cuthbert, B., Garvey, M., Heinssen, R., Pine, D. S., Quinn, K., et al. (2010). Research domain criteria (RDoC): Toward a new classification framework for research on mental disorders. *American Journal of Psychiatry, 167*(7), 748–751.

Insel, T. R. (2009). Translating scientific opportunity into public health impact: A strategic plan for research on mental illness. *Archives of General Psychiatry, 66*(2), 128–133.

Jacobs, B. L., & Fornal, C. A. (1999). Activity of serotonergic neurons in behaving animals. *Neuropsychopharmacology, 21*(Suppl. 2), 9S–15S.

Jarnum, H., Eskildsen, S. F., Steffensen, E. G., Lundbye-Christensen, S., Simonsen, C. W., Thomsen, I. S., et al. (2011). Longitudinal MRI study of cortical thickness, perfusion, and metabolite levels in major depressive disorder. *Acta Psychiatrica Scandinavica, 124*(6), 435–446.

Jasinska, A. J., Lowry, C. A., & Burmeister, M. (2012). Serotonin transporter gene, stress and raphe–raphe interactions: A molecular mechanism of depression. *Trends in Neurosciences, 35*(7), 395–402.

Johnstone, T., van Reekum, C. M., Urry, H. L., Kalin, N. H., & Davidson, R. J. (2007). Failure to regulate: Counterproductive recruitment of top-down prefrontal–subcortical circuitry in major depression. *Journal of Neuroscience, 27*, 8877–8884.

Kagan, J. (2007). A trio of concerns. *Perspectives on Psychological Science, 2*(4), 361–376.

Kapur, S., Phillips, A. G., & Insel, T. R. (2012). Why has it taken so long for biological psychiatry to develop clinical tests and what to do about it? *Molecular Psychiatry, 17*(12), 1174–1179.

Keedwell, P. A., Andrew, C., Williams, S. C., Brammer, M. J., & Phillips, M. L. (2005). A double dissociation of ventromedial prefrontal cortical responses to sad and happy stimuli in depressed and healthy individuals. *Biological Psychiatry, 58*(6), 495–503.

Kempton, M. J., Salvador, Z., Munafo, M. R., Geddes, J. R., Simmons, A., Frangou, S., et al. (2011). Structural neuroimaging studies in major depressive disorder: Meta-analysis and comparison with bipolar disorder. *Archives of General Psychiatry, 68*(7), 675–690.

Kendler, K. S. (2008). Explanatory models for psychiatric illness. *American Journal of Psychiatry, 165*(6), 695–702.

Kendler, K. S., Karkowski, L. M., & Prescott, C. A. (1999). Causal relationship between stressful life events and the onset of major depression. *American Journal of Psychiatry, 156*(6), 837–841.

Kessler, R. C. (1997). The effects of stressful life events on depression. *Annual Review of Psychology, 48,* 191–214.

Kim, J. S., Schmid-Burgk, W., Claus, D., & Kornhuber, H. H. (1982). Increased serum glutamate in depressed patients. *Archiv fur Psychiatrie und Nervenkrankheiten, 232*(4), 299–304.

Klimek, V., Schenck, J. E., Han, H., Stockmeier, C. A., & Ordway, G. A. (2002). Dopaminergic abnormalities in amygdaloid nuclei in major depression: A postmortem study. *Biological Psychiatry, 52*(7), 740–748.

Klimke, A., Larisch, R., Janz, A., Vosberg, H., Muller-Gartner, H. W., & Gaebel, W. (1999). Dopamine D2 receptor binding before and after treatment of major depression measured by [123I]IBZM SPECT. *Psychiatry Research, 90*(2), 91–101.

Kondo, D. G., Hellem, T. L., Sung, Y. H., Kim, N., Jeong, E. K., Delmastro, K. K., et al. (2011). Review: Magnetic resonance spectroscopy studies of pediatric major depressive disorder. *Depression Research and Treatment, 2011,* 650450. Available at *www.hindawi.com/journals/drt/2011/650450/.*

Koolschijn, P. C., van Haren, N. E., Lensvelt-Mulders, G. J., Hulshoff Pol, H. E., & Kahn, R. S. (2009). Brain volume abnormalities in major depressive disorder: A meta-analysis of magnetic resonance imaging studies. *Human Brain Mapping, 30*(11), 3719–3735.

Kring, A. M., & Sloan, D. M. (Eds.). (2010). *Emotion regulation and psychopathology: A transdiagnostic approach to etiology and treatment.* New York: Guilford Press.

Kumar, P., Waiter, G., Ahearn, T., Milders, M., Reid, I., & Steele, J. D. (2008). Abnormal temporal difference reward-learning signals in major depression. *Brain, 131*(Pt. 8), 2084–2093.

Laasonen-Balk, T., Kuikka, J., Viinamaki, H., Husso-Saastamoinen, M., Lehtonen, J., & Tiihonen, J. (1999). Striatal dopamine transporter density in major depression. *Psychopharmacology, 144*(3), 282–285.

Liao, Y., Huang, X., Wu, Q., Yang, C., Kuang, W., Du, M., et al. (2013). Is depression a disconnection syndrome?: Meta-analysis of diffusion tensor imaging studies in patients with MDD. *Journal of Psychiatry and Neuroscience, 38*(1), 49–56.

Luscher, B., Shen, Q., & Sahir, N. (2010). The GABAergic deficit hypothesis of major depressive disorder. *Molecular Psychiatry, 16*(4), 383–406.

Luykx, J. J., Laban, K. G., van den Heuvel, M. P., Boks, M. P., Mandl, R. C., Kahn, R. S., et al. (2011). Region and state specific glutamate downregulation in major depressive disorder: A meta-analysis of (1)H-MRS findings. *Neuroscience and Biobehavioral Reviews, 36*(1), 198–205.

Malone, D. A., Jr., Dougherty, D. D., Rezai, A. R., Carpenter, L. L., Friehs, G. M., Eskandar, E. N., et al. (2009). Deep brain stimulation of the ventral capsule/ventral striatum for treatment-resistant depression. *Biological Psychiatry, 65*(4), 267–275.

Martinot, M., Bragulat, V., Artiges, E., Dolle, F., Hinnen, F., Jouvent, R., et al. (2001). Decreased presynaptic dopamine function in the left caudate of depressed patients with affective flattening and psychomotor retardation. *American Journal of Psychiatry, 158*(2), 314–316.

Matsuo, K., Glahn, D. C., Peluso, M. A., Hatch, J. P., Monkul, E. S., Najt, P., et al. (2007). Prefrontal hyperactivation during working memory task in untreated individuals with major depressive disorder. *Molecular Psychiatry, 12*(2), 158–166.

Matthews, S. C., Strigo, I. A., Simmons, A. N., Yang, T. T., & Paulus, M. P. (2008). Decreased functional coupling of the amygdala and supragenual cingulate is related to increased depression in unmedicated individuals with current major depressive disorder. *Journal of Affective Disorders, 111*(1), 13–20.

Mayberg, H. S., Lozano, A. M., Voon, V., McNeely, H. E., Seminowicz, D., Hamani, C., et al. (2005). Deep brain stimulation for treatment-resistant depression. *Neuron, 45*(5), 651–660.

McEwen, B. S. (2007). Physiology and neurobiology of stress and adaptation: Central role of the brain. *Physiological Reviews, 87*(3), 873–904.

McGrath, C. L., Kelley, M. E., Holtzheimer, P. E., Dunlop, B. W., Craighead, W. E., Franco, A. R., et al. (2013). Toward a neuroimaging treatment selection biomarker for major depressive disorder. *Journal of the American Medical Association Psychiatry, 70,* 1–9.

McKinnon, M. C., Yucel, K., Nazarov, A., & MacQueen, G. M. (2009). A meta-analysis examining clinical predictors of hippocampal volume in patients with major depressive disorder. *Journal of Psychiatry and Neuroscience, 34*(1), 41–54.

McNab, F., Varrone, A., Farde, L., Jucaite, A., Bystritsky, P., Forssberg, H., et al. (2009). Changes in cortical dopamine D1 receptor binding associated with cognitive training. *Science, 323,* 800–802.

Merkl, A., Schubert, F., Quante, A., Luborzewski, A., Brakemeier, E. L., Grimm, S., et al. (2010). Abnormal cingulate and prefrontal cortical neurochemistry in major depression after electroconvulsive therapy. *Biological Psychiatry, 69*(8), 772–779.

Meyer, J. H., Kruger, S., Wilson, A. A., Christensen, B. K., Goulding, V. S., Schaffer, A., et al. (2001). Lower dopamine transporter binding potential in striatum during depression. *NeuroReport, 12,* 4121–4125.

Mitterschiffthaler, M. T., Kumari, V., Malhi, G. S., Brown, R. G., Giampietro, V. P., Brammer, M. J., et al. (2003). Neural response to pleasant stimuli in anhedonia: An fMRI study. *NeuroReport, 14*(2), 177–182.

Mitterschiffthaler, M. T., Williams, S. C., Walsh, N. D., Cleare, A. J., Donaldson, C., Scott, J., et al. (2008). Neural basis of the emotional Stroop interference effect in major depression. *Psychological Medicine, 38*(2), 247–256.

Ochsner, K. N., Ray, R. D., Cooper, J. C., Robertson, E. R., Chopra, S., Gabrieli, J. D., et al. (2004). For better or for worse: Neural systems supporting the cognitive down- and up-regulation of negative emotion. *NeuroImage, 23*(2), 483–499.

Parsey, R. V., Oquendo, M. A., Zea-Ponce, Y., Rodenhiser, J., Kegeles, L. S., Pratap, M., et al. (2001). Dopamine D(2) receptor availability and amphetamine-induced dopamine release in unipolar depression. *Biological Psychiatry, 50*(5), 313–322.

Petty, F., & Schlesser, M. A. (1981). Plasma GABA in affective illness: A preliminary investigation. *Journal of Affective Disorders, 3*(4), 339–343.

Petty, F., & Sherman, A. D. (1981). GABAergic modulation of learned helplessness. *Pharmacology, Biochemistry and Behavior, 15*(4), 567–570.

Pizzagalli, D. A. (2011). Frontocingulate dysfunction in depression: Toward biomarkers of treatment response. *Neuropsychopharmacology, 36*(1), 183–206.

Pizzagalli, D. A. (in press). Depression, stress, and anhedonia: Toward a synthesis and integrated model. *Annual Review of Clinical Psychology.*

Pizzagalli, D. A., Holmes, A. J., Dillon, D. G., Goetz, E. L., Birk, J. L., Bogdan, R., et al. (2009). Reduced caudate and nucleus accumbens response to rewards in unmedicated individuals with major depressive disorder. *American Journal of Psychiatry, 166*(6), 702–710.

Pizzagalli, D. A., Iosifescu, D., Hallett, L. A., Ratner, K. G., & Fava, M. (2008). Reduced hedonic capacity in major depressive disorder: Evidence from a probabilistic reward task. *Journal of Psychiatric Research, 43*(1), 76–87.

Plomin, R., Haworth, C. M., & Davis, O. S. (2009). Common disorders are quantitative traits. *Nature Reviews. Genetics, 10,* 872–878.

Portella, M. J., de Diego-Adelino, J., Gomez-Anson, B., Morgan-Ferrando, R., Vives, Y., Puigdemont, D., et al. (2010). Ventromedial prefrontal spectroscopic abnormalities over the course of depression: A comparison among first episode, remitted recurrent and chronic patients. *Journal of Psychiatric Research, 45*(4), 427–434.

Radley, J. J., Gosselink, K. L., & Sawchenko, P. E. (2009). A discrete GABAergic relay mediates medial prefrontal cortical inhibition of the neuroendocrine stress response. *Journal of Neuroscience, 29,* 7330–7340.

Radley, J. J., & Sawchenko, P. E. (2011). A common substrate for prefrontal and hippocampal inhibition of the neuroendocrine stress response. *Journal of Neuroscience, 31,* 9683–9695.

Rahmim, A., & Zaidi, H. (2008). PET versus SPECT: Strengths, limitations and challenges. *Nuclear Medicine Communications, 29*(3), 193–207.

Rose, A. J., Carlson, W., & Waller, E. M. (2007). Prospective associations of co-rumination with friendship and emotional adjustment: Considering the socioemotional trade-offs of co-rumination. *Developmental Psychology, 43*(4), 1019–1031.

Salamone, J. D., & Correa, M. (2012). The mysterious motivational functions of mesolimbic dopamine. *Neuron, 76*(3), 470–485.

Saleh, K., Carballedo, A., Lisiecka, D., Fagan, A. J., Connolly, G., Boyle, G., et al. (2012). Impact of family history and depression on amygdala volume. *Psychiatry Research, 203*(1), 24–30.

Sanacora, G., Treccani, G., & Popoli, M. (2012). Towards a glutamate hypothesis of depression: An emerging frontier of neuropsychopharmacology for mood disorders. *Neuropharmacology, 62*(1), 63–77.

Sanislow, C. A., Pine, D. S., Quinn, K. J., Kozak, M. J., Garvey, M. A., Heinssen, R. K., et al. (2010). Developing constructs for psychopathology research: Research domain criteria. *Journal of Abnormal Psychology, 119*(4), 631–639.

Sapolsky, R. M. (2000). Glucocorticoids and hippocampal atrophy in neuropsychiatric disorders. *Archives of General Psychiatry, 57*(10), 925–935.

Sarchiapone, M., Carli, V., Camardese, G., Cuomo, C., Di Giuda, D., Calcagni, M. L., et al. (2006). Dopamine transporter binding in depressed patients with anhedonia. *Psychiatry Research, 147*(2–3), 243–248.

Savitz, J. B., & Drevets, W. C. (2013). Neuroreceptor imaging in depression. *Neurobiology of Disease, 52*, 49–65.

Schildkraut, J. J. (1965). The catecholamine hypothesis of affective disorders: A review of supporting evidence. *American Journal of Psychiatry, 122*(5), 509–522.

Schlegel, A. A., Rudelson, J. J., & Tse, P. U. (2012). White matter structure changes as adults learn a second language. *Journal of Cognitive Neuroscience, 24*(8), 1664–1670.

Schultz, W. (2007). Behavioral dopamine signals. *Trends in Neuroscience, 30*(5), 203–210.

Shah, P. J., Ogilvie, A. D., Goodwin, G. M., & Ebmeier, K. P. (1997). Clinical and psychometric correlates of dopamine D2 binding in depression. *Psychological Medicine, 27*(6), 1247–1256.

Sherdell, L., Waugh, C. E., & Gotlib, I. H. (2011). Anticipatory pleasure predicts motivation for reward in major depression. *Journal of Abnormal Psychology, 121*, 51–80.

Siegle, G. J., Steinhauer, S. R., Thase, M. E., Stenger, V. A., & Carter, C. S. (2002). Can't shake that feeling: Event-related fMRI assessment of sustained amygdala activity in response to emotional information in depressed individuals. *Biological Psychiatry, 51*(9), 693–707.

Siegle, G. J., Thompson, W., Carter, C. S., Steinhauer, S. R., & Thase, M. E. (2007). Increased amygdala and decreased dorsolateral prefrontal BOLD responses in unipolar depression: Related and independent features. *Biological Psychiatry, 61*(2), 198–209.

Smith, D. F., & Jakobsen, S. (2013). Molecular neurobiology of depression: PET findings on the elusive correlation with symptom severity. *Frontiers in Psychiatry, 4*, 8.

Stone, L. B., Hankin, B. L., Gibb, B. E., & Abela, J. R. Z. (2011). Co-rumination predicts the onset of depressive disorders during adolescence. *Journal of Abnormal Psychology, 120*(3), 752–757.

Surguladze, S., Brammer, M. J., Keedwell, P., Giampietro, V., Young, A. W., Travis, M. J., et al. (2005). A differential pattern of neural response toward sad versus happy facial expressions in major depressive disorder. *Biological Psychiatry, 57*(3), 201–209.

Treadway, M. T., Bossaller, N. A., Shelton, R. C., & Zald, D. H. (2012). Effort-based decision-making in major depressive disorder: A translational model of motivational anhedonia. *Journal of Abnormal Psychology, 121*(3), 553–558.

Treadway, M. T., & Pizzagalli, D. A. (in press). Imaging the pathophysiology of major depressive disorder—from localist models to circuit-based analysis. *Biology of Mood and Anxiety Disorders*.

Treadway, M. T., & Zald, D. H. (2011). Reconsidering anhedonia in depression: Lessons from translational neuroscience. *Neuroscience and Biobehavioral Reviews, 35*(3), 537–555.

Treadway, M. T., & Zald, D. H. (2013). Parsing anhedonia translational models of reward-processing deficits in psychopathology. *Current Directions in Psychological Science, 22*(3), 244–249.

van Eijndhoven, P., van Wingen, G., van Oijen, K., Rijpkema, M., Goraj, B., Jan Verkes, R., et al. (2009). Amygdala volume marks the acute state in the early course of depression. *Biological Psychiatry, 65*(9), 812–818.

van Praag, H. M., Korf, J., & Schut, D. (1973). Cerebral monoamines and depression: An investigation with the Probenecid technique. *Archives of General Psychiatry, 28*(6), 827–831.

Victor, T. A., Furey, M. L., Fromm, S. J., Ohman, A., & Drevets, W. C. (2010). Relationship between amygdala responses to masked faces and mood state and treatment in major depressive disorder. *Archives of General Psychiatry, 67*(11), 1128–1138.

Villoslada, P., Steinman, L., & Baranzini, S. E. (2009). Systems biology and its application to the understanding of neurological diseases. *Annals of Neurology, 65*(2), 124–139.

Wagner, G., Sinsel, E., Sobanski, T., Kohler, S., Marinou, V., Mentzel, H. J., et al. (2006). Cortical inefficiency in patients with unipolar depression: An event-related FMRI study with the Stroop task. *Biological Psychiatry, 59*(10), 958–965.

Willner, P. (1983). Dopamine and depression: A review of recent evidence: I. Empirical studies. *Brain Research, 287*(3), 211–224.

Yang, Y. K., Yeh, T. L., Yao, W. J., Lee, I. H., Chen, P. S., Chiu, N. T., et al. (2008). Greater availability of dopamine transporters in patients with major depression: A dual-isotope SPECT study. *Psychiatry Research, 162*(3), 230–235.

Yucel, K., McKinnon, M. C., Chahal, R., Taylor, V. H., Macdonald, K., Joffe, R., et al. (2008). Anterior cingulate volumes in never-treated patients with major depressive disorder. *Neuropsychopharmacology, 33*(13), 3157–3163.

Yuksel, C., & Ongur, D. (2010). Magnetic resonance spectroscopy studies of glutamate-related abnormalities in mood disorders. *Biological Psychiatry, 68*(9), 785–794.

Zarate, C. A., Jr., Singh, J. B., Carlson, P. J., Brutsche, N. E., Ameli, R., Luckenbaugh, D. A., et al. (2006). A randomized trial of an N-methyl-D-aspartate antagonist in treatment-resistant major depression. *Archives of General Psychiatry, 63*(8), 856–864.

CHAPTER 12

Early Adverse Experiences and Depression

SHERRYL H. GOODMAN *and* CARA M. LUSBY

Researchers and clinicians have long considered early adverse experiences as having potentially great etiological significance in the development of depression. In this chapter, we take a developmental psychopathology perspective to provide an overview of the current state of knowledge and ongoing issues in the understanding of associations between early adverse experiences and depression, with the aims of informing etiological mechanisms, revealing modifiable mechanisms of transmission, and clarifying for whom the associations are strongest. In addressing these aims, we emphasize timing of exposures and take into consideration biological systems, the attachment system, cognitive diathesis, and emotion, as well as potential additive or interacting or transactional influences among such systems.

EXPERIENCES DURING FETAL DEVELOPMENT

Maternal Stress, Anxiety, and Depression

Studies of both animals and humans reveal that mothers' stress during pregnancy contributes to risk for the development of a range of behavioral disturbances in their offspring, with etiological significance for depression. For example, prenatal anxiety was associated with 4- and 7-year-olds' elevated levels of emotional problems even after controlling for other risks and postpartum anxiety and depression (O'Connor, Heron, Golding, & Glover, 2003). Prenatal depression predicts a range of poor outcomes in neonates (e.g., prematurity, low birthweight, excessive fussiness) and infants (e.g., less positive affect, higher cortisol; as reviewed in Field, 2011). Furthermore, although depression is highly comorbid with anxiety and stress in pregnant women (Goodman & Tully, 2009), the effects of depression, anxiety, and stress on offspring outcomes may differ (e.g., Brennan et al., 2008), suggesting either independent or moderated relations.

There is both theoretical and empirical support for fetal development and later outcomes being differently affected based on the timing of prenatal exposure (Martin &

Dombrowski, 2008), including stress. Early to midpregnancy exposure, compared with prepregnancy and third-trimester exposure to the stressors, was associated with emotional and behavioral problems through age 11 years in Project Ice Storm (King, Liau, Brunet, Schmitz, & Laplante, 2011). In contrast, third-trimester exposure to maternal depression, controlling for first- and second-trimester exposure, significantly predicted infant state organization and irritability (Goodman, Rouse, Long, Ji, & Brand, 2011).

Researchers from several different theoretical perspectives have attempted to identify how maternal stress, anxiety, and depression alter fetal development in ways that might place infants at risk for the later development of depression. Next, we review theory and research on six proposed mechanisms: (1) neuroendocrine abnormalities, (2) reduced blood flow to the fetus, (3) altered fetal neurobehavioral development, (4) poor health behaviors, (5) mothers' use of antidepressant medications, and (6) genetics.

Neuroendocrine Abnormalities

A fetus's first transactions with the mother occur at gestational day 13 or 14, when *in utero* blood flow is established; thus fetal exposure to the neuroendocrine correlates of the mother's stress or depression begins early and could potentially influence all aspects of fetal development. In particular, fetal exposure to hypersecretion of corticotropin-releasing factor (CRF), the prime regulator of the endocrine stress response that coordinates behavioral and biological responses to stress, could precipitate the development of abnormal biological, behavioral, and affective systems that are implicated in the etiology of depression (Davidson, Pizzagalli, Nitschke, & Putnam, 2002) and may be particular vulnerabilities to stress-induced depression (see Monroe, Slavich, & Georgiades, Chapter 16, this volume). Consequently, it has been important to determine whether prenatal stress, anxiety, or depression is associated with women's higher levels of cortisol and whether maternal cortisol is then circulated to the fetus.

Some earlier findings supported associations between fluctuations in women's prenatal stress/anxiety or depression and their cortisol levels (e.g. Field et al., 2004). By contrast, recent findings have yielded little support for this association (Evans, Myers, & Monk, 2008; Shea et al., 2007; Voegtline et al., 2013), suggesting that maternal cortisol is unlikely to be a mechanism in associations between mothers' prenatal psychological state and infant outcomes. Nonetheless, cortisol has been found to cross the placenta to the fetus: at 20–36 weeks of pregnancy, maternal levels of cortisol accounted for 50% of the variance in the fetal cortisol levels (Glover, Teixeira, Gitau, & Fisk, 1999). Thus maternal cortisol may directly influence offspring outcomes associated with the later development of depression (Shea et al., 2007).

Reduced Blood Flow to the Fetus

Reduced blood flow to the fetus might also explain risk for the later development of depression in offspring of prenatally distressed mothers, although findings have been contradictory. Glover and colleagues found maternal trait anxiety to be associated with impaired uterine blood flow in healthy third-trimester pregnant women (Teixeira, Fisk, & Glover, 1999). Since this initial finding, results of other studies have been mixed (Mendelson, DiPietro, Costigan, Chen, & Henderson, 2011; Monk et al., 2012). However, as with prenatal cortisol levels, reduced uterine blood flow may still be an early adverse experience for infants, given its association with lower birthweight and prematurity (Teixeira et al., 1999) and low birthweight having been found to predict later depression, at least in females, controlling for other early adversities (Costello, Worthman, Erkanli, & Angold, 2007).

Altered Fetal Neurobehavioral Development

Researchers have consistently shown links between maternal higher levels of stress and anxiety during pregnancy and indices of fetal neurobehavioral development, including greater fetal motor activity, higher levels of heart rate variability, and steeper incline in motor-heart coupling as gestational age increases, each of which is an index of neurological maturation (as reviewed in DiPietro, 2012). Despite these seemingly beneficial outcomes associated with maternal distress, the findings have negative implications for emotional regulation later in life, as evidenced by higher fetal activity by 36 weeks' gestation predicting infants' greater fussiness, unadaptability, unpredictability, and activity, as well as lower distress to limitations at age 1 year and lower behavioral inhibition at age 2 years. Moreover, DiPietro (2012) cautions that the facilitative aspects of maternal distress are likely to be constrained to relatively healthy, more advantaged women relative to women with clinical depression or anxiety or women dealing with poverty. In addition, findings from experimental studies suggest reason for concern. For example, fetuses of mothers with anxiety disorders had greater increases in heart rate after exposure to a mild stressor, compared with fetuses of mothers without anxiety disorders (Monk et al., 2004).

Poor Health Behaviors

A fetus may be at risk for the later development of depression because of the distressed pregnant mother's inadequate health care and engagement in risky behaviors, which may endanger healthy fetal development. For example, depression during pregnancy has been associated with less frequent and less adequate prenatal care, more unhealthy eating and sleeping patterns, and more smoking (e.g. Marcus, Flynn, Blow, & Barry, 2003). Although these maternal behaviors have most often been associated with offspring's risk for externalizing disorders (Milberger, Biederman, Faraone, Chen, & Jones, 1996), externalizing disorders predicted the duration of comorbid dysthymia in children who were experiencing their first major depressive episode or instance of dysthymia (Kovacs, Obrosky, Gatsonis, & Richards, 1997).

Mothers' Use of Antidepressant Medications

Given that antidepressant medication is the primary approach to treating depression, even in pregnancy (Dietz et al., 2007), many fetuses are exposed *in utero* to these antidepressant medications, which are known to cross the placental barrier (Loughhead et al., 2006). See Gitlin (Chapter 26, this volume). Drawing conclusions from studies of infant outcomes associated with antidepressant exposure has been constrained by methodological shortcomings, for example, self-report, retrospective data, outcome assessment not blinded to maternal status, and no control for depression severity. In one study that accounted for these issues and measured offspring outcomes relevant to the later development of depression, prenatal exposure to selective serotonin reuptake inhibitors (SSRIs) was associated with poorer neonatal outcomes even after controlling for maternal prenatal mood symptoms, although moderated by the serotonin transporter promoter genotype (Oberlander, Bonaguro, et al., 2008). In addition, 3-month-old infants prenatally exposed to SSRIs displayed lower baseline cortisol levels than infants who were not exposed, even after controlling for pre- and postnatal maternal mood (Oberlander, Grunau, et al., 2008). Furthermore, genetics may help to explain differential effects of antidepressant exposure on infant outcomes (Devane et al., 2006).

Genetics

Genetic contributions to depression are discussed in other chapters in this volume. It is noteworthy that prenatal and early postnatal environments can influence epigenetic programming, whereby epigenetic changes mediate the association between environment and gene expression, including the risk of later disorder (Kofink, Boks, Timmers, & Kas, 2013). In particular, prenatal stress has been found to decrease placental 11β hydroxysteroid dehydrogenase 2 (11 11β-HSD2) and reduce DNA methylation in the hippocampus and amygdala at the corticotropin-releasing hormone (CRH) gene (Mueller, Brocke, Fries, Lesch, & Kirschbaum, 2010). Both, in turn, alter responsiveness of the hypothalamic–pituitary–adrenocortical (HPA) axis, which may represent early vulnerability to the later development of psychopathology (Kofink et al., 2013). This genetic programming of offspring's stress sensitivity may also be sex-specific (Mueller & Bale, 2008).

EXPERIENCES DURING INFANCY AND EARLY CHILDHOOD

Early Life Experiences

The predominant aspect of early life experiences of infants and young children associated with risk for depression is inadequate parenting, which may be associated with children's risk for the later development of depression by: (1) failing to provide for infants' and young children's stage-salient needs; (2) exposing children to maladaptive models of social skills and affective expression; and (3) stressing infants through over- or understimulation. Infants and young children who experience inadequate parenting may develop problems such as emotion dysregulation, poorer interpersonal skills, and dysfunctional stress response, each of which may predispose children to the later development of depression. Humans have the capacity to respond to stress as early as the neonatal period (Graham, Heim, Goodman, Miller, & Nemeroff, 1999), such as with high levels of stress hormones potentially damaging still-developing neurons (Hane & Fox, 2006), which underscores the importance of studies of stressors in infancy.

Unresponsive or Neglectful Parenting

In face-to-face interactions with their infants, depression in mothers is associated with higher levels of disengaged parenting (as reviewed by Lovejoy, Graczyk, O'Hare, & Neuman, 2000), and infants of disengaged mothers, especially boys, display more negative affect and more self-regulatory behaviors (Weinberg, Olson, Beeghly, & Tronick, 2006). Thus persistent exchanges with a withdrawn, unresponsive caregiver both fail to provide the help infants need to learn to manage arousal and also socialize depression-like affective expressions. Moreover, from a social learning theory perspective (Bandura, 1986), infants and young children who experience low levels of contingent responsiveness to their initiatives may fail to learn healthy patterns of self-reward and adaptive attributional styles.

Intrusive, Harsh, or Coercive Parenting

Some parents, including some mothers with depression, have been observed to be intrusive, interfering, hostile, and irritable, as well as to report greater physical and psychological aggression toward their young children (Turney, 2011). In turn, maternal hostility and intrusiveness with infants has been cross-sectionally associated with infant fussiness and avoidance, especially in girls (Weinberg, Beeghly, Olson, & Tronick, 2008), and longitudinally predictive of children's internalizing problems 2 (Mäntymaa, Puura, Luoma, Salmelin, & Tamminen, 2004) and 5 years later (Mäntymaa et al., 2012). Intrusive or hostile mothers may interfere with their infants' development of autonomous functioning or contribute to a developing sense of helplessness and a tendency to view themselves as having little control over outcomes (Egeland, Pianta, & O'Brian, 1993). Each of these sets of beliefs, and their associated behavior patterns, increases children's vulnerability to depression (Chorpita, 2001).

Abuse

Physical or sexual abuse or neglect of a child by a parent represents the extreme of inadequate parenting and adverse early life experiences. Parents who abuse their children often also suffer from depression, substance abuse, high stress levels, social isolation, or an abusive partner relationship, each of which may independently or interactively increase children's risk for depression (Gelles, 1998). Infants and toddlers are the most frequently reported victims of physical abuse (Gelles, 1998), and, not surprisingly, these early abuse victims have high rates of depression in childhood and beyond (as reviewed by Jaffee & Maikovich-Fong, 2013). Maltreatment is also associated with vulnerabilities to depression such as lower self-esteem, difficulty relating to peers, insecure attachment relationships, dysfunctional attributions, social-cognitive biases (Romens & Pollak, 2012), and neuroendocrine and other biological abnormalities predictive of the development of depression (as reviewed by Cicchetti, 2013). The specific neurobiological sequelae have been found to vary based on the type of abuse, showing that the effects are influenced by many factors (Neigh, Gillespie, & Nemeroff, 2009).

Loss

The early experience of loss, particularly a parent's death and the associated grief, has long been considered a risk for depression. Recent studies, which included careful matching of risk and control samples, support links between the childhood experience of parental death and later depressive disorders (Gray, Weller, Fristad, & Weller, 2011; Schmiege, Khoo, Sandler, Ayers, & Wolchik, 2006), with the association especially strong with parental suicide or accidental death (Brent, Melhem, Donohoe, & Walker, 2009), when the loss is associated with ongoing disruptions in children's environment and routine, with depression in the surviving parent, and with the unavailability of supportive others (Brent et al., 2009; Schmiege et al., 2006).

Deprived Environments (Institutional Rearing)

For some children, loss of parents is followed by severe deprivation. In particular, international conflicts have left many children orphaned, some of whom are raised in sparse, institutional orphanages; others are adopted, either early or later in childhood; and some experience international adoptions. Researchers consistently find that whereas children who were adopted earlier (prior to 4 months of age) did not significantly differ from matched controls, children who were adopted later (especially after 2 years of age) show attachment disorders, behavioral problems, blunted circadian rhythms, elevated cortisol levels, larger amygdala volume, and more false alarms to negative but not positive expressions on a go/no-go task, demonstrating difficulties with emotion regulation, with some of these outcomes present several years later (Gunnar, Van Dulmen, & International Adoption Project Team, 2007; O'Connor, Rutter, & the English & Romanian Adoptees Study Team, 2000; Rutter et al., 2007; Tottenham, 2012).

Family Functioning

A number of more common aspects of family functioning have also been conceptualized as early adverse experiences that may contribute to maladaptive patterns of coping, beliefs, and interpersonal styles, leaving children vulnerable to depression. Examples include: (1) parents who set overly stringent reward criteria, thus rewarding their children at low rates, which may lead children to internalize those standards and contingencies for reinforcement (Cole & Rehm, 1986); (2) parents' high level of emotional overinvolvement, which has been associated with children's onset of depression independent of mothers' history of depression (Tompson et al., 2010); (3) interparental conflict, which has been associated with children's later development of depression, particularly if the conflict is intense, aggressive, and unresolved; if children are exposed repeatedly and at early ages (Davies, Cicchetti, & Martin, 2012; Davies & Cummings, 1994); and if the conflict spills over to parenting practices (Sturge-Apple, Cicchetti, Davies, & Suor, 2013).

Cumulative Stress

As Sameroff and others have long noted, childhood adversities often co-occur (Sameroff, Gutman, Peck, & Luthar, 2003). For example, children who are sexually abused may also be physically abused, witness interparental violence, and be exposed to their parents' alcohol problems. In a prospective longitudinal study of urban children, the more adverse events to which children had been exposed, the more negative outcomes they experienced at adolescence (Appleyard, Egeland, van Dulmen, & Sroufe, 2005). Promising new directions for exploring cumulative stress are emerging from the paradigm of allostatic load, an approach to considering the consequences of multiple adversities on the body (McEwen, 2012). Childhood adversities are linked to allostatic overload of the HPA axis, which in turn has implications for the later development of depression (Essex et al., 2011; Wilkinson & Goodyer, 2011).

Conceptual Models to Explain the Role of Early Experiences

Biological Systems

NEUROENDOCRINE: STRESS HORMONES AND THE SEROTONERGIC SYSTEM
AND NEUROPEPTIDES

Two biological systems with strong links to depression are HPA axis activity (stress hormones) and the serotonin system (5-HT functioning). The HPA system coordinates behavioral, immunological, endocrinological, and autonomic responses to stress (Arborelius, Owens, Plotsky, & Nemeroff, 1999). Cortisol is the primary steroid hormone produced by the HPA system in humans in response to stress. By the age of 3 months, human infants have adult-equivalent levels of cortisol and are capable of responding to stress.

Brief elevations of cortisol levels in response to acute stressors reflect enhanced physiological and behavioral ability to manage stress. In contrast, prolonged hyperactivity of the HPA axis (persistently elevated cortisol levels) has been associated with negative effects on physiological and behavioral systems. Early life stress is likely to predispose children to at least transient, if not permanent, alterations in the CRF system, interfering with their ability to respond adaptively to later stressors (Gunnar & Vazquez, 2001). Early life stress, particularly perinatal, may also reprogram the regulation of the HPA system through epigenetic processes, altering the expression of the genes that are essential for the function of the HPA system (Booij, Wang, Levesque, Tremblay, & Szyf, 2013). Consistent with this model are findings on associations between infant exposure to maternal depression and preschool-age children's abuse and institutional-rearing histories and children's higher cortisol levels and higher levels of behavior problems in middle childhood through adolescence, although whether cortisol evidenced hyper- or hypoarousal varied with the nature of the early life stress (Essex et al., 2011).

The serotonergic system also has strong empirical support as a biological system that explains associations between early adverse experiences and the later development of depression. The *5-HTT* or *SERT* transporter gene plays a central role in the neurotransmission of 5-HT; alterations in the gene in humans have also been implicated in both the development and functioning of brain regions involved in emotion regulation (Munafo, Brown, & Hariri, 2008). As reviewed by Booij and colleagues (2013), the alteration of 5-HT function following early life stressors is likely to be stable and persistent. Of particular concern is knowledge that the DNA methylation pattern is formed during gestation and is "highly vulnerable to environmental exposures" (Booij et al., 2013), as discussed earlier. Several studies have now shown that early trauma is associated with DNA methylation levels in candidate genes, both HPA-axis stress-related genes and the *SLC6A4* (*5-HTT* transporter) gene (e.g., Frodl & O'Keane, 2013).

It should be noted that the neurohormones oxytocin (OT) and arginine vasopressin (AVP) are also implicated in links between early life stressors and the later development of depression (Carter, 2005; Murgatroyd & Nephew, 2013). For example, orphanage-reared children who had been living in their adoptive homes for an average of 35 months, compared with children reared by their biological parents, had lower levels of overall AVP, and their OT levels did not increase after physical contact with their mothers (Wismer Fries, Ziegler, Kurian, Jacoris, & Pollak, 2005). This finding suggests that early stress may inhibit the development of the AVP system, although it is not yet known whether these alterations in hormonal functioning are predictive of the later development of depression.

NERVOUS SYSTEM: CARDIAC VAGAL TONE

Porges, Doussard-Roosevelt, Portales, and Greenspan (1996) and Porges and Furman (2010) put forth two roles for vagal tone: (1) to maintain homeostasis (baseline vagal tone) and (2) to act as a brake that regulates cardiac output in response to environmental challenge (vagal suppression). Greater baseline vagal tone and vagal suppression are more adaptive and represent more capacity for self-regulation and actual emotional regulation, respectively. Field, Pickens, Fox, Nawrocki, and Gonzalez (1995) found that infants of mothers with depression have lower vagal tone and fail to show expected developmental increases, as compared with infants of mothers without depression. More broadly, lower baseline vagal tone and vagal suppression may index vulnerability in a transactional model of pathways to depression (Porges & Furman, 2010).

FRONTAL LOBE DEVELOPMENT AND FUNCTIONING

Postnatal brains undergo significant continued development beyond that which occurs during fetal development. Of particular concern with regard to potential influence on depression is the rapid development during the first year of life of the frontal lobes, the interhemispheric connections, and the neurotransmitter systems that mediate emotional behavior (Chugani, Phelps, & Mazziotta, 2002). Each of these structures or systems is related to the experience and regulation of affect such that they may increase risk for depression. For example, in studies of unselected infants and adults, right-brain activation is associated with the experience of negative emotions, whereas left-brain activation is associated with positive emotions (Davidson & Fox, 1982). Increasing evidence indicates that early adverse experiences relate to the manner in which these structures or systems develop. For example, institutional rearing and maternal depression have been linked to the same hemispheric asymmetries, as measured by electroencephalogram (EEG), that are associated with depression (e.g., Dawson et al., 1999; Feng et al., 2012; McLaughlin, Fox, Zeanah, & Nelson, 2011). In our own lab, we (Lusby, Goodman, Bell, & Newport, 2014) found that among 3- and 6-month-old infants, infants of mothers with stably high depressive symptoms pre- and postnatally were especially likely to show relative right frontal EEG asymmetry.

Early adverse experiences such as maltreatment and institutionalization have also been linked to smaller volume in the hippocampus (Buss et al., 2007), medial prefrontal cortex (van Harmelen et al., 2010), and orbitofrontal cortex (Pollak et al., 2010) but greater amygdalar volume (Tottenham, 2012; Tottenham et al., 2010). Other studies support links between volume in these brain areas and emotion regulation problems, suggesting vulnerabilities to depression (Mayberg, 2003). Knowledge that different brain regions mature at different rates (Tau & Peterson, 2010) may contribute to an understanding of sensitive periods for the effects of early adverse experiences.

INHERITED VULNERABILITIES AND EPIGENETICS

Genetics undoubtedly plays a role in explaining the risk for depression in association with early experience. There are several possible roles of genetics. Until recently, most studies emphasized heritability of depression per se. Chapters in this volume attest to the heritability of depression in adults and adolescents, and somewhat less for children. An alternative to the notion that children may inherit likelihood for depression per se is that children inherit affective, cognitive, and interpersonal vulnerabilities to depression. Support has been found for heritability of behavioral inhibition and shyness (Eley et al., 2003), low self-esteem (Raevuori et al., 2007), neuroticism (Tellegen et al., 1988), sociability (Plomin et al., 1993), subjective well-being (Lykken & Tellegen, 1996), negative affectivity (Lemery-Chalfant, Kao, Swann, & Goldsmith, 2013), and even the likelihood of negative events (Kendler & Baker, 2007). Research on such vulnerabilities is being pursued with the study of endophenotypes (Kendler & Neale, 2010) and the domains proposed by the Research Domain Criteria (RDoC), such as the positive valence system (Bogdan & Pizzagalli, 2009).

Epigenetics—referring to changes in gene expression and behavior, either DNA methylation or histone modification, caused by mechanisms other than DNA sequence changes—are another way that early life stress may "get under the skin," a kind of biological embedding of early life experiences that then interact with potential change from experiences that occur over the lifespan (McEwen, 2012). Rutter (2012) proposed methodological and conceptual challenges to guide research attempting to clarify epigenetic mechanisms whereby early adverse experiences are associated with the later development of depression.

Attachment System

Disturbances in the attachment relationship have also been suggested as mechanisms explaining associations between early adverse experiences and vulnerability to the development of depression (Cummings & Cicchetti, 1990; Sroufe, Coffino, & Carlson, 2010). Insecure attachment, relative to secure attachment, is associated with more negative expectancies for relationships and negative self-perceptions (as reviewed by Groh, Roisman, van IJzendoorn, Bakermans-Kranenburg, & Fearon, 2012) and is predictive of depression in children and adolescents (Duggal, Carlson, Sroufe, & Egeland, 2001). Disorganized attachment is also associated with elevated risk for the later development of internalizing problems, even relative to insecurely attached infants (Sroufe et al., 2010). Among the adverse experiences associated with insecure or disorganized attachment are clinically significant early maternal depression (Martins & Gaffan, 2000; Tharner et al., 2012b), physical abuse of infants by their caregivers (Cicchetti & Barnett, 1991), and the number of preadoption placements among international adoptees (Niemann & Weiss, 2012).

In terms of the role that attachment might play in associations between early adverse experiences and risk for the development of depression, support for a moderating model is building. That is, attachment security either exacerbates or buffers associations between early adverse experiences and infant outcomes associated with the development of depression (Luijk et al., 2010; Tharner et al., 2012a, 2013). No studies were found to support attachment as a mediator of associations between early adverse experiences and risk for the development of depression.

Cognitive Vulnerabilities and Self-System

Early adverse experiences may also be linked to later depression through the mechanism of depressogenic cognitions. Early childhood, beginning in the second year of life, is a critical period for the construction of the sense of self and self in relation to others and the world (Thompson, 2006), which is fostered by warm, responsive parenting. In contrast, early adverse experiences are associated with cognitive distortions, such as a sense of oneself as unlovable and as unlikely to get one's needs met, hopelessness and helplessness, and having unrealistically high standards for self-reinforcement (Garber & Martin, 2002). These depressotypic cognitions may play either a meditational role in the association between early adversities and the development of depression (Hankin, 2005) or a moderating role, with cognitive vulnerability interacting with stress to predict depression (Lakdawalla, Hankin, & Mermelstein, 2007).

Affect: Emotional Expression and Regulation

Problems in emotional expression or regulation may also at least partially explain associations between early adverse experiences and the later emergence of depression. Emotion dysregulation is a prominent feature of depression in children (Garber, Braafladt, & Zeman, 1991; Kovacs, Joormann, & Gotlib, 2008), as well as of many of the biological and behavioral vulnerabilities in infancy that have been associated with early adverse experiences.

Children of mothers with depression have been found to use less adaptive styles of emotion regulation compared with children of mothers who never had depression (Silk, Shaw, Skuban, Oland, & Kovacs, 2006) and are of particular concern given findings that: (1) infants imitate the negative affects of mothers with depression (Bendell et al., 1994); (2) mothers with depression less often reinforce their infants' positive affect with displays of interest relative to mothers without depression (Pickens & Field, 1993), and (3) mothers with a history of depression respond to their children's negative emotions with more magnification, neglect, and punishment than mothers who never had depression, which prospectively predicted children's internalizing symptoms (Silk et al., 2011).

Integrative Models: Vulnerability

Clearly, early adverse experiences do not directly or inevitably predict depression in a main effects–type model. Thus integrative models have been developed that take into account the likely complexities. In vulnerability models, individuals inherit or acquire deficits or dysfunctions or abnormalities as a function of early adverse experience, which then increase their likelihood of developing psychopathology, though they are unlikely to be singular, linear causes of depression. The vulnerability model serves as a basis for two other models that generate testable hypotheses and yield supportive findings: diathesis–stress models and transactional models.

DIATHESIS–STRESS MODELS

As reviewed by Monroe and Simons (1991), diathesis–stress models explain that a vulnerability manifests itself only in the context of stress or, more broadly, maladaptive environments, and they propose conditions under which a vulnerability, or diathesis, would or would not lead to disorder. The model has been proposed as a way to explain why some people with the diathesis develop disorder (exacerbating factors) whereas others do not (resilience or protective factors) and why some people remain disorder-free until a certain point in time and then emerge with the disorder. In such a model, early adverse experiences are associated with the development of diatheses for depression (e.g. dysregulated HPA system), and stress is a moderator variable. Children who acquire one or more of the diatheses would be expected to be more sensitive to the effects of additional stressors relative to their less vulnerable counterparts. Conversely, children with the diatheses may benefit from high-quality environments. For example, in parallel to findings that alterations in maternal care may explain the effects of maternal separation on rat pups' HPA-axis response to stress (Kaffman & Meaney, 2007), higher maternal prenatal depression was found to be associated with decreased physiological adaptability and increased negative emotionality only when mothers reported lower instances of stroking their infants (Sharp et al., 2012). Moreover, the diatheses might be considered the equivalent of an active/evocative gene; that is, they might be expressed in ways that evoke particular reactions, such as harshness or withdrawal, from others. Gene-by-environment interactions are a form of diathesis–stress model, with genetic factors as the primary diatheses (Klengel & Binder, 2013).

TRANSACTIONAL MODELS

Goodman and Gotlib (1999) asserted the need for a transactional model of risk for depression in children of mothers with depression, and such a model is also implicated with regard to other early adverse experiences. Transactional models describe the processes of child and environment mutually influencing each other over time (Sameroff, 2009), such that environmental characteristics influence the child's course of development and the child's characteristics influence the nature of the environment. For example, children with a pattern of frontal EEG asymmetries are likely to experience a predominance of negative emotions, and in turn they may engage with the environment less actively or less positively. Conversely, others are likely to interact with the child in ways that are evoked by the child's affective, behavioral, and cognitive styles.

The transactional model provides a theoretical context within which alternative courses of development of children who are exposed early to adverse experiences can be explored. Although the model early on was constrained by limits on how to study it, newer statistical approaches enable stringent tests of transactional models (Sameroff, 2009). For example, Nicholson, Deboeck, Farris, Boker, and Borkowski (2011) used dynamical systems to model time continuously and found that over the course of early development, as mothers' depressive symptoms became more (or less) severe, children's behavior problems increased (or decreased) in a reciprocal manner.

DIFFERENTIAL SUSCEPTIBILITY

A developmental psychopathology perspective also considers that development includes individuals adapting to their unique environmental conditions. As applied to developmental psychopathology, terms such as *experience-adaptive programming effects* (Rutter, O'Connor, & the English & Romanian Adoptees Study Team, 2004), *developmental plasticity* (Bateson et al., 2004), and *differential susceptibility* (Belsky, Bakermans-Kranenburg, & van IJzendoorn, 2007; Ellis, Boyce, Belsky, Bakermans-Kranenburg, & Van IJzendoorn, 2011) explain that individuals are born having been programmed to deal with certain conditions and are at a disadvantage if later exposed to different conditions. Findings consistent with this theory are promising. Important next steps will be moving beyond correlational studies to experimental manipulations of implicated aspects of the environment (see a review and commentary by van IJzendoorn & Bakermans-Kranenburg, 2012).

Alternative Developmental Pathways

Consistent with a developmental psychopathology perspective, individuals show tremendous heterogeneity in both short- and long-term response to early adverse experiences; thus early adverse experiences may link with the later emergence of depression and other outcomes by following many different pathways (Rutter, 2012). Furthermore, such pathways may relate to the nature of any depression that emerges (Cicchetti & Toth, 1998). That is, there is great variability both (1) within groups of individuals with depression, all of whom experienced early adverse experiences, and (2) between individuals with depression who experienced early adversities and those who did not.

First, some of the alternative pathways reflect the tremendous differences in the nature of any of the adverse experiences described in this chapter. In particular, severity of early adverse experiences increases risk for depression in adults in a dose–response relationship (Chapman et al., 2004), and chronicity increases the likelihood of a sensitizing effect relative to transient, especially if mild, adverse experiences (Rutter, 2013). Second, development matters in numerous ways, a theme that is woven through this chapter, with a particular emphasis on age at the time of exposures. Third, gender may matter in the effects of early adverse experiences or in the mechanisms that might explain those effects (Brummelte, Lieblich, & Galea, 2012). Fourth, the transactional processes that unfold over time add even more variation in alternative pathways.

FUTURE DIRECTIONS

Considering the role of early adverse experience in the emergence of depression within an integrative, developmentally sensitive, transactional model raises many important questions requiring further study. A few examples are mentioned here. First, given common comorbidity and co-occurrences among the various adversities, future studies may benefit from tests of moderated or additive (cumulative) relations in the prediction of later depression. Second, findings have supported associations between early life stressors and numerous vulnerabilities; however, there are many unanswered questions about mechanisms. Third, the role of normative developmental changes in associations between early adversity and later depression are still not well understood. For example, do moderating processes operate similarly over the course of development? In addition, it will be important to explore the persistence of adaptation or maladaptation over time (Clark, Caldwell, Power, & Stansfeld, 2010). Further study of resilience is also warranted. For example, the same brain systems implicated in adverse outcomes associated with exposure to early life stress are also sufficiently plastic to enable the capacity for resilience or for such effects to be mitigated later in life (Karatoreos & McEwen, 2013). Fourth, more understanding is needed of multifinality to understand the degree of specificity of depression as the outcome associated with early adversities (Cicchetti & Rogosch, 1996).

Finally, although not the emphasis of this chapter, the ideas presented here have important implications for interventions, including the idea of experimental interventions as tests of models of risk. For example, research that furthers our understanding of the neurobiology of the stress response could lead to the development of interventions that target stress response systems, such as the psychosocial intervention that normalized a biological regulatory process in infants exposed to early adverse experience (e.g., Cicchetti, Rogosch, Toth, & Sturge-Apple, 2011). Two clear implications are that: (1) the goal of preventive and early interventions needs to be to decrease vulnerability to the development of depression, focusing on the vulnerabilities that have been identified in pathways between early adversities and depression; and (2) treatments for depression must recognize the role that early adversities and subsequent developmental pathways play in the etiology of that depression (e.g., Nemeroff et al., 2003).

ACKNOWLEDGMENTS

We acknowledge the contribution of Sarah Brand to the version of this chapter that appeared in the second edition.

REFERENCES

Appleyard, K., Egeland, B., van Dulmen, M. H. M., & Sroufe, L. A. (2005). When more is not better: The role of cumulative risk in child behavior outcomes. *Journal of Child Psychology and Psychiatry and Allied Disciplines, 46*(3), 235–245.

Arborelius, L., Owens, M. J., Plotsky, P. M., & Nemeroff, C. B. (1999). The role of corticotropin-releasing factor in depression and anxiety disorders. *Journal of Endocrinology, 160*(1), 1–12.

Bandura, A. (1986). *Social foundations of thought and action: A social cognitive theory.* Englewood Cliffs, NJ: Prentice-Hall.

Bateson, P., Barker, D., Clutton-Brock, T., Deb, D., D'Udine, B., Foley, R. A., et al. (2004). Developmental plasticity and human health. *Nature, 430,* 419–421.

Belsky, J., Bakermans-Kranenburg, M. J., & van IJzendoorn, M. H. (2007). For better and for worse: Differential susceptibility to environmental influences. *Current Directions in Psychological Science, 16*(6), 300–304.

Bendell, D., Field, T., Yando, R., Lang, C., Martinez, A., & Pickens, J. (1994). "Depressed" mothers' perceptions of their preschool children's vulnerability. *Child Psychiatry and Human Development, 24*(3), 183–190.

Bogdan, R., & Pizzagalli, D. A. (2009). The heritability of hedonic capacity and perceived stress: A twin study evaluation of candidate depressive phenotypes. *Psychological Medicine, 39*(2), 211–218.

Booij, L., Wang, D. S., Levesque, M. L., Tremblay, R. E., & Szyf, M. (2013). Looking beyond the DNA sequence: The relevance of DNA methylation processes for the stress–diathesis model of depression. *Philosophical Transactions of the Royal Society B: Biological Sciences, 368,* 20120251. Available at *http://rstb.royalsocietypublishing.org/content/368/1615/20120251. abstract.*

Brennan, P. A., Pargas, R., Walker, E. F., Green, P., Newport, D. J., & Stowe, Z. (2008). Maternal depression and infant cortisol: Influences of timing, comorbidity and treatment. *Journal of Child Psychology and Psychiatry, 49*(10), 1099–1107.

Brent, D., Melhem, N., Donohoe, M. B., & Walker, M. (2009). The incidence and course of depression in bereaved youth 21 months after the loss of a parent to suicide, accident, or sudden natural death. *American Journal of Psychiatry, 166*(7), 786–794.

Brummelte, S., Lieblich, S. E., & Galea, L. A. M. (2012). Gestational and postpartum corticosterone exposure to the dam affects behavioral and endocrine outcome of the offspring in a sexually-dimorphic manner. *Neuropharmacology, 62*(1), 406–418.

Buss, C., Lord, C., Wadiwalla, M., Hellhammer, D. H., Lupien, S. J., Meaney, M. J., et al. (2007). Maternal care modulates the relationship between prenatal risk and hippocampal volume in women but not in men. *Journal of Neuroscience, 27*(10), 2592–2595.

Carter, C. S. (2005). The chemistry of child neglect: Do oxytocin and vasopressin mediate the effects of early experience? *Proceedings of the National Academy of Sciences of the USA, 102,* 18247–18248.

Chapman, D. P., Whitfield, C. L., Felitti, V. J., Dube, S. R., Edwards, V. J., & Anda, R. F. (2004). Adverse childhood experiences and the risk of depressive disorders in adulthood. *Journal of Affective Disorders, 82*(2), 217–225.

Chorpita, B. F. (2001). *Control and the development of negative emotion.* New York: Oxford University Press.

Chugani, H. T., Phelps, M. E., & Mazziotta, J. C. (2002). Positron emission tomography study of human brain functional development. *Brain development and cognition: A reader* (2nd ed., pp. 101–116). Malden, MA: Blackwell.

Cicchetti, D. (2013). Annual Research Review: Resilient functioning in maltreated children: Past, present, and future perspectives. *Journal of Child Psychology and Psychiatry, 54*(4), 402–422.

Cicchetti, D., & Barnett, D. (1991). Attachment organization in maltreated preschoolers. *Development and Psychopathology, 3,* 397–411.

Cicchetti, D., & Rogosch, F. A. (1996). Equifinality and multifinality in developmental psychopathology. *Development and Psychopathology, 8,* 597–600.

Cicchetti, D., Rogosch, F. A., Toth, S. L., & Sturge-Apple, M. L. (2011). Normalizing the development of cortisol regulation in maltreated infants through preventive interventions. *Development and Psychopathology, 23*(3), 789–800.

Cicchetti, D., & Toth, S. (1998). The development of depression in children and adolescents. *American Psychologist, 53*, 221–241.

Clark, C., Caldwell, T., Power, C., & Stansfeld, S. A. (2010). Does the influence of childhood adversity on psychopathology persist across the lifecourse?: A 45-year prospective epidemiologic study. *Annals of Epidemiology, 20*(5), 385–394.

Cole, D. A., & Rehm, L. P. (1986). Family interaction patterns and childhood depression. *Journal of Abnormal Child Psychology, 14*, 297–314.

Costello, E. J., Worthman, C., Erkanli, A., & Angold, A. (2007). Prediction from low birth weight to female adolescent depression: A test of competing hypotheses. *Archives of General Psychiatry, 64*(3), 338–344.

Cummings, E. M., & Cicchetti, D. (1990). Toward a transactional model of relations between attachment and depression. In M. T. Greenberg, D. Cicchetti, & E. M. Cummings (Eds.), *Attachment in the preschool years: Theory, research, and intervention* (pp. 339–372). Chicago: University of Chicago Press.

Davidson, R. J., & Fox, N. (1982). Asymmetrical brain activity discriminates between positive and negative affective stimuli in human infants. *Science, 218*, 1235–1237.

Davidson, R. J., Pizzagalli, D., Nitschke, J. B., & Putnam, K. (2002). Depression: Perspectives from affective neuroscience. *Annual Review of Psychology, 53*, 545–574.

Davies, P. T., Cicchetti, D., & Martin, M. J. (2012). Toward greater specificity in identifying associations among interparental aggression, child emotional reactivity to conflict, and child problems. *Child Development, 83*(5), 1789–1804.

Davies, P. T., & Cummings, E. M. (1994). Marital conflict and child adjustment: An emotional security hypothesis. *Psychological Bulletin, 116*(3), 387–411.

Dawson, G., Frey, K., Self, J., Panagiotides, H., Hessl, D., Yamada, E., et al. (1999). Frontal brain electrical activity in infants of depressed and nondepressed mothers: Relation to variations in infant behavior. *Development and Psychopathology, 11*, 589–605.

Devane, C. L., Stowe, Z. N., Donovan, J. L., Newport, D. J, Pennell, P. B., Ritchie, J. C., et al. (2006). Therapeutic drug monitoring of psychoactive drugs during pregnancy in the genomic era: Challenges and opportunities. *Journal of Psychopharmacology, 20*(Suppl. 4), 54–59.

Dietz, P. M., Williams, S. B., Callaghan, W. M., Bachman, D. J., Whitlock, E. P., & Hornbrook, M. C. (2007). Clinically identified maternal depression before, during, and after pregnancies ending in live births. *American Journal of Psychiatry, 164*(10), 1515–1520.

DiPietro, J. A. (2012). Maternal stress in pregnancy: Considerations for fetal development. *Journal of Adolescent Health, 51*(2), S3–S8.

Duggal, S., Carlson, E. A., Sroufe, L. A., & Egeland, B. (2001). Depressive symptomatology in childhood and adolescence. *Development and Psychopathology, 13*(01), 143–164.

Egeland, B., Pianta, R., & O'Brian, M. (1993). Maternal intrusiveness in infancy and child maladaptation in early school years. *Development and Psychopathology, 5*, 359–370.

Eley, T. C., Bolton, D., O'Connor, T. G., Perrin, S., Smith, P., & Plomin, R. (2003). A twin study of anxiety-related behaviours in pre-school children. *Journal of Child Psychology and Psychiatry, 44*(7), 945–960.

Ellis, B. J., Boyce, W. T., Belsky, J., Bakermans-Kranenburg, M. J., & Van IJzendoorn, M. H. (2011). Differential susceptibility to the environment: An evolutionary– neurodevelopmental theory. *Development and Psychopathology, 23*(1), 7–28.

Essex, M. J., Shirtcliff, E. A., Burk, L. R., Ruttle, P. L., Klein, M. H., Slattery, M. J., et al. (2011). Influence of early life stress on later hypothalamic–pituitary–adrenal axis functioning and its covariation with mental health symptoms: A study of the allostatic process from childhood into adolescence. *Development and Psychopathology, 23*, 1039–1058.

Evans, L. M., Myers, M. M., & Monk, C. (2008). Pregnant women's cortisol is elevated with anxiety and depression—but only when comorbid. *Archives of Women's Mental Health, 11*, 239–248.

Feng, X., Forbes, E., Kovacs, M., George, C. J., Lopez-Duran, N. L., Fox, N. A., & Cohn, J. F.

(2012). Children's depressive symptoms in relation to EEG frontal asymmetry and maternal depression. *Journal of Abnormal Child Psychology, 40*(2), 265–276.

Field, T. (2011). Prenatal depression effects on early development: A review. *Infant Behavior and Development, 34*(1), 1–14.

Field, T., Diego, M., Dieter, J., Hernandez-Reif, M., Schanberg, S., Kuhn, C., et al. (2004). Prenatal depression effects on the fetus and the newborn. *Infant Behavior and Development, 27*(2), 216–229.

Field, T., Pickens, J., Fox, N. A., Nawrocki, T., & Gonzalez, J. (1995). Vagal tone in infants of depressed mothers. *Development and Psychopathology, 7,* 227–231.

Frodl, T., & O'Keane, V. (2013). How does the brain deal with cumulative stress?: A review with focus on developmental stress, HPA axis function and hippocampal structure in humans. *Neurobiology of Disease, 52,* 24–37.

Garber, J., Braafladt, N., & Zeman, J. (1991). The regulation of sad affect: An information-processing perspective. In J. Garber & K. A. Dodge (Eds.), *The development of emotion regulation and dysregulation* (pp. 208–242). Cambridge, UK: Cambridge University Press.

Garber, J., & Martin, N. C. (2002). Negative cognitions in offspring of depressed parents: Mechanisms of risk. In S. H. Goodman & I. H. Gotlib (Eds.), *Children of depressed parents: Mechanisms of risk and implications for treatment* (pp. 121–154). Washington, DC: American Psychological Association.

Gelles, R. J. (1998). The youngest victims: Violence toward children. In R. K. Berger (Ed.), *Issues in intimate violence* (pp. 5–24). Thousand Oaks, CA: Sage.

Glover, V., Teixeira, J., Gitau, R., & Fisk, N. M. (1999). Mechanisms by which maternal mood in pregnancy may affect the fetus. *Contemporary Reviews in Obstetrics and Gynecology, 11,* 155–160.

Goodman, S. H., Rouse, M. H., Long, Q., Ji, S., & Brand, S. R. (2011). Deconstructing antenatal depression: What is it that matters for neonatal behavioral functioning? *Infant Mental Health Journal, 32*(3), 1–12.

Goodman, S. H., & Tully, E. C. (2009). Recurrence of depression during pregnancy: Psychosocial and personal functioning correlates. *Depression and Anxiety, 26*(6), 557–567.

Graham, Y. P., Heim, C., Goodman, S. H., Miller, A. H., & Nemeroff, C. B. (1999). The effects of neonatal stress on brain development: Implications for psychopathology. *Development and Psychopathology, 11,* 545–565.

Gray, L. B., Weller, R. A., Fristad, M., & Weller, E. B. (2011). Depression in children and adolescents two months after the death of a parent. *Journal of Affective Disorders, 135*(1–3), 277–283.

Groh, A. M., Roisman, G. I., van IJzendoorn, M. H., Bakermans-Kranenburg, M. J., & Fearon, R. P. (2012). The significance of insecure and disorganized attachment for children's internalizing symptoms: A meta-analytic study. *Child Development, 83*(2), 591–610.

Gunnar, M. R., Van Dulmen, M. H., & International Adoption Project Team. (2007). Behavior problems in postinstitutionalized internationally adopted children. *Development and Psychopathology, 19*(1), 129–148.

Gunnar, M. R., & Vazquez, D. M. (2001). Low cortisol and a flattening of expected daytime rhythm: Potential indices of risk in human development. *Development and Psychopathology, 13,* 515–538.

Hane, A. A., & Fox, N. A. (2006). Ordinary variations in maternal caregiving influence human infants' stress reactivity. *Psychological Science, 17*(6), 550–556.

Hankin, B. L. (2005). Childhood maltreatment and psychopathology: Prospective tests of attachment, cognitive vulnerability, and stress as mediating processes. *Cognitive Therapy and Research, 29*(6), 645–671.

Jaffee, S. R., & Maikovich-Fong, A. K. (2013). Child maltreatment and risk for psychopathology. In T. Beauchaine & S. Hinshaw (Eds.), *Child and adolescent psychopathology* (2nd ed., pp. 171–196). New York: Wiley.

Kaffman, A., & Meaney, M. J. (2007). Neurodevelopmental sequelae of postnatal maternal care in rodents: Clinical and research implications of molecular insights. *Journal of Child Psychology and Psychiatry, 48*(3–4), 224–244.

Karatoreos, I. N., & McEwen, B. S. (2013). Annual Research Review: The neurobiology and physiology of resilience and adaptation across the life course. *Journal of Child Psychology and Psychiatry, 54*(4), 337–347.

Kendler, K. S., & Baker, J. H. (2007). Genetic influences on measures of the environment: A systematic review. *Psychological Medicine, 37*(5), 615–626.

Kendler, K. S., & Neale, M. C. (2010). Endophenotype: A conceptual analysis. *Molecular Psychiatry, 15*(8), 789–797.

King, S., Liau, X., Brunet, A., Schmitz, N., & Laplante, D. P. (2011, September). *Prenatal maternal stress from a natural disaster predicts internalizing and externalizing problems through age 11½ years: Project Ice Storm.* Paper presented at the annual meeting of the Society for Research in Psychopathology, Boston.

Klengel, T., & Binder, E. B. (2013). Gene–environment interactions in major depressive disorder. *Canadian Journal of Psychiatry, 58*(2), 76–83.

Kofink, D., Boks, M. P., Timmers, H. T., & Kas, M. J. (2013). Epigenetic dynamics in psychiatric disorders: Environmental programming of neurodevelopmental processes. *Neuroscience and Biobehavioral Reviews, 37*(5), 831–845.

Kovacs, M., Joormann, J., & Gotlib, I. H. (2008). Emotion (dys)regulation and links to depressive disorders. *Child Development Perspectives, 2*(3), 149–155.

Kovacs, M., Obrosky, D. S., Gatsonis, C., & Richards, C. (1997). First-episode major depressive and dysthymic disorder in childhood: Clinical and sociodemographic factors in recovery. *Journal of the American Academy of Child and Adolescent Psychiatry, 36*(6), 777–784.

Lakdawalla, Z., Hankin, B. L., & Mermelstein, R. (2007). Cognitive theories of depression in children and adolescents: A conceptual and quantitative review. *Clinical Child and Family Psychology Review, 10*(1), 1–24.

Lemery-Chalfant, K., Kao, K. R., Swann, G., & Goldsmith, H. H. (2013). Childhood temperament: Passive gene–environment correlation, gene–environment interaction, and the hidden importance of the family environment. *Development and Psychopathology, 25*(1), 51–63.

Loughhead, A. M., Stowe, Z. N., Newport, D. J., Ritchie, J. C., DeVane, C. L., & Owens, M. J. (2006). Placental passage of tricyclic antidepressants. *Biological Psychiatry, 59*(3), 287–290.

Lovejoy, M. C., Graczyk, P. A., O'Hare, E., & Neuman, G. (2000). Maternal depression and parenting behavior: A meta-analytic review. *Clinical Psychology Review, 20*(5), 561–592.

Luijk, M. P. C. M., Saridjan, N., Tharner, A., van IJzendoorn, M. H., Bakermans-Kranenburg, M. J., Jaddoe, V. W. V., et al. (2010). Attachment, depression, and cortisol: Deviant patterns in insecure-resistant and disorganized infants. *Developmental Psychobiology, 52*(5), 441–452.

Lusby, C. M., Goodman, S. H., Bell, M. A., & Newport, D. J. (2014). Electroencephalogram patterns in infants of depressed mothers. *Developmental Psychobiology, 56*(3), 459–473.

Lykken, D. T., & Tellegen, A. (1996). Happiness is a stochatic phenomenon. *Psychological Science, 7*, 186–189.

Mäntymaa, M., Puura, K., Luoma, I., Latva, R., Salmelin, R., & Tamminen, T. (2012). Predicting internalizing and externalizing problems at five years by child and parental factors in infancy and toddlerhood. *Child Psychiatry and Human Development, 43*(2), 153–170.

Mäntymaa, M., Puura, K., Luoma, I., Salmelin, R. K., & Tamminen, T. (2004). Early mother–infant interaction, parental mental health and symptoms of behavioral and emotional problems in toddlers. *Infant Behavior and Development, 27*(2), 134–149.

Marcus, S. M., Flynn, H. A., Blow, F. C., & Barry, K. L. (2003). Depressive symptoms among pregnant women screened in obstetrics settings. *Journal of Women's Health, 12*(4), 373–380.

Martin, R. P., & Dombrowski, S. C. (2008). *Prenatal exposures: Psychological and educational consequences for children.* New York: Springer.

Martins, C., & Gaffan, E. (2000). Effects of early maternal depression on patterns of infant–mother attachment: A meta-analytic investigation. *Journal of Child Psychology and Psychiatry, 41*(6), 737–746.

Mayberg, H. S. (2003). Modulating dysfunctional limbic-cortical circuits in depression: Towards development of brain-based algorithms for diagnosis and optimised treatment. *British Medical Bulletin, 65*, 193–207.

McEwen, B. S. (2012). Brain on stress: How the social environment gets under the skin. *Proceedings of the National Academy of Sciences of the USA, 109*, 17180–17185.

McLaughlin, K. A., Fox, N. A., Zeanah, C. H., & Nelson, C. A. (2011). Adverse rearing environments and neural development in children: The development of frontal electroencephalogram asymmetry. *Biological Psychiatry, 70*(11), 1008–1015.

Mendelson, T., DiPietro, J. A., Costigan, K. A., Chen, P., & Henderson, J. L. (2011). Associations of maternal psychological factors with umbilical and uterine blood flow. *Journal of Psychosomatic Obstetrics and Gynecology, 32*(1), 3–9.

Milberger, S., Biederman, J., Faraone, S. V., Chen, L., & Jones, J. (1996). Is maternal smoking during pregnancy a risk factor for attention deficit hyperactivity disorder in children? *American Journal of Psychiatry, 153*, 1138–1142.

Monk, C., Newport, D. J., Korotkin, J. H., Long, Q., Knight, B., & Stowe, Z. N. (2012). Uterine blood flow in a psychiatric population: Impact of maternal depression, anxiety, and psychotropic medication. *Biological Psychiatry, 72*(6), 483–490.

Monk, C., Sloan, R. P., Myers, M. M., Ellman, L., Werner, E., Jeon, J., et al. (2004). Fetal heart rate reactivity differs by women's psychiatric status: An early marker for developmental risk? *Journal of the American Academy of Child and Adolescent Psychiatry, 43*, 283–290.

Monroe, S. M., & Simons, A. D. (1991). Diathesis–stress theories in the context of life-stress research: Implications for depressive disorders. *Psychological Bulletin, 110*, 406–425.

Mueller, A., Brocke, B., Fries, E., Lesch, K.-P., & Kirschbaum, C. (2010). The role of the serotonin transporter polymorphism for the endocrine stress response in newborns. *Psychoneuroendocrinology, 35*(2), 289–296.

Mueller, B. R., & Bale, T. L. (2008). Sex-specific programming of offspring emotionality after stress early in pregnancy. *Journal of Neuroscience, 28*, 9055–9065.

Munafo, M. R., Brown, S. M., & Hariri, A. R. (2008). Serotonin transporter (5-HTTLPR) genotype and amygdala activation: A meta-analysis. *Biological Psychiatry, 63*(9), 852–857.

Murgatroyd, C. A., & Nephew, B. C. (2013). Effects of early life social stress on maternal behavior and neuroendocrinology. *Psychoneuroendocrinology, 38*(2), 219–228.

Neigh, G. N., Gillespie, C. F., & Nemeroff, C. B. (2009). The neurobiological toll of child abuse and neglect. *Trauma, Violence, and Abuse, 10*(4), 389–410.

Nemeroff, C. B., Heim, C. M., Thase, M. E., Klein, D. N., Rush, A. J., Schatzberg, A. F., et al. (2003). Differential responses to psychotherapy versus pharmacotherapy in patients with chronic forms of major depression and childhood trauma. *Proceedings of the National Academy of Sciences of the USA, 100*, 14293–14296.

Nicholson, J. S., Deboeck, P. R., Farris, J. R., Boker, S. M., & Borkowski, J. G. (2011). Maternal depressive symptomatology and child behavior: Transactional relationship with simultaneous bidirectional coupling. *Developmental Psychology, 47*(5), 1312–1323.

Niemann, S., & Weiss, S. (2012). Factors affecting attachment in international adoptees at 6 months post adoption. *Children and Youth Services Review, 34*(1), 205–212.

Oberlander, T. F., Bonaguro, R. J., Misri, S., Papsdorf, M., Ross, C. J. D., & Simpson, E. M. (2008). Infant serotonin transporter (SLC6A4) promoter genotype is associated with adverse neonatal outcomes after prenatal exposure to serotonin reuptake inhibitor medications. *Molecular Psychiatry, 13*(1), 65–73.

Oberlander, T. F., Grunau, R., Mayes, L., Riggs, W., Rurak, D., Papsdorf, M., et al. (2008). Hypothalamic–pituitary–adrenal (HPA) axis function in 3-month-old infants with prenatal selective serotonin reuptake inhibitor (SSRI) antidepressant exposure. *Early Human Development, 84*(10), 689–697.

O'Connor, T. G., Heron, J., Golding, J., & Glover, V. (2003). Maternal antenatal anxiety and behavioural/emotional problems in children: A test of a programming hypothesis. *Journal of Child Psychology and Psychiatry, 44*(7), 1025–1036.

O'Connor, T. G., Rutter, M., & the English & Romanian Adoptees Study Team. (2000). Attachment disorder behavior following early severe deprivation: Extension and longitudinal follow-up. *Journal of the American Academy of Child and Adolescent Psychiatry, 39*, 703–712.

Pickens, J., & Field, T. (1993). Facial expressivity in infants of "depressed" mothers. *Developmental Psychology, 29*, 986–988.

Plomin, R., Emde, R. N., Braungart, J. M., Campos, J., Corley, R. P., Fulker, D. W., et al. (1993). Genetic change and continuity from fourteen to twenty months: The MacArthur Longitudinal Twin Study. *Child Development, 64*, 1354–1376.

Pollak, S. D., Nelson, C. A., Schlaak, M. F., Roeber, B. J., Wewerka, S. S., Wiik, K. L., et al. (2010). Neurodevelopmental effects of early deprivation in postinstitutionalized children. *Child Development, 81*(1), 224–236.

Porges, S. W., Doussard-Roosevelt, J. A., Portales, A. L., & Greenspan, S. I. (1996). Infant regulation of the vagal "brake" predicts child behavior problems: A psychobiological model of social behavior. *Developmental Psychobiology, 29*, 697–712.

Porges, S. W., & Furman, S. A. (2010). The early development of the autonomic nervous system provides a neural platform for social behavior: A polyvagal perspective. *Infant and Child Development, 20*(1), 106–118.

Raevuori, A., Dick, D. M., Keski-Rahkonen, A., Pulkkinen, L., Rose, R. J., Rissanen, A., et al. (2007). Genetic and environmental factors affecting self-esteem from age 14 to 17: A longitudinal study of Finnish twins. *Psychological Medicine, 37*(11), 1625–1633.

Romens, S. E., & Pollak, S. D. (2012). Emotion regulation predicts attention bias in maltreated children at risk for depression. *Journal of Child Psychology and Psychiatry, 53*(2), 120–127.

Rutter, M. (2012). Achievements and challenges in the biology of environmental effects. *Proceedings of the National Academy of Sciences of the USA, 109*, 17149–17153.

Rutter, M. (2013). Annual Research Review: Resilience—clinical implications. *Journal of Child Psychology and Psychiatry, 54*(4), 474–487.

Rutter, M., Colvert, E., Kreppner, J., Beckett, C., Castle, J., Groothues, C., et al. (2007). Early adolescent outcomes for institutionally-deprived and non-deprived adoptees: I. Disinhibited attachment. *Journal of Child Psychology and Psychiatry, 48*(1), 17–30.

Rutter, M., O'Connor, T. G., & the English & Romanian Adoptees Study Team. (2004). Are there biological programming effects for psychological development?: Findings from a study of Romanian adoptees. *Developmental Psychology, 40*(1), 81–94.

Sameroff, A. (2009). The transactional model. In A. Sameroff (Ed.), *The transactional model of development: How children and contexts shape each other* (pp. 3–21). Washington, DC: American Psychological Association.

Sameroff, A., Gutman, L. M., Peck, S. C., & Luthar, S. S. (2003). Adaptation among youth facing multiple risks: Prospective research findings. In S. S. Luthar (Ed.), *Resilience and vulnerability: Adaptation in the context of childhood adversities* (pp. 364–391). New York: Cambridge University Press.

Schmiege, S. J., Khoo, S. T., Sandler, I. N., Ayers, T. S., & Wolchik, S. A. (2006). Symptoms of internalizing and externalizing problems: Modeling recovery curves after the death of a parent. *American Journal of Preventive Medicine, 31*(6, Suppl. 1), 152–160.

Sharp, H., Pickles, A., Meaney, M., Marshall, K., Tibu, F., & Hill, J. (2012). Frequency of infant stroking reported by mothers moderates the effect of prenatal depression on infant behavioural and physiological outcomes. *PLoS One, 7*(10), e45446.

Shea, A. K., Streiner, D. L., Fleming, A., Kamath, M. V., Broad, K., & Steiner, M. (2007). The effect of depression, anxiety and early life trauma on the cortisol awakening response during pregnancy: Preliminary results. *Psychoneuroendocrinology, 32*, 1013–1020.

Silk, J. S., Shaw, D. S., Prout, J. T., O'Rourke, F., Lane, T. J., & Kovacs, M. (2011). Socialization of emotion and offspring internalizing symptoms in mothers with childhood-onset depression. *Journal of Applied Developmental Psychology, 32*(3), 127–136.

Silk, J. S., Shaw, D. S., Skuban, E. M., Oland, A. A., & Kovacs, M. (2006). Emotion regulation strategies in offspring of childhood-onset depressed mothers. *Journal of Child Psychology and Psychiatry, 47*(1), 69–78.

Sroufe, L. A., Coffino, B., & Carlson, E. A. (2010). Conceptualizing the role of early experience: Lessons from the Minnesota Longitudinal Study. *Developmental Review, 30*(1), 36–51.

Sturge-Apple, M. L., Cicchetti, D., Davies, P. T., & Suor, J. H. (2013). Differential susceptibility in spillover between interparental conflict and maternal parenting practices: Evidence for OXTR and 5-HTT genes. *Journal of Family Psychology, 26*(3), 431–442.

Tau, G. Z., & Peterson, B. S. (2010). Normal development of brain circuits. *Neuropsychopharmacology, 35*(1), 147–168.

Teixeira, J. M., Fisk, N. M., & Glover, V. (1999). Association between maternal anxiety in pregnancy and increased uterine artery resistance index: Cohort-based study. *British Medical Journal, 318*, 153–157.

Tellegen, A., Lykken, D. T., Bouchard, T. J., Wilcox, K. J., Segal, N. L., & Rich, S. (1988). Personality similarity in twins reared apart and together. *Journal of Personality and Social Psychology, 54*, 1031–1039.

Tharner, A., Dierckx, B., Luijk, M. P. C. M., van IJzendoorn, M. H., Bakermans-Kranenburg, M. J., van Ginkel, J. R., et al. (2013). Attachment disorganization moderates the effect of maternal postnatal depressive symptoms on infant autonomic functioning. *Psychophysiology, 50*(2), 195–203.

Tharner, A., Luijk, M. P. C. M., van IJzendoorn, M. H., Bakermans-Kranenburg, M. J., Jaddoe, V. W. V., Hofman, A., et al. (2012a). Infant attachment, parenting stress, and child emotional and behavioral problems at age 3 years. *Parenting: Science and Practice, 12*(4), 261–281.

Tharner, A., Luijk, M. P. C. M., van IJzendoorn, M. H., Bakermans-Kranenburg, M. J., Jaddoe, V. W. V., Hofman, A., et al. (2012b). Maternal lifetime history of depression and depressive symptoms in the prenatal and early postnatal period do not predict infant–mother attachment quality in a large, population-based Dutch cohort study. *Attachment and Human Development, 14*(1), 63–81.

Thompson, R. A. (2006). The development of the person: Social understanding, relationships, conscience, self. In W. Damon, R. M. Lerner, & N. Eisenberg (Eds.), *Handbook of child psychology: Vol. 3. Social, emotional, and personality development* (6th ed., pp. 24–98). Hoboken, NJ: Wiley.

Tompson, M. C., Pierre, C. B., Boger, K. D., McKowen, J. W., Chan, P. T., & Freed, R. D. (2010). Maternal depression, maternal expressed emotion, and youth psychopathology. *Journal of Abnormal Child Psychology, 38*(1), 105–117.

Tottenham, N. (2012). Human amygdala development in the absence of species-expected caregiving. *Developmental Psychobiology, 54*(6), 598–611.

Tottenham, N., Hare, T. A., Quinn, B. T., McCarry, T. W., Nurse, M., Gilhooly, T., et al. (2010). Prolonged institutional rearing is associated with atypically large amygdala volume and difficulties in emotion regulation. *Developmental Science, 13*(1), 46–61.

Turney, K. (2011). Labored love: Examining the link between maternal depression and parenting behaviors. *Social Science Research, 40*(1), 399–415.

van Harmelen, A. L., van Tol, M. J., van der Wee, N. J., Veltman, D. J., Aleman, A., Spinhoven, P., et al. (2010). Reduced medial prefrontal cortex volume in adults reporting childhood emotional maltreatment. *Biological Psychiatry, 68*(9), 832–838.

van IJzendoorn, M. H., & Bakermans-Kranenburg, M. J. (2012). Differential susceptibility experiments: Going beyond correlational evidence—Comment on beyond mental health, differential susceptibility articles. *Developmental Psychology, 48*(3), 769–774.

Voegtline, K. M., Costigan, K. A., Kivlighan, K. T., Laudenslager, M. L., Henderson, J. L., & DiPietro, J. A. (2013). Concurrent levels of maternal salivary cortisol are unrelated to self-reported psychological measures in low-risk pregnant women. *Archives of Women's Mental Health, 16*(2), 101–108.

Weinberg, M. K., Beeghly, M., Olson, K. L., & Tronick, E. (2008). Effects of maternal depression and panic disorder on mother–infant interactive behavior in the face-to-face still-face paradigm. *Infant Mental Health Journal, 29*(5), 472–491.

Weinberg, M. K., Olson, K. L., Beeghly, M., & Tronick, E. Z. (2006). Making up is hard to do, especially for mothers with high levels of depressive symptoms and their infant sons. *Journal of Child Psychology and Psychiatry, 47*(7), 670–683.

Wilkinson, P. O., & Goodyer, I. M. (2011). Childhood adversity and allostatic overload of the hypothalamic–pituitary–adrenal axis: A vulnerability model for depressive disorders. *Development and Psychopathology, 23*, 1017–1037.

Wismer Fries, A. B., Ziegler, T. E., Kurian, J. R., Jacoris, S., & Pollak, S. D. (2005). Early experience in humans is associated with changes in neuropeptides critical for regulating social behavior. *Proceedings of the National Academy of Sciences of the USA, 102*, 17237–17240.

CHAPTER 13

Children of Parents
with Depression

IAN H. GOTLIB *and* NATALIE L. COLICH

O ver the past three decades, researchers have studied the offspring of parents with depression in order to gain a better understanding of factors involved in the onset of major depressive disorder (MDD). The impetus for investigating this population came from findings that having a parent with depression significantly increases children's risk of developing MDD (e.g., Goodman, Adamson, Riniti, & Cole, 1994; Weissman et al., 1987). More recently, however, investigators have moved beyond simply characterizing the association between familial depression and symptomatology in offspring to studying the mechanisms that underlie the intergenerational transmission of risk for depression. This shift in focus has significant implications for increasing our understanding of the biological underpinnings of MDD and for developing prevention and intervention programs for children at familial risk for depression.

Given the higher prevalence of depression in women than in men (see Hilt & Nolen-Hoeksema, Chapter 19, this volume), most investigators have focused on the effects of having a mother with depression. In addition, because women are at the highest risk for developing depression during their childbearing years (Evans, Heron, Francomb, Oke, & Golding, 2001), it is likely that maternal depression will occur during the formative years of children's development. It is important to note, however, that researchers have also documented adverse effects of paternal depression on internalizing and externalizing disorders in offspring (for a meta-analysis, see Kane & Garber, 2004). Moreover, there appears to be a linear increase in children's risk for developing psychopathology as a function of having none, one, or two parents who have experienced diagnosable episodes of depression (Weissman et al., 1984).

In this chapter we operationalize familial risk for depression as having at least one parent with a clinical diagnosis of depression during the child's lifetime. We briefly review the impact of parental depression on the functioning of young children and adolescents and then discuss psychobiological mechanisms that may underlie risk for depression in these offspring. Given estimates that the heritability of depression is 37% (Sullivan, Neale, & Kendler, 2000), it is likely that the transmission of risk for MDD involves more than a genetic predisposition to developing depression. In this context, therefore, we discuss both biological factors that may increase susceptibility to depression (including dysfunctional regulatory mechanisms that influence emotion regulation and stress reactivity) and psychological and social factors that may contribute to the familial transmission of risk for depression (including stressful family environments and cognitive vulnerabilities such as negative information-processing biases).

Before we begin, there are several methodological issues that should be considered in examining research on the intergenerational transmission of risk for depression. Perhaps most important, it is clear that there are bidirectional effects of parent and child psychopathology (see Pardini, 2008). Thus, in order to understand the developmental progression of risk for depression, it is important that researchers study samples of offspring of parents with depression before the children experience their first episode of diagnosable psychopathology. As we discuss, some studies include offspring who have already experienced an episode of MDD; indeed, in the absence of a comprehensive assessment of the history of parental MDD, it is possible that depression in the child led to or exacerbated depression in the parent. Clearly, long-term longitudinal studies are required to characterize the causal nature of the relation between parental depression and child psychopathology, as well as the trajectory of the development of MDD in the offspring of parents with depression.

In addition to assessing the time course of depression in the parent and, potentially, in the child, it is also important to document history of parental treatment for the disorder. Investigators have found that treatment attenuates the negative consequences of parental depression in the children; in fact, remission of maternal depression has been found to be associated with a significant reduction in the rates of depression in offspring (Weissman et al., 2006). Similarly, researchers have posited that there are different risk profiles for offspring of mothers who have experienced depression prior to pregnancy, during pregnancy (perinatal), or at multiple periods in the child's lifetime (Brennan et al., 2008; Goodman et al., 2011). This formulation highlights the importance of understanding the course of disorder in the parent in studies of children at risk for psychopathology. Unfortunately, few studies provide details about the nature of the parents' psychopathology beyond the fact that they have experienced depression; as we note later, this lack of detail makes it difficult to account for discrepant findings in the literature.

OUTCOMES OF CHILDREN OF PARENTS WITH DEPRESSION

Parental depression has been documented to have significant adverse consequences for children, starting as early as the first months of life. Studies of prenatal and postpartum depression consistently report adverse social and emotional effects on the infant. The quality of the mother–infant relationship is crucial for the development of adaptive social and emotional regulation in the infant and young child; indeed, parents play the primary role in regulating affect during this period (Eisenberg et al., 2001), which makes depression in a parent particularly problematic at early developmental stages.

Effects of Parental Depression in Infants and Preschool-Age Children

Negative consequences of having a parent with depression are apparent early in life; many studies have demonstrated a range of adverse effects of parental depression in infants and preschool-age children. In a recent meta-analysis, Goodman and colleagues (2011) found that effect sizes for the association between maternal depression and children's internalizing and externalizing behaviors, general psychopathology, and negative affect and behavior were stronger for younger than for older children. Thus there may be an early critical period during which children are particularly vulnerable to the negative effects of having a mother with depression. In this context, it is likely that very young children who are exposed to depression are more exclusively dependent on their caregivers than are older children. As children develop, they are better able to regulate their emotions and emotional experiences, which helps to buffer the adverse effects of having a parent with depression. Similarly, children's social worlds also expand, exposing them to role models other than their parents and to other support figures. Nevertheless, it is clear that parental depression early in development has detrimental effects and likely plays an important role in the subsequent onset of disorder in children.

Researchers have documented negative effects of having a mother with depression on infants almost immediately after birth. For example, infants of mothers with depression have been found to exhibit anomalous psychobiological emotion regulation functioning, including elevated heart rate (Allister, Lester, Carr, & Liu, 2001), increased basal cortisol level (Lundy et al., 1999), and more negative affect in interactions with their mothers and with adults without depression (see Field, Diego, & Hernandez-Reif, 2006, for a review). This psychophysiological profile suggests that the intergenerational transmission of risk for depression begins as early as the prenatal period and, as we document later, continues throughout childhood and adolescence.

Negative effects of parental depression have also been documented in preschool-age children; toddlers of parents with depression exhibit less secure attachment patterns with their caretakers (Coyl, Roggman & Newland, 2002), anomalous HPA-axis functioning (Dougherty et al., 2011), and increased internalizing and externalizing behaviors (Connell & Goodman, 2002). Not all studies, however, are consistent in reporting a main effect of parental depression on children's internalizing and externalizing behavior problems. Researchers have posited that moderators influence the association between maternal depression and toddler's problem behaviors, including the child's emotion regulation strategies (Silk, Shaw, Forbes, Lane, & Kovacs, 2006), the presence of paternal depression (Dietz, Jennings, Kelley, & Marshal, 2009), and high levels of parental expressed emotion (Gravener et al., 2012).

Effects of Parental Depression in School-Age Children and Adolescents

Adverse effects of parental depression have also been documented in school-age children and adolescents, a developmental period during which several forms of psychopathology emerge. In an early study, Lee and Gotlib (1989) followed four groups of mothers and their 7- to 13-year-old children through late childhood and adolescence: mothers with clinical depression, psychiatric patients without depression, medical patients without depression, and healthy controls. Offspring of women with depression in this study were rated by clinicians as having more behavioral difficulties, but were similar in their level of difficulties to the psychiatric group without depression, suggesting that behavioral problems in early adolescence are a nonspecific consequence of maternal psychopathology. In a 10-month follow-up, Lee and Gotlib (1991) found that children who had experienced maternal psychopathology continued to show increased internalizing and externalizing problems and high levels of mood symptoms and somatic complaints, regardless of whether the mother had recovered from MDD.

Murray, Halligan, Adams, Patterson, and Goodyer (2006) followed 91 mother–child pairs for 13 years to examine the effects of postpartum depression on socioemotional development through childhood and adolescence. They found that daughters whose mothers had experienced postpartum depression were more emotionally sensitive than were both sons of mothers with depression and boys and girls in the control group. Furthermore, this emotional sensitivity was related to insecure attachment in infancy. Murray and colleagues (2006) also found higher rates of depression in daughters whose mothers had experienced postpartum depression, but only if the mother developed additional depressive episodes later in the child's life, highlighting the importance of chronicity of maternal depression in influencing risk for MDD. These findings were replicated by Pawlby, Hay, Sharp, Waters, and O'Keane (2009), who found that children who were exposed to prenatal depression were almost five times more likely to develop depression than were control children and that this effect was mediated by chronicity of maternal depression. Interestingly, Hammen and Brennan (2003) found that severity of maternal depression was more important than chronicity in contributing to risk for depression in offspring of mothers with depression; thus further research is needed to continue to examine this issue.

MECHANISMS OF EFFECTS OF PARENTAL DEPRESSION

It is clear from this brief review that parental depression is associated with a range of negative outcomes in children from infancy to adolescence and beyond. These adverse effects are likely due to a variety of factors that are associated with depression. In addition to heredity, potential mechanisms underlying the intergenerational transmission of risk for depression include altered prenatal environments, exposure to dysfunctional and stressful family contexts, negative cognitive biases, anomalous endocrine response to stress, and aberrant neurobiological functioning. It is critical that we elucidate these psychobiological mechanisms both in order to understand the onset of the disorder in vulnerable children and to reduce the adverse effects of these factors before the development of depression.

Prenatal Effects of Maternal Depression

The intergenerational transmission of risk for depression has been posited to begin as early as the prenatal period. The fetuses of women with depression have been found to exhibit elevated heart rates while their mothers undergo an acute stress task (Monk et al., 2004); furthermore, this increased heart rate appears to be related to high levels of maternal cortisol (Fink et al., 2010; Monk et al., 2011). Pregnant mothers with depression are hypothesized to experience more stress throughout pregnancy than do their counterparts without depression (Field, Hernandez-Reif, & Diego, 2006), which may alter the prenatal environment because of the higher levels of cortisol that have been reported in stressed pregnant women and their newborns (for a review, see Field, 2010). Mood states that are often associated with depression, such as maternal anxiety and anger, have also been shown to adversely affect newborns when experienced throughout pregnancy. Thus risk for depression may be transmitted through the development of aberrant stress and emotion regulation systems in the infant (for a more detailed examination of this issue, see Goodman & Lusby, Chapter 12, this volume).

Family Environments of Children of Parents with Depression

In addition to an adverse prenatal environment, researchers have found that offspring of parents with depression experience more stressful home environments and more negative parenting behaviors than do children of parents without depression. Consistent with a diathesis–stress model, early life stress may alter the cognitive and socioemotional development of children of parents with depression, increasing their vulnerability for developing disorder. As Goodman (2007) noted, several environmental mechanisms may help to explain the association between maternal depression and depression in offspring, including social modeling/learning of depressotypic cognitions, affect and behaviors, inadequate parenting, and exposure to depression-related stressors in the mother. In this section we briefly discuss studies that have documented the impact of maternal depression on parenting behaviors and the exposure of children to stress and stress generation of their mothers with depression (for more detailed reviews, see Goodman & Lusby, Chapter 12, this volume; Joormann, Eugène, & Gotlib, 2008).

One mechanism through which early exposure to parental depression may have a significant impact on children's development trajectory involves the early caregiver–child relationship. In particular, attachment style has been posited to predict children's ability to develop emotion regulation skills and form stable relationships throughout childhood and beyond (see Ainsworth, Blehar, Waters, & Wall, 1978). In this context, children of mothers with depression have been found to exhibit disrupted patterns of early childhood attachment. In a meta-analysis examining attachment patterns of infants with mothers with clinical depression, Martins and Gaffan (2000) reported that offspring of mothers with depression are less likely to be securely attached than are offspring of mothers with no psychiatric history. Similarly, Gravener and colleagues (2012) found that 2-year-old children of mothers with depression exhibited high levels of insecure attachment and high rates of internalizing and externalizing behaviors. They also found that these maladaptive behaviors were mediated by the mothers' criticism both of themselves and of their children, suggesting that criticism mediates the relation between insecure attachment and the development of psychopathology.

A large body of research indicates that both maternal and paternal depression are associated with maladaptive parenting behaviors. Compared with mothers without depression, mothers with depression are less affectionate and more anxious and display less verbal and play interaction with their infants (for a review, see Field, 2010). Furthermore, mothers with depression exhibit fewer repairs of interrupted interactions; not surprisingly, therefore, toddlers of mothers with depression have been found to be less able to maintain interactions than toddlers of mothers without depression (Jameson, Gelfand, Kulcsar, & Teti, 1997). These impoverished interactions with infants throughout the first 3 months of life are associated with higher rates of depressive symptoms at 19 years of age (Schmid et al., 2011), suggesting that poor mother–child interactions contribute to the development of depression in later adolescence.

Similarly, infants and young children of parents with depression are exposed to greater levels of negative affect from their caregivers. For instance, when interacting with infants and young children, mothers with depression display more negative, sad, and irritable affect and less positive affect than do mothers without depression (Cohn, Campbell, Matias, & Hopkins, 1990; Goodman et al., 1994). Parents with depression are also less consistent in their parenting strategies, alternating between being unavailable and demonstrating less parental control and engaging in authoritarian parenting behaviors (Pelaez, Field, Pickens, & Hart, 2008; Righetti-Veltema, Bousquet, & Manzano,

2003). In a meta-analysis examining the association between maternal depression and parenting behaviors, Lovejoy, Graczyk, O'Hare, and Neuman (2000) found that mothers with depression exhibit more negative parenting behaviors than do mothers without depression; although not found as consistently, mothers with depression also disengage or withdraw from their children. Thus chronic exposure to negative parental attitudes and parenting strategies in offspring of parents with depression appears to be an important mechanism underlying the transmission of risk for MDD.

In addition to the stresses associated with negative parenting behaviors, researchers have documented high levels of marital conflict in families with one or two parents with depression (see Davila, Stroud, & Starr, Chapter 22, this volume), indicating that this is an additional stressor for offspring. In reviewing the literature examining the effects of depression on family relationships, Burke (2003) described women with depression as likely to marry men with psychiatric illnesses and to experience marital disharmony. Interestingly, in a sample of mothers with depression and their children, Pilowsky, Wickramaratne, Nomura, and Weissman (2006) found that greater family instability in adolescence due to parental depression predicted the development of depression and substance abuse over the next 20 years. Similarly, in a study of more than 14,000 families, Hanington, Heron, Stein, and Ramchandani (2012) found that marital conflict partially mediated the relation between the experience of parental depression in early childhood and the subsequent development of psychopathology.

Finally, Hammen and her colleagues reported that chronic familial stress, combined with negative parenting behaviors such as high expressed emotion and criticism, mediated the relation between parental depression and depression in their children (e.g., Hammen, Brennan, & Shih, 2004; Hammen, Shih, & Brennan, 2004). These findings suggest that the presence of a stressful family environment and negative parental behaviors significantly increase the risk for depression in the offspring of parents with depression. This elevated risk may be due to chronic exposure to stress in the offspring (and, therefore, to chronic activation of the HPA axis) or to the parent modeling negative affect, behaviors, and cognitions for their children.

Cognitive Vulnerabilities in Offspring of Parents with Depression

Depression in adults and adolescents has been found to be characterized by negative information-processing biases. Consistent with Beck's (1976) cognitive model of depression, individuals with depression attend to, interpret, and recall stimuli in the environment in a manner consistent with their sad/negative mood state while minimizing the processing of positive stimuli. These biases are posited to be activated by stressful events and to contribute to both the onset and the maintenance of the disorder by maintaining negative affective states and impeding recovery from stressors (see Joormann & Arditte, Chapter 14, this volume). Importantly, negative information-processing biases similar to those documented in adults and adolescents with depression have been reported in never-disordered offspring of parents with depression, suggesting that these biases are a vulnerability factor for the development of depression. For example, in an early study Garber, Robinson, and Valentiner (1997) found that, compared with children in a control group, offspring of mothers with mood disorders were characterized by more negative cognitive styles, including negative attribution biases and lower self-worth, even after controlling for current levels of depressive symptomatology.

More recently, investigators have moved beyond the use of self-report measures to assess the cognitive functioning of offspring of parents with depression and have used more sophisticated methods to assess biases in information processing. For instance, Joormann, Talbot, and Gotlib (2007) administered a dot-probe task to examine attentional biases to emotional stimuli in daughters of mothers with recurrent depression. Joormann and colleagues found that, following a negative mood induction (used to activate negative schemas in vulnerable individuals), daughters of mothers with depression selectively attended to sad faces. In contrast, daughters of healthy control mothers selectively attended to happy faces. Dearing and Gotlib (2009) found that these daughters of mothers with depression interpreted ambiguous words and stories more negatively than did the control daughters, and Joormann, Gilbert, and Gotlib (2010) reported that the high-risk daughters required greater emotional intensity of expression in order to identify sad faces and labeled low-intensity angry faces as sad faces. In sum, therefore, findings that negative biases in the processing of emotional information are observable in high-risk children before the onset of significant depressive symptomatology or disorder suggest that negative schemas of vulnerable adolescents increase their risk for developing psychopathology.

Genetics

Although investigators have examined numerous candidate genes in the search for the etiology of MDD (see Lau et al., Chapter 9, this volume), perhaps not surprisingly given the heterogeneity of MDD, this search has not yielded a specific gene or set of genes that is associated reliably with depression or that is implicated in parental transmission of risk for this disorder. Nevertheless, Sullivan and colleagues (2000) found in a meta-analysis that 26–42% of the variance in MDD is due to genetic effects, with the highest rates of heritability in children of parents with depression. Therefore, we present findings involving the most frequently studied candidate for the genetic transmission of risk for the development of depression. We argue here that it is not the disorder itself that is heritable but rather the traits and characteristics that confer risk for the development of MDD.

The largest literature on the genetics of depression involves the repeat polymorphism located in the promoter region of *5-HTTLPR*—the serotonin transporter gene. This variation in the promoter region functionally alters transcription of the serotonin transporter protein that removes serotonin from the synapse. The short or long alleles of this promoter region decrease and increase transcription rates, respectively, allowing more or less serotonin to remain in the synapse. Interest in this polymorphism and its relation to depression has increased in the past decades because of the effectiveness of selective serotonin reuptake inhibitors (SSRIs) in treating major depression (see Gitlin, Chapter 26, this volume). Consistent with a diathesis–stress formulation, a number of investigators have found that individuals who carry one or two copies of the *5-HTTLPR* short allele exhibit more depressive symptoms following a stressful life event than do individuals who are homozygous for the long allele (e.g., Caspi et al., 2003). In a study of the transmission of depression across three generations, Talati, Weissman, and Hamilton (2013) found a fourfold increase in the rates of homozygous short-allele carriers in the high-risk group (defined as having a grandparent or parent who has experienced major depression). Importantly, however, allele length did not differentiate individuals who had or had not experienced a major depressive episode. Thus this genetic polymorphism may serve as a risk factor that, when combined with exposure to stress, leads to the development of MDD. Indeed, Hammen, Brennan, Keenan-Miller, Hazel, and Najman (2010) reported higher rates of depression in 20-year-old females who carried one or two *5-HTTLPR* short alleles *and* who reported having experienced chronic family stress at age 15.

Interestingly, this gene-by-environment interaction was not significant for acute stressors, suggesting that this genetic polymorphism increases individuals' susceptibility to chronic or recurrent stressors, such as those associated with having a mother with depression (e.g., decreased parental bonding, increased marital discord). Gotlib, Joormann, Minor, and Hallmayer (2008) found that girls with two copies of the *5-HTTLPR* short allele showed higher and more prolonged cortisol secretion in response to a laboratory stressor than did girls with at least one long allele, thus linking this polymorphism with a biological stress response that has been implicated in MDD. As Lau and colleagues (Chapter 9, this volume) note, however, recent meta-analyses of the relation between *5-HTTLPR* and depression have failed to support these findings of a gene-by-environment interaction (e.g., Risch et al., 2009), arguably due in part to selective reviews and inclusion of relevant studies and considerable variability in how investigators have assessed and quantified environmental variables. In fact, in a more inclusive meta-analysis, Karg, Burmeister, Shedden, and Sen (2011) found strong support for the association between *5-HTTLPR* and MDD and suggested that discrepancies in the results of meta-analyses are due to methodological differences among studies rather than to a veridical lack of support for this gene–environment interaction.

As Goodman and Gotlib (1999) and Joormann and colleagues (2008) note, it is unlikely that a single genetic polymorphism accounts for risk for depression; instead, heritability of maladaptive traits or characteristics likely increase individuals' risk for developing MDD. In fact, there are a number of relevant traits or characteristics that have been found to be highly heritable, including behavioral inhibition or shyness (Cherny, Fulker, Corley, Plomin, & DeFries, 1994), neuroticism (Tellegen et al., 1988), expression of negative affect (Plomin et al., 1993), and subjective feelings of well-being (Lykken & Tellegen, 1996). High rates of heritability have also been documented for measures of stress reactivity, such as basal levels of cortisol, and, in particular, cortisol awakening response (CAR; Bartels, de Geus, Kirschbaum, Sluyter, & Boomsma, 2003). Together, these findings suggest that the genetic transmission of risk for depression involves the inheritance of depressogenic cognitive, affective, and psychobiological vulnerabilities.

Stress Reactivity

Researchers have documented an association between stressful life circumstances, including separation from caregivers and insufficient caregiving behavior, and altered HPA-axis function in both animals and humans (Gunnar, Morison, Chisholm, & Schuder, 2001; Suomi, 1999). The HPA system and its production of cortisol indexes individuals' psychophysiological stress response and has been examined in two primary contexts. Individuals release cortisol throughout the day (basal, or diurnal, cortisol), as well as in response to threat or stress (cortisol reactivity); importantly, alterations in both of these patterns of cortisol secretion have been linked to depression in adults. For example, investigators have found that adults diagnosed with MDD are characterized by elevated basal levels of cortisol (Knorr, Vinberg, Kessing, & Wetterslev, 2010) and by blunted levels of cortisol following a laboratory stress task, although findings in this area have been equivocal (for a review, see Burke, Davis, Otte, & Mohr, 2005). This pattern of results suggests that individuals with depression experience difficulties coping with, or regulating the effects of, stressful circumstances.

Recently, researchers have begun to examine whether these anomalies in HPA-axis functioning are not merely a symptom of MDD but also serve as a biological marker of risk for development of the disorder. Goodman and Gotlib (1999) postulated that one consequence of maternal depression is the chronic activation of the HPA axis in the child as a result of the stress of living with a parent with depression. This HPA-axis activation likely reflects an impaired ability to cope effectively with stress and to regulate negative affect. Similarly, Walker, Walder, and Reynolds (2001) proposed that an increase in levels of basal cortisol with puberty is implicated in the higher incidence of emotional disorders following this developmental milestone. Thus dysregulated HPA-axis functioning might contribute to the increased risk for MDD in offspring of parents with depression. Several studies have supported this formulation; researchers have found increased levels of basal cortisol in children with a parent with depression (for a review, see Guerry & Hastings, 2011). Essex, Klein, Cho, and Kalin (2002) found that preschool children who were exposed to high levels of maternal stress in infancy and early development had significantly higher cortisol levels than did children in less stressful environments; moreover, severity of maternal depression during infancy was the strongest predictor of children's subsequent cortisol levels. A specific aspect of diurnal cortisol, CAR, not only has been found to be elevated in adolescents with a familial history of depression (Mannie, Harmer, & Cowen, 2007) but also to predict levels of depressive symptomatology in later adolescence (Adam et al., 2010). Finally, Halligan, Herbert, Goodyer, and Murray (2007) showed that morning cortisol levels at age 13 mediated the relation between maternal depression and youth depression symptoms 3 years later, implicating CAR in the intergenerational transmission of risk for depression.

In addition to having increased levels of morning and diurnal cortisol, offspring of parents with depression have also been found to have aberrant cortisol reactivity. For instance, Feldman and colleagues (2009) found that infants of mothers with depression had higher levels of cortisol following a fear-induction paradigm than did infants of mothers without a history of psychopathology, indicating that disrupted HPA-axis functioning is present in early stages of development.

It is instructive to note that high levels of cortisol resulting from chronic activation of the HPA axis can disrupt functioning in regions of the brain that have been implicated in the regulation of emotion (e.g., the prefrontal cortex [PFC], the anterior cingulate cortex [ACC], and the amygdala). This, too, therefore, may be a mechanism through which HPA-axis activation is related to children's ability to cope with stress. Interestingly, these same neural regions have been found to be functionally and/or structurally abnormal in the children of parents with depression (e.g., Gotlib et al., 2010; Joormann, Cooney, Henry, & Gotlib, 2012), further implicating these neurobiological systems of emotion regulation in the intergenerational transmission of risk for depression.

Neurobiological Functioning

Researchers have also identified abnormalities in neural structure and function in individuals diagnosed with MDD in brain regions that have been implicated in the processing and regulation of emotional stimuli (see Pizzagalli & Treadway, Chapter 11, this volume). Recent meta-analyses suggest that adults with depression have structural abnormalities in gray matter volumes of the hippocampus, amygdala, ACC, and dorsolateral PFC (dlPFC; e.g., Hamilton, Siemer, & Gotlib, 2008; Kempton et al., 2011). Anomalies in neural function, reflected in patterns of brain activation, have also been reported in adults with depression, most frequently involving increased activation in subcortical emotion-processing regions, such as the amygdala and limbic circuits, combined with attenuated activation in cognitive control regions, such as the dlPFC. This pattern of activation has been posited to underlie the increased negative affect that characterizes depression (Hamilton et al., 2012). As we discussed earlier, the role of these abnormalities in neural structure and function in the onset of depression is not clear. To address this question, researchers have begun to examine whether children and adolescents at risk for depression exhibit neural abnormalities before the onset of a depressive episode in the same brain regions that have been documented in adults with depression.

Although few studies have been conducted to date, anomalies in both neural structure and function similar to those documented in adults with depression have been identified in never-disordered offspring of parents with depression (see Foland-Ross, Hardin, and Gotlib, 2013, for a detailed review of this literature). For example, mirroring findings of reduced hippocampal volume in adults and adolescents with depression, as well as in individuals who were exposed to early life stress (e.g., McKinnon, Nazarov, & MacQueen, 2009), researchers have found attenuated hippocampal volume in never-disordered offspring of parents with depression (Chen, Hamilton, & Gotlib, 2010; Rao et al., 2010). In fact, Rao and colleagues (2010) found in a mediation analysis that hippocampal volume partially accounted for the relation between early life stress and depressive symptoms assessed at a longitudinal follow-up, suggesting that volumetric abnormalities in hippocampal development represent a biomarker for the development of MDD.

Studies of adults with depression have documented anomalous structure and function of the amygdala (see Pizzagalli & Treadway, Chapter 11, this volume). Importantly, similar abnormalities have also been reported in children and adolescents with a family history of depression. Lupien and colleagues (2011) found larger bilateral amygdala volume in 10-year-old children of mothers with recurrent depression than in children of healthy mothers. Furthermore, this increased amygdala volume was positively correlated with mothers' mean depression scores over the child's lifetime, suggesting that mothers' depressive symptomatology is intimately linked to their children's amygdala development. Interestingly, this finding replicates results of studies with orphanage-reared children who experienced early maternal separation or poor maternal caretaking (Mehta et al., 2009; Tottenham et al., 2010). Furthermore, compared with children of healthy parents, children of parents with depression have also been found to exhibit anomalous patterns of neural activation in response to affective stimuli, exhibiting greater amygdala activation both to sad emotion faces (Monk et al., 2008) and to sad film clips (Joormann et al., 2012).

Offspring of parents with depression have also been found to show patterns of structural and functional aberrations in prefrontal regions responsible for emotion regulation and cognitive control similar to those that have been documented in adults with depression (Foland-Ross et al., 2013). For example, Peterson and colleagues (2009) found cortical thinning in the right dorsal and inferior frontal gyrus in both children and adults who had a first- or second-degree relative with severe depression. Patterns of hypoactivity in children of parents with depression have also been documented using measures of electrophysiology (both electroencephalography [EEG] and event-related potential [ERP]), reflecting decreased activation in regions of the PFC (Perez-Edgar, Fox, Cohn, & Kovacs, 2006; Tomarken, Dichter, Garber, & Simien, 2004). Similarly attenuated functional recruitment of the dlPFC has been found in high-risk children as they viewed negative faces (Mannie, Taylor, Harmer, Cowen, & Norbury, 2011) and as they attempted to repair or regulate negative mood states by recalling positive memories (Joormann et al., 2012).

Gotlib and colleagues (2010) documented attenuated striatal activation, indexed by decreased activation in putamen and left insula, in children of mothers with depression as they anticipated and received rewards. Importantly, adults with depression have also been found to exhibit aberrant neural responses to both the anticipation and the receipt of rewarding stimuli, including attenuated responses in striatal regions, such as the caudate and nucleus accumbens (Knutson, Bhanji, Cooney, Atlas, & Gotlib, 2008; Pizzagalli et al., 2009). These findings suggest that altered development of reward circuitry is a risk factor for the onset of depression; further studies are necessary, however, to corroborate the role of the striatum in the transmission of this risk. Considered collectively, these findings of anomalies in neural function and structure in children of parents with depression, even before the onset of an episode of depression, indicate that neural abnormalities may be vulnerability factors for developing MDD, playing a critical role in the familial transmission of risk for depression.

MODERATORS OF THE EFFECTS OF PARENTAL DEPRESSION

As we reviewed earlier in this chapter, investigators have documented consistent associations between parental depression and adverse child outcomes. Importantly, however, the outcomes examined in this research are varied and are often not specific to having a parent with depression. Children of parents with depression and of parents with various other forms of psychopathology have been found to exhibit elevated levels of internalizing and externalizing behaviors, as well as other forms of disturbed functioning. The diversity in outcomes may be due in part to factors that moderate the relation between parental psychopathology and children's development. Understanding the effects of these moderators is critical if research is to move forward in elucidating the nature of intergenerational transmission of risk for depression and in understanding the development of risk and resilience in the offspring of parents with depression.

Across multiple studies, investigators have reported that having two parents with depression confers greater risk for depression and for other forms of psychopathology than does having only one parent with depression (e.g., Brennan, Hammen, Katz, & Le Brocque, 2002; Landman-Peeters et al., 2008). Not all investigators have found this increased risk, however (e.g., Lieb, Isensee, Hofler, Pfister, & Wittchen, 2002), suggesting that there are intricacies involved in the effects of having one versus two parents with depression that we do not yet understand. Similarly, findings concerning the differential effects of maternal versus paternal depression are also mixed. In a meta-analysis, Connell and Goodman (2002) found that although depression in either the mother or father was associated with increased internalizing and externalizing behavior difficulties in the offspring, the strongest association was between maternal depression and child internalizing behavior problems. Finally, several researchers have found a heightened risk for anxiety disorders in offspring of mothers with depression, but not of fathers with depression, highlighting the importance of conducting differential diagnoses in children of parents with depression (Brennan et al., 2002; Landman-Peeters et al., 2008). Clearly, investigators should continue to examine mechanisms through which risk for various forms of psychopathology may be transmitted differentially by mothers and fathers to their sons and daughters.

Another moderator that likely affects the intergenerational transmission of risk for depression is the history of the parents' depression during the child's lifetime. More specifically, the severity, chronicity, comorbidity, and timing of parental depressive episodes can influence how risk for depression, and for other forms of psychopathology, is transmitted from parents to their offspring. Investigators have demonstrated relatively consistently that more chronic and severe parental depression increases the risk that the children will develop depressive symptoms and other forms of psychopathology (e.g., Hammen & Brennan, 2003; Mars et al., 2011). And recently, Apter-Levy, Feldman, Vakart, Ebstein, and Feldman (2013) reported that variation in a polymorphism of the oxytocin receptor gene moderated the adverse effects of the chronicity of maternal depression on young children's functioning. Nevertheless, additional research is needed to increase our understanding of the effects of the timing of depressive episodes in parents on risk for depression in offspring. For example, as we noted earlier, some investigators have found that exposure to maternal depression in the first 2 years of life confers greater risk for offspring than does exposure later in childhood or adolescence (Goodman et al., 2011); in contrast, however, other researchers have reported that the chronicity of depressive episodes in parents has a stronger effect on the functioning offspring than does the timing of the episodes (e.g., Hammen & Brennan, 2003; Pilowsky et al., 2006). Importantly, however as Hammen and Brennan (2003) note, chronicity and timing are likely confounded in many studies, given that early onset of MDD is associated with chronic, recurrent, depressive episodes.

Finally, socioeconomic status (SES) has been posited to moderate the intergenerational transmission of risk for depression. Goodman and colleagues (2011) noted that low SES can be a proxy for a range of stressors, including discrimination, poverty, and limited access to health care and resources (Krieger, 1999; Sue, Capodilupo, & Holder, 2008). Based on this formulation, Goodman and colleagues hypothesized that the relation between maternal depression and psychopathology in offspring would be stronger in low- than in high-SES families. They conducted a meta-analysis of 193 studies and, confirming their prediction, found that the effect sizes for reports of internalizing problems, externalizing problems, and general psychopathology were greater for low-income than for middle- or high-income families. Given the significant effects of SES on health outcomes and behaviors, it is important that future research examine more explicitly how this construct may moderate the intergenerational transmission of risk for depression.

CONCLUSIONS AND FUTURE DIRECTIONS

Researchers have clearly documented that the presence of parental depression has significant negative consequences for infants, children, and adolescents, including heightened stress reactivity, impaired emotion regulation strategies, and increased risk for the development of depression. The specific mechanisms that underlie the intergenerational transmission of risk for MDD in these offspring, however, are less clear. We have reviewed evidence indicating that there are multiple factors that may lead children of parents with depression to develop depression themselves, including altered prenatal development, exposure to stressful parenting behaviors and family environments, cognitive vulnerabilities, genetic predispositions, anomalous HPA-axis functioning, and aberrant neural function and structure. As we note subsequently, however, much work remains to be done to gain a more comprehensive understanding of these mechanisms and their interactions with other risk factors and to examine how specific moderators affect the transmission of risk for depression from parent to child.

For example, it is important that investigators attempt to develop and test integrative models of risk rather than exploring potential mechanisms that underlie risk in isolation. Our models of transmission of risk for depression should develop as our research methods and designs become more sophisticated, our understanding of psychobiological processes increases, and available technology advances. Goodman and Gotlib's (1999) model of risk for depression posits that four factors contribute to risk for depression in the offspring of individuals with depression: heritability of depression; innate dysfunctional neuroregulatory mechanisms; exposure to negative maternal cognitions, behaviors, and affect; and the presence of stressful life events. The authors highlight the transactional nature of this model, emphasizing that these factors do not operate in isolation but, rather, interact in complex ways. Future research should focus on incorporating advances in our understanding of both the psychological and biological contributions of risk in order to further refine this model. For instance, advances in the study of epigenetics suggest that gene expression can be altered by environmental influences, such as early exposure to life stress (Murgatroyd et al., 2009; Roth, Lubin, Funk, & Sweatt, 2009; see Lau et al., Chapter 9, this volume). Thus examining environmental risk factors and genetic influences on behavior, as well as their interrelations, is crucial to building our understanding of the transmission of risk for MDD.

Future studies should also attempt to rectify the lack of attention given to understanding risk for depression in different social groups. The majority of studies focus on unselected groups of parents with depression—largely middle-class Caucasian samples; as we noted previously, however, many individuals who develop depression are working-class, low-income, and/or unemployed mothers with young children (Weissman et al., 2004), who experience a broad range of stressors. Being a member of an ethnic minority group can similarly be associated with exposure to a variety of stressors. Indeed, researchers have documented higher levels of risk for depression in the offspring of minority mothers with depression, suggesting that this is a particularly vulnerable population with respect to the transmission of risk for MDD (Goodman et al., 2011). Although it is likely that it is largely the accumulated life stressors associated with minority status that place these children, adolescents, and adults at elevated risk for the development of depression, the fact remains that we know little about the transmission of risk in minority samples.

Examining the transition to puberty in the context of risk for depression is also important in attempting to understand why some offspring of parents with depression are at greater risk than others for developing depression. The greater prevalence of depression in females than in males begins by the age of 10–14 years (see Hilt & Nolen-Hoeksema, Chapter 19, this volume), and pubertal status has been found to be a better predictor of depression than is chronological age (Angold, Costello, & Worthman, 1998). These findings suggest that changes that occur with puberty have differential effects for males and females. We know little, however, about social and endocrine factors that differentially affect males and females throughout puberty. To address this issue, investigators need to conduct a comprehensive examination of pubertal status and the psychobiological functioning of offspring of parents with depression during this transition period, including an assessment of the contribution of gonadal hormones to risk for depression.

Finally, there is clearly heterogeneity not only in the presentation of depression in parents, but in the functioning of their offspring as well. We know virtually nothing about the differential impact of various symptoms or subtypes of depression (e.g., psychomotor retardation, anhedonia) on the functioning of offspring. Similarly, children of parents with depression are typically treated as a homogeneous group, even though we know that (only) half will go on to develop an episode of depression. We desperately need strong longitudinal studies that will help us to understand more precisely the nature of the relation between parental depression and child psychopathology, the trajectory of the development of MDD in the offspring of parents with depression, and factors that contribute to resilience in high-risk children who do not experience depression.

REFERENCES

Adam, E. K., Doane, L. D., Zinbarg, R. E., Mineka, S., Craske, M. G. & Griffith, J. W. (2010). Prospective prediction of major depressive disorder from cortisol awakening response in adolescence. *Psychoneuroendocrinology, 35*(6), 921–931.

Ainsworth, M. S., Blehar, M. C., Waters, E., & Wall, S. (1978). *Patterns of attachment: A psychological study of the strange situation.* Oxford, UK: Erlbaum.

Allister, L., Lester, B. M., Carr, S., & Liu, J. (2001). The effects of maternal depression on fetal heart rate response to vibroacoustic stimulation. *Developmental Neuropsychology, 20,* 639–651.

Angold, A., Costello, E. J., & Worthman, C. M. (1998). Puberty and depression: The roles of age, pubertal status and pubertal timing. *Psychological Medicine, 28*(1), 51–61.

Apter-Levy, Y., Feldman, M., Vakart, A., Ebstein, R. P., & Feldman, R. (2013). Impact of maternal depression across the first 6 years of life on the child's mental health, social engagement, and empathy: The moderating role of oxytocin. *American Journal of Psychiatry, 170*(10), 1161–1168.

Bartels, M., de Geus, E. J. C., Kirschbaum, C., Sluyter, F., & Boomsma, D. I. (2003). Heritability of daytime cortisol levels in children. *Behavior Genetics, 33*(4), 421–433.

Beck, A. T. (1976). *Cognitive therapy and the emotional disorder.* New York: Meridian.

Brennan, P. A., Hammen, C., Katz, A. R., & Le Brocque, R. M. (2002). Maternal depression, paternal psychopathology, and adolescent diagnostic outcomes. *Journal of Consulting and Clinical Psychology, 70*(5), 1075–1085.

Brennan, P. A., Pargas, R., Walker, E. F., Green, P., Newport, D. J., & Stowe, Z. (2008). Maternal depression and infant cortisol: Influences of timing, comorbidity and treatment. *Journal of Child Psychology and Psychiatry, 49*(10), 1099–1107.

Burke, H. M., Davis, M. C., Otte, C., & Mohr, D. C. (2005). Depression and cortisol responses to psychological stress: A meta-analysis. *Psychoneuroendocrinology, 30*(9), 846–856.

Burke, L. (2003). The impact of maternal depression on familial relationships. *International Review of Psychiatry, 15,* 243–255.

Caspi, A., Sugden, K., Moffitt, T. E., Taylor, A., Craig, I. W., Harrington, H., et al. (2003). Influence of life stress on depression: Moderation by a polymorphism in the *5-HTT* gene. *Science, 301,* 386–389.

Chen, M. C., Hamilton, J. P., & Gotlib, I. H. (2010). Decreased hippocampus volume in healthy girls at risk for depression. *Archives of General Psychiatry, 67*(3), 270–276.

Cherny, S. S., Fulker, D. W., Corley, R. P., Plomin, R., & DeFries, J. C. (1994). Continuity and change in infant shyness from 14 to 20 months. *Behavioral Genetics, 24,* 365–379.

Cohn, J. F., Campbell, S. B., Matias, R., & Hopkins, J. (1990). Face-to-face interactions of postpartum depressed and nondepressed mother–infant pairs at 2 months. *Developmental Psychology, 26*(1), 15–23.

Connell, A. M., & Goodman, S. H. (2002). The association between psychopathology in fathers versus mothers and children's internalizing and externalizing behavior problems: A meta-analysis. *Psychological Bulletin, 128*(5), 746–773.

Coyl, D. D., Roggman, L. A., & Newland, L. A. (2002). Stress, maternal depression, and negative mother–infant interactions in relation to infant attachment. *Infant Mental Health Journal, 23,* 145–163.

Dearing, K., & Gotlib, I. H. (2009). Interpretation of ambiguous information in girls at risk for depression. *Journal of Abnormal Child Psychology, 37*(1), 79–91.

Dietz, L. J., Jennings, K. D., Kelley, S. A., & Marshal, M. (2009). Maternal depression, paternal psychopathology, and toddlers' behavioral problems. *Journal of Clinical Child and Adolescent Psychology, 38*(1), 48–61.

Dougherty, L. R., Klein, D. N., Rose, S., & Laptook, R .S. (2011). Hypothalamic–pictuitary–adrenal axis reactivity in the preschool-age offspring of depressed parents: Moderation by early parenting. *Psychological Science, 22*(5), 650–658.

Eisenberg, N., Losoya, S., Fabes, R. A., Guthrie, I. K., Reiser, M., Murphy, B., et al. (2001). Parental socialization of children's dysregulated expression of emotion and externalizing problems. *Journal of Family Psychology, 15*(2), 183–205.

Essex, M. J., Klein, M. H., Cho, E., & Kalin, N. H. (2002). Maternal stress beginning in infancy may sensitize children to later stress exposure: Effects on cortisol and behavior. *Biological Psychiatry, 52*(8), 776–784.

Evans, J., Heron, J., Francomb, H., Oke, S., & Golding, J. (2001). Cohort study of depressed mood during pregnancy and after childbirth. *British Medical Journal, 323*, 257–260.

Feldman, R., Granat, A., Pariente, C., Kanety, H., Kuint, J., & Gilboa-Schechtman, E. (2009). Maternal depression and anxiety across the postpartum year and infant social engagement, fear regulation, and stress reactivity. *Journal of the American Academy of Child and Adolescent Psychiatry, 48*(9), 919–927.

Field, T. (2010). Postpartum depression effects on early interactions, parenting, and safety practices: A review. *Infant Behavior and Development, 33*(1), 1–6.

Field, T., Diego, M., & Hernandez-Reif, M. (2006). Prenatal depression effects on the fetus and newborn: A review. *Infant Behavior and Development, 29*, 445–455.

Field, T., Hernandez-Reif, M., & Diego, M. (2006). Risk factors and stress variables that differentiate depressed from nondepressed pregnant women. *Infant Behavior and Development, 29*, 169–174.

Fink, N. S., Urech, C., Berger, C. T., Hoesli, I., Holzgreve, W., Bitzer J., et al. (2010). Maternal laboratory stress influences fetal neurobehavior: Cortisol does not provide all answers. *Journal of Maternal–Fetal and Neonatal Medicine, 23*(6), 488–500.

Foland-Ross, L. C., Hardin, M. G., & Gotlib, I. H. (2013). Neurobiological marks of familial risk for depression. *Current Topics in Behavioral Neuroscience, 14*, 181–206.

Garber, J., Robinson, N. S., & Valentiner, D. (1997). The relation between parenting and adolescent depression: Self-worth as a mediator. *Journal of Adolescent Research, 12*(1), 12–33.

Goodman, S. H. (2007). Depression in mothers. *Annual Review of Clinical Psychology, 3*, 107–135.

Goodman, S. H., Adamson, L. B., Riniti, J., & Cole, S. (1994). Mothers' expressed attitudes: Associations with maternal depression and children's self-esteem and psychopathology. *Journal of the American Academy of Child and Adolescent Psychiatry, 33*, 1265–1274.

Goodman, S. H., & Gotlib, I. H. (1999). Risk for psychopathology in the children of depressed mothers: A developmental model for understanding mechanisms of transmission. *Psychological Review, 106*, 458–490.

Goodman, S. H., Rouse, M. H., Connell, A. M., Robbins Broth, M., Hall, C. M., & Heyward, D. (2011). Maternal depression and child psychopathology: A meta-analytic review. *Clinical Child and Family Psychology Review, 14*, 1–27.

Gotlib, I. H., Hamilton, J. P., Cooney, R. E., Singh, M. K., Henry, M. L., & Joormann, J. (2010). Neural processing of reward and loss in girls at risk for depression. *Archives of General Psychiatry, 67*(4), 380–387.

Gotlib, I. H., Joormann, J., Minor, K. L. & Hallmayer, J. (2008). HPA-axis reactivity: A mechanism underlying the associations among *5-HTTLPR*, stress, and depression. *Biological Psychiatry, 63*(9), 847–851.

Gravener, J. A., Rogosch, F. A., Oshri, A., Narayan, A. J., Cicchetti, D., & Toth, S. L. (2012). The relations among maternal depressive disorder, maternal expressed emotion, and toddler behavior problems and attachment. *Journal of Abnormal Child Psychology, 40*, 803–813.

Guerry, J. D., & Hastings, P. D. (2011). In search of HPA axis dysregulation in child and adolescent depression. *Clinical Child and Family Psychology Review, 14*(2), 135–160.

Gunnar, M. R., Morison, S. J., Chisholm, K., & Schuder, M. (2001). Salivary cortisol levels in children adopted from Romanian orphanages. *Development and Psychopathology, 13*, 611–628.

Halligan, S. L., Herbert, J., Goodyer, I., & Murray, L. (2007). Disturbances in morning cortisol secretion in association with maternal postnatal depression predicts depressive symptomatology in adolescence. *Biological Psychiatry, 62*, 40–46.

Hamilton, J. P., Etkin, A., Furman, D. J., Lemus, M. G., Johnson, R. F., & Gotlib, I. H. (2012). Functional neuroimaging of major depressive disorder: A meta-analysis and new integration of baseline activation and neural response data. *American Journal of Psychiatry, 169*(7), 693–703.

Hamilton, J. P., Siemer, M., & Gotlib, I. H. (2008). Amygdala volume in major depressive disorder: A meta-analysis of magnetic resonance imaging studies. *Molecular Psychiatry, 13*(11), 993–1000.

Hammen, C., & Brennan, P. A. (2003). Severity, chronicity, and timing of maternal depression and risk for adolescent offspring diagnoses in a community sample. *Archives of General Psychiatry, 60*, 253–258.

Hammen, C., Brennan, P. A., Keenan-Miller, D., Hazel, N. A., & Najman, J. M. (2010). Chronic and acute stress, gender, and serotonin transporter gene–environment interactions predicting depression symptoms in youth. *Journal of Child Psychology and Psychiatry, 51*(2), 180–187.

Hammen, C., Brennan, P., & Shih, J. (2004). Family discord and stress predictors of depression and other disorders in adolescent children of depressed and nondepressed women. *Journal of the American Academy of Child and Adolescent Psychiatry, 43*, 994–1002.

Hammen, C., Shih, J., & Brennan, P. (2004). Intergenerational transmission of depression: Test of an interpersonal stress model in a community sample. *Journal of Consulting and Clinical Psychology, 72*(3), 511–522.

Hanington, L., Heron, J., Stein, A., & Ramchandani, P. (2012). Parental depression and child outcomes: Is marital conflict the missing link? *Child: Care, Health and Development, 38*(4), 520–529.

Jameson, P. B., Gelfand, D. M., Kulcsar, E., & Teti, D. M. (1997). Mother–toddler interaction patterns associated with maternal depression. *Development and Psychopathology, 9*, 537–550.

Joormann, J., Cooney, R. E., Henry, M. L., & Gotlib, I. H. (2012). Neural correlates of automatic mood regulation in girls at high risk for depression. *Journal of Abnormal Psychiatry, 51*(5), 575–582.

Joormann, J., Eugène, F., & Gotlib, I. H. (2008). Parental depression: Impact on offspring and mechanisms underlying transmission of risk. In S. Nolen-Hoeksema & L. M. Hilt (Eds.), *Handbook of adolescent depression* (pp. 441–472). New York: Taylor & Francis.

Joormann, J., Gilbert, K., & Gotlib, I. H. (2010). Emotion identification in girls at high risk for depression. *Journal of Child Psychology and Psychiatry, 51*(5), 575–582.

Joormann, J., Talbot, L., & Gotlib, I. H. (2007). Biased processing of emotional information in girls at risk for depression. *Journal of Abnormal Psychology, 116*(1), 135–143.

Kane, P., & Garber, J. (2004). The relations among depression in fathers, children's psychopathology, and father–child conflict: A meta-analysis. *Clinical Psychology Review, 24*, 339–360.

Karg, K., Burmeister, M., Shedden, K., & Sen, S. (2011). The serotonin transporter promoter variant (*5-HTTLPR*), stress, and depression meta-analysis revisited: Evidence of genetic moderation. *Archives of General Psychiatry, 68*(5), 444–454.

Kempton, M. J., Salvador, Z., Munafo, M. R., Geddes, J. R., Simmons, A., Frangou, S., et al. (2011). Structural neuroimaging studies in major depressive disorder: Meta-analysis and comparison with bipolar disorder. *Archives of General Psychiatry, 68*(7), 675–690.

Knorr, U., Vinberg, M., Kessing, L. V., & Wetterslev, J. (2010). Salivary cortisol in depressed patients versus control persons: A systematic review and meta-analysis. *Psychoneuroendocrinology, 35*(9), 1275–1286.

Knutson, B., Bhanji, J. P., Cooney, R. E., Atlas, L. Y., & Gotlib, I. H. (2008). Neural responses to monetary incentives in major depression. *Biological Psychiatry, 63*(7), 686–692.

Krieger, N. (1999). Embodying inequality: A review of concepts, measures, and methods for studying health consequences of discrimination. *International Journal of Health Services, 29*, 295–352.

Landman-Peeters, K. M., Ormel, J., Van Sonderen, E. L., Den Boer, J. A., Minderaa, R. B., & Hartman, C. A. (2008). Risk of emotional disorder in offspring of depressed parents: Gender differences in the effect of a second emotionally affected parent. *Depression and Anxiety, 25*(8), 653–660.

Lee, C. M., & Gotlib, I. H. (1989). Maternal depression and child adjustment: A longitudinal analysis. *Journal of Abnormal Psychology, 98*(1), 78–85.

Lee, C. M., & Gotlib, I. H. (1991). Adjustment of children of depressed mothers: A 10-month follow-up. *Journal of Abnormal Psychology, 100*(4), 473–477.

Lieb, R., Isensee, B., Hofler, M., Pfister, H., & Wittchen, U. H. (2002). Parental major depression and the risk of depression and other mental disorders in offspring: A prospective-longitudinal community study. *Archives of General Psychiatry, 59*, 365–374.

Lovejoy, M. C., Graczyk, P. A., O'Hare, E., & Neuman, G. (2000). Maternal depression and parenting behavior: A meta-analytic review. *Clinical Psychology Review, 20*(5), 561–592.

Lundy, B., Jones, N., Field, T., Nearing, G., Davalos, M., Pietro, P., et al. (1999). Prenatal depression effects on neonates. *Infant Behavioral Development, 22*, 119–129.

Lupien, S. J., Parent, S., Evans, A. C., Tremblay, R. E., Zelazo, P. D., Corbo, V., et al. (2011). Larger amygdala but no change in hippocampal volume in 10-year-old children exposed to maternal depressive symptomatology since birth. *Proceedings of the National Academy of Sciences of the USA, 108*(34), 14324–14329.

Lykken, D. T., & Tellegen, A. (1996). Happiness is a stochastic phenomenon. *Psychological Science, 7*, 186–189.

Mannie, Z. N., Harmer, C. J., & Cowen, P. J. (2007). Increased waking salivary cortisol levels in young people at familial risk of depression. *American Journal of Psychiatry, 164*(4), 617–621.

Mannie, Z. N., Taylor, M. J., Harmer, C. J., Cowen, P. J., & Norbury, R. (2011). Frontolimbic responses to emotional faces in young people at familial risk of depression. *Journal of Affective Disorders, 130*(1–2), 127–132.

Mars, B., Collishaw, S., Smith, D., Thapar, A., Potter, R., Sellers, R., et al. (2011). Offspring of parents with recurrent depression: Which features of parental depression index risk for offspring psychopathology? *Journal of Affective Disorders, 136*, 44–53.

Martins, C., & Gaffan, E. A. (2000). Effects of early maternal depression on patterns of infant–mother attachment. *Journal of Child Psychology and Psychiatry, 41*(6), 737–746.

McKinnon, M. C., Nazarov, Y. K., & MacQueen, G. M. (2009). A meta-analysis examining clinical predictors of hippocampal volume in patients with major depressive disorder. *Journal of Psychiatry and Neuroscience, 34*, 41–54.

Mehta, M. A., Golembo, N. I., Nosarti, C., Colvert, E., Mota, A., Williams, S. C., et al. (2009). Amygdala, hippocampal and corpus callosum size following severe early institutional deprivation: The English and Romanian adoptees study pilot. *Journal of Child Psychology and Psychiatry, 50*(8), 943–951.

Monk, C., Fifer, W. P., Myers, M. M., Bagiella, E., Duong, J. K., Chen, I. S., Leotti, L., et al. (2011). Effects of maternal breathing rate, psychiatric status, and cortisol on fetal heart rate. *Developmental Psychobiology, 53*, 221–233.

Monk, C., Sloan, R. P., Myers, M. M., Ellman, L., Werner, E., Jeon, J., et al. (2004). Fetal heart rate reactivity differs by women's psychiatric status: An early marker for developmental risk? *Journal of the American Academy of Child and Adolescent Psychiatry, 43*(3), 283–290.

Monk, C. S., Klein, R. G., Telzer, E. H., Schroth, E. A., Mannuzza, S., Moulton, J. L., III, et al. (2008). Amygdala and nucleus accumbens activation to emotional facial expressions in children and adolescents at risk for major depression. *American Journal of Psychiatry, 165*(1), 90–98.

Murgatroyd, C., Patchev, A. V., Wu, Y., Micale, V., Bockmuhl, Y., Fischer, D., et al. (2009). Dynamic DNA methylation programs persistent adverse effects of early-life stress. *Nature Neuroscience, 12*, 1559–1566.

Murray, L., Halligan, S. L., Adams, G., Patterson, P., & Goodyer, I. M. (2006). Socioemotional development in adolescents at risk for depression: The role of maternal depression and attachment style. *Development and Psychopathology, 18*(2), 489.

Pardini, D. A. (2008). Novel insights into longstanding theories of bidirectional parent–child influences: Introduction to the special section. *Journal of Abnormal Child Psychology, 36*, 627–631.

Pawlby, S., Hay, D. F., Sharp, D., Waters, C. S., & O'Keane, V. (2009). Antenatal depression predicts depression in adolescent offsring: Prospective longitudinal community-based study. *Journal of Affective Disorders, 113*, 236–243.

Pelaez, M., Field, T., Pickens, J. N., & Hart, S. (2008). Disengaged and authoritarian parenting behavior of depressed mothers with their toddlers. *Infant Behavior and Development, 31*, 145–148.

Perez-Edgar, K., Fox, N. A., Cohn, J. F., & Kovacs, M. (2006). Behavioral and electrophysiological markers of selective attention in children of parents with a history of depression. *Biological Psychiatry, 60*(10), 1131–1138.

Peterson, B. S., Warner, V., Bansal, R., Zhu, H., Hao, X., Liu, J., et al. (2009). Cortical thinning in persons at increased familial risk for major depression. *Proceedings of the National Academy of Sciences of the USA, 106*(15), 6273–6278.

Pilowsky, D. J., Wickramaratne, P., Nomura, Y., & Weissman, M. M. (2006). Family discord, parental depression, and psychopathology in offspring: 20-year follow-up. *Journal of the American Academy of Child and Adolescent Psychiatry, 45*(4), 452–460.

Pizzagalli, D. A., Holmes, A. J., Dillon, D. G., Goetz, E. L., Birk, J. L., Bogdan, R., et al. (2009). Reduced caudate and nucleus accumbens response to rewards in unmedicated subjects with major depressive disorder. *American Journal of Psychiatry, 166*, 702–710.

Plomin, R., Emde, R. N., Braungart, J. M., Campos, J., Corley, R. P., Fulker, D. W., et al. (1993). Genetic change and continuity from fourteen to twenty months: The MacArthur Longitudinal Twin Study. *Child Development, 64*, 1354–1376.

Rao, U., Chen, L. A., Bidesi, A. S., Shad, M. U., Thomas, M. A., & Hammen, C. L. (2010). Hippocampal changes associated with early-life adversity and vulnerability to depression. *Biological Psychiatry, 67*(4), 357–364.

Righetti-Veltema, M., Bousquet, A., & Manzano, J. (2003). Impact of postpartum depressive symptoms on mother and her 18-month-old infant. *European Child and Adolescent Psychiatry, 12*(2), 75–83.

Risch, N., Herrell, R., Lehner, T., Liang, K., Eaves, L., Hoh, J., et al. (2009). Interaction between the serotonin transporter gene (*5-HTTLPR*), stressful life events, and risk of depression: A meta-analysis. *Journal of the American Medical Association, 301*(23), 2462–2471.

Roth, T. L., Lubin, F. D., Funk, A. J., & Sweatt, D. (2009). Lasting epigenetic influence of early-life adversity on the BDNF gene. *Biological Psychiatry, 65*(9), 760–769.

Schmid, B., Blomeyer, D., Buchmann, A. F., Trautmann-Villalba, P., Zimmermann, U. S., Schmidt, M. H., et al. (2011). Quality of early mother–child interaction associated with depressive psychopathology in the offspring: A prospective study from infancy to adulthood. *Journal of Psychiatric Research, 45*, 1387–1394.

Silk, J. S., Shaw, D. S., Forbes, E. E., Lane, T. L., & Kovacs, M. (2006). Maternal depression and child internalizing: The moderating role of child emotion regulation. *Journal of Clinical Child and Adolescent Psychology, 35*(1), 116–126.

Sue, D. W., Capodilupo, C. M., & Holder, A. M. B. (2008). Racial microaggressions in the life experience of Black Americans. *Professional Psychology: Research and Practice, 39*(3), 329–336.

Sullivan, P. F., Neale, M. C., & Kendler, K. S. (2000). Genetic epidemiology of major depression: Review and meta-analysis. *American Journal of Psychiatry, 157*, 1552–1562.

Suomi, S. J. (1999). Conflict and cohesion in rhesus monkey family life. In M. Cox & J. Brooks-Gunn (Eds.), *Conflict and cohesion in families* (pp. 283–299). Mahwah, NJ: Erlbaum.

Talati, A., Weissman, M. M., & Hamilton, S. P. (2013). Using the high-risk family design to identify biomarkers for major depression. *Philosophical Transactions of the Royal Society,* *368,* 1–10.

Tellegen, A., Lykken, D. T., Bouchard, T. J., Wilcox, K. J., Segal, N. L., & Rich, S. (1988). Personality similarity in twins reared apart and together. *Journal of Personality and Social Psychology, 54,* 1031–1039.

Tomarken, A. J., Dichter, G. S., Garber, J., & Simien, C. (2004). Resting frontal brain activity: Linkages to maternal depression and socioeconomic status among adolescents. *Biological Psychiatry, 67,* 77–102.

Tottenham, N., Hare, T. A., Quinn, B. T., McCarry, T. W., Nurse, M., Gilhooly, T., et al. (2010). Prolonged institutional rearing is associated with atypically large amygdala volume and difficulties in emotion regulation. *Developmental Science, 13*(1), 46–61.

Walker, E. F., Walder, D. J., & Reynolds, F. (2001). Developmental changes in cortisol secretion in normal and at-risk youth. *Development and Psychopathology, 13,* 721–732.

Weissman, M. M., Feder, A., Pilowsky, D. J., Olfson, M., Fuentes, M., Blanco, C., et al. (2004). Depressed mothers coming to primary care: Maternal reports of problems with their children. *Journal of Affective Disorders, 78*(2), 93–100.

Weissman, M. M., Gammon, D., John, K., Merikangas, K. R., Warner, V., Prusoff, B. A., et al. (1987). Children of depressed parents: Increased psychopathology and early onset of major depression. *Archives of General Psychiatry, 44,* 847–853.

Weissman, M. M., Pilowsky, D. J., Wickramarantne, P. J., Talati, A., Wisniewski, S. R., Fava, M., et al. (2006). Remission in maternal depression and child psychopathology: A STAR*D-Child report. *Journal of the American Medical Association, 295*(12), 1389–1398.

Weissman, M. M., Prusoff, B. A., Gammon, G. D., Merikangas, K. R., Leckman, J. F., & Kidd, K. K. (1984). Psychopathology in the children (ages 6–18) of depressed and normal parents. *Journal of the American Academy of Child Psychiatry, 23,* 78–84.

CHAPTER 14

Cognitive Aspects of Depression

JUTTA JOORMANN *and* KIMBERLY ARDITTE

One of the most important topics in depression research concerns the issue of vulnerability versus resilience. How can we explain why some people respond to seemingly minor stressors with increasingly negative affect that can spiral into a full-blown depressive episode, whereas others seem never to become depressed, even when they face major adversity? Cognitive theories of depression propose that people's thoughts, inferences, and attitudes, as well as the ways in which they attend to, interpret, and recall emotion-eliciting events, determine their emotional responses. Consequently, cognitions are thought to play a crucial role in influencing the extent to which people are affected by negative experiences and in determining whether stressful events will be followed by quick recovery or by recurring depressive episodes. Cognitive theories rely on the assumption that investigating the content of one's thoughts and the nature of one's cognitive processes, particularly in the context of stressful life events, is crucial to our understanding of depression.

Studies investigating the interaction of cognition and emotion have a long tradition in depression research. Early research focused primarily on demonstrating that the thought content differs between people with and without depression and that individuals with depression exhibit cognitive deficits and biased processing of emotional material. These studies employed a variety of self-report measures and experimental tasks and generally provided consistent evidence that depression is characterized by negative, automatic thoughts about the self, the future, and the world (e.g., Ingram, Miranda, & Segal, 1998; Mathews & MacLeod, 2005). Indeed, one of the most successful interventions for depression, cognitive-behavioral therapy, focuses on modifying dysfunctional automatic thoughts (Beck, 1976; Hollon & Dimidjian, Chapter 27, this volume). Theorists have also implicated cognitive biases as possible vulnerability markers for depression (e.g., Ingram et al., 1998). Fewer studies, however, have explicitly tested the underlying vulnerability–stress model or examined how general cognitive deficits and biased processing of negative emotional material are related to each other and, more importantly, to the hallmark feature of depression—sustained negative affect.

In this chapter, we provide a brief review of the literature on cognition in unipolar depression. We discuss the major models for explaining the role of cognition in this disorder and review evidence indicating that depression is characterized by both the preferential processing of negative material and general cognitive deficits. In addition, we summarize recent research focusing on mechanisms that might underlie depression-related changes in cognitive content and processing and highlight the consequences of these changes for depressive affect.

COGNITIVE MODELS OF DEPRESSION

Cognitive Styles and Depressive Schemas

Research on cognition in depression has largely been guided by the *helplessness model*, which was later refined to take into account attributional style and is now referred to as the *hopelessness model* (Abramson, Metalsky, & Alloy, 1989; Alloy, Abramson, Walshaw, & Neeren, 2006), the *response styles theory* (Nolen-Hoeksema, 1991), and Beck's (1976) *schema theory of depression*. The helplessness/hopelessness model of depression has its roots in Seligman's (1975) concept of *learned helplessness*, which states that expectancies about the lack of control over events lead to depressive episodes. This model was refined by Abramson and colleagues (1989), who proposed that *hopelessness* (i.e., the expectation that highly desired outcomes will not occur and/or that highly aversive outcomes are certain) is a proximal sufficient cause of depressive symptoms and may be the consequence of attributing negative life events to stable and global causes. Moreover, attributing these events to internal causes is likely to lead to lowered self-esteem and feelings of worthlessness, which may further strengthen the symptoms of depression. Abramson and colleagues point out that the hopelessness model may not apply to all forms of depression; rather, it may represent an important subtype of depressive disorders (e.g., Alloy et al., 2006).

Another cognitive style that has been related to heightened depression risk is rumination. Rumination is defined as repetitive thinking that focuses one's attention on one's depressive symptoms and on the implications, causes, and meanings of these symptoms (Nolen-Hoeksema, Wisco, & Lyubomirsky, 2008). The response style theory of depression proposes that rumination is a trait-like response to negative affect (Nolen-Hoeksema, 1991) that exacerbates sad mood and predicts future depressive episodes (Nolen-Hoeksema et al., 2008). What characterizes rumination and differentiates it from negative automatic thoughts is that it is a *style* of thought rather than just negative *content* (Nolen-Hoeksema, 1991; Nolen-Hoeksema et al., 2008). Thus rumination is defined by the process of recurring thoughts and ideas, often described as a "recycling" of thoughts, and not necessarily by the content of these recurring thoughts.

Beck (1976) postulates that individuals use existing representations of stimuli, ideas, or experiences (i.e., *schemas*) to filter and process information from the environment. Although reliance on our schemas is often adaptive, processing information in a manner congruent with dysfunctional schemas may contribute to the onset or exacerbation of depression symptoms. Schemas of persons with depression often include themes of loss, separation, failure, worthlessness, and rejection; consequently, individuals with depression often exhibit systematic schema-congruent biases in the processing of environmental stimuli. People with depression may attend selectively to dysphoric stimuli in their environment and interpret neutral and ambiguous stimuli in a negative way. Similarly, people with depression may demonstrate biased recall of semantic information and auto-biographical memories that are consistent with their moods and/or schemas. Because dysfunctional schemas and processing biases appear to endure beyond the depressive episode, they are thought to represent stable vulnerability factors for depression onset and recurrence.

Importantly, schemas can remain latent, which means that they are less accessible and are unlikely to influence affect. Yet, when activated by stressors, dysfunctional schemas may lead to specific negative cognitions. These automatic cognitions typically involve pessimistic views of the self, the world, and the future—the cognitive triad. Schema-influenced negative thoughts and related processing biases initiate and maintain depressed mood through a vicious cycle of increasingly negative thinking and negative affect.

In sum, these models each provide an account of how depression symptoms may develop and maintain over time. Still, the theories have important differences that should not be overlooked. Whereas the hopelessness model makes assumptions about the content of depressive cognition, the response style theory and Beck's theory add assumptions about cognitive processes that include attention, memory, and reasoning. In addition, the response style theory emphasizes individual differences in responding to negative affect and in the regulation of emotion as a risk factor for depression. Finally, because these biases and cognitive styles are thought to endure beyond acute episodes of depression, they are thought to characterize the functioning of individuals who are vulnerable to experiencing episodes of depression.

Resource Allocation and Affective Interference

The theories discussed thus far have primarily focused on the preferential processing of mood-congruent stimuli. However, other theories emphasize two distinct patterns of cognition documented in depressed and dysphoric samples. Although people with depression can easily concentrate on negative, self-focused thoughts and exhibit enhanced processing of mood-congruent information, they also report impairment in the processing of stimuli that is mood-incongruent (i.e., neutral or positive; Burt, Zembar, & Niederehe, 1995). In general, researchers have either examined the biased processing of emotional information or the valence-nonspecific "cognitive symptoms" of depression (e.g., general difficulties with concentration or decision making); relatively few attempts have been made to integrate the findings obtained in these separate lines of research.

The *resource allocation hypothesis* postulates that there is a limit on the amount of resources available for cognitive operations and that depression either occupies or functionally reduces these resources (Ellis & Ashbrook, 1988). As a result, individuals with depression exhibit deficits when engaging in other effortful cognitive procedures. Moreover, it has been suggested that rumination is a key mechanism that drains cognitive resources among people with depression and impairs or prevents them from engaging in controlled tasks that require focused attention (Hertel, 1998; Levens, Muhtadie, & Gotlib, 2009). Thus, compared with healthy controls, persons with depression have demonstrated greater emotional distraction in response to negative, but not positive, stimuli and poorer performance on a working memory task containing negative distractors (e.g., Segrave et al., 2012).

Similarly, the *affective interference hypothesis* posits that persons with depression are preoccupied with the processing of emotional material. Thus their performance on tasks will not be impaired if they need to process emotional stimuli but will be impaired when they must disengage from emotional aspects of a stimulus in order to process other aspects (Siegle, Ingram, & Matt, 2002). For example, if individuals with depression are required to make valence judgments about words, their tendency to prioritize the processing of emotional material will aid them. If, however, they are instructed to ignore the emotional content of words while making a lexical decision judgment, their processing priorities will interfere, and their performance will be impaired (Siegle et al., 2002).

Deficits in Cognitive Control in Depression

As noted earlier, a key and often troubling aspect of depression is the frequent occurrence of ruminative, unintentional, and often uncontrollable negative thoughts and memories. Rumination has been found to increase the risk of depression onset, to maintain depressive episodes, and to elevate risk for symptom recurrence. But why do people ruminate? Examining deficits in executive functioning among people with depression is thought to be essential to our understanding of the dysfunctional cognitive processes, such as rumination, that may underlie prolonged negative affect in depression.

Overriding prepotent responses and inhibiting the processing of irrelevant material that captures attention are core abilities that allow us to respond flexibly and to adjust our behavior and emotional responses to changing situations. Cognitive control is related to the functioning of executive control processes such as inhibition, disengagement, and updating in working memory (Miyake & Friedman, 2012). Working memory is a limited-capacity system that provides temporary access to a select set of representations in the service of current cognitive processes (Cowan, 1999). Thus working memory reflects the focus of attention and the temporary activation of representations that are the contents of awareness. Given the capacity limitation of this system, it is important that the contents of working memory be updated efficiently, a task that is controlled by executive processes. Executive processes must selectively gate access to working memory, shielding it from intrusion of irrelevant material, as well as discarding information that is no longer relevant. In this context, individual differences in the experience and resolution of interference are likely to affect cognitive and emotional functioning, and several researchers have suggested that rumination and depression are associated with such deficits in executive functioning (Joormann, 2010; Whitmer & Gotlib, 2012).

According to Baddeley (2013), for example, persons with depression may maintain representations of symptoms in their working memory. These representations serve to amplify, rather than minimize, the experience of subsequent depression symptoms. Furthermore, cognitive inhibition has been proposed to play an important role in difficulties in emotion regulation in depression (Joormann, 2010). If changes in mood are associated with activations of mood-congruent material in working memory, impairment in the ability to control the contents of working memory by inhibiting mood-congruent content may be expected to play an important role in the development of rumination and, therefore, in recovery from negative mood.

Other research suggests that depressive ruminators can often be characterized by trait-level mental inflexibility that impairs performance on cognitive tasks that require shifting ability (Altamirano, Miyake, & Whitmer, 2010). Finally, Hertel (2004) has proposed that depression is characterized by an impaired ability to override automatic, prepotent response tendencies, including rumination and negative, self-focused thoughts. Because the ability to override prepotent responses and focus attention on the demands of a current task is associated with inhibitory processes, depression-related dysfunction in this area may explain the lack of self-controlled attention to the task at hand.

Considered collectively, these models propose that individuals who exhibit impaired executive functioning are vulnerable to rumination and subsequent depression. Moreover, it appears that the constructs of updating working memory, shifting, and inhibition may be important in explaining both general cognitive deficits in depression and the preferential processing of depression-relevant material.

EMPIRICAL TESTS OF COGNITIVE MODELS OF DEPRESSION

Cognitive Styles and Depressive Schemas

Most studies investigating the role of dysfunctional attitudes and attributional styles have relied on self-report measures, such as the Dysfunctional Attitudes Scale (DAS; Weissman & Beck, 1978), the Cognitive Styles Questionnaire (CSQ; modified from Peterson et al.'s 1982 Attributional Styles Questionnaire), and the Young Schema Questionnaire (YSQ; Young, 1999). Numerous cross-sectional studies using these questionnaires have found associations among dysfunctional attitudes, attributional styles, maladaptive schemas, and other negative cognitions in individuals with current depression (Alloy, Abramson, & Francis, 1999; Leahy, Tirch, & Melwani, 2012).

Although these findings are interesting, examining cognitive styles in cross-sectional studies of people with current depression makes it impossible to determine whether participants endorse such cognitions because they have current depression or whether these cognitions precipitate the onset of depression and thus play a role in increasing vulnerability to depression. To investigate this question, a number of studies have used remission designs to look for evidence of continued cognitive dysfunction beyond the scope of a depressive episode. In a review of early studies, Haaga, Dyck, and Ernst (1991) stated that there was only limited evidence that depressive cognitions remain stable after depression symptoms have remitted (see also Ingram et al., 1998; Just, Abramson, & Alloy, 2001). However, vulnerability–stress models hypothesize that prior activation of latent dysfunctional schemas is necessary before negative cognitions can be observed. Therefore, some studies have used mood inductions or have heightened self-focus/self-relevance to activate negative schemas before assessing dysfunctional cognitions in remitted participants. This research has painted a more positive picture (for a review, see Scher, Ingram, & Segal, 2005). For example, compared with participants who never had depression, participants who formerly had depression demonstrate a greater change in dysfunctional attitudes after a negative mood induction (e.g., Gemar, Segal, Sagrati, & Kennedy, 2001).

Yet remission designs have also been criticized because they cannot differentiate between vulnerability factors and consequences or "scars" of having experienced a past depressive episode (e.g., Just et al., 2001). More promising are longitudinal studies that examine the ability of self-report measures to predict recovery and improvements in symptom severity. Results from such studies have produced mixed findings. Research suggests that specific subscales of the DAS and YSQ demonstrate moderate test–retest reliability over long periods of time (e.g., 9 years) and are predictive of depression relapse (Halvorsen, Wang, Eisemann, & Waterloo, 2010; Wang, Halvorsen, Eisemann, & Waterloo, 2010). Thus such subscales are thought to measure stable, trait-level vulnerability factors. Still, other subscales of the DAS and YSQ are found to fluctuate greatly over time and may be best conceptualized as state-level markers of depression symptom severity. Other prospective studies have investigated the prediction of depression onset. Gibb, Beevers, Andover, and Holleran (2006), for example, reported that negative attributional style in interaction with negative events predicted subsequent depressive symptoms. Similarly, Lewinsohn, Joiner, and Rohde (2001) reported that dysfunctional attitudes interacted with stress to predict onset of a depressive episode during a 1-year interval, and Seeds and Dozois (2010) found that more strongly activated negative self-schemas and, conversely, more diffuse positive self-schemas were associated with elevations in depression following stressful life events.

Finally, longitudinal studies have focused on high-risk samples. These studies are particularly promising, as they prospectively assess participants before the initial onset of psychopathology. There are different ways of identifying someone as at "high risk for depression." High-risk samples can be relatives of persons with depression or individuals at high risk because of other factors (e.g., socioeconomic status or cognitive profile). Abela and Skitch (2007) found an interaction between daily hassles and DAS scores in children at high risk for depression due to their parents' psychopathology (see Dunbar et al., 2013, for a similar finding). Alloy and colleagues (2006) recruited never-depressed college students who demonstrated depressive cognitive styles, defined by elevated scores on the DAS and the CSQ. In a 30-month follow-up, these investigators found that individuals who exhibited negative attributional styles and dysfunctional attitudes were more likely than were participants who scored low on measures of cognitive vulnerability to experience first onsets of depression. Indeed, the risk of depression in the high-risk group was about seven times higher than it was in the low-risk group (Alloy et al., 2006). Therefore, longitudinal studies largely support the formulation that cognitive factors interact with acute stressors to play an important role in the onset, maintenance, and recurrence of depressive episodes.

Self-reported levels of ruminative response style have been found to predict higher levels of dysphoria over time in prospective studies with nonclinical samples, even after controlling for initial differential depression levels (e.g., Nolen-Hoeksema & Morrow, 1991). Moreover, studies have shown that rumination predicts higher levels of depressive symptoms and onset of major depressive episodes and mediates the gender difference in depressive symptoms (Nolen-Hoeksema, 2000; Nolen-Hoeksema et al., 2008). Research also indicates that rumination enhances cognitive biases in information-processing tasks and impairs mood regulation, resulting in sustained negative mood states (e.g., Lyubomirsky & Nolen-Hoeksema, 1995). Thus dysphoric participants who were induced to ruminate endorsed more negative interpretations of hypothetical situations, generated less effective problem-solving strategies (Lyubormirsky & Nolen-Hoeksema, 1995), and showed increased recall of negative autobiographical memories (Lyubomirsky, Caldwell, & Nolen-Hoeksema, 1998).

Cognitive Processing Biases in Depression

Theoretical models, especially Beck's schema theory, emphasize that individuals with depression exhibit cognitive biases in all aspects of information processing, including memory, interpretation, and attention (Mathews & MacLeod, 2005). Although such theoretical predictions are straightforward, the empirical results are not always so clear. More specifically, there is strong evidence for biased memory among individuals with depression but controversy over the existence and presentation of interpretation and attentional biases in depression. Of note, the following summary discusses extant literature on each cognitive bias as a unique factor associated with depression and depression vulnerability. Whereas the *combined cognitive bias hypothesis* purports that biases may interact to produce depressive affect, initial research has provided conflicting support for this hypothesis (see Everaert, Koster, & Derakshan, 2012).

Cognitive Biases in Memory

Enhanced memory for negative, relative to positive, information is perhaps the most robust cognitive bias associated with major depression (Matt, Vázquez, & Campbell, 1992). In a meta-analysis of studies assessing recall performance, Matt and colleagues found that people with major depression remembered 10% more negative words than positive words. Research has also found a bias for the recall of negative autobiographical memories (e.g., Whalley, Rugg, & Brewin, 2012). For example, using the Autobiographical Memory Task, participants with depression were better able to generate specific memories in response to negative cues than in response to positive cues (Gupta & Kar, 2012). Interestingly, persons with depression also differ from their counterparts without depression in that they do not appear to display a memory bias for positive information (Matt et al., 1992). In a recent study examining memory biases using a matching task with both positive and negative words, Gotlib, Jonides, Buschkuehl, and Joormann (2011) found that participants without depression turned over (i.e., searched for) more positive than negative words and matched more positive than negative pairs within the first 5 minutes of the task. In contrast, participants with depression were equally as likely to turn over negative words as they were to turn over positive words and matched significantly fewer positive pairs within the first 5 minutes of the task than did participants without depression.

There is also emerging evidence to indicate that memory biases persist even after depression symptoms have remitted. Following a sad mood induction, participants with remitted depression were found to recall more vivid, self-defining negative memories and less emotionally intense, self-defining positive memories than did either participants with remitted depression who had undergone a neutral mood induction or never-depressed participants who had received either induction (Werner-Seidler & Moulds, 2012). Moreover, even when individuals with remitted depression and those who had never had depression do not differ in their memory performance, functional magnetic resonance imaging (fMRI) research suggests that individuals with remitted depression require greater recruitment of brain regions, such as the cingulate gyrus, right inferior- and left-medial frontal gyrus, the right anterior hippocampus, and the amygdala in order to successfully encode positively valenced stimuli (Arnold et al., 2011; see Pizzagalli & Treadway, Chapter 11, this volume). Taken together, such findings suggest that biased memory represents a vulnerability factor that predisposes individuals to recurrence of depressive episodes. However, as we noted earlier, prospective studies are needed to examine vulnerability to an initial onset of major depressive disorder (MDD).

Depression is associated not only with enhanced recall of negative events and difficulties encoding positive material but also with the recall of rather generic memories despite instructions to recall specific events (i.e., overgeneral memory; see Williams et al., 2007, for a review). Importantly, this research has demonstrated that overgeneral memories are associated with difficulties in problem solving and in imagining future events, as well as with delayed recovery from episodes of depression (Dalgleish, Spinks, Yiend, & Kuyken, 2001; Peeters, Wessel, Merckelbach, & Boon-Vermeeren, 2002; Raes et al., 2005). Moreover, overgeneral memories remain stable outside of episodes of the disorder (Mackinger, Pachinger, Leibetseder, & Fartacek, 2000) and have been shown to predict later onset of depressive episodes (Rawal & Rice, 2012; van Minnen, Wessel, Verhaak, & Smeenk, 2005). Williams and colleagues (2007) proposed that individual differences in cognitive control, and specifically in inhibitory dysfunction, may underlie overgeneral recall in depression. In support of this hypothesis, Dalgleish and colleagues (2007) conducted a series of experiments that demonstrated that deficits in executive control and cognitive inhibition were associated with overgeneral memory deficits in depression. These authors propose that reduced specificity is the result of deficits in executive control and inhibition, leading to impoverished retrieval strategies during memory search and/or problems with inhibiting inappropriate candidate memory responses in the Autobiographical Memory Task. Indeed, the authors found a significant relation between reduced specificity of autobiographical memories in depression and poor performance on tasks assessing executive control. An important explanation of this relation is that a reduced ability to inhibit prepotent responses (i.e., negative self-referent, ruminative responses) makes it difficult for individuals to focus on the goal of retrieving a specific event. In addition, studies have shown that rumination may maintain overgeneral memory in patients with depression (Watkins & Teasdale, 2004). Therefore, understanding overgeneral memory in the context of emotion regulation in depression is an important goal for future research. One particularly promising study found that training dysphoric individuals to be more concrete and less overgeneral in their thinking led to a significant reduction in depressive symptoms and rumination (Watkins, Baeyens, & Read, 2009).

Cognitive Biases in Interpretation and Attention

Research with depressed and dysphoric samples has produced some evidence of biased interpretation of negative stimuli. When presented with ambiguous scenarios, participants with clinical depression ranked negative interpretations as more probable than other interpretations (Butler & Mathews, 1983). In addition, research assessing interpretation biases via sentence completion tasks (e.g., Scrambled Sentences Test) has found evidence that persons with depression lack a positive bias (Moser, Huppert, Foa, & Simons, 2012), as well as an association between negative biases and increases in depressive symptoms over time (Rude, Wenzlaff, Gibbs, Vane, & Whitney, 2002). However, the assessment of interpretation biases using response latencies has produced mixed findings. Whereas some studies have found that participants with depression and dysphoria do not differ from participants without depression in their reaction times to a target word (Lawson & MacLeod, 1999; Sears, Bisson & Neilsen, 2011), others have found quicker reaction times among participants with than among those without dysphoria when associating a negative word with an ambiguous sentence (Cowden Hindash & Amir, 2012). Furthermore, a recent study reported a negative interpretation bias in daughters of mothers with depression who had never had a disorder themselves, providing evidence for a role of these biases in increasing risk for depression onset (Dearing & Gotlib, 2009). Clearly, further research is needed to elucidate these conflicting results.

Evidence for the existence of depression-related attentional biases has also been mixed. One possible explanation for such findings is that depression is not associated with all aspects of attention for mood-congruent material. Studies using the Modified Stroop Task have not typically found differences between participants with depression and controls (e.g., Mogg, Bradley, Williams, & Mathews, 1993). Similarly, research using attentional allocation paradigms (e.g., the dot-probe task) has often failed to find evidence for attentional biases among persons with depression (for a review, see Mathews & MacLeod, 2005). However, more recent research suggests that depression-related attentional biases may not be present within the context of initial orientation to negative stimuli but rather are observed under conditions of maintained attentional engagement (see Armstrong & Olatunji, 2012, for a meta-analytic review). Indeed, dot-probe tasks that have included conditions of longer stimulus exposure have produced evidence for selective attention in depression (e.g., Joormann & Gotlib, 2007). Studies utilizing eye-tracking technology have further supported the notion that persons with depression maintain attention toward negatively valenced stimuli over time. In fact, when eye movement is tracked over a period of time, participants with depression and dysphoria appear to fixate on dysphoric images more frequently (Kellough, Beevers, Ellis, & Wells, 2008) and for longer durations (Eizenman et al., 2003) than do control participants, and they have difficulty disengaging from negative stimuli when instructed to do so (Sánchez, Vazquez, Marker, LeMoult, & Joormann, 2013; Sears, Thomas, LeHuquet, & Johnson, 2010). Eye-tracking research has also produced preliminary evidence to suggest that individuals with depression and dysphoria lack an attentional bias for positive stimuli (e.g., Armstrong & Olantuji, 2012; Sears et al., 2010; Sears, Newman, Ference, & Thomas, 2011).

Studies have replicated results supporting depression-related attentional biases in samples of adults with remitted depression (Joormann & Gotlib, 2007) and girls at high risk for depression (Joormann, Talbot, & Gotlib, 2007; see also Kujawa et al., 2011). These findings suggest that, rather than being simply a symptom of depression or a scar from a previous depressive episode, attentional biases may play an important role in the vulnerability to depression, perhaps through their link with emotion dysregulation. Indeed, experimental research has found that, among individuals with depression, biased attention for dysphoric stimuli is associated with impaired ability to repair mood following a sad mood induction (Clasen, Wells, Ellis, & Beevers, 2013).

Taken together, results suggest that depression is characterized by an attentional bias for negative information but that this bias does not operate throughout all aspects of selective attention. Individuals with depression may not automatically orient attention toward negative information in the environment, but once such information has become the focus of attention, they may have greater difficulty disengaging from it.

Cognitive Control Deficits

Recent research points strongly to the existence of depression-related deficits in executive control. In particular, depression has been found to be related to impairment in the ability to inhibit irrelevant material, update working memory, and shift between stimulus sets. For example, persons with MDD have shown impairment in cognitive inhibition, as evidenced by more errors on the Prose Distraction Task (PDT) and the Hayling Sentence Completion Test and slower response times on the Trail Making Test and Stroop Task (Ardal & Hammer, 2011). Moreover, inhibitory deficits appear to persist beyond the scope of the depressive episode and for as long as 10 years after depression remission (Ardal & Hammer, 2011; Preiss et al., 2009; Wekking, Bockting, Koeter, & Schene, 2012). These findings indicate that deficits in inhibitory capacity may represent a marker of depression vulnerability, though Wekking and colleagues (2012) did not find direct relations between neuropsychological performance and recurrence of depressive episodes over a 24-month follow-up period.

There is also some evidence of impairment in the ability of persons with depression to shift between task sets. De Lissnyder and colleagues (2012) found that participants with MDD demonstrated poorer performance on an internal shift task than participants without depression. This impaired performance did not appear to be influenced by emotional valence of task stimuli but was associated with increased levels of rumination. Additionally, persons with depression who were instructed to ruminate demonstrated poorer switching ability than did persons with depression who were instructed to distract and healthy controls receiving either rumination or distraction instructions (Whitmer & Gotlib, 2012).

Finally, depression-related deficits in executive control may be more apparent in highly demanding contexts, such as within dual-task paradigms. Indeed, Doumas, Smolders, Brunfaut, Bouckaert, and Krampe (2012) found that participants with MDD performed more poorly than did a sample of age-matched controls and that depression-related deficits in working memory increased as a second task (i.e., a task of postural control) was added and as this task became more difficult (i.e., standing on a moving rather than a stable platform). Similarly, Levens and colleagues (2009) found that although persons with depression did not differ from persons without depression in a low-interference condition of a dual-task version of a recency probes task, participants with depression performed significantly more poorly than did controls in the high-interference condition of the task.

Cognitive Control of Affective Stimuli

Beyond general depression-related deficits in executive control, persons with depression may demonstrate impaired control in response to mood-congruent stimuli. For example, Murphy, Michael, and Sahakian (2012) found that the ability of persons with depression to flexibly shift their attention was unimpaired when assessed with a task using neutral stimuli but was significantly poorer than that of persons without depression when the same task included emotional stimuli. As discussed earlier, theorists have proposed that persons with or at risk for depression demonstrate particular difficulty keeping negative content from entering or remaining in their working memories (Joormann, 2010). Mood-congruent inhibitory deficits may result in prolonged processing of negative, goal-irrelevant aspects of presented information, thereby hindering recovery from negative mood and leading to the sustained negative affect that characterizes depressive episodes. Moreover, it has been suggested that deficits in cognitive inhibition lie at the heart of memory and attention biases in depression and set the stage for ruminative responses to negative events and negative mood states. In the past decade, increasing attention has been paid to the identification of such deficits, using a number of experimental paradigms, including the negative affective priming (NAP) task and other measures of interference control and working memory.

The NAP task was designed to assess inhibition in the processing of emotional information (Joormann, 2004). This task assesses response times to positive and negative material that participants are instructed to ignore. Joormann and Gotlib (2010) found that participants with depression exhibited an impaired ability to inhibit negative words; these participants responded faster when a negative target was presented after a negative distractor on the previous trial. As predicted, no group difference was found for the inhibition of positive words. Negative priming tasks assess only one aspect of inhibition, that is, the ability to control the access of relevant and irrelevant material to working memory. Although these studies suggest that depression involves difficulties in keeping irrelevant emotional information from *entering* working memory, studies have also examined whether depression is associated with difficulties in *removing* previously relevant negative material from working memory. Difficulties in inhibiting the processing of negative material that was, but is no longer, relevant might explain why people respond to negative mood states and negative life events with recurring, uncontrollable, and unintentional negative thoughts.

To test this hypothesis, Joormann and Gotlib (2008) used a modified Sternberg Task that combined a short-term recognition task with instructions to ignore a previously memorized list of words. They found that participants with MDD exhibited difficulties in removing irrelevant negative material from working memory. Specifically, compared with never-depressed controls, individuals with depression exhibited longer decision latencies to an intrusion probe (i.e., a probe from the irrelevant list) than to a new probe (i.e., a completely new word), reflecting the strength of the residual activation of the contents of working memory that were declared to be no longer relevant. Importantly, this pattern was not found for positive material. Similar findings have been reported in directed-forgetting tasks (Bjork, 1972). Using positive and negative words, Power, Dalgleish, Claudio, Tata, and Kentish (2000), reported differential directed-forgetting effects for participants with and without depression. Specifically, the participants with depression exhibited a facilitation effect for negative words after the "forget" instruction.

Interestingly, research has begun to examine neural correlates of emotion-specific inhibitory deficits and has started to examine samples at risk for future depressive episodes. Analyzing fMRI data, healthy individuals with a first-degree relative with MDD appear to demonstrate inhibitory dysfunction in response to negative, but not positive or neutral, images, as measured by increased activation of the right middle cingulate cortex and the left caudate nucleus in comparison with healthy individuals not at risk for depression (Lisiecka et al., 2012). In addition, using a cued emotional conflict task, individuals with remitted depression, compared with never-depressed controls, demonstrated slower reaction times and reduced N450 event-related potential amplitude on trials that required discarding negative images from working memory in order to respond to instructions to identify the *opposite* emotion (Vanderhasselt et al., 2012).

In summary, these findings suggest that depression is associated with difficulties in inhibiting negative irrelevant material. As inhibitory processes are the central function of working memory, their impairment might have severe cognitive and emotional consequences, including rumination and depressive affect.

Summary and Future Directions

Studies examining cognitive aspects of depression are beginning to elucidate the nature of the relations among cognition, emotion regulation, and depression. Individuals with depression have difficulties disengaging from negative material; consequently, they exhibit sustained processing and increased elaboration of negative content. Because the experience of negative mood states is associated with the activation of mood-congruent cognitions in working memory, the ability to control the contents of working memory may be critical in differentiating people who recover easily from negative affect from those who initiate a vicious cycle of increasingly negative ruminative thinking and deepening sad mood. Investigating individual differences in executive functioning and, specifically, in the inhibitory control of the contents of working memory has the potential to provide important insights concerning the maintenance of negative affect and vulnerability to experience depressive episodes.

Though recent research has looked to identify underlying mechanisms of depressive cognition, more work will be necessary to fully elucidate cognitive vulnerability to depression onset, maintenance, and recurrence. Aside from work on cognitive biases, executive functioning, and rumination, other important areas of future research include studies on developmental aspects of depressive cognition in high-risk populations and on the transmission of cognitive vulnerabilities from parents with depression to their offspring. Prospective studies, particularly in high-risk samples, seem especially critical for examining these questions more closely.

Future research should also examine the causal relations among biased processing, difficulties in emotion regulation, and depression onset and maintenance. Recent studies examining the effects of cognitive bias modification and cognitive control training seem particularly promising. Most of these studies have been conducted in anxiety disorders, but at least two recent papers have provided encouraging data that cognitive bias modification may also apply to depression (Baert, Koster, & De Raedt, 2011; Wells & Beevers, 2010). Of special importance is a recent study that showed improvement in cognitive control after a training of executive control. Specifically, cognitive control training yielded transferable gains to improved control over affective stimuli (Schweizer, Hampshire, & Dalgleish, 2011). A similar training showed effects on thought control over intrusive memories (Bomyea & Amir, 2011). Furthermore, training studies have shown that modifications in cognitive biases affect stress reactivity and recovery and emotion regulation (Schweizer, Grahn, Hampshire, Mobbs, & Dalgleish, 2013). Cognitive bias modification provides a unique method with which to examine the causal role of cognition in psychopathology; future research is needed, however, to understand the mechanisms underlying the effectiveness of bias modification and moderators of these effects. This work could have important implications for the development of new interventions that focus on cognitive aspects of depression and their relation to emotion dysregulation.

In addition, further integration of biological and psychological research will be important for improving our understanding of the links among cognitive vulnerability factors, emotion dysregulation, and depressive disorders. For example, researchers have recently begun to explore potential neural mechanisms underlying Beck's schema theory (for reviews, see Auerbach, Webb, Gardiner, & Pechtel, 2013; Disner, Beevers, Haigh, & Beck, 2011). Reviewing findings from neuroimaging studies, these authors propose an integrated cognitive-biological model composed of two key processes. First, a bottom-up process characterized by hyperactivity in the amygdala, thalamus, nucleus accumbens, hippocampus, caudate, putamen, and the anterior cingulate cortex is thought to be associated with quick, low-level processing of affective stimuli and may initiate cognitive biases. Second, attenuated cognitive control in individuals with depression may represent a dysfunctional top-down process that maintains cognitive biases and, subsequently, negative mood states. Patterns of hypoactivity in ventral, dorsal, and medial areas of the prefrontal cortex may be particularly important in understanding the neural mechanisms associated with diminished cognitive control in depression.

Investigation into the cognitive aspects of emotion and mood regulation continues to be an exciting area of research. Recent studies show not only that people with depression are prone to using particularly maladaptive emotion regulation strategies such as suppression and rumination but, furthermore, that depression is also associated with difficulties implementing effective regulation strategies such as reappraisal and mood-incongruent recall (see Joormann & Siemer, 2013, for a recent review). Many of the cognitive deficits and biases discussed in this chapter may contribute to these difficulties in emotion regulation. Koster, de Lissnyder, Derakshan, and De Raedt (2011), for example, posited that rumination underlies the relation between attentional disengagement and emotional responding. In addition, contemporary accounts of neural aspects of emotion regulation posit a top-down modulation of ventral limbic structures, such as the amygdala, by more dorsal structures, such as the dorsolateral prefrontal cortex (e.g., Ochsner & Gross, 2005). Interestingly, these regions are also activated by tasks that involve cognitive inhibition (e.g., Disner et al., 2011). Taken together, these findings have led researchers to propose that an overlapping set of prefrontal regions play an important role in the cognitive control of emotional responding. Importantly, investigators have also identified abnormalities in limbic and prefrontal cortical areas in depression that largely overlap with regions implicated in emotion regulation (see Pizzagalli & Treadway, Chapter 11, this volume). This suggests that limbic–cortical dysregulation results in sustained negative affect, rumination, and impaired reward processing—formulations that parallel behavioral findings in depression (e.g., biased processing of negative information and a lack of responsivity to positive stimuli). These findings represent first steps toward a more comprehensive model of how psychological and biological factors interact to facilitate or hinder emotion regulation, thereby affecting individuals' vulnerability to experiencing depressive episodes.

REFERENCES

Abela, J. R. Z., & Skitch, S. A. (2007). Dysfunctional attitudes, self-esteem, and hassles: Cognitive vulnerability to depression in children of affectively ill parents. *Behaviour Research and Therapy, 45,* 1127–1140.

Abramson, L. Y., Metalsky, G. I., & Alloy, L. B. (1989). Hopelessness depression: A theory-based subtype of depression. *Psychological Review, 96,* 358–372.

Alloy, L. B., Abramson, L. Y., & Francis, E. L. (1999). Do negative cognitive styles confer vulnerability to depression? *Current Directions in Psychological Science, 8,* 128–132.

Alloy, L. B., Abramson, L. Y., Walshaw, P. D., & Neeren, A. M. (2006). Cognitive vulnerability to unipolar and bipolar mood disorders. *Journal of Social and Clinical Psychology, 25,* 726–754.

Altamirano, L. J., Miyake, A., & Whitmer, A. J. (2010). When mental inflexibility facilitates executive control: Beneficial side effects of ruminative tendencies on goal maintenance. *Psychological Science, 21,* 1377–1382.

Ardal, G., & Hammar, A. (2011). Is impairment in cognitive inhibition in the acute phase of major depression irreversible?: Results from a 10-year follow-up study. *Psychology and Psychotherapy: Theory, Research, and Practice, 84,* 141–150.

Armstrong, T., & Olatunji, B. O. (2012). Eye tracking of attention in the affective disorders: A meta-analytic review and synthesis. *Clinical Psychology Review, 32,* 704–723.

Arnold, J. F., Fitzgerald, D. A., Fernández, G., Rijpkema, M., Rinck, M., Eling, P. A. T. M., et al.(2011). Rose or black-coloured glasses?: Altered neural processing of positive events during memory formation is a trait marker of depression. *Journal of Affective Disorders, 131,* 214–223.

Auerbach, R. P., Webb, C. A., Gardiner, C. K., & Pechtel, P. (2013). Behavioral and neural mechanisms underlying cognitive vulnerability models of depression. *Journal of Psychotherapy Integration, 23*(3), 222–235.

Baddeley, A. (2013). Working memory and emotion: Ruminations on a theory of depression. *Review of General Psychology, 17,* 20–27.

Baert, S., Koster, E. H. W., & De Raedt, R. (2011). Modification of information processing biases in emotional disorders: Clinically relevant developments in experimental psychopathology. *International Journal of Cognitive Therapy, 4,* 208–222.

Beck, A. T. (1976). *Cognitive therapy and the emotional disorders.* New York: International Universities Press.

Bjork, R. A. (1972). Theoretical implications of directed forgetting. In A. W. Melton & E. Martin (Eds.), *Coding processes in human memory.* Washington, DC: Winston.

Bomyea, J., & Amir, N. (2011). The effect of an executive functioning training program on working memory capacity and intrusive thoughts. *Cognitive Therapy and Research, 35,* 529–535.

Burt, D. B., Zembar, M. J., & Niederehe, G. (1995). Depression and memory impairment: A meta-analysis of the association, its pattern, and specificity. *Psychological Bulletin, 117,* 285–305.

Butler, G., & Mathews, A. (1983). Cognitive processes in anxiety. *Advances in Behaviour Research and Therapy, 5,* 51–62.

Clasen, P. C., Wells, T. T., Ellis, A. J., & Beevers, C. G. (2013). Attentional biases and the persistence of sad mood in major depressive disorder. *Journal of Abnormal Psychology, 122,* 74–85.

Cowan, N. (1999). An embedded-processes model of working memory. In A. Miyake & P. Shah (Eds.), *Models of working memory: Mechanisms of active maintenance and executive control* (pp. 62–101). New York: Cambridge University Press.

Cowden Hindash, A. H., & Amir, N. (2012). Negative interpretation bias in individuals with depressive symptoms. *Cognitive Therapy and Research, 36,* 502–511.

Dalgleish, T., Spinks, H., Yiend, J., & Kuyken, W. (2001). Autobiographical memory style in seasonal affective disorder and its relationship to future symptom remission. *Journal of Abnormal Psychology, 110,* 335–340.

Dalgleish, T., Williams, J. M. G., Golden, A. M. J., Perkins, N., Barrett, L. F., Barnard, P. J., et al. (2007). Reduced specificity of autobiographical memory and depression: The role of executive control. *Journal of Experimental Psychology: General, 136,* 23–42.

Dearing, K. F., & Gotlib, I. H. (2009). Interpretation of ambiguous information in girls at risk for depression. *Journal of Abnormal Child Psychology, 37,* 79–91.

de Lissnyder, E., Koster, E. H. W., Everaert, J., Schacht, R., Van den Abbele, D., & de Raedt, R. (2012). Internal cognitive control in clinical depression: General but no emotion-specific impairments. *Psychiatry Research, 199,* 124–130.

Disner, S. G., Beevers, C. G., Haigh, E. A. P., & Beck, A. T. (2011). Neural mechanisms of the cognitive model of depression. *Nature Reviews: Neuroscience, 12,* 465–477.

Doumas, M., Smolders, C., Brunfaut, E., Bouckaert, F., & Krampe, R. T. (2012). Dual task performance of working memory and postural control in major depressive disorder. *Neuropsychology, 26,* 110–118.

Dunbar, J. P., McKee, L., Rakow, A., Watson, K. H., Forehand, R., & Compas, B. E. (2013). Coping, negative cognitive style and depressive symptoms in children of depressed parents. *Cognitive Therapy and Research, 37,* 18–28.

Eizenman, M., Yu, L. H., Grupp, L., Eizenman, E., Ellenborgen, M., Gemar, M., et al. (2003). A naturalistic visual scanning approach to assess selective attention in major depressive disorder. *Psychiatry Research, 118,* 117–128.

Ellis, H. C., & Ashbrook, P. W. (1988). Resource allocation model of the effects of depressed mood states on memory. In K. Fiedler & J. P. Forgas (Eds.), *Affect, cognition, and social behavior* (pp. 25–43). Göttingen, Germany: Hogrefe.

Everaert, J., Koster, E. H. W., & Derakshan, N. (2012). The combined cognitive bias hypothesis in depression. *Clinical Psychology Review, 32,* 413–424.

Gemar, M. C., Segal, Z. V., Sagrati, S., & Kennedy, S. J. (2001). Mood-induced changes on the Implicit Association Test in recovered depressed patients. *Journal of Abnormal Psychology, 110,* 282–289.

Gibb, B. E., Beevers, C. G., Andover, M. S., & Holleran, K. (2006). The hopelessness theory of depression: A prospective multi-wave test of the vulnerability–stress hypothesis. *Cognitive Therapy and Research, 30,* 763–772.

Gotlib, I. H., Jonides, J., Buschkuehl, M., & Joormann, J. (2011). Memory for affectively valenced and neutral stimuli in depression: Evidence from a novel matching task. *Cognition and Emotion, 25,* 1246–1254.

Gupta, R., & Kar, B. R. (2012). Attention and memory biases as stable abnormalities among currently depressed and currently remitted individuals with unipolar depression. *Frontiers in Psychiatry, 3,* 1–7.

Haaga, D. A., Dyck, M. J., & Ernst, D. (1991). Empirical status of cognitive theory of depression. *Psychological Bulletin, 110,* 215–236.

Halvorsen, M., Wang, C. E., Eisemann, M., & Waterloo, K. (2010). Dysfunctional attitudes and early maladaptive schemas as predictors of depression: A 9-year follow-up study. *Cognitive Therapy and Research, 34,* 368–379.

Hertel, P. T. (1998). The relationship between rumination and impaired memory in dysphoric moods. *Journal of Abnormal Psychology, 107,* 166–172.

Hertel, P. T. (2004). Memory for emotional and nonemotional events in depression: A question of habit? In D. Reisberg & P. Hertel (Eds.), *Memory and emotion* (pp. 186–216). New York: Oxford University Press.

Ingram, R. E., Miranda, J. & Segal, Z. V. (1998). *Cognitive vulnerability to depression.* New York: Guilford Press.

Joormann, J. (2004). Attentional bias in dysphoria: The role of inhibitory processes. *Cognition and Emotion, 18,* 125–147.

Joormann, J. (2010). Cognitive inhibition and emotion regulation in depression. *Current Directions in Psychological Science, 19,* 161–166.

Joormann, J., & Gotlib, I. H. (2007). Selective attention to emotional faces following recovery from depression. *Journal of Abnormal Psychology, 116,* 80–85.

Joormann, J., & Gotlib, I. H. (2008). Updating the contents of working memory in depression: Interference from irrelevant negative material. *Journal of Abnormal Psychology, 117,*182–192. Joormann, J., & Gotlib, I. H. (2010). Emotion regulation in depression: Relation to cognitive inhibition. *Cognition and Emotion, 24,* 281–298.

Joormann, J., & Siemer, M. (2013). Emotion regulation in mood disorders. In J. J. Gross (Ed.), *Handbook of emotion regulation* (pp. 413–427). New York: Guilford Press.

Joormann, J., Talbot, L., & Gotlib, I. H. (2007). Biased processing of emotional information in girls at risk for depression. *Journal of Abnormal Psychology, 116,* 135–143.

Just, N., Abramson, L. Y., & Alloy, L. B. (2001). Remitted depression studies as tests of the cognitive vulnerability hypotheses of depression onset: A critique and conceptual analysis. *Clinical Psychology Review, 21,* 63–83.

Kellough, J. L., Beevers, C. G., Ellis, A. J., & Wells, T. T. (2008). Time course of selective attention in clinically depressed young adults: An eye tracking study. *Behaviour Research and Therapy, 46,* 1238–1243.

Koster, E. W., De Lissnyder, E., Derakshan, N., & De Raedt, R. (2011). Understanding depressive rumination from a cognitive science perspective: The impaired disengagement hypothesis. *Clinical Psychology Review, 31,* 138–145.

Kujawa, A. J., Torpey, D., Kim, J., Hajcak, G., Rose, S., Gotlib, I. H., et al. (2011). Attentional biases for emotional faces in young children of mothers with chronic or recurrent depression. *Journal of Abnormal Child Psychology, 39,* 125–135.

Lawson, C., & MacLeod, C. (1999). Depression and the interpretation of ambiguity. *Behaviour Research and Therapy, 37,* 463–474.

Leahy, R. L., Tirch, D. D., & Melwani, P. S. (2012). Processes underlying depression: Risk aversion, emotional schemas, and psychological flexibility. *International Journal of Cognitive Therapy, 5,* 362–379.

Levens, S. M., Muhtadie, L., & Gotlib, I. H. (2009). Rumination and impaired resource allocation in depression. *Journal of Abnormal Psychology, 118,* 757–766.

Lewinsohn, P. M., Joiner, T. E. Jr., & Rohde, P. (2001). Evaluation of cognitive diathesis–stress models in predicting major depressive disorder in adolescents. *Journal of Abnormal Psychology, 110,* 203–215.

Lisiecka, D. M., Carballedo, A., Fagan, A. J., Connolly, G., Meaney, J., & Frodl, T. (2012). Altered inhibition of negative emotions in subjects at family risk of major depressive disorder. *Journal of Psychiatric Research, 46,* 181–188.

Lyubomirsky, S., Caldwell, N. D., & Nolen Hoeksema, S. (1998). Effects of ruminative and distracting responses to depressed mood on retrieval of autobiographical memories. *Journal of Personality and Social Psychology, 75,* 166–177.

Lyubomirsky, S., & Nolen-Hoeksema, S. (1995). Effects of self-focused rumination on negative thinking and interpersonal problem solving. *Journal of Personality and Social Psychology, 69,* 176–190.

Mackinger, H. F., Pachinger, M. M., Leibetseder, M. M., & Fartacek, R. R. (2000). Autobiographical memories in women remitted from major depression. *Journal of Abnormal Psychology, 109,* 331–334.

Mathews, A., & MacLeod, C. (2005). Cognitive vulnerability to emotional disorders. *Annual Review of Clinical Psychology, 1,* 167–195

Matt, G. E., Vázquez, C., & Campbell, W. K., (1992). Mood-congruent recall of affectively toned stimuli: A meta-analytic review. *Clinical Psychology Review, 12,* 227–255.

Miyake, A., & Friedman, N. P. (2012). The nature and organization of individual differences in executive functions: Four general conclusions. *Current Directions in Psychological Science, 21,* 8–14.

Mogg, K., Bradley, B. P., Williams, R., & Mathews, A. (1993). Subliminal processing of emotional information in anxiety and depression. *Journal of Abnormal Psychology, 102,* 304–311.

Moser, J. S., Huppert, J. D., Foa, E. B., & Simons, R. F. (2012). Interpretation of ambiguous social scenarios in social phobia and depression: Evidence from event-related brain potentials. *Biological Psychology, 89,* 387–397.

Murphy, F. C., Michael, A., & Sahakian, B. J. (2012). Emotion modulates cognitive flexibility in patients with major depression. *Psychological Medicine, 42,* 1373–1382.

Ochsner, K. N., & Gross, J. J. (2005). Putting the "I" and the "Me" in emotion regulation: Reply to Northoff. *Trends in Cognitive Sciences, 9,* 409–410.

Nolen-Hoeksema, S. (1991). Responses to depression and their effects on the duration of depressive episodes. *Journal of Abnormal Psychology, 100,* 569–582.

Nolen Hoeksema, S. (2000). The role of rumination in depressive disorders and mixed anxiety/depressive symptoms. *Journal of Abnormal Psychology, 109,* 504–511.

Nolen-Hoeksema, S., & Morrow, J. (1991). A prospective study of depression and posttraumatic stress symptoms after a natural disaster: The 1989 Loma Prieta earthquake. *Journal of Personality and Social Psychology, 61,* 115–121.

Nolen-Hoeksema, S., Wisco, B. E., & Lyubomirsky, S. (2008). Rethinking rumination. *Perspectives on Psychological Science, 3,* 400–424.

Peeters, F., Wessel, I., Merckelbach, H., & Boon Vermeeren, M. (2002). Autobiographical memory specificity and the course of major depressive disorder. *Comprehensive Psychiatry, 43,* 344–350.

Peterson, C., Semmel, A., von Baeyer, C., Abramson, L. Y., Metalsky, G. I., & Seligman, M. E. P. (1982). The Attributional Style Questionnaire. *Cognitive Therapy and Research, 6,* 287–299.

Power, M. J., Dalgleish, T., Claudio, V., Tata, P., & Kentish, J. (2000). The directed forgetting task: Application to emotionally valent material. *Journal of Affective Disorders, 57,* 147–157

Preiss, M., Kucerova, H., Lukavsky, J., Stepankova, H., Sos, P., & Kawaciukova, R. (2009). Cognitive deficits in the euthymic phase of unipolar depression. *Psychiatry Research, 169,* 235–239.

Raes, F., Hermans, D., Williams, J. M. G., Demyttenaere, K., Sabbe, B., Pieters, G., et al. (2005). Reduced specificity of autobiographical memory: A mediator between rumination and ineffective social problem-solving in major depression? *Journal of Affective Disorders, 87,* 331–335.

Rawal, A., & Rice, F. (2012). A longitudinal study of processes predicting the specificity of autobiographical memory in the adolescent offspring of depressed parents. *Memory, 20,* 518–526.

Rude, S. S., Wenzlaff, R. M., Gibbs, B., Vane, J., & Whitney, T. (2002). Negative processing biases predict subsequent depressive symptoms. *Cognition and Emotion, 16*, 423–440.

Sánchez, A., Vazquez, C., Marker, C., LeMoult, J., & Joormann, J. (2013). Attentional disengagement predicts stress recovery in depression: An eye-tracking study. *Journal of Abnormal Psychology, 122*(2), 303–313.

Scher, C. D., Ingram, R. E., & Segal, Z. V. (2005). Cognitive reactivity and vulnerability: Empirical evaluation of construct activation and cognitive diatheses in unipolar depression. *Clinical Psychology Review, 25*, 487–510.

Schweizer, S., Grahn, J., Hampshire, A., Mobbs, D., & Dalgleish, T. (2013). Training the emotional brain: Improving affective control through emotional working memory training. *Journal of Neuroscience, 33*, 5301–5311.

Schweizer, S., Hampshire, A., & Dalgleish, T. (2011). Extending brain-training to the affective domain: Increasing cognitive and affective executive control through emotional working memory training. *PLoS ONE, 6*(9), e24372.

Sears, C. R., Bisson, M. A. S., & Nielsen, K. E. (2011). Dysphoria and the immediate interpretation of ambiguity: Evidence for a negative interpretation bias in error rates but not response latencies. *Cognitive Therapy and Research, 35*, 469–476.

Sears, C. R., Newman, K. R., Ference, J. D., & Thomas, C. L. (2011) Attention to emotional images in previously depressed individuals: An eye-tracking study. *Cognitive Therapy and Research, 35*, 517–528.

Sears, C. R., Thomas, C. L., LeHuquet, J. M., & Johnson, J. C. S. (2010). Attentional biases in dysphoria: An eye-tracking study of the allocation and disengagement of attention. *Cognition and Emotion, 24*, 1349–1368.

Seeds, P. M., & Dozois, D. J. A. (2010). Prospective evaluation of a cognitive vulnerability stress model for depression: The interaction of schema self-structures and negative life events. *Journal of Clinical Psychology, 66*, 1307–1323.

Segrave, R. A., Thomson, R. H., Cooper, N. R., Croft, R. J., Sheppard, D. M. & Fitzgerald, P. B. (2012). Emotive interference during cognitive processing in major depression: An investigation of lower alpha 1 activity. *Journal of Affective Disorders, 141*, 185–193.

Seligman, M. E. P. (1975). *Helplessness: On depression, development, and death.* New York: Freeman/Times Books/Holt.

Siegle, G. J., Ingram, R. E., & Matt, G. E. (2002). Affective interference: An explanation for negative attention biases in dysphoria? *Cognitive Therapy and Research, 26*, 73–87.

van Minnen, A., Wessel, I., Verhaak, C., & Smeenk, J. (2005). The relationship between autobiographical memory specificity and depressed mood following a stressful life event: A prospective study. *British Journal of Clinical Psychology, 44*, 405–415.

Vanderhasselt, M., De Raedt, R., Dillon, D. G., Dutra, S. J., Brooks, N., & Pizzagalli, D. A. (2012). Decreased cognitive control in response to negative information in patients with remitted depression: An event-related potential study. *Journal of Psychiatry and Neuroscience, 37*, 250–258.

Wang, C. E. A., Halvorsen, M., Eisemann, M., & Waterloo, K. (2010). Stability of dysfunctional attitudes and early maladaptive schemas: A 9-year follow-up study of clinically depressed subjects. *Journal of Behavior Therapy and Experimental Psychiatry, 41*, 389–396.

Watkins, E., Baeyens, C. B., & Read, R. (2009). Concreteness training reduces dysphoria: Proof-of-principle for repeated cognitive bias modification in depression. *Journal of Abnormal Psychology, 118*, 55–64.

Watkins, E., & Teasdale, J. D. (2004). Adaptive and maladaptive self-focus in depression. *Journal of Affective Disorders, 82*, 1–8.

Weissman, A. N., & Beck, A. T. (1978, November). *Development and validation of the Dysfunctional Attitude Scale: A preliminary investigation.* Paper presented at the annual meeting of the Association for Advanced Behavior Therapy, Chicago.

Wekking, E. M., Bockting, C. L. H., Koeter, M. W. J., & Schene, A. H. (2012). Cognitive functioning in euthymic recurrently depressed patients: Relationship with future relapses and prior course of disease. *Journal of Affective Disorders, 141,* 300–307.

Wells, T. T., & Beevers, C. G. (2010). Biased attention and dysphoria: Manipulating selective attention reduces subsequent depressive symptoms. *Cognition and Emotion, 24,* 719–728.

Werner-Seidler, A., & Moulds, M. L. (2012). Characteristics of self-defining memory in depression vulnerability. *Memory, 20,* 935–948.

Whalley, M. G., Rugg, M. D., & Brewin, C. R. (2012). Autobiographical memory in depression: An fMRI study. *Psychiatry Research: Neuroscience, 201,* 98–106.

Whitmer, A. J., & Gotlib, I. H. (2012). Switching and backward inhibition in major depressive disorder: The role of rumination. *Journal of Abnormal Psychology, 121,* 570–578.

Williams, J. M. G., Barnhofer, T., Crane, C., Herman, D., Raes, F., Watkins, E., et al. (2007). Autobiographical memory specificity and emotional disorder. *Psychological Bulletin, 133*(1), 122–148.

Young, J. E. (1999). *Cognitive therapy for personality disorders: A schema-focused approach* (3rd ed.). Sarasota, FL: Professional Resource Press/Professional Resource Exchange.

CHAPTER 15

Depression and Interpersonal Processes

Constance L. Hammen *and* Josephine Shih

F or most people depression is a disorder of dysfunctional responses to stressors and stressful circumstances, perhaps most commonly about the loss of, frustrated access to, or failure to attain something that the individual believes is essential to his or her sense of worth and competence. Often, it is the loss of an important interpersonal relationship.

Both the depressive symptoms themselves and the vulnerabilities to respond to stress with depression may contribute to dysfunctional interactions with the social world. The internal etiological processes of neurobiological, genetic, emotional, cognitive, and personality vulnerabilities intersect with the interpersonal and environmental context in which persons function in their daily roles as mates, family members, parents, workers, and friends. The relations of the person with depression or who is vulnerable to depression with others are affected in ways that may create further social stressors and provoke depressive responses. Indeed, several of the defining features of the course of depression are related to aspects of the *interpersonal context of depression*: It is far more prevalent in women than men; it can be a self-perpetuating disorder for many individuals with resulting chronic and recurring episodes; it can be self-propagating from one generation to another in the context of dysfunctional patterns of family processes, vulnerabilities, stressors, and depression. Dynamic, transactional processes affecting close relationships are woven through all elements of our understanding of depression. This chapter explores research on the interpersonal elements of depression—the interpersonal consequences of depression, interpersonal risk and vulnerability factors, and possible origins of such vulnerabilities.

INTERPERSONAL CORRELATES AND CONSEQUENCES OF DEPRESSION

At the most basic level of the effects of depression, the *symptoms* of depression may contribute to difficulties in close relationships. Irritability, loss of energy and enjoyment, sensitivity to criticism, or pessimistic or even suicidal thoughts may initially elicit concern from others but eventually may seem burdensome, unreasonable, or even willfully per-petuated by failure to take the steps others think would resolve them. Coyne (1976a) observed that interactions with people with depression are aversive to others and, in turn, often frustrating for the sufferer, who feels misunderstood and rejected. Many early experimental studies demonstrated negative attitudes and rejection in response to expres-sions of depression (reviewed in Hammen & Watkins, 2008) and robust evidence of "contagion"—depression that induces depressive symptoms in others (Joiner & Katz, 1999). Not surprisingly, social interactional and communication skills may be impaired when the person is in a depressive state (Segrin & Abramson, 1994). However, there also appear to be relatively stable traits and behaviors, such as rejection sensitivity, depen-dency, and reassurance seeking, that are not confined to depressive states and that may contribute to vicious cycles of interpersonal stress and depression. Several such character-istics are reviewed in a subsequent section.

In this section, the focus is on the interactions of people with depression in personal relationships, illustrating the reality that depression takes a toll on others as well as on the sufferer. Because of variations and limitations in designs and methodologies, research on social interactions associated with depression cannot easily be classified according to whether the depression is the cause of the impaired social pattern or whether both are due to a third (vulnerability/risk) variable or are simply a correlate; indeed, find-ings commonly implicate reciprocal effects between depression and social dysfunction. In particular, considerable research has identified marital, parental, and social difficulties associated with depression.

Marital Functioning and Depression

Depression has a negative impact on marriage and romantic relationships. At the very least, depression in one spouse (associated with lack of interest in social activities; sui-cidal, helpless, and hopeless thoughts; low energy) is a significant burden for the other spouse, often creating substantial psychological distress in the "well" spouse (Coyne et al., 1987). As Coyne (1976b) noted in his classic formulations about the negative impact of depression on others, there may be a deteriorating marital process in which initial con-cern and caring on the part of the well spouse for the spouse with depression eventually is replaced by resentment and impatience—reactions likely perceived by the person with depression as rejection and lack of sympathy, provoking further depression. The bidi-rectional association between depression and marital instability/discord has been exten-sively noted (e.g., Whisman, 2007). Breslau and colleagues (2011) reported that depres-sion has the largest population-attributable risk for divorce of all disorders and is also associated with one of the lowest likelihoods of marriage, based on a multinational study of mental disorders, marriage, and divorce. Current depression has also been shown to be associated with significantly higher rates of marital dissatisfaction with partners com-pared with groups of people without illness and with other psychiatric diagnoses in an epidemiological sample (Zlotnick, Kohn, Keitner, & Della Grotta, 2000). Marital dissat-isfaction is not only apparent when the person is currently depressed but is also evident in adults who formerly had depression but did not currently compared with women who had never had depression, according to both wives' and their husbands' reports (Ham-men & Brennan, 2002).

Depressive disorders and symptoms in youth also have been shown in longitudinal studies to predict romantic relationship difficulties (Vujeva & Furman, 2011), including romantic partners' reports of relationship dissatisfaction and poor conflict resolution

(Rao, Hammen, & Daley, 1999). Gotlib, Lewinsohn, and Seeley (1998) found that depression in adolescence predicted higher rates of marital distress in early adulthood. Research also documents the adverse effects of marital conflict on children's adjustment; for example, the link between parent and child depression may be mediated in part by marital discord (e.g., Cummings, Keller, & Davies, 2005). Marital and family functioning impairments of depressed adults and youth are extensively described in Chapter 22 by Davila, Stroud, and Starr in this volume.

Parenting and Depression

Parental depression is one of the strongest predictors of depression and other disorders in children, and dysfunctions in parenting behaviors are prominent among the many mechanisms accounting for intergenerational transmission of depression (see Gotlib & Colich, Chapter 13, this volume, on children of parents with depression). Observational studies of parenting behaviors of mothers with current depression (e.g., those reviewed in Lovejoy, Graczyk, O'Hare, & Neuman, 2000) suggest patterns of relatively more negative/hostile/critical and withdrawn or disengaged parenting, as well as less positive behaviors. Similar findings have been reported in the less extensive literature on parenting behaviors in fathers with depression (Wilson & Durbin, 2010). Chapters in this volume on early adversity and depression (Goodman & Lusby, Chapter 12) and on children of parents with depression (Gotlib & Colich, Chapter 13) specifically detail evidence of harsh, intrusive, or unresponsive parenting behaviors of women with depression who have infants and children and the effects of such maladaptive responses on the children. Retrospective reports by adults with depression (Alloy, Abramson, Smith, Gibb, & Neeren, 2006; Parker & Gladstone, 1996), as well as studies of parents of children with depression (McLeod, Weisz, & Wood, 2007), similarly indicate maladaptive parent–child interactions characterized by hostility, detachment, low warmth, and overcontrol. For instance, McLeod and colleagues (2007) found that the strongest link between parent behavior and child functioning was between parental hostility toward the child and the child's depression.

Social and Peer Behavior

The social behaviors and quality of social relationships of individuals with depression are typically impaired (e.g., Brown & Harris, 1978; Weissman & Paykel, 1974). In the classic Medical Outcomes Study, Wells and colleagues (1989) found that social functioning (defined as the extent to which the condition interferes with social activities such as visiting friends or relatives in the preceding month) was significantly worse among adults with depressive disorders or symptoms compared with those who had any of eight chronic medical problems.

The availability of interpersonal relationships that serve as coping resources has been posited to be an important determinant of the likelihood that stressors will lead to depressive reactions. To the extent that individuals with depression and who are vulnerable to depression either perceive that their relationships are unsupportive and/or actually have fewer social and family connections with supportive others, they are likely to experience depression. However, rather than functioning as a buffering factor in which availability reduces the likelihood of depressive outcomes following stress, much of the research demonstrates that low availability of supportive relationships is actually a main-effect predictor of depressive episodes (Burton, Stice, & Seeley, 2004; Kendler, Myers, &

Prescott, 2005); indeed, the buffering effect was disconfirmed in both of these large-scale prospective studies. Wildes, Harkness, and Simons (2002) found that a lower number of social relations predicted increases in women's depressive symptoms over a 1-year period. Eberhart and Hammen (2006) also found that more dysfunctional peer relationships predicted increases in high school women's depressive symptoms over time. Moreover, depression may serve to erode support, as shown in a study of adolescent women, at least while the youth were depressed (Stice, Ragan, & Randall, 2004). Much of the research on social support has focused on female samples, but it is interesting to note that Kendler and colleagues (2005) found in a study of male and female adults that women reported higher levels of support than did men and that depression was more strongly related to perceived support in women than it was in men.

With regard to social functioning, adolescents with depression exhibited significantly poorer functioning in peer, best friend, and romantic relationship roles than did youth without depression (Hammen & Brennan, 2001). Poorer social functioning appears to be a risk factor that predicts depression. It is likely that depression itself may color individuals' perceptions of the quality of their social relations, especially when studies employ subjective measures of perceived support. For example, Stice, Rohde, Gau, and Ochner (2011) found that successful treatment of depression in adolescents (e.g., cognitive-behavioral therapy) resulted in greater increases in perceived support from friends. However, there is also evidence of stable impairments in friendship relations, as well as marital and parenting quality, with women who formerly but not currently had depression displaying more negative interactions than women who had never had depression (but less than women who currently had depression; Hammen & Brennan, 2002).

The importance of peer relations in the lives of children and adolescents highlights the salience of the social antecedents of depression. Furthermore, the effects of depression on social functioning in youth likely interfere with the development of socially skillful behaviors and attitudes with long-term implications. For example, Agoston and Rudolph (2013) tested a model in which depressive symptoms predicted social helplessness, which in turn predicted neglect and even rejection of children in middle school and young adolescence by their peers. Deficits in peer relationships in youth may specifically reflect excessive reassurance seeking, social withdrawal, and ineffective social problem solving that predict depression (e.g., Agoston & Rudolph, 2011). For a fuller account of interpersonal processes in depression in children and adolescents, see Rudolph and Flynn, Chapter 21, this volume.

Stress Generation and Depression

As evidenced by the maladaptive interactional behaviors in relationships and families, it is not surprising that individuals with depression contribute to stressful circumstances that may exceed their coping capabilities and lead to further depression. Marital discord and problematic relationships with children, for example, include both ongoing frustration and tension but likely also the acute stressors of arguments, conflicts, and breaches of the relationships, as well as stormy and difficult relationships outside of the immediate family. Considerable evidence has accumulated to support the idea that adults with depression histories, but also adolescents and children, contribute to the occurrence of stressful life events and circumstances (e.g., "stress generation"; Hammen, 1991; reviewed in Hammen, 2006; Liu & Alloy, 2010). The occurrence of stressful life events that are dependent on individuals' characteristics, actions, and circumstances, even when they are not currently in a depressive episode, suggests that in addition to depressive symptoms and behaviors that might contribute to stress generation, additional stable vulnerability factors also contribute (and are discussed in later sections). To a great extent, although not exclusively, stress generation in depression involves events with interpersonal content (e.g., Hammen, 1991), often involving conflict with spouses/partners, children, and family members, as well as coworkers and friends. Some studies have observed that stress generation patterns are more pronounced in depressed female than male samples (e.g., Shih, Eberhart, Hammen, & Brennan, 2006). Although patterns of stress generation do not occur exclusively in those with depression histories, given that most forms of psychological disorder have deleterious effects on social functioning, major depression may have a particularly prominent association with stress generation. Conway, Hammen, and Brennan (2012) found that a broadband internalizing factor aggregated across all diagnoses predicted an association with interpersonal events caused in part by the person (such as conflict with another person), whereas an externalizing factor (disruptive and substance abuse disorders) was associated with noninterpersonal events caused by the person (such as getting fired from a job for poor performance). Furthermore, when variance due to the broad internalizing factor and to individual diagnoses was partialed out, major depressive episode was the only diagnosis associated with an incremental prediction of interpersonal dependent events.

A key implication of stress generation is the likelihood of promoting chronic and recurring depression. Hammen (2009) elaborated on an additional, broader perspective on stress generation—the creation of stressful life contexts that by definition are enduring and likely stressful on a daily basis, promoting continuing risk of dysphoria and depression. Analyses of a large community sample of adolescents at risk for depression illustrate the concept. In one study, Keenan-Miller, Hammen, and Brennan (2007) found that being a victim of severe intimate partner violence (requiring legal and/or medical intervention) by age 20 was predicted by having had depression by age 15 and by being female. Furthermore, selecting into a problematic (higher conflict, less marital satisfaction as reported both by the youth and the partner) but committed romantic relationship by age 20 was shown to be an outcome of having a mother with depression, mediated by poor quality parent–child relations at age 15 (Katz, Hammen, & Brennan, 2013). In an additional project, Hammen, Brennan, and LeBrocque (2011) found that early (teenage) childbirth occurred more often in young women with histories of depression diagnoses than among women who had never had depression and was accompanied typically by lack of both educational attainment and financial independence. Young women also had high rates of current depression in the role of mother and of parenting impairment as rated by both the young woman and her mother. In these illustrations of the generation of chronic stress—likely also punctuated by related acute stressors—the young woman chose a partner or elected childbirth associated with conditions that portend enduring stress and challenge and likely future depression. "Selection" does not imply a conscious, deliberate, or single choice, but rather is probably a product of complex personal characteristics and environmental circumstances, and it involves actions that may affect the individual's life—and those of others—for lengthy periods with ongoing stress and thus continuing potential for depression. Such choices of life trajectories would be especially likely in adolescence and during the transition to adulthood as decisions affecting adult roles become normative.

Consistent with stress generation associated with selecting into difficult, possibly entrapping circumstances, assortative mating studies have shown that people with depression tend to marry other people with psychological problems, thus increasing the chances of marital disharmony (Mathews & Reus, 2001). Research on nonpatient samples similarly shows spouse similarity for depressive disorders (e.g., Galbaud du Fort, Bland, Newman, & Boothroyd, 1998; Hammen & Brennan, 2002) and wives' major depression associated with husbands' antisocial personality disorder (Galbaud du Fort et al., 1998). Although the possible reasons for nonrandom mating are beyond the scope of this chapter, the implications are clear: Relationships in which both partners experience symptoms and vulnerabilities to disorder may contribute to stressful home environments, and the partners may have limited skills for resolving interpersonal disputes. For individuals with depression, such partner choices may portend further depression and stress.

INTERPERSONAL RISK AND VULNERABILITY FACTORS

Two general conditions are relevant to understanding the role of interpersonal features in depression: human sociality and gender effects. Humans are fundamentally social beings, born requiring the caring and protection of others and created to form bonds with others to ensure survival. It is assumed that humans both possess inborn biological systems that support attachment, love, protection, loyalty, and cooperation that nourish social bonds and also experience continuing socialization through learning and modeling to affirm the values and behaviors that ensure sociality. Studies of gender differences in social behaviors and emotional reactions to negative social experiences (e.g., Rudolph, 2002; Shih et al., 2006) support the view that, compared with males, females are particularly programmed through socialization and biology to value and engage in social connectedness and to experience greater emotional distress in the face of threats to their own relationships or to the well-being of those to whom they are attached (e.g., Cyranowski, Frank, Young, & Shear, 2000). Therefore, it is likely that a good portion of the higher rate of depression in women compared with men originates in women's greater investment in and nurturance of social relations, their greater exposure to stressful circumstances, and their greater emotional reactivity to interpersonal losses, threats, and perceived difficulties in their own lives or those of their more extensive family and friendship networks (see Hilt & Nolen-Hoeksema, Chapter 19, this volume, for a comprehensive discussion of gender differences in depression).

Interpersonal vulnerability factors for depression may be broadly categorized into (1) interpersonal styles and traits (e.g., interpersonal dependency) derived from personality theories and (2) interpersonal behaviors (e.g., excessive reassurance seeking)—although clearly these categories overlap. Much of the work on interpersonal vulnerability factors has examined direct main effects as predictors of depression and in some cases has conceptualized the vulnerabilities as moderators of the link between stress and depression in a diathesis–stress framework. In recent years, researchers have also examined a complementary stress generation mediation pathway in which particular interpersonal styles may generate stressful life events that in turn trigger depression. The following section briefly reviews research on interpersonal vulnerabilities as predictors of depression, as moderators of the stress–depression relation, and as predictors of stress generation.

Traits and Temperament

Are there particular temperament traits relevant to sociality that are predictive of depression? Research suggests that early childhood manifestations of traits of social withdrawal (social inhibition, reticence) predict depression in early adulthood. Caspi, Moffitt, Newman, and Silva (1996) found that inhibited traits in 3-year-olds predicted depressive (but not anxiety) disorders at 21. Katz, Conway, Hammen, Brennan, and Najman (2011) reported that social withdrawal traits at age 5 (controlling for internalizing symptoms) predicted depressive symptoms at age 20, and the effect was mediated by dysfunctional social relationships at 15. Shyness is a temperament that describes discomfort with social novelty and shares considerable conceptual overlap with constructs such as behavioral inhibition and social withdrawal (Karevold, Ystrom, Coplan, Sanson, & Mathiesen, 2012). Several studies have demonstrated that shyness, in conjunction with peer exclusion (Gazelle & Ladd, 2003) or low social support (Joiner, 1997), predicted increases in depressive symptoms.

Fundamental personality and temperament traits, such as neuroticism/negative emotionality (N/NE) and extraversion/positive emotionality (E/PE), have been shown to predict depressive disorders; high N/NE and low E/PE, especially in interaction, predict depression in children and adults (reviewed in Klein, Kotov, & Bufferd, 2011; see also Watson, Gamez, & Simms, 2005). Although not explicitly predictive of social motivations and behaviors, the traits reflect characteristics that doubtless affect level of approach motivation and energy, attitudes and expectations, emotional reactivity, and related constructs of rumination, dependency, and self-criticism (Klein et al., 2011)—all of which are likely to affect the quality of social engagement. These authors review evidence that high N/NE is associated with the generation of stressful life events and both N/NE and low E/PE with poorer quality of functioning in close relationships.

Dependency/Sociotropy

Theorists from different schools of thought have converged on conceptually similar traits of dependency (Blatt, 1990), sociotropy (Beck, 1983), and interpersonal dependency (Hirschfeld et al., 1977) as an interpersonal vulnerability for depression. Sociotropy refers to the excessive need for close interpersonal relationship with others such that individuals base their self-worth excessively on such relationships. Dependency also describes a preoccupation with interpersonal relatedness involving concerns about abandonment and wanting to be close to others. Interpersonal dependency is similarly defined as emotional reliance on important others. Both sociotropy and dependency have been hypothesized to put individuals at particularly greater risk for depression in the face of interpersonal stressors or interpersonal loss. Several studies have provided support for a diathesis–stress model in which the match between interpersonal vulnerability and interpersonal stressors predicted depressive symptoms (e.g., Priel & Shahar, 2000).

Support for dependency predicting diagnosable depression comes from a twin study using a slightly different conceptualization, defining interpersonal dependency as emotional reliance on others (Sanathara, Gardner, Prescott, & Kendler, 2003) and demonstrating that it predicted lifetime depression risk in both men and women. Research has also demonstrated that sociotropy predicted the generation of interpersonal stress in women that in turn predicted higher levels of depressive symptoms (Shih, 2006). Shih's (2006) findings suggest a double bind for highly sociotropic individuals: Not only are they more likely to experience depressive symptoms in reaction to interpersonal stressors, but they may also be contributing to the very interpersonal stressors to which they are reactive. Nevertheless, two other studies using sociotropy and dependency found that these constructs predicted *lower* interpersonal stress (Shih, Abela, & Starrs, 2009; Shih & Auerbach, 2010). These seemingly contradictory findings suggest that whereas for some individuals, investment in interpersonal relationships may lead to behaviors that foster positive relationships, for others this investment may lead to more maladaptive behaviors. Shahar (2008) noted that interpersonal dependency is a multifaceted construct with adaptive and maladaptive components of relatedness and neediness. Future research would benefit from a clearer differentiation of adaptive and maladaptive components of dependency/sociotropy.

Attachment Security

Bowlby's (1973) attachment theory has been extensively studied as a risk factor for depression. Although some have speculated that it overlaps with traits of dependency (Coyne & Whiffen, 1995), the extensive volume of research merits separate discussion. Attachment theory holds that the quality of attachment to caregivers in infancy forms the basis of attitudes (representations, working models) about the worth of the self and the expectations of the responsiveness and availability of others, guiding social development and interpersonal behaviors into adulthood. Care that is inconsistently available, unresponsive, and insensitive interferes with development of a positive sense of an autonomous self and a sense of security about managing in the world, with expectations that others are untrustworthy and unavailable or unreliable. A meta-analysis demonstrated that attachment is relatively stable across the lifespan (Fraley, 2002).

There is solid evidence that insecure attachment, measured in diverse ways, predicts depression and internalizing symptomatology in infants, children, and adults (e.g., Duggal, Carlson, Sroufe, & Egeland, 2001; Eberhart & Hammen, 2006; Groh, Roisman, van IJzendoorn, Bakermans-Kranenburg, & Fearon, 2012; Morley & Moran, 2011). Its effects operate in part through the acquired cognitive representations of the self as inadequate, with negative expectations of unstable care and low warmth from others (e.g., Morley & Moran, 2011). Attachment representations also appear to moderate the link between early adverse experiences and later depression, as discussed by Goodman and Lusby (Chapter 12, this volume).

Insecure attachment also predicts stress generation. Hankin, Kassel, and Abela (2005) demonstrated that both avoidant and anxious attachment predicted prospective increases in depressive symptoms over a 2-year period. Eberhart and Hammen (2010) studied women in romantic relationships and showed that anxious attachment style contributed to higher rates of romantic conflict stressors over a longitudinal period. This interpersonal stress generation process further predicted increases in depressive symptoms.

Classical attachment theory hypothesized that attachment resulted from the nature and quality of the caring bond between infant and caretaker, but it is important to note that recent research has supported an additional contribution by biological and genetic factors. For example, in a meta-analysis, Gervai (2009) concluded that effects of parenting are modified by genetic factors, particularly noting research on genes of monoamine transmission (see also Kendler & Baker, 2007, on genetic contributions to parenting).

Rejection Sensitivity

Another related interpersonal vulnerability is rejection sensitivity, the disposition to anxiously expect, readily perceive, and intensely react to rejection (e.g., Downey & Feldman, 1996). Studies have shown that relational stressors predict depression and that the association is strongest for those who also have high levels of rejection sensitivity (Chango, McElhaney, Allen, Schad, & Marston, 2012). Moreover, consistent with stress generation, high levels of rejection sensitivity may elicit hostility and aggression, provoking the very rejection the individual fears; higher levels of rejection sensitivity predicted the occurrence of higher rates of romantic relationship breakups for both men and women in a longitudinal field study of couples (Downey, Freitas, Michaelis, & Khouri, 1998). Romero-Canyas, Downey, Berensen, Ayduk, and Kang (2010) outline a model of rejection sensitivity as a socially learned defensive response that also includes cognitive bias toward exaggeration and misattribution of rejection cues.

Excessive Reassurance Seeking

Coyne's (1976b) original interpersonal theory proposed that individuals with depression may act in ways that elicit rejection, further maintaining their depression. Joiner, Alfano, and Metalsky (1992) proposed that excessive reassurance seeking (ERS), in which individuals seek reassurances from close others that they truly care for and love them, is one way in which individuals with depression may provoke rejecting responses. In a meta-analysis, Starr and Davila (2008) concluded that ERS is associated with concurrent depressive symptoms and interpersonal rejection. More recently, investigators have studied ERS not only as a correlate but also as a predictor of depression symptoms (e.g., Davila, 2001). Furthermore, there has been support for ERS as a predictor of interpersonal stress generation in multiple studies and samples, beyond the effects of depressive symptoms (e.g., Shih & Auerbach, 2010).

Negative Feedback Seeking

In addition to excessive reassurance seeking, depressed individuals have also been hypothesized to engage in more negative feedback seeking (NFS). Derived from Swann's (1990) self-verification theory, NFS is defined as the tendency to solicit criticism from others about oneself due to the desire to seek evidence that is consistent with one's negative self-concept. It is proposed that when individuals with depression seek negative feedback, the negative feedback in turn increases their negative affect. Borelli and Prinstein (2006) undertook the most rigorous study of NFS to date. They found a prospective association between NFS and depressive symptoms in adolescent girls, which remained significant even while controlling for effects of social anxiety and self-esteem. Of note, frequency of NFS was not higher among girls, but NFS prospectively predicted depressive symptoms only in girls.

Corumination

Nolen-Hoeksema (1991) identified the ruminative response style as a risk factor for depression, especially in women. Rose (2002) extended the research to include corumination, an interpersonal ruminative process in which individuals within a dyad engage in non-solution-focused discussions of problems focusing primarily on details of the problems and the negative feelings associated with them. Extending the research to adolescent same-sex best friendships, Rose demonstrated that although adolescents with more corumination reported higher friendship quality, they also had more depressive symptoms. Stone, Hankin, Gibb, and Abela (2010) conducted one of the most rigorous longitudinal tests of corumination as a risk factor for depression to date. Using a 2-year longitudinal design with adolescents, they demonstrated that corumination predicted first-onset major depressive episodes, shorter time to episode, and longer, more severe episodes of depression. Of note, gender did not moderate this finding, suggesting that when adolescent boys do coruminate, corumination also confers a risk of depression for them. Hankin, Stone, and Wright (2010) further explicated the roles of corumination and depressive symptoms by demonstrating in a multiwave study a transactional relationship between corumination, dependent interpersonal stress, and depressive symptoms. Corumination predicted increases in internalizing symptoms through interpersonal stress generation, while internalizing symptoms and stressors also predicted increases in corumination over time. White and Shih (2012) extended these findings by also demonstrating that corumination moderates the effect of daily stressful life events to predict within-day worsening in mood.

Despite being a relatively new construct, corumination has been shown to be an important interpersonal risk factor for depression, exerting its impact on depression directly, via stress generation, and moderating the effect of stressful life events on depressive symptoms. Most recently, it has also been implicated in a depression contagion effect in adolescent friendships. Schwartz-Mette and Rose (2009) demonstrated that it is not self-disclosure by the adolescents with depression that predicted depression contagion in the friend; rather, it was corumination in particular that mediated the depression contagion effect in dyadic friend pairs.

SOURCES OF INTERPERSONAL RISK AND VULNERABILITIES FOR DEPRESSION

Throughout this chapter, interpersonal aspects of depression have been discussed variously as consequences or correlates of or contributors to depression. In this final section, we briefly speculate about sources of interpersonal vulnerabilities to depression.

A key source of interpersonal styles and behaviors is, of course, the family context. In an earlier section, the link between parenting dysfunction in parents with depression and children's maladaptive outcomes was noted. Alloy and colleagues (2006) present an extensive review and critical analyses of the research on the more general link between harsh parenting and depression. The authors note that whereas depression research generally focuses on the combination of parental low warmth and high control, "affectionless control," the empirical evidence most strongly supports low caring (low warmth, hostility) as the parenting difficulty that is most strongly related to depressive outcomes in the offspring. These authors (see also Morley & Moran, 2011) propose that the effect of negative parenting on depression is mediated in part by cognitive vulnerability, noting evidence of low self-esteem, self-criticism, dysfunctional attitudes, and negative inferential style associated with negative parenting—all of which may lead to interpersonally relevant negative attributions and expectations of the behaviors of loved ones that in turn may potentially elicit rejecting behaviors from others.

In addition to effects of parenting as such, the quality of marital interactions in the family of origin is also a strong predictor of quality of intimate relationships experienced in adolescence and adulthood. Parents' marital discord is highly predictive of offspring relationship discord (Amato & Booth, 2001), whereas positive family engagement in adolescence predicts positive quality marital outcomes for the offspring and their partners nearly 20 years later (Ackerman et al., 2013). Ackerman and colleagues (2013) have hypothesized that intergenerational transmission of marital quality results from both observational learning and direct socialization experiences within the family. Thus youth exposed to early evidence of parental conflict may not only experience early depression (e.g., Cummings et al., 2005) but may also create their own stressful marital relationships, predicting continued stress–depression cycles. Both harsh parenting and marital dysfunction also expose children to highly stressful situations for which they fail to learn effective coping skills and that likely overwhelm the coping capabilities that they do have. Thus direct learning of dysfunctional interpersonal skills and cognitions in the context of family life are profoundly likely to create diverse vulnerabilities, including those that specifically prepare children for depressing experiences and reactions.

Neural and Genetic Contributions to Interpersonal Risks for Depression

Some of the strongest and most consistent findings of neural correlates of depression involve structures and circuits of the brain that have to do with perception and recognition of emotional faces (Cusi, Nazarov, Holshausen, MacQueen, & McKinnon, 2012). These authors suggest that the substantial disruptions in interpersonal functioning observed in individuals with depression are due to underlying deficits in social cognition, evidenced by processing biases that involve enhanced recognition and responding to negatively valenced faces, mislabeling of positively valenced faces as sad, or amplification of the amount of negative emotion seen in faces. As also detailed by Pizzagalli and Treadway (Chapter 11, this volume), such patterns are associated with heightened responsivity of the limbic system (especially the amygdala) accompanied by hypoactivation of prefrontal areas (e.g., dorsolateral prefrontal cortex) in tasks requiring attention to nonemotional aspects of the stimuli. Deficits in cognitive control of emotion during processing of emotionally salient stimuli suggest both elevated activity and altered connectivity in the circuits during depressive states. However, research suggests that with symptom remission, levels of activation appear to return to levels seen in healthy controls (Cusi et al., 2012), although associations of dysfunctional processing with course of illness (severity, number of episodes) remain to be clarified. Many other questions remain to be answered about the influence of stress-related brain changes (e.g., hippocampal volume) and genetic contributors to neural development and susceptibility to neural processes that may be trait markers of vulnerability to maladaptive social-affective processing.

Genetic contributions to depression indicate moderate heritability (and are detailed by Lau et al., Chapter 9, this volume), and apparently represent an aggregation of small effects of multiple genes. A great deal of interest has focused on genes associated with neuroticism or negative emotionality (NE) and other traits and risk indicators associated with anxiety, introversion, reward dependency, and harm avoidance. Such heritable personality-related putative risk factors and endophenotypes are likely to affect interpersonal behaviors and vulnerabilities (see Ebstein, 2006). Genetic factors have long been known to influence so-called environmental variables such as parenting and relationship dysfunction (e.g., Kendler & Baker, 2007).

Recent research has attempted to translate general heritability estimates into specific genetic predictors, with significant efforts to examine the moderating effects of environmental experiences on the influence of genetic factors. Perhaps the most widely studied candidate gene for depression is the *5-HTTLPR* polymorphism in the promoter region of the serotonin transporter gene, the short allele of which predicts depression under conditions of exposure to stress (e.g., Caspi et al., 2003). The association of this genotype with interpersonal risk stems from its effects interpreted as reflecting sensitivity to the environment, with strong gene–environment interaction (G x E) effects in the context of maltreatment and chronic family discord (e.g., reviewed in Caspi, Hariri, Holmes, Uher, & Moffitt, 2010; Karg, Burmeister, Shedden, & Sen, 2011). Obviously, depression is not limited to the triggering effects of only *interpersonal* stressors in individuals at risk due to short alleles of *5-HTTLPR*, but there is strong and consistent evidence of dysfunctional family/parenting conditions in the backgrounds of individuals with depression, suggesting heightened depression reactivity to such negative conditions in those at genetic risk.

Other candidate genes have also been examined in relation to heightened likelihood of depressive responses to social stress or prediction of the quality of social behaviors. Functions of the neuropeptide oxytocin have been shown to be associated with psychological disorders involving impairments in social behavior and social cognition (e.g., Kumsta & Heinrichs, 2013). The gene coding for the oxytocin receptor, *OXTR*, has been implicated in a range of social behaviors such as trust, parenting sensitivity, empathy, positive affect, and sensitivity to social support or support seeking during stress. In one example of G X E with *OXTR*, Bradley and colleagues (2011) observed that the relations between childhood maltreatment and emotional dysregulation and attachment style were moderated by a single nucleotide polymorphism (SNP) of *OXTR*. The fact that genetic variation in OXTR influences sensitivity to social context makes it highly relevant to depression and to the effects of parents with depression on children (e.g., Thompson, Parker, Hallmayer, Waugh, & Gotlib, 2011). Another example of a candidate gene relevant to social functioning is the μ_1 opioid receptor, *OPRM1*, which has been shown to be associated with dispositional differences in rejection sensitivity. Eisenberger, Lieberman, and Williams (2003) have shown that social pain such as exclusion and rejection are associated with neural regions also activated by physical pain, particularly the dorsal anterior cingulate cortex, and Way, Taylor, and Eisenberger (2009) showed that carriers of G alleles of *OPRM1* exhibited both higher self-reported levels of rejection sensitivity in daily life and greater neural responses to being socially excluded in controlled laboratory settings.

Brain-derived neurotropic factor is also potentially relevant to depressive sensitivity to the social environment. For example, self-reported childhood adversity had a greater impact on adult depressive symptoms among Met-allele carriers than non-Met-allele carriers (e.g., Carver, Johnson, Joormann, LeMoult, & Cuccaro, 2011). Numerous other candidate genes, such as those regulating HPA-axis mechanisms of stress responses, are also emerging as targets of study in depression (e.g., Bradley et al., 2008). The burgeoning research findings on G × E often have been inconsistent, replete with inadequately sized samples and statistical errors, and applied with measures of the social environment that vary considerably in quality. However, such studies provide a promise of steadily improving methods, helping to clarify the enormously complex associations among contextual and intraindividual predictors of depressive symptoms and syndromes.

CONCLUSIONS AND FUTURE DIRECTIONS

Depression has an enormous and generally negative impact on relationships with others, and many of the vulnerabilities that put a person at risk for developing depression may be the same ones that contribute to interpersonal difficulties. As a result, patterns of recurring stress and depression cycles are common, and depression has a strong likelihood of being propagated from parents to children and their offspring—all attributable in great measure to interpersonal difficulties associated with depression. Moreover, pervasive gender differences in depression are due in part to women's greater sensitivities and investments in close relationships and, hence, vulnerability to disruptions and threats to relationships. Despite all that is known about interpersonal aspects of depression, however, the term is far too vague to be maximally useful unless efforts are made to address the many conceptual and practical gaps in our understanding of the interpersonal side of depression.

One important gap is our understanding of fundamental processes of intimate relationships, with limited models of how relational needs, proclivities, and skills develop, change, and affect interactions—their basic elements, both biological and experiential, as well as mechanisms and processes that eventuate in successful or unsuccessful adaptations in intimate relationships. Clearly, these questions transcend traditional psychopathology research. Attachment theory is one organizing model, but seemingly additional systematic understanding is needed in order to develop and disseminate a language for describing interactions among multiple levels of analysis relevant to interpersonal processes, including but not limited to cognitive, emotional, genetic, and neurobiological factors, and how these unfold over development along different pathways shaped by experience and environmental resources. The very fundamental relational, developmental, and environmental parameters that are *not* currently well represented in the new Research Domain Criteria (RDoC) initiative (Sanislow et al., 2010) are precisely the kinds of issues that need to be fleshed out—perhaps in support of understanding of all forms of psychopathology, but certainly for depression. By necessity, an interpersonal perspective on depression promotes a transactional, dynamic approach to understanding both the effects of the social environment on the person and the individual's effect on the environment.

Relatedly, there are significant limitations of research that are induced by heterogeneous diagnostic phenotypes such as "depression" and compounded by diagnostic comorbidity. The concerns are widely acknowledged. There are certainly questions of specificity: Which interpersonal difficulties are particularly germane to depression, if any, compared with other forms of maladaptive behavior and impaired emotional reactivity? Perhaps broader transdiagnostic approaches to defining broad but fairly homogenous phenotypes will help to refine knowledge and advance the field; in addition, many have called for greater focus on intermediate phenotypes that are more narrowly but precisely defined and studied and tied more closely to causal mechanisms. In interpersonal approaches to depression, perhaps there are relational phenotypes to be defined and pursued for relevance to depressive or internalizing psychopathology, such as conflict, interpersonal patterns of disregard or disconfirmation in intimate relationships, or relational insecurity, among many possibilities. Distilling essential components and links to other important constructs in depression is crucial. For example, there are diverse vulnerability constructs studied in depression that may be similar and in need of integration and refinement, such as sociotropy, dependence, and excessive reassurance seeking. Can such complex constructs be boiled down to component parts that are shared or unique? Similarly, what are the differences and overlapping features among neuroticism, negative cognitive styles, and rumination, and what is their relation to maladaptive interpersonal behaviors that promote or perpetuate depression? How are depression-relevant intermediate phenotypes such as reward dependency or negative valence systems, for example, related to interpersonal behaviors and quality of relationships? These questions would be especially usefully studied if there were an improved and well-disseminated language of understanding, characterizing, and measuring intimate relationship behaviors.

Most of these theoretical and empirical gaps also lead to limitations in treatment and prevention strategies. One practical gap in knowledge involves the question of how we can best identify individuals with relationship risk factors for targeted prevention efforts. Although much is known about the predictive utility of risk factors (such as being female, having a parent with depression, harsh parenting, insecure attachment, experiencing prior depression, and others), little is known about the threshold of risk for making individual decisions. How much attachment insecurity or harsh parenting increases risk; what combinations of predictors can identify those likely to benefit from targeted prevention? If depression and depression vulnerability contribute to the occurrence of stressful life events, how can this dysfunctional cycle be broken? How can individuals be helped to choose, make, and maintain constructive relationships, to be effective in interpreting and responding to the needs and behaviors of intimates, to get their own needs met and also solve mutual relational problems? Even beyond helping individuals with depression or those vulnerable to depression, significant issues such as repairing abusive parenting or deflecting the formation of maladaptive romantic relationships would clearly benefit from advances in relationship science. Obviously, treatment options and therapeutic success for those already identified as having depression and seeking help would benefit from further refinements in understanding relational pathology relevant to depression and from examining how to change dysfunctional patterns of beliefs about the self and others in the social world, social behavioral interactions, and social problem solving. Just as new developments in imaging techniques and the mapping of the human genome created enormous and evolving bodies of knowledge relevant to human affective disorders, so too are significant new developments and paradigms eagerly awaited in characterizing the social environments of individuals with depression.

REFERENCES

Ackerman, R., Kashy, D., Donnellan, M. B., Neppl, T., Lorenz, F., & Conger, R. D. (2013). The interpersonal legacy of a positive family climate in adolescence. *Psychological Science, 24,* 243–250.

Agoston, A. M., & Rudolph, K. D. (2011). Transactional associations between youths' responses to peer stress and depression: The moderating roles of sex and stress exposure. *Journal of Abnormal Child Psychology, 39,* 159–171.

Agoston, A. M., & Rudolph, K. D. (2013). Pathways from depressive symptoms to low social status. *Journal of Abnormal Child Psychology, 41,* 295–308.

Alloy, L., Abramson, L., Smith, J., Gibb, B., & Neeren, A. (2006). Role of parenting and maltreatment histories in unipolar and bipolar mood disorders: Mediation by cognitive vulnerability to depression. *Clinical Child and Family Psychology Review, 9,* 23–64.

Amato, P., & Booth, A. (2001). The legacy of parents' marital discord: Consequences for children's marital quality. *Journal of Personality and Social Psychology, 81,* 627–638.

Beck, A. T. (1983). Cognitive therapy of depression: New perspectives. In P. J. Clayton & J. E. Barrett (Eds.), *Treatment of depression: Old controversies and new approaches* (pp. 265–290). New York: Raven Press.

Blatt, S. J. (1990). Interpersonal relatedness and self-definition: Two personality configurations and their implication for psychopathology and psychotherapy. In J. Singer (Ed.), *Repression: Defense mechanism and personality* (pp. 299–335). Chicago: University of Chicago Press.

Borelli, J. L., & Prinstein, M. J. (2006). Reciprocal, longitudinal associations between adolescents' negative feedback-seeking, depressive symptoms, and friendship perceptions. *Journal of Abnormal Child Psychology, 34,* 159–169.

Bowlby, J. (1973). *Attachment and loss: Vol. 2. Separation: Anxiety and anger.* New York: Basic Books.

Bradley, B., Westen, D., Mercer, K. B., Binder, E. B., Jovanovic, T., Crain, D., et al. (2011). Association between childhood maltreatment and adult emotional dysregulation in a low-income, urban, African American sample: Moderation by oxytocin receptor gene. *Developmental Psychopathology, 23,* 439–452.

Bradley, R., Binder, E. B., Epstein, M. P., Tang, Y., Nair, H. P., Liu, W., et al. (2008). Influence of child abuse on adult depression: Moderation by the corticotropin-releasing hormone receptor gene. *Archives of General Psychiatry, 65*, 190–200.

Breslau, N., Miller, E., Jin, R., Sampson, N. A., Alonso, J., Andrade, L. H., et al. (2011). A multinational study of mental disorders, marriage, and divorce. *Acta Psychiatrica Scandinavica, 124*, 474–486.

Brown, G. W., & Harris, T. O. (1978). *Social origins of depression*. New York: Free Press.

Burton, E., Stice, E., & Seeley, J. (2004). A prospective test of the stress-buffering model of depression in adolescent girls: No support once again. *Journal of Consulting and Clinical Psychology, 72*, 689–697.

Carver, C. S., Johnson, S. L., Joormann, J., LeMoult, J., & Cuccaro, M. L. (2011). Childhood adversity interacts separately with 5-HTTLPR and BDNF to predict lifetime depression diagnosis. *Journal of Affective Disorders, 132*, 89–93.

Caspi, A., Hariri, A., Holmes, A., Uher, R., & Moffitt, T. (2010). Genetic sensitivity to the environment: The case of the serotonin transporter gene and its implications for studying complex diseases and traits. *American Journal of Psychiatry, 167*, 509–527.

Caspi, A., Moffitt, T. E., Newman, D. L., & Silva, P. A. (1996). Behavioral observations at age 3 predict adult psychiatric disorders: Longitudinal evidence from a birth cohort. *Archives of General Psychiatry, 53*, 1033–1039.

Caspi, A., Sugden, K., Moffitt, T. E., Taylor, A., Craig, I. W., Harrington, H., et al. (2003). Influence of life stress on depression: Moderation by a polymorphism in the 5-HTT gene. *Science, 301*(5631), 386–389.

Chango, J., McElhaney, K., Allen, J., Schad, M., & Marston, E. (2012). Relational stressors and depressive symptoms in late adolescence: Rejection sensitivity as a vulnerability. *Journal of Abnormal Child Psychology, 40*, 369–379.

Conway, C., Hammen, C., & Brennan, P. (2012). Expanding stress generation theory: Test of a transdiagnostic model. *Journal of Abnormal Psychology, 121*, 754–766.

Coyne, J. C. (1976a). Depression and the response of others. *Journal of Abnormal Psychology, 85*, 186–193.

Coyne, J. C. (1976b). Toward an interactional description of depression. *Psychiatry: Journal for the Study of Interpersonal Processes, 39*, 28–40.

Coyne, J. C. (1999). Thinking interactionally about depression: A radical restatement. In T. Joiner & J. C. Coyne (Eds.), *The interactional nature of depression: Advances in interpersonal approaches* (pp. 365–392). Washington, DC: American Psychological Association.

Coyne, J. C., Kessler, R. C., Tal, M., Turnbull, J., Wortman, C. B., & Greden, J. F. (1987). Living with a depressed person. *Journal of Consulting and Clinical Psychology, 55*, 347–352 .

Coyne, J. C., & Whiffen, V. E. (1995). Issues in personality as diathesis for depression: The case of sociotropy-dependency and autonomy-self-criticism. *Psychological Bulletin, 188*, 358–378.

Cummings, E. M., Keller, P. S., & Davies, P. T. (2005). Towards a family process model of maternal and paternal depressive symptoms: Exploring multiple relations with child and family functioning. *Journal of Child Psychology and Psychiatry, 46*, 479–489.

Cusi, A., Nazarov, A., Holshausen, K., MacQueen, G., & McKinnon, M. (2012). Systematic review of the neural basis of social cognition in patients with mood disorders. *Journal of Psychiatry and Neuroscience, 37*, 154–169.

Cyranowski, J. M., Frank, E., Young, E., & Shear, K. (2000). Adolescent onset of the difference in lifetime rates of depression. *Archives of General Psychiatry, 57*, 21–27.

Davila, J. (2001). Refining the association between excessive reassurance seeking and depressive symptoms: The role of related interpersonal constructs. *Journal of Social and Clinical Psychology, 20*, 538–559.

Downey, G., & Feldman, S. (1996). Implications of rejection sensitivity for intimate relationships. *Journal of Personality and Social Psychology, 70*, 1327–1343.

Downey, G., Freitas, A., Michaelis, B., & Khouri, H. (1998). The self-fulfilling prophecy in close relationships: Rejection sensitivity and rejection by romantic partners. *Journal of Personality and Social Psychology, 75*, 545–560.

Duggal, S., Carlson, E. A., Sroufe, L. A., & Egeland, B. (2001). Depressive symptomatology in childhood and adolescence. *Development and Psychopathology, 13*(01), 143–164.

Eberhart, N., & Hammen, C. (2006). Interpersonal predictors of onset of depression during the transition to adulthood. *Personal Relationships, 13*, 195–206.

Eberhart, N., & Hammen, C. (2010). Interpersonal style, stress, and depression: An examination of transactional and diathesis–stress models. *Journal of Social and Clinical Psychology, 29*(1), 23–38.

Ebstein, R. P. (2006). The molecular genetic architecture of human personality: Beyond self-report questionnaires. *Molecular Psychiatry, 11*, 427–445.

Eisenberger, N., Lieberman, M., & Williams, K. (2003). Does rejection hurt? An fMRI study of social exclusion. *Science, 302*, 290–292.

Fraley, R. C. (2002). Attachment stability from infancy to adulthood: Meta-analysis and dynamic modeling of developmental mechanisms. *Personality and Social Psychology Review, 6*, 123–151.

Galbaud du Fort, G., Bland, R. C., Newman, S. C., & Boothroyd, L. J. (1998). Spouse similarity for lifetime psychiatric history in the general population. *Psychological Medicine, 28*, 789–803.

Gazelle, H., & Ladd, G. W. (2003). Anxious solitude and peer exclusion: A diathesis–stress model of internalizing trajectories in children. *Child Development, 74*, 257–278.

Gervai, J. (2009). Environmental and genetic influences on early attachment. *Child and Adolescent Psychiatry and Mental Health, 3*, 25.

Gotlib, I., Lewinsohn, P., & Seeley, J. (1998). Consequences of depression during adolescence: Marital status and marital functioning in early adulthood. *Journal of Abnormal Psychology, 107*, 686–690.

Groh, A., Roisman, G., van IJzendoorn, M., Bakermans-Kranenburg, M., & Fearon, R. (2012). The significance of insecure and disorganized attachment for children's internalizing symptoms: A meta-analytic study. *Child Development, 83*, 591–610.

Hammen, C. (1991). The generation of stress in the course of unipolar depression. *Journal of Abnormal Psychology, 100*, 555–561.

Hammen, C. (2006). Stress generation in depression: Reflections on origins, research, and future directions. *Journal of Clinical Psychology, 62*, 1065–1082.

Hammen, C. (2009). Adolescent depression: Stressful interpersonal contexts and risk for recurrence. *Current Directions in Psychological Science, 18*, 200–204.

Hammen, C., & Brennan, P. (2001). Depressed adolescents of depressed and nondepressed mothers: Tests of an interpersonal impairment hypothesis. *Journal of Consulting and Clinical Psychology, 69*, 284–294.

Hammen, C. & Brennan, P. (2002). Interpersonal dysfunction in depressed women: Impairments independent of depressive symptoms. *Journal of Affective Disorders, 72*, 145–156.

Hammen, C., Brennan, P., & Le Brocque, R. (2011). Youth depression and early childrearing: Stress generation and intergenerational transmission of depression. *Journal of Consulting and Clinical Psychology, 79*, 353–363.

Hammen, C., & Watkins, E. (2008). *Depression* (2nd ed.). London: Psychology Press/Taylor & Francis.

Hankin, B. L., Kassel, J. D., & Abela, J. R. Z. (2005). Adult attachment dimensions and specificity of emotional distress symptoms: Prospective investigations of cognitive risk and interpersonal stress generation as mediating mechanisms. *Personality and Social Psychology Bulletin, 31*, 136–151.

Hankin, B. L., Stone, L., & Wright, P. A. (2010). Corumination, interpersonal stress generation, and internalizing symptoms: Accumulating effects and transactional influences in a multiwave study of adolescents. *Development and Psychopathology, 22*, 217–235.

Hirschfeld, R. M. A., Klerman, G. L., Gough, H. R., Barrett, J., Lorchin, S. J., & Chodoff, P. (1977). A measure of interpersonal dependency. *Journal of Personality Assessment, 41*, 610–618.

Joiner, T. E. (1997). Shyness and low social support as interactive diatheses, with loneliness as mediator: Testing an interpersonal–personality view of vulnerability to depressive symptoms. *Journal of Abnormal Psychology, 106,* 386–394.

Joiner, T. E., Alfano, M. S., & Metalsky, G. I. (1992). When depression breeds contempt: Reassurance seeking, self-esteem, and rejection of depressed college students by roommates. *Journal of Abnormal Psychology, 101,* 165–173.

Joiner, T. E., & Katz, J. (1999). Contagion of depressive symptoms and mood: Meta-analytic review and explanations from cognitive, behavioral, and interpersonal viewpoints. *Clinical Psychology: Science and Practice, 6,* 149–164.

Karevold, E., Ystrom, E., Coplan, R. J., Sanson, A. V., & Mathiesen, K. S. (2012). A prospective longitudinal study of shyness from infancy to adolescence: Stability, age-related changes and prediction of socio-emotional functioning. *Journal of Abnormal Child Psychology, 40,* 1167–1177.

Karg, K., Burmeister, M., Shedden, K., & Sen, S. (2011). The serotonin transporter promoter variant (5-HTTLPR), stress, and depression meta-analysis revisited: Evidence of genetic moderation. *Archives of General Psychiatry, 68*(5), 444–454.

Katz, S., Conway, C., Hammen, C., Brennan, P., & Najman, J. (2011). Childhood social withdrawal, interpersonal impairment, and young adult depression: A mediational model. *Journal of Abnormal Child Psychology, 39*(8), 1227–1238.

Katz, S., Hammen, C., & Brennan, P. (2013). Maternal depression and the intergenerational transmission of relational impairment. *Journal of Family Psychology, 27,* 86–95.

Keenan-Miller, D., Hammen, C., & Brennan, P. (2007). Adolescent psychosocial risk factors for severe intimate partner violence in young adulthood. *Journal of Consulting and Clinical Psychology, 75,* 456–463.

Kendler, K., & Baker, J. (2007). Genetic influences on measures of the environment: A systematic review. *Psychological Medicine, 37,* 615–626.

Kendler, K., Myers, J., & Prescott, C. (2005). Sex differences in the relationship between social support and risk for major depression: A longitudinal study of opposite-sex twin pairs. *American Journal of Psychiatry, 162,* 250–256.

Klein, D. N., Kotov, R., & Bufferd, S. J. (2011). Personality and depression: Explanatory models and review of the evidence. *Annual Review of Clinical Psychology, 7,* 269–295.

Kumsta, R., & Heinrichs, M. (2013). Oxytocin, stress and social behavior: Neurogenetics of the human oxytocin system. *Current Opinion in Neurobiology, 23,* 11–16.

Lovejoy, M. C., Graczyk, P. A., O'Hare, E., & Neuman, G. (2000). Maternal depression and parenting behavior: A meta-analytic review. *Clinical Psychology Review, 20,* 561–592.

Liu, R. T., & Alloy, L. B. (2010). Stress generation in depression: A systematic review of the empirical literature and recommendations for future study. *Clinical Psychology Review, 30,* 582–593.

Mathews, C. A., & Reus, V. I. (2001). Assortative mating in the affective disorders: A systematic review and meta-analysis. *Comprehensive Psychiatry, 42,* 257–262.

McLeod, B. D., Weisz, J. R., & Wood, J. J. (2007). Examining the association between parenting and childhood depression: A meta-analysis. *Clinical Psychology Review, 27,* 986–1003.

Morley, T. E., & Moran, G. (2011). The origins of cognitive vulnerability in early childhood: Mechanisms linking early attachment to later depression. *Clinical Psychology Review, 31,* 1071–1082.

Nolen-Hoeksema, S. (1991). Responses to depression and their effect on the duration of depressive episodes. *Journal of Abnormal Psychology, 100,* 569–582.

Parker, G., & Gladstone, G. (1996). Parental characteristics as influences on adjustment in adulthood. In G. R. Pierce, B. R. Sarason, & I. G. Sarason (Eds.), *Handbook of social support and the family* (pp. 195–218). New York: Plenum Press.

Priel, B., & Shahar, G. (2000). Dependency, self-criticism, social context and distress: Comparing moderating and mediating models. *Personality and Individual Differences, 28,* 515–525.

Rao, U., Hammen, C., & Daley, S. (1999). Continuity of depression during the transition to adulthood: A 5-year longitudinal study of young women. *Journal of the American Academy of Child and Adolescent Psychiatry, 38*, 908–915.

Romero-Canyas, R., Downey, G., Berenson, K., Ayduk, O., & Kang, N. (2010). Rejection sensitivity and the rejection–hostility link in romantic relationships. *Journal of Personality, 78*, 119–148.

Rose, A. J. (2002). Co-rumination in the friendships of girls and boys. *Child Development, 73*, 1830–1843.

Rudolph, K. D. (2002). Gender differences in emotional responses to interpersonal stress during adolescence. *Journal of Adolescent Health, 30*(Supp.), 3–13.

Sanathara, V., Gardner, C. O., Prescott, C. A., & Kendler, K. S. (2003). Interpersonal dependence and major depression: Aetiological inter-relationship and gender differences. *Psychological Medicine, 33*, 927–932.

Sanislow, C., Pine, D., Quinn, K., Kozak, M., Garvey, M., Heinssen, R., et al. (2010). Developing constructs for psychopathology research: Research Domain Criteria. *Journal of Abnormal Psychology, 119*, 631–639.

Schwartz-Mette, R. A., & Rose, A. J. (2009). Conversational self-focus in adolescent friendships: Observational assessment of an interpersonal process and relations with internalizing symptoms and friendship quality. *Journal of Social and Clinical Psychology, 28*, 1263–1297.

Segrin, C., & Abramson, L. Y. (1994). Negative reactions to depressive behaviors: A communication theories analysis. *Journal of Abnormal Psychology, 103*, 655–668.

Shahar, G. (2008). What measure of interpersonal dependency predicts changes in social support? *Psychological Assessment, 90*, 61–65.

Shih, J. H. (2006). Sex differences in stress generation: An examination of sociotropy/autonomy. *Personality and Social Psychology Bulletin, 32*, 434–446.

Shih, J. H., Abela, J. R. Z., & Starrs, C. (2009). Cognitive and interpersonal predictors of stress generation in children of affectively ill parents. *Journal of Abnormal Child Psychology, 37*, 195–208.

Shih, J. H., & Auerbach, R. P. (2010). Gender differences and stress generation: An examination of interpersonal predictors. *International Journal of Cognitive Therapy, 3*, 332–344.

Shih, J. H., Eberhart, N., Hammen, C., & Brennan, P. A. (2006). Differential exposure and reactivity to interpersonal stress predict sex differences in adolescent depression. *Journal of Clinical Child and Adolescent Psychology, 35*, 103–115.

Starr, L. R., & Davila, J. (2008). Clarifying co-rumination: Associations with internalizing symptoms and romantic involvement among adolescent girls. *Journal of Adolescence, 32*, 19–37.

Stice, E., Ragan, J., & Randall, P. (2004). Prospective relations between social support and depression: Differential direction of effects for parent and peer support? *Journal of Abnormal Psychology, 113*, 155–159.

Stice, E., Rohde, P., Gau, J., & Ochner, C. (2011). Relation of depression to perceived social support: Results from a randomized adolescent depression prevention trial. *Behaviour Research and Therapy, 49*, 361–366.

Stone, L. B., Hankin, B. L., Gibb, B. E., & Abela, J. R. Z. (2010). Co-rumination predicts the onset of depressive disorders during adolescence. *Journal of Abnormal Psychology, 120*, 752–757.

Swann, W. B. (1990). To be known or to be adored: The interplay between self-enhancement and self-verification. In E. T. Higgins & R. M. Sorrentino (Eds.), *Handbook of motivation and cognition: Vol. 2. Foundations of social behavior* (2nd ed., pp. 408–448). New York: Guilford Press.

Thompson, R. J., Parker, K. J., Hallmayer, J. F., Waugh, C. E., & Gotlib, I. H. (2011). Oxytocin receptor gene polymorphism (rs2254298) interacts with familial risk for psychopathology to predict symptoms of depression and anxiety in adolescent girls. *Psychoneuroendocrinology, 36*, 144–147.

Vujeva, H., & Furman, W. (2011). Depressive symptoms and romantic relationship qualities from adolescence through emerging adulthood: A longitudinal examination of influences. *Journal of Clinical Child and Adolescent Psychology, 40*, 123–135.

Watson, D., Gamez, W., & Simms, L. (2005). Basic dimensions of temperament and their relation to anxiety and depression: A symptom-based perspective. *Journal of Research in Personality, 39,* 46–66.

Way, B. M., Taylor, S. E., & Eisenberger, N. I. (2009). Variation in the mu-opioid receptor gene (OPRM1) is associated with dispositional and neural sensitivity to social rejection. *Proceedings of the National Academy of Sciences of the USA, 106,* 15079–15084.

Weissman, M. M., & Paykel, E. S. (1974). *The depressed woman: A study of social relationships.* Chicago: University of Chicago Press.

Wells, K., Stewart, A., Hays, R., Burnam, M. A., Rogers, W., Daniels, M., et al. (1989). The functioning and well-being of depressed patients: Results from the Medical Outcomes Study. *Journal of the American Medical Association, 262,* 914–919.

Whisman, M. A. (2007). Marital distress and DSM-IV psychiatric disorders in a population-based national survey. *Journal of Abnormal Psychology, 116,* 638–643.

White, M. E., & Shih, J. H. (2012). A daily diary study of co-rumination, stressful life events, and depressed mood in late adolescents. *Journal of Clinical Child and Adolescent Psychology, 41,* 598–610.

Wildes, J., Harkness, K., & Simons, A. (2002). Life events, number of social relationships, and twelve-month naturalistic course of major depression in a community sample of women. *Depression and Anxiety, 16,* 104–113.

Wilson, S., & Durbin, E. (2010). Effects of paternal depression on fathers' parenting behaviors: A meta-analytic review. *Clinical Psychology Review, 30,* 167–180.

Zlotnick, C., Kohn, R., Keitner, G., & Della Grotta, S. A. (2000). The relationship between quality of interpersonal relationships and major depressive disorder: Findings from the National Comorbidity Survey. *Journal of Affective Disorders, 59,* 205–215.

CHAPTER 16

The Social Environment and Depression

The Roles of Life Stress

SCOTT M. MONROE, GEORGE M. SLAVICH,
and KATHOLIKI GEORGIADES

Patients, clinicians, researchers, and the general public commonly assume that depression is inexorably intertwined with the material and social worlds of the person with depression. There can be little doubt that when bad things happen, people become distressed and unhappy. When very bad things happen, some people become clinically depressed. Once a person has developed depression, his or her social and material worlds are altered, often in adverse ways that compound and perpetuate the original problem, outlast the depressive episode, and perhaps contribute to future recurrences of the disorder. A better understanding of depression, its origins and long-term course, requires enlarging the scope of inquiry to take into account the interplay of social-environmental factors and life stress with depression over the course of an episode, as well as over the lifetime of the individual.

We begin this chapter with an overview of issues involving concepts and measures of life stress. This discussion provides a platform from which we then review research that addresses how life stress relates to onset of depression and subsequently how life stress is associated with the clinical course, lifetime course, and heterogeneity of depression. We focus on key theoretical debates, unresolved issues, and empirical gaps, along with the methodological implications for research on life stress and depression. We conclude with a discussion of directions for future research.

CONCEPTUALIZATION AND MEASUREMENT OF LIFE STRESS

Psychological stress represents an intuitively attractive and socially legitimated explanation for all varieties of unwanted emotional and physical conditions. Biases toward stress explanations confound research practices, permitting seemingly plausible but incorrect results to be enthusiastically embraced and elude critical commentary. The challenge is to translate the potentially productive ideas about psychological stress into more precise concepts, definitions, and operational procedures, thereby preventing such biases and providing an appropriate empirical basis for scientific inquiry (Monroe & Slavich, 2007). We illustrate how these concerns can influence measurement practices in the next two sections.

Self-Report Scales

Research on life stress proliferated in the late 1960s and 1970s as a result of innovations in the assessment of life changes and the development of life event self-report checklists (Holmes & Rahe, 1967; Monroe & Yoder, in press). This novel approach promised the potential to measure stress in a standardized and objective manner and, in this format, to do so simply, with relatively little time, expense, or investigator effort.

Innovation and expediency, however, outweighed wisdom in the early development of these methods, and serious deficiencies in the self-report checklist approach became increasingly recognized. These deficiencies included the aforementioned potential bias of respondents to "explain away" (i.e., incorrectly attribute) their mental or medical problems to stress. However, the deficiencies also included the confounding between life events and symptoms of depression (e.g., inclusion of items such as change in sleeping and eating habits) and confounding between life events as consequences (as opposed to causes) of depression (e.g., trouble with boss, divorce, being fired from a job). With such approaches, too, it was difficult to accurately establish the objective severity of the event. Despite early recognition of these major limitations by some in the field (Brown, 1974; Paykel, 2001), as well as of the mounting evidence documenting other fundamental problems with self-report checklists (Dohrenwend, 2006), measures of this type continue to predominate in research on life stress and depression (Monroe, 2008).

Interview-Based Systems

Other investigators appreciated the promise of measuring stress by focusing on recent life events and developed methods for doing so with more scientifically sound procedures (Brown & Harris, 1978; Dohrenwend, 2006; Hammen, 1991; Paykel, 2001). Probably the most elaborate system for assessing, defining, and rating life stress is the Life Events and Difficulties Schedule (LEDS; Brown & Harris, 1978). The LEDS incorporates explicit rules and operational criteria for defining acute and chronic stressors, for distinguishing between complex constellations of such stressors, and for rating these experiences using a comprehensive manual. This system provides "contextual ratings" for each life event, wherein the individual's unique biographical circumstances are taken into account to evaluate the likely meaning of the event for that particular individual. The information from the interview can be presented in a separate meeting to independent raters who are blind to other clinical and study data and possible respondent biases. This is an important methodological procedure to prevent confounding of the severity ratings with depression status or with other known risk factors for depression (e.g., whether the person became depressed following the event or has other vulnerabilities for depression, such as a personal history of depression or family history of depression). The approach yields consensually agreed-upon objective ratings of the person's recent life events and chronic difficulties that are informed by his or her biographical circumstances and not dependent on his or her perceptions of stress or current mental health status.

Alternative investigator-based systems have been developed that are consistent with the LEDS philosophy and that incorporate many of the same procedural advantages (Dohrenwend, 2006; Hammen, 1991; Paykel, 2001). Importantly, these investigator-based approaches have been found to be superior to self-report measures with respect to their psychometric properties, ability to control potential sources of bias, and capacity to predict depression (Brown & Harris, 1989; Hammen, 2005; Mazure, 1998; Paykel, 2003; Tennant, 2002). Given the resource-intensive nature of these systems, recent efforts have also been aimed at developing automated interviewing systems for assessing life stress (Slavich & Epel, 2010). These systems are not substitutes for intensive investigator-based procedures but rather are intended to combine the sophistication of an interview-based measure of stress with the simplicity of a self-report instrument. One such instrument, the Stress and Adversity Inventory (STRAIN), inquires about 96 different types of acute and chronic stress that are assessed by the LEDS. The online "interview" takes 25–35 minutes to complete and generates more than 115 stress exposure scores and life charts that summarize respondents' exposure to stress over the lifespan (Slavich & Epel, 2010).

LIFE STRESS AND THE ONSET OF DEPRESSION

Reviews of research on life stress and depression unequivocally conclude that major life events precede the onset of many, if not most, depressive episodes. Depending on the type of sample under study (e.g., inpatient, outpatient, community cases), approximately 50–80% of individuals with depression report an acute, severe life event prior to onset (Brown & Harris, 1989; Hammen, 2005; Mazure, 1998; Paykel, 2003). A conservative estimate, based on a patient sample and restricted to events that are entirely independent of the person's actions ("fateful" severe events), is that persons with depression have a 2.5-fold greater likelihood of having experienced a severe life event prior to onset compared with controls (Mazure, 1998; Shrout et al., 1989). A more liberal estimate based on a nonclinical sample raises the risk of depression onset following a severe life event severalfold (e.g., odds ratio of 9.38 for a first lifetime onset of depression; Kendler, Thornton, & Gardner, 2000). Most intriguing, multifactorial research that simultaneously evaluates a number of risk factors indicates that recent severe life events emerge as the most powerful indicator (Kendler, Gardner, & Prescott, 2002). Substantial evidence, too, indicates that these associations reflect causal influences for the onset of depression (Kendler & Gardner, 2010; Kendler, Karkowksi, & Prescott, 1999).

The Significance of Life Event Severity

It is important to emphasize that these findings are based on research involving acute, highly aversive life events occurring within about 3 months prior to onset of depression. In a review of more than 20 studies on the topic, Mazure (1998) observed that the consistency and strength of the association between life stress and depression is not simply a generic stress effect but is specifically related to "occurrences that are defined as *undesirable, major* life events" (p. 294; original emphasis). Kessler (1997) came to a similar conclusion, stating that "There is a consistently documented association between exposure to major stressful life events and subsequent onset of episodes of major depression" (p. 193). Kessler further noted that associations between life stress and depression are "generally stronger when 'contextual' measures are used rather than simple life event checklists" (p. 193).

One class of life events that has been found to be most strongly associated with depression onset is specifically termed "severe events" (Brown & Harris, 1978, 1989). These are major life events that are rated high on long-term contextual threat (i.e., events likely to have an enduring negative impact). This class of events represents intensely negative experiences, involving events such as serious threats to or losses of core relationships or occupations, acute adverse economic or health changes, humiliation and entrapment (Brown, Harris, & Hepworth, 1995; Kendler, Hettema, Butera, Gardner, & Prescott, 2003), and targeted rejection and social exclusion (Slavich, Thornton, Torres, Monroe, & Gotlib, 2009). Several studies have found that risk for depression increases dramatically for life events with the highest ratings on long-term contextual threat (see Kendler, Kuhn, Vittum, Prescott, & Riley, 2005). As such, severe life events represent a very significant focal point for advancing theory and research (Kendler et al., 2002; Monroe & Hadjiyannakis, 2002).

Theoretical Debates, Unresolved Issues, and Empirical Gaps

The empirical picture is consistent and robust in demonstrating that many, if not most, individuals who develop an episode of major depression do so following a severe life event. What it might be about severe events in particular that potentiates the risk for depression, however, remains unclear. There are several issues for research that may help fill this gap.

Major Life Stress and Onset of Depression

Why is there a lack of interest in how this class of severe life events is particularly strongly associated with onset of a depressive episode? Although there is great interest in the cognitive and biological correlates of stress, there has been relatively little specific interest or research using severe events as a focal point for investigating cognitive or biological aspects of depression (cf. Monroe, Slavich, Torres, & Gotlib, 2007b). Perhaps researchers in the field are inclined to interpret a strong association between life stress and onset of depression as an obvious outcome; such an association makes convincing intuitive sense. Although many if not most people with depression (i.e., 50–80%) have had recent (i.e., pre-onset) severe life stress, only about 20% of individuals who are exposed to severe life events subsequently develop depression (Brown & Harris, 1978). Thus depression is not an obvious or normative outcome—it is a relatively infrequent one. Very little is known, too, about the 80% of people exposed to severe stressors who do not become depressed. Perhaps "stress" has been too readily embraced as a sufficient, self-contained explanation, without probing more deeply into the matter (Monroe, 2008).

One way to stimulate discussion would be for investigators to refine the types of severe events that are particularly virulent and often lead to depression. As indicated previously, research suggests that specific types of contextually rated adverse experiences are especially potent for precipitating a depressive episode. What might it be about this class of events that makes them so potentially depressogenic? Might there be contextual factors that are particularly influential (e.g., lack of support, past failures with similar experiences)? By deepening understanding of the psychological potency of these key markers for depression, it may help to elucidate the cognitive and biological consequences that collectively precipitate depression.

The "downstream" consequences and mediators of severe events represent other topics with potential to help understand why some people with these experiences become depressed whereas others do not. Although both psychosocial and biological approaches to depression invoke the importance of stress as a key mechanism translating environmental adversity into biological processes involved with depression, there is remarkably little research with severe events that attempts to link the two domains. What biological processes initiated by severe events might be important for initiating depression? Three promising areas of research involve regulation of the hypothalamic–pituitary–adrenal (HPA) axis, regulation of the immune system, and genetic influences.

Severe Life Events and the Biology of Depression

HPA-AXIS REGULATION

One of the most consistently replicated biological findings in psychiatry is the overactivity of the HPA axis in patients with depression (see Goodwin & Jamison, 2007; Jarcho, Slavich, Tylova-Stein, Wolkowitz, & Burke, 2013). At a general level, research on human life stress and the human neuroendocrine system appear to converge: One might expect cortisol, a major stress hormone, to be elevated in persons with depression suffering from recent major stress. Indeed, estimates of the proportion of the depressed samples reporting prior stress (50–80%) aligns nicely with the proportion of patients with HPA-axis dysregulation and excessively elevated cortisol levels (20–80%; Stetler & Miller, 2011).

However, the literature on naturally occurring severe life events and HPA-axis function in depression provides little clarity on the matter (van Praag, de Kloet, & van Os, 2004). In fact, very few studies have directly examined the association between severe life events and cortisol function in patients with depression. At least one study reported cortisol to be elevated for persons with depression and with recent major stress (Dolan, Calloway, Fonagy, De Souza, & Wakeling, 1985). In contrast, at least one study reported HPA-axis dysfunction for persons with depression *without* recent stress (Roy, Pickar, Linnoila, Doran, & Paul, 1986). Other, more recent research also has yielded discrepant findings regarding cortisol's relation to life events and depression onset (Hammen, 2005). Inconsistencies in this literature could be attributable to several factors, including differences across studies in how life stress was assessed, how HPA functioning was assessed, the types of individuals with depression who were sampled (e.g., community cases vs. inpatients), or in the timing of the index episode in the life course of the individual (e.g., first onset vs. fourth recurrence; Stetler & Miller, 2011).

Clarifying how severe life events and HPA-axis disturbances are related represents an obvious next step for research. For example, if individuals with a severe life event exhibit a more dysregulated pattern of HPA-axis functioning, is this due to continuation of the environmental stress or due to a centrally mediated "breakdown" in regulation of the HPA axis? Alternatively, if the high-stress group exhibits fewer HPA irregularities, conventional thinking on the stress–biology relations in depression would be challenged and require explanation. Because HPA-axis hyperactivity is often found to be greater among melancholic and endogenous subtypes of depression that often appear to report less stress, such an outcome is reasonable to entertain (Stetler & Miller, 2011). Given the theoretical importance of stress and cortisol, as well as the adverse effects of excessive cortisol on the brain structure and function, all possible contributing factors to HPA-axis overdrive merit exploration (Sapolsky, 2000).

IMMUNE SYSTEM FUNCTION AND INFLAMMATION

One of the most recent and potentially important insights on the biology of stress and depression concerns the recognition that components of the immune system involved in inflammation may promote depression (Slavich & Irwin, 2014). Although inflammation is typically thought of as the body's primary response to tissue damage or bacterial infection, a large body of research has now accumulated demonstrating that stress can also trigger significant increases in systemic inflammatory activity (i.e., in the absence of illness or injury; Segerstrom & Miller, 2004). Markers of inflammation that have been found to be influenced by stress include the pro-inflammatory cytokines interleukin-1, interleukin-6 (IL-6), and tumor necrosis factor-α, which are key mediators of inflammation, and C-reactive protein, a key biomarker of inflammation that is synthesized in the liver in response to IL-6. In addition, one study has also shown that recent severe life stress is associated with the activation of intracellular signaling pathways that regulate inflammation (Murphy, Slavich, Rohleder, & Miller, 2013). Levels of inflammation, in turn, have been found to be elevated in individuals with depression compared to those without depression (who are otherwise healthy; Dowlati et al., 2010). In addition, experimental studies in animal models and in humans have shown that immunological challenges that acutely upregulate inflammation (e.g., endotoxin administration) can evoke clinically significant episodes of depression (DellaGioia & Hannestad, 2010). As a result, there exists (at least in principle) a biologically plausible pathway by which life stress may evoke depression.

Given the recency of these findings, many unanswered questions remain. For example, does inflammation mediate the link between severe life stress and depression? Is inflammation relevant for all depressive symptoms or forms of depression, or only for certain symptoms or depressive subtypes? And are elevated levels of inflammation sufficient for onset of depression, or do other vulnerability factors need to be present for depression to occur? Given that inflammation has been implicated in a variety of physical disease conditions—including obesity, diabetes, arthritis, and cardiovascular disease—there also exists the possibility that inflammation may serve as a common biological mechanism linking stress with both major depression and other disorders that frequently co-occur with depression (Slavich & Irwin, 2014). However, much more research is needed to examine this hypothesis.

GENETIC FACTORS

One explanation for the fact that some people develop depression in the face of life stress whereas others do not involves specific vulnerability genes. Gene–environment research has become quite popular over the past decade, given advances in mapping of the human genome and the development of powerful molecular genetics techniques for detecting specific allelic variations in genes. In a landmark study, Caspi and colleagues (2003) reported that individuals with one or two copies of the short allele (i.e., 5-HTTLPR) of the serotonin transporter gene were especially susceptible to developing depression following stressful life events. As a result of these findings, a new generation of studies was spawned on life stress, genes, and depression.

Unfortunately, the majority of studies attempting to replicate the original study of Caspi and colleagues (2003) have used varied and often questionable procedures for assessing and defining life stress (Monroe & Reid, 2008). Recent reviews and meta-analyses arrive at opposing conclusions depending on how the quality of stress measurement is taken into consideration (Risch et al., 2009; Uher & McGuffin, 2010). At present, it appears that studies with high-quality stress measures that assess major (i.e., severe) life events often replicate the gene–environment interaction, whereas studies without such quality measures and indicators of stress do not (Karg, Burmeister, Shedden, &

Sen, 2011). Progress in gene–environment research will depend on proper specification of both the genetic and environmental components of the proposed interaction.

Although focusing on severe types of life events represents one promising approach for future research on life stress and depression, it begs the question of why some people become depressed without apparent major stress prior to onset. How are these cases to be explained? This next topic may be the singularly most pressing unresolved issue at the present time for research on life stress and depression.

Nonsevere Life Stress and Onset of Depression

Without question, not all people who become depressed do so following an acute, severe life event (Monroe & Harkness, 2011). Two lines of evidence substantiate this point: (1) major life stress does not always precede onset of a depressive episode, and (2) major life stress frequently precedes first or early lifetime episodes, and less often recurrences of depression. Specifically, it is estimated that about 20–50% of people with depression overall do not report recent severe stress and that an even greater percentage of people with recurrent episodes of depression do not report recent severe stress (Mazure, 1998; Monroe & Harkness, 2005). These data indicate that a substantial proportion of major depressive episodes cannot be accounted for by a severe life event.

In the absence of severe stress prior to onset of depression, investigators commonly have inferred that some individuals are especially sensitive to stress and, consequently, that less severe forms of stress trigger onset of depression for these highly vulnerable individuals (see Monroe & Harkness, 2005). Sensitization to stress can be conceptualized in terms of many factors, including influences of genes, early adversity, cognitive predisposition, and prior experiences of depression. For example, some people may be cognitively prone to perceive relatively benign or ambiguous life events as if the events were more severe (Abramson, Metalsky, & Alloy, 1989). A key assumption is that, for the complement of people who become depressed without severe stress prior to onset of depression, some form of stress is still believed to be of causal importance, albeit at lower degrees of severity and in conjunction with particular vulnerabilities. This is a pivotal assumption, and to our knowledge an assumption that has not been addressed directly. It is also a very challenging assumption to test scientifically, and if the research is not properly conducted, progress could be impeded by inconsistent findings for years to come.

Unlike the situation concerning severe life events that are defined objectively by interview-based methods and for which there is a theoretically credible and empirically well-established reference point, no such clear reference point exists for life events that fall beneath this severity threshold. And the domain of nonsevere stress is vast. There are no guiding principles as to how to carve out the particular life events and chronic life conditions that might be capable of triggering depression in the purportedly predisposed. Most people have many stressors in their lives of varied types and levels of severity. People move, change jobs, make friends, lose friends, get raises, lose money, have altercations at home or at work, go on vacations, are robbed, become ill, renovate homes, have babies, get traffic tickets, have accidents, have pets that come and go, and so on. Respondents also are acquainted with many other people who may have similar experiences and may even have severe events (e.g., a brother's divorce, a sister's brain tumor, a best friend's loss of work, a spouse fired from a job), all of which the respondents themselves may report upon, too. The sheer number of life events in people's lives that are likely unrelated to depression almost certainly will compromise the ability to detect any meaningful associations between nonsevere stress and depression. As a consequence, conceptualizations of stress in this nonsevere domain are generic, nonspecific, and inconsistent.

These conceptual shortcomings represent methodological obstacles for operationalizing nonsevere life stress. Without theoretical guidance, it will prove challenging to reliably unpack or meaningfully aggregate the flow of daily experiences involving nonsevere stressors, which vary in timing, degree, duration, and psychological content. The problem is compounded by the tendency of many researchers to opt for expedient methods and employ *ad hoc* measures that are neither reliable nor validated (Monroe & Reid, 2008). This situation could yield a patchwork of published findings that are loosely linked only by the most generic underlying notion of "stress." One needs only to turn to the depression literature on life stress and the serotonin transporter gene to appreciate that these concerns are not unfounded (Monroe & Reid, 2008; Uher & McGuffin, 2010).

Promising leads have recently appeared that point to the potential of productively investigating nonsevere forms of stress in relation to heightened susceptibility to depression (e.g., Espejo et al., 2006; Hammen, Henry, & Daley, 2000; Kendler et al., 2005; Monroe et al., 2006; Slavich, Monroe, & Gotlib, 2011; Stroud, Davila, Hammen, & Vrshek-Schallhorn, 2011). Although these efforts are in the early stages of development, they have already demonstrated alternatives in how stress is conceptualized, assessed, and operationalized in relation to depression. Research on nonsevere forms of stress will require hard thinking to avoid soft measurement practices and ultimately unproductive outcomes. We discuss these matters further in the section titled "Future Directions."

When Stress Is Absent and Depression Occurs

Not all people who become clinically depressed necessarily experience *any* changes in their life circumstances prior to onset. Furthermore, some of these people do not appear to have any detectable adversity—at all. In other words, people who do not have recent severe stress do not *ipso facto* have moderate or even necessarily even mild stress. Yet research practices have tended to treat them as such, as if they are hyperresponsive to stress. Depression for people without any detectable stress appears to come "out of the blue." Such cases have a venerable clinical history but a correspondingly uneven research record with regard to validating a distinctive subtype of depression (see the upcoming subsection titled "Life Stress and Subtypes of Depression"). The field may have mistakenly forced some cases of depression to fit within a stress framework. Biases toward invoking stress foster creative thinking about how moderate or relatively minor experiences "could" have major consequences for highly sensitized individuals. Inclusion of cases without any stress in research, too, would impede the ability of the study design to detect stress sensitization. Stress in its *absence* may represent as important a finding and useful focal point for enlarging understanding of depression as is the presence of severe life stress (Monroe & Reid, 2009).

It is likely, though, that after examining the preceding discussion, many readers will conjure up thoughts of how a pleasant vacation, a nice raise in pay (without added effort or responsibilities), or a child graduating from the eighth grade (and/or all three) just *might* work its inimical way into some predisposed person's psyche and set the stage for depression's onset. (Or perhaps a severe event went undetected. Or perhaps it was the stress of boredom reflected by no events whatsoever. Perhaps . . .) We hope readers will give equal and impartial thought to how unproductive such extended and unbounded efforts to resurrect stress as an explanation can be, and to how prone we are to resort to this mode of thinking.

LIFE STRESS, CLINICAL CHARACTERISTICS, AND CLINICAL COURSE OF DEPRESSION

A general challenge facing depression researchers is how to explain why individuals with depression often exhibit such varied constellations of signs and symptoms and why only some individuals have a persistent, or recurrent, long-term course. A full account of depression should be capable of explaining these core questions. These concerns are the subject of studies of: (1) symptom severity, symptom profiles, and depression subtypes; and (2) the course of depression over an episode and a lifetime.

Life Stress, Symptom Severity, Symptom Profiles, and Depression Subtypes

Life Stress, Symptom Severity, and Symptom Profiles

People with depression who experience recent severe life stress prior to onset of depression have greater levels of depressive symptoms compared to people with depression without such stress (e.g., Monroe, Harkness, Simons, & Thase, 2001; Muscatell, Slavich, Monroe, & Gotlib, 2009; Tennant, 2002). Research suggests that stress-severity associations often hold for symptoms assessed with the Beck Depression Inventory (BDI; Beck et al., 1988), but not for symptoms assessed with the Hamilton Rating Scale for Depression (HRSD; Hamilton, 1960). Due to the different loadings of cognitive (BDI) versus somatic (HRSD) symptoms on these two instruments, the findings suggest some degree of symptom specificity.

Monroe and colleagues (2001) found life stress to be associated principally with cognitive-affective symptoms. Across different assessment methods, there also was a consistent positive association between severe life events and suicidal ideation. Muscatell and colleagues (2009) examined both acute and chronic stressors in relation to BDI scores in a sample of participants with depression. They found that the acute, severe events predicted symptom severity in general and, more specifically, severity of cognitive and somatic symptoms (as well as lower levels of global functioning); importantly, chronic difficulties were not predictive of the current depressive symptomatology. Overall, research on life stress and the symptoms of depression is relatively sparse. However, existing work suggests that it may be a useful approach for clarifying the role of life stress in the expression of depression and more generally in explaining some of the heterogeneity of depressive signs and symptoms.

Life Stress and Subtypes of Depression

Historically, many early accounts of depression refer to a syndrome of "sadness without reason" (Klibansky, Panofsky, & Saxl, 1979; Monroe & Depue, 1991). Kraepelin (1921) suggested that some forms of depression "may be to an astonishing degree largely *independent of external influences*" (p. 181, italics in the original). Still others, invoking similar concepts, employ terms such as *excessive depression, unjustified depression*, and *depression disproportionate to causative factors* (Jackson, 1986, p. 316). All of these observations reflect the same central theme that some forms of depression appear to arise independent of social circumstances and life stress. As a result of these ideas, it is often assumed that an "endogenous" or "melancholic" subtype of depression exists that is fundamentally biologically driven, arising unconnected with environmental circumstances. This type of depression is typically contrasted with depressions that are presumed to result from adverse social circumstances, indicative of a separate "reactive" form of the disorder (Jackson, 1986).

Several reviews of the literature from the past 25 years have indicated that life stress is more commonly present prior to the onset of almost *any* depressive subtype based on symptomatic differences (relative to the rate for nondepressed populations; Mazure, 1998). Some of these studies also suggest that there is a weak relationship between life stress and a particular depressive subtype (Mazure, 1998; Monroe & Depue, 1991; Tennant, 2002). Although most recent attempts to validate the endogenous or melancholic subtype have not provided promising leads (Hadzi-Pavlovic & Boyce, 2012; Wakefield, 2012), these questions have typically been posed without due attention to the lifetime course of depression. There are good reasons to suspect that by taking into account the lifetime course of depression (rather than focusing on the "index" episode), greater clarity regarding life stress and depressive subtypes might be attained (e.g., Brown, Harris, & Hepworth, 1994; Monroe & Harkness, 2005). We examine this topic further in the next section.

Life Stress and Clinical Course of Depression

A number of studies have examined associations between life stress, the short-term course of a depressive episode, and the long-term course of the disorder over a lifetime. Whereas research on life stress and onset of depression has one focal point (i.e., onset), research on life stress and the clinical and life course of depression has many points of interest over time (e.g., remission, relapse, recurrence, chronicity). And whereas the timing of life stress with regard to depression onset is fixed by the nature of the question (i.e., stress precedes onset), questions about the clinical course of a depressive episode involve ongoing stress at any point in time, pre- and post-onset. In contrast to the large literature on stress and depression onset, research on these related topics in relation to life stress is sparse. Although relatively unexplored, these topics could have great clinical utility and potential theoretical value.

Recovery

Given that severe life stress often precedes onset of a depressive episode, the question arises as to whether or not such circumstances might have prognostic utility with regard to differences in timing or rates of recovery. Although some research has addressed this topic, the variability in methods and the heterogeneity of depressed populations involved complicates the picture. Methodological differences in the timing of life stress (e.g., pre-onset vs. post-onset), the type of life stress (e.g., severe life events vs. other indices of stress), the population of participants studied (e.g., first onset, recurrences, severity, age), and treatment status (e.g., natural course, psychotherapy, pharmacotherapy) contribute to the discrepant findings.

With regard to *time to recovery*, some research suggests a more rapid resolution of depression following recent pre-onset stress (e.g., Kendler, Walters, & Kessler, 1997; Parker & Blignault, 1985), whereas other research suggests a slower response time to remission (Karp et al., 1993). With respect to life stress *after* onset, major life events exacerbate symptomatology (Brown & Harris, 1978), and recovery can be delayed considerably when stressors occur during treatment (e.g., Monroe, Roberts, Kupfer, & Frank, 1996). Again, however, caution is warranted owing to the relatively few studies on the topic and the diversity of methods, definitions, designs, and patient samples employed.

Research on life stress and the overall likelihood of eventual recovery has been some-what more plentiful, but not necessarily more consistent. Some studies report that life events prior to onset of depression forecast a better clinical prognosis, yet other studies suggest a worse outcome (Mazure, 1998; Paykel, 2003; Tennant, 2002). Major events occurring during the course of the episode may interfere with recovery (Mazure, 1998). Some of the discrepancies in this literature again are likely due to difference in methods and populations studied. For example, some studies suggest that life stress prior to onset forecasts a lower likelihood of recovery for people with severe forms of depression (e.g., recurrent depression) compared with those with less severe forms (e.g., first onset; Monroe et al., 1996). Also, although the presence of chronic stressors has rarely been taken into account (Hammen, 2005), such forms of stress have been found to impair improve-ment and make timely recovery less likely (Brown & Rosellini, 2011; Tennant, 2002). Overall, many questions about pre-onset events, chronic stressors, and the clinical course of depression remain unanswered, whereas there is more consistency about the adverse effects of concurrent stressors on overall recovery.

Relapse

Once recovery is attained, the person with a history of depression is at high risk for devel-oping depression again. When this happens shortly following recovery, it is assumed that the person is slipping back into the prior episode (Monroe & Harkness, 2011). Can life stress help to explain why some individuals relapse whereas others do not during this vul-nerable period? For example, does a stress-related episode imply that, while recovering, the psychobiological system is more or less susceptible to depression reemerging? Or can stress occurring after onset of depression be a factor in falling back into depression? With regard to pre-onset stressors, the evidence is once again mixed (Mazure, 1998; Paykel, 2003, Tennant, 2002). Life stress prior to the onset of a depressive episode, though, may forecast continuing stress, particularly given that persons with depression often generate life events (even when not actively depressed; Hammen, 2005). Thus the continuation of pre-onset stressors, the occurrence of new stressors, or the presence of chronic stressors all could be factors in promoting relapse. Research to date has not taken into consid-eration these different processes over time, even though such information could be of considerable clinical and theoretical value.

Recurrence

Over the past 25 years, attention to the long-term course of depression has shifted from the periphery to the center stage of clinical and research interest. Previously viewed as an acute, time-limited condition, major depression is presently seen as a recurrent, persistent disorder over the life course. For example, in the recently released DSM-5 (American Psy-chiatric Association, 2013), it is stated, "A diagnosis based on a single episode is possible, although the disorder is a recurrent one in the majority of cases" (p. 155).

The latest research, however, suggests that the pendulum has swung too far toward viewing depression as *primarily* a recurrent condition (Monroe & Harkness, 2011). Recent longitudinal research on population-based samples indicates that approximately 50%, perhaps up to 60%, of individuals who become depressed for the first time never suffer another episode and certainly do not suffer a lifetime riven by repeated recurrences (Eaton et al., 2008; Moffitt et al., 2010). One of the most intriguing questions and major gaps in the literature pertains to the role of life stress in relation to these two dramatically different trajectories over the life course for people who develop depression for the first time.

A consistent finding from research on life stress and recurrence of depression is that major life events precede onset of initial and early lifetime episodes more commonly than later recurrences of depression (Monroe & Harkness, 2005; Monroe, Slavich, Torres, & Gotlib, 2007a; Stroud, Davila, & Moyer, 2008). Post (1992) proposed the "kindling" hypothesis to explain these observations, arguing that the relations of major stress to subsequent episodes of depression changes over time, such that progressively less severe doses of stress are required to bring about onset. Eventually, after many episodes, recurrences may appear spontaneously, independent of psychosocial origins. These intriguing ideas are derived from animal laboratory studies on electrophysiological kindling and behavioral sensitization, paradigms that demonstrate the plausibility of transitions from precipitated episodes to episodes apparently arising independent, or autonomous, of the original triggering stimulus conditions.

Awareness that depression is not always a chronic and recurrent condition and that major stress plays a different role in the initiation of first episodes versus recurrences raises intriguing questions and reveals important gaps in our understanding of these complex matters. These two issues, also, are intertwined with the previously discussed concepts and concerns regarding measurement of nonsevere life stress. We turn to these timely topics next.

THEORETICAL DEBATES, UNRESOLVED ISSUES, AND EMPIRICAL GAPS

As noted, the emphasis upon recurrence and chronicity of depression over the past decades has diverted attention from the corollary statistic indicating that not all incident cases of depression are followed by recurrences (minimum estimates, 40–50%), and, indeed, perhaps even the majority of people who become depressed for the first time never suffer a recurrence (maximum estimate, 60%). This realization points directly to a very important empirical gap: Who are these people who become depressed once, but apparently never again? How can someone who is proven to be capable of depression escape further episodes? How might these people with a single lifetime episode of depression differ from less fortunate individuals who experience an initial episode but who go on to suffer multiple recurrences (Monroe & Harkness, 2011)?

One obvious empirical gap pertains to possible initial difference between these two groups, particularly with regard to life stress. Might they differ in terms of the type or degree of stress prior to the initial onset? Might they differ in terms of ongoing stressors that are not resolved and that perpetuate problems or propagate new problems (Hammen, 2006)? Or might they differ in terms of early adversity and genetics (Brown, 2012; Brown & Harris, 2008)? It would appear that life stress, in its presence or absence, may be a key component for beginning to understand why some people may have but one lifetime episode while others have many.

Another theoretical distinction and unresolved issue complicates this quest to understand differences between those who are recurrence prone and those who are not at the time of their first lifetime onset of depression. This concerns what the "changing role" of life stress over repeated recurrences signifies. Because almost all research on this topic has been cross-sectional, two interpretations currently are tenable: (1) A person becomes more and more susceptible to stress and recurrences with repeated stress and recurrences of depression; and (2) a recurrence-prone person develops depression for the first and subsequent episodes without any major stress (and may or *may not* require nonsevere stress to develop depression again). With regard to the latter hypothesis, the role of major stress appears to change only as these recurrent-prone cases become increasingly represented in the recurrence distribution as lifetime total number of recurrences rises. In essence, this hypothesis maintains that there is a distinct recurrent subtype of depression that is detectable very early on in the life course of depression and that stress—either in its presence or absence—may be an important tool for detecting individuals with and without high propensity to recurrence (Burcusa & Iacono, 2007; Monroe & Harkness, 2011).

FUTURE DIRECTIONS, QUESTIONS, AND RECOMMENDATIONS

Life stress can play many roles in furthering understanding of the origins and course of major depression. Given the numerous possibilities, what might be the best way to prioritize the future research agenda? We suggest that new insights are most likely to be gained with a continued focus on severe life events. By using these types of experiences as a cornerstone for research, the role of stress and its importance in the context of other risk factors can be systematically probed in relation to the causes, consequences, and long-term course of major depression.

With respect to etiology, it is firmly established that major, severe life events represent one of the strongest available indicators of an impending depressive episode. The risk of depression increases dramatically at the highest levels of ratings for long-term contextual threat. There are reasonably well-established procedures available for defining and assessing these potentially uniquely informative types of stress. Although these interview-based assessment procedures are more costly in terms of labor, time, and expense, they are indispensible. It does not make scientific sense to adopt unreliable methods simply for the sake of expediency. (Otherwise, the research literature would be awash with self-report measures of genetic polymorphisms, amygdala activity, HPA-axis function, and so on!) Investigators interested in the causes of depression and its recurrences are well advised to use this empirical reference point in developing better models of the causes of depression.

For example, there are many risk factors for depression that need to be integrated with the findings on severe life events. We suspect that individual differences in, for instance, genetic predisposition, early adversity, cognitive vulnerability, personality, and social support will be of great value in explaining why some people develop depression following a severe life event and others do not. But if investigators in these related areas are interested in life stress, it is very important to evaluate their predictions in the specific context of severe life events first (before turning to less well-established stress indices such as moderate or minor stressors). The current debates about gene–environment interactions with the serotonin transporter polymorphisms might have been avoided had such a recommendation been adopted initially (Karg et al., 2011; Risch et al., 2009; Uher & McGuffin, 2010).

Adopting such integrative approaches with severe life events can help address contemporary questions about multicausality and concerns about the heterogeneity of major depression. How the different risk indicators "go with" severe events can inform investigators about the additive or multiplicative nature of the proposed models (Kendler & Eaves, 1986; Monroe & Simons, 1991). For example, are genetic or family history factors more or less influential given the presence of a severe life event (Monroe, Slavich, & Gotlib, 2014)? Do cognitive vulnerabilities "build on" a severe event to distinguish those who go on to develop depression, or does greater cognitive vulnerability amplify lower degrees of stress to cause depression (Abramson et al., 1989)? Is HPA-axis dysregulation during an episode of depression characteristic of people who do or do not have a severe life event prior to onset? Does the role of severe life events change over successive episodes of depression, or is there a distinctive recurrent subtype in which people become depressed independent of life stress (Burcusa & Iacono, 2007; Monroe & Harkness, 2011)? These questions, guided by a focus on severe life events, we believe are of pressing importance and in theory can be addressed in the coming years.

We view severe events as the bright side of current stress theory and research in depression, the best present starting point from which to move forward. But obviously there is much more to "stress" than severe events, and, as we have emphasized, not all persons with depression have experienced severe life events just prior to onset of their condition. A core challenge remains in explaining depression's origins for people who do not have a severe event prior to onset. This is where the empirical literature on severe stress leaves off and the theoretical premise of stress sensitization fills in.

Nonsevere forms of stress currently represent the dark side of stress theory and research on depression. Can moderate or low levels of stress contribute to the onset of a depressive episode? Might such forms of stress be particularly relevant for recurrences? There is optimism about what stress sensitization has to offer the field, and there are promising leads. But at present, theory on stress sensitization and nonsevere forms of stress for individuals with depression has been presumed more than affirmed. The framework of ideas involved has not been fully articulated or scrutinized, and the methods required to test them have not been sufficiently developed. As a consequence, nonsevere forms of stress are dark in the sense that they are relatively unknown, but also in the sense that there is something vaguely foreboding about them.

As we have indicated, a major challenge is how to extract the potentially nonsevere forms of stress from the "sea" of stress that might contribute to onset of a depressive episode. One place to start would be to take clues from the literature on severe life events and prioritize life events of lesser magnitude that possess similar potentially depressogenic themes for the participant. For example, there are a number of experiences that are consistent with a depressogenic motif, events that might harbor particular meanings of relevance for depression (e.g., loss, hopelessness, humiliation, interpersonal rejection; Abramson et al., 1989; Beck, 1983; Brown & Harris, 1978; Slavich et al., 2009). Life events that are "fateful," that are beyond the control of the individual, also may be of particular interest (Monroe et al., 2006; Shrout et al., 1989). But there are likely to be other substantial methodological issues for researchers to attend to and work through that do not translate directly from the research on severe life events. For example, the time scale for an event to trigger a depressive episode might well differ between severe and nonsevere life events (e.g., if sensitized, it is plausible that the depression would develop more quickly and implausible that an event 3 months prior would suddenly trigger an episode). Perhaps most foreboding, though, are questions about the limits of stress sensitization. At what point, under what circumstances, and for which people with depression might researchers refute or abandon the stress premise?

Stress sensitization represents a theoretical premise that could be important for understanding depression and its recurrences and worthy of continued research. Indeed, one of the most promising lines of future research on stress sensitization and depression involves identifying the range of mechanisms at different levels of analysis (e.g., neural, physiological, molecular, genomic) that may become aberrant and underpin depressive symptoms, either in the face of minor stressors or, perhaps, in the absence of detectable life stress altogether (Cuthbert & Insel, 2013; Sanislow et al., 2010; Slavich & Irwin, 2014). Given the conceptual and practical challenges for conducting research on this topic just noted, however, investigators should be circumspect and proceed with caution.

In light of some 35 years of research documenting the special role of severe life events in relation to the onset of depression (Brown & Harris, 1978), we recommend that researchers maintain an active focus centered on these types of stressors. We hope that important advances may come from attention to severe life events as a window into the lives of persons with depression and a reference point for understanding the collective processes through which depression may take hold.

REFERENCES

Abramson, L. Y., Metalsky, G. I., & Alloy, L. B. (1989). Hopelessness depression: A theory-based subtype of depression. *Psychological Review, 96*, 358–372.

American Psychiatric Association. (2013). *Diagnostic and statistical manual of mental disorders* (5th ed.). Washington, DC: Author.

Beck, A. T. (1983). Cognitive therapy of depression: New perspectives. In P. J. Clayton & J. E. Barrett (Eds.), *Treatment of depression: Old controversies and new approaches* (pp. 265–290). New York: Raven Press.

Beck, A. T., Steer, R. A., & Garbin, M. G. (1988). Psychometric properties of the Beck Depression Inventory: Twenty-five years of evaluation. *Clinical Psychology Review, 8*, 77–100.

Brown, G. W. (1974). Meaning, measurement, and stress of life events. In B. S. Dohrenwend & B. P. Dohrenwend (Eds.), *Stressful life events: Their nature and effects* (pp. 217–243). New York: Wiley.

Brown, G. W. (2012). The promoter of the serotonin transporter genotype, environment and depression: A hypothesis supported? *Journal of Affective Disorders, 137*, 1–3

Brown, G. W., & Harris, T. O. (1978). *Social origins of depression: A study of psychiatric disorder in women*. New York: Free Press.

Brown, G. W., & Harris, T. O. (Eds.). (1989). *Life events and illness*. New York: Guilford Press.

Brown, G. W., & Harris, T. O. (2008). Depression and the serotonin transporter 5-HTTLPR polymorphism: A review and a hypothesis concerning gene–environment interaction. *Journal of Affective Disorders, 111*, 1–12.

Brown, G. W., Harris, T. O., & Hepworth, C. (1994). Life events and endogenous depression: A puzzle reexamined. *Archives of General Psychiatry, 51*, 525–534.

Brown, G. W., Harris, T. O., & Hepworth, C. (1995). Loss, humiliation and entrapment among women developing depression: A patient and non-patient comparison. *Psychological Medicine, 25*, 7–21.

Brown, T. A., & Rosellini, A. J. (2011). The direct and interactive effects of neuroticism and life stress on the severity and longitudinal course of depressive symptoms. *Journal of Abnormal Psychology, 122*, 105–110.

Burcusa, S. L., & Iacono, W. G. (2007). Risk for recurrence in depression. *Clinical Psychology Review, 27*, 959–985.

Caspi, A., Sugden, K., Moffitt, T. E., Taylor, A., Craig, I. W., Harrington, H., et al. (2003). Influence of life stress on depression: Moderation by a polymorphism in the *5-HTT* gene. *Science, 301*, 386–389.

Cuthbert, B. N., & Insel, T. R. (2013). Toward the future of psychiatric diagnosis: The seven pillars of RDoC. *BMC Medicine, 11*, 126.

DellaGioia, N., & Hannestad, J. (2010). A critical review of human endotoxin administration as an experimental paradigm of depression. *Neuroscience and Biobehavioral Reviews, 34,* 130–143.

Dohrenwend, B. P. (2006). Inventorying stressful life events as risk factors for psychopathology: Toward resolution of the problem of intracategory variability. *Psychological Bulletin, 132,* 477–495.

Dolan, R. J., Calloway, S. P., Fonagy, P., De Souza, F. V., & Wakeling, A. (1985). Life events, depression and hypothalamic–pituitary–adrenal axis function. *British Journal of Psychiatry, 147,* 429–433.

Dowlati, Y., Herrmann, N., Swardfager, W., Liu, H., Sham, L., Reim, E. K., et al. (2010). A meta-analysis of cytokines in major depression. *Biological Psychiatry, 67,* 446–457.

Eaton, W. W., Shao, H., Nestadt, G., Lee, H. B., Lee, B. H., Bienvenu, O. J., et al. (2008). Population-based study of first onset and chronicity in major depressive disorder. *Archives of General Psychiatry, 65,* 513–520.

Espejo, E. P., Hammen, C. L., Connolly, N. P., Brennan, P. A., Najman, J. M., & Bjor, W. (2006). Stress sensitization and adolescent depressive severity as a function of childhood adversity: A link to anxiety disorders. *Journal of Abnormal Child Psychology, 35,* 287–299.

Goodwin, F. K., & Jamison, K. R. (2007). *Manic-depressive illness: Bipolar disorders and recurrent depression* (2nd ed.). New York: Oxford University Press.

Hadzi-Pavlovic, D., & Boyce, P. (2012). Melancholia. *Current Opinion in Psychiatry, 25,* 14–18.

Hamilton, M. (1960). A rating scale for depression. *Journal of Neurology, Neurosurgery, and Psychiatry, 23,* 56–62.

Hammen, C. (1991). Generation of stress in the course of unipolar depression. *Journal of Abnormal Psychology, 100,* 555–561.

Hammen, C. (2005). Stress and depression. *Annual Review of Clinical Psychology, 1,* 293–319.

Hammen, C. (2006). Stress generation in depression: Reflections on origins, research, and future directions. *Journal of Clinical Psychology, 62,* 1065–1082.

Hammen, C., Henry, R., & Daley, S. E. (2000). Depression and sensitization to stressors among young women as a function of childhood adversity. *Journal of Consulting and Clinical Psychology, 68,* 782–787.

Holmes, T. H., & Rahe, R. H. (1967). The Social Readjustment Rating Scale. *Journal of Psychosomatic Research, 11,* 213–218.

Jackson, S. W. (1986). *Melancholia and depression.* New Haven, CT: Yale University Press.

Jarcho, M. R., Slavich, G. M., Tylova-Stein, H., Wolkowitz, O. M., & Burke, H. M. (2013). Dysregulated diurnal cortisol pattern is associated with glucocorticoid resistance in women with major depressive disorder. *Biological Psychology, 93,* 150–158.

Karg, K., Burmeister, M., Shedden, K., & Sen, S. (2011). The serotonin transporter promoter variant (5-HTTLPR), stress, and depression meta-analysis revisited: Evidence of genetic moderation. *Archives of General Psychiatry, 68,* 444–454.

Karp, J. F., Frank, E., Anderson, B., George, C. J., Reynolds, C. F. I., Mazumdar, S., et al. (1993). Time to remission in late-life depression: Analysis of effects of demographic, treatment, and life-events measures. *Depression, 1,* 250–256.

Kendler, K. S., & Eaves, L. J. (1986). Models for the joint effect of genotype and environment liability to psychiatric illness. *American Journal of Psychiatry, 143,* 279–289.

Kendler, K. S., & Gardner, C. O. (2010). Dependent stressful life events and prior depressive episodes in the prediction of major depression: The problem of causal inference in psychiatric epidemiology. *Archives of General Psychiatry, 67,* 1120.

Kendler, K. S., Gardner, C. O., & Prescott, C. A. (2002). Toward a comprehensive developmental model for major depression in women. *American Journal of Psychiatry, 159,* 1133–1145.

Kendler, K. S., Hettema, J. M., Butera, F., Gardner, C. O., & Prescott, C. A. (2003). Life event dimensions of loss, humiliation, entrapment, and danger in the prediction of onsets of major depression and generalized anxiety. *Archives of General Psychiatry, 60,* 789–796.

Kendler, K. S., Karkowski, L. M., & Prescott, C. A. (1999). Causal relationship between stressful life events and the onset of major depression. *American Journal of Psychiatry, 156,* 837–841.

Kendler, K. S., Kuhn, J. W., Vittum, J., Prescott, C. A., & Riley, B. (2005). The interaction of stressful life events and a serotonin transporter polymorphism in the prediction of episodes of major depression: A replication. *Archives of General Psychiatry, 62,* 529–535.

Kendler, K. S., Thornton, L. M., & Gardner, C. O. (2000). Stressful life events and previous episodes in the etiology of major depression in women: An evaluation of the "kindling" hypothesis. *American Journal of Psychiatry, 157,* 1243–1251.

Kendler, K. S., Walters, E. E., & Kessler, R. C. (1997). The prediction of length of major depressive episodes: Results from an epidemiological of female twins. *Psychological Medicine, 27,* 107–117.

Kessler, R. C. (1997). The effects of stressful life events on depression. *Annual Review of Psychology, 48,* 191–214.

Klibansky, R., Panofsky, E., & Saxl, E. (1979). *Saturn and melancholy: Studies in natural philosophy, religion and art.* Nendeln, Liechtenstein: Kraus Reprint.

Kraepelin, E. (1921). *Manic-depressive insanity and paranoia.* Edinburgh, UK: Livingstone.

Mazure, C. M. (1998). Life stressors as risk factors in depression. *Clinical Psychology: Science and Practice, 5,* 291–313.

Moffitt, T. E., Caspi, A., Taylor, A., Kokaua, J., Milne, B. J., Polanczyk, G., et al. (2010). How common are common mental disorders?: Evidence that lifetime prevalence rates are doubled by prospective versus retrospective ascertainment. *Psychological Medicine, 40,* 899–909.

Monroe, S. M. (2008). Modern approaches to conceptualizing and measuring life stress. *Annual Review of Clinical Psychology, 4,* 33–52.

Monroe, S. M., & Depue, R. A. (1991). Life stress and depression. In J. Becker & A. Kleinman (Eds.), *Psychosocial aspects of depression* (pp. 101–130). New York: Erlbaum.

Monroe, S. M., & Hadjiyannakis, K. (2002). The social environment and depression: Focusing on severe life stress. In I. H. Gotlib & C. L. Hammen (Eds.), *Handbook of depression* (pp. 314–340). New York: Guilford Press.

Monroe, S. M., & Harkness, K. L. (2005). Life stress, the "kindling" hypothesis, and the recurrence of depression: Considerations from a life stress perspective. *Psychological Review, 112,* 417–445.

Monroe, S. M., & Harkness, K. L. (2011). Recurrence in major depression: A conceptual analysis. *Psychological Review, 118,* 655–674.

Monroe, S. M., Harkness, K., Simons, A. D., & Thase, M. E. (2001). Life stress and the symptoms of major depression. *Journal of Nervous and Mental Disease, 189,* 168–175.

Monroe, S. M., & Reid, M. W. (2008). Gene–environment interactions in depression: Genetic polymorphisms and life stress polyprocedures. *Psychological Science, 19,* 947–956.

Monroe, S. M., & Reid, M. W. (2009). Life stress and major depression. *Current Directions in Psychological Science, 18,* 68–72.

Monroe, S. M., Roberts, J. E., Kupfer, D. J., & Frank, E. (1996). Life stress and treatment course of recurrent depression: II. Postrecovery associations with attrition, symptom course, and recurrence over 3 years. *Journal of Abnormal Psychology, 105,* 313–328.

Monroe, S. M., & Simons, A. D. (1991). Diathesis–stress in the context of life stress research: Implications for the depressive disorders. *Psychological Bulletin, 110,* 406–425.

Monroe, S. M., & Slavich, G. M. (2007). Psychological stressors, overview. In G. Fink (Ed.), *Encyclopedia of stress* (2nd ed., Vol. 3, pp. 278–284). Oxford, UK: Academic Press.

Monroe, S. M., Slavich, G. M., & Gotlib, I. H. (2014). Life stress and family history for depression: The moderating role of past depressive episodes. *Journal of Psychiatric Research, 49,* 90–95.

Monroe, S. M., Slavich, G. M., Torres, L. D., & Gotlib, I. H. (2007a). Major life events and major chronic difficulties are differentially associated with history of major depressive episodes. *Journal of Abnormal Psychology, 116,* 116–124.

Monroe, S. M., Slavich, G. M., Torres, L. D., & Gotlib, I. H. (2007b). Severe life events predict specific patterns of change in cognitive biases in major depression. *Psychological Medicine, 37,* 863–871.

Monroe, S. M., Torres, L. D., Guillaumot, J., Harkness, K. L., Roberts, J. E., Frank, E., et al. (2006). Life stress and the long-term treatment course of recurrent depression: III. Nonsevere life events predict recurrence for medicated patients over 3 years. *Journal of Consulting and Clinical Psychology, 74,* 112–120.

Monroe, S. M., & Yoder, A. (in press). Measuring life events. In R. Cautin & S. Lilienfeld (Eds.), *The encyclopedia of clinical psychology.* Hoboken, NJ: Wiley-Blackwell.

Murphy, M. L. M., Slavich, G. M., Rohleder, N., & Miller, G. E. (2013). Targeted rejection triggers differential pro- and anti-inflammatory gene expression in adolescents as a function of social status. *Clinical Psychological Science, 1,* 30–40.

Muscatell, K. A., Slavich, G. M., Monroe, S. M., & Gotlib, I. H. (2009). Stressful life events, chronic difficulties, and the symptoms of clinical depression. *Journal of Nervous and Mental Disease, 197,* 154–160.

Parker, G., & Blignault, I. (1985). Psychosocial predictors of outcome in subjects with untreated depressive disorder. *Journal of Affective Disorders, 8,* 73–81.

Paykel, E. S. (2001). The evolution of life events research in psychiatry. *Journal of Affective Disorders, 62,* 141–149.

Paykel, E. S. (2003). Life events and affective disorders. *Acta Psychiatrica Scandinavica, 108*(Suppl. 418), 61–66.

Post, R. (1992). Transduction of psychosocial stress into the neurobiology of recurrent affective disorder. *American Journal of Psychiatry, 149,* 999–1010.

Risch, N., Herrell, R., Lehner, T., Liang, K.-Y., Eaves, L., Hoh, J., et al. (2009). Interaction between the serotonin transporter gene (5-HTTLPR), stressful life events, and risk of depression. *Journal of the American Medical Association, 301,* 2462–2471.

Roy, A., Pickar, D., Linnoila, M., Doran, A. R., & Paul, S. M. (1986). Cerebrospinal fluid monoamine and monoamine metabolite levels and the dexamethasone suppression test in depression: Relationship to life events. *Archives of General Psychiatry, 43,* 356–360.

Sanislow, C. A., Pine, D. S., Quinn, K. J., Kozak, M. J., Garvey, M. A., Heinssen, R. K., et al. (2010). Developing constructs for psychopathology research: Research Domain Criteria. *Journal of Abnormal Psychology, 119,* 631–639.

Sapolsky, R. M. (2000). Glucocorticoids and hippocampal atrophy in neuropsychiatric disorders. *Archives of General Psychiatry, 57,* 925–935.

Segerstrom, S. C., & Miller, G. E. (2004). Psychological stress and the human immune system: A meta-analytic study of 30 years of inquiry. *Psychological Bulletin, 130,* 601–630.

Shrout, P. E., Link, B. G., Dohrenwend, B. P., Skodol, A. E., Stueve, A., & Mirotznik, J. (1989). Characterizing life events as risk factors for depression: The role of fateful loss. *Journal of Abnormal Psychology, 98,* 460–467.

Slavich, G. M., & Epel, E. S. (2010). *The Stress and Adversity Inventory (STRAIN): An automated system for assessing cumulative stress exposure.* Los Angeles: University of California.

Slavich, G. M., & Irwin, M. R. (2014). From stress to inflammation and major depressive disorder: A social signal transduction theory of depression. *Psychological Bulletin, 140,* 774–815.

Slavich, G. M., Monroe, S. M., & Gotlib, I. H. (2011). Early parental loss and depression history: Associations with recent life stress in major depressive disorder. *Journal of Psychiatric Research, 45,* 1146–1152.

Slavich, G. M., Thornton, T., Torres, L. D., Monroe, S. M., & Gotlib, I. H. (2009). Targeted rejection predicts hastened onset of major depressive disorder. *Journal of Social and Clinical Psychology, 28,* 223–243.

Stetler, C., & Miller, G. E. (2011). Depression and hypothalamic–pituitary–adrenal activation: A quantitative summary of four decades of research. *Psychosomatic Medicine, 73,* 114–126.

Stroud, C. B., Davila, J., Hammen, C., & Vrshek-Schallhorn, S. (2011). Severe and nonsevere events in first onsets versus recurrences of depression: Evidence for stress sensitization. *Journal of Abnormal Psychology, 120,* 142–154.

Stroud, C. B., Davila, J., & Moyer, A. (2008). The relationship between stress and depression in first onsets versus recurrences: A meta-analytic review. *Journal of Abnormal Psychology, 117,* 206–213

Tennant, C. (2002). Life events, stress and depression: A review of recent findings. *Australian and New Zealand Journal of Psychiatry, 36,* 173–182.

Uher, R., & McGuffin, P. (2010). The moderation by the serotonin transporter gene of environmental adversity in the etiology of depression: 2009 update. *Molecular Psychiatry, 15,* 18–22.

van Praag, H. M., de Kloet, E. R., & van Os, J. (2004). *Stress, the brain and depression.* New York: Cambridge University Press.

Wakefield, J. C. (2012). Mapping melancholia: The continuing typological challenge for major depression. *Journal of Affective Disorders, 138,* 180–182.

CHAPTER 17

Risk Factors for Bipolar Disorder

SHERI L. JOHNSON, AMY K. CUELLAR, *and* ANDREW D. PECKHAM

The goal of this chapter is to review risk factors for bipolar disorder. We begin by reviewing major biological models. Biological vulnerability, though, helps explain who develops the disorder, rather than why symptoms and episodes occur at a given point in time. Extensive research documents that psychosocial factors can trigger symptom expression, and so we review that literature as well.

Before beginning, it is worth noting some limits to the scope of our review. As discussed by Youngstrom and Algorta (Chapter 8, this volume), DSM includes multiple bipolar diagnoses, including cyclothymia, bipolar II disorder, and bipolar I disorder. Although it is believed that bipolar II disorder and cyclothymia are more common than bipolar I disorder (Merikangas et al., 2007), these milder bipolar spectrum disorders have received less research attention. Beyond diagnoses, there is increasing support for considering vulnerability to mania as a continuum. Multiple measures are available to characterize the frequency and intensity of manic symptoms, including the General Behavior Inventory and the Hypomanic Personality Scale. Both scales have been shown to robustly predict the onset of bipolar disorder (Depue et al., 1981; Kwapil et al., 2000). A large literature has focused on the psychosocial correlates of elevations on these scales, and the findings have been remarkably consistent with findings regarding the correlates of mania within bipolar disorder. Reviewing the literature on bipolar spectrum disorders and subsyndromal mania, though, is outside the scope of this chapter. Hence, we focus on bipolar I disorder (which we abbreviate as BD).

We also are limited in our ability to cover one of the more fascinating aspects of BD: the remarkable heterogeneity in functional outcomes. Most readers will be familiar with the oft-cited statistics that people with BD are at high risk for suicidality (Angst, Angst, Gerber-Werder, & Gamma, 2005) and poor psychosocial function (Fagiolini et al., 2005). Despite these frequently noted poor outcomes, some people with BD seem to do extremely well, often surpassing the levels of accomplishment observed in the general population (Lobban, Taylor, Murray, & Jones, 2012). The growing literature on functioning, though, is beyond the scope of this review.

Within our narrow focus on the risk factors for bipolar symptoms, we focus on differentiating mania and depression. Although clinical lore and the very name of the disorder suggest that BD necessarily involves depression, this is not the case. In community samples, as many as 20–33% of individuals with BD report no lifetime episode of major depression (cf. Karkowski & Kendler, 1997). Even among the people with BD who do experience depressive episodes, there is dramatic variability in the expression of depression. For some, depressive symptoms can be quite chronic and severe. Among 146 patients with BD followed for more than 12 years, depressive symptoms were present on average for about one-third of weeks (Judd et al., 2002). Although manic symptoms are the defining feature of BD, depressive symptoms trigger more help seeking than do manic symptoms (Fagiolini et al., 2005) and are related to suicide risk (Angst et al., 2005) and impaired functioning (Fagiolini et al., 2005). Our review, then, focuses on psychosocial variables that trigger depressive symptoms, as well as those that trigger manic symptoms within BD.

Although differentiating risk factors for mania versus depression might seem straightforward, this goal raises a set of methodological issues. Imagine the person who experiences a manic episode and whose behaviors during that episode lead to a breakdown of his or her marriage, a loss of his or her job, and significant financial debt. That person might demonstrate a profile of poor social support, high life stress, and negative cognitions about him- or herself. Despite the likelihood of such a profile in BD, a key question is whether elevations on those indices are mere artifacts of the episode or can help predict the course of future symptoms. Only prospective research can define which variables will predict manic symptoms and which will predict depressive symptoms. Given this fact, we focus on prospective research.

Although some neurobiological research has considered whether findings are more relevant to depressive versus manic symptoms, less is known about this topic. For this reason, our chapter consists of three major sections: neurobiological correlates of BD, psychosocial predictors of depression, and psychosocial predictors of mania. Where research is available comparing the neurobiology of BD to unipolar depression, we note this.

BIOLOGICAL VULNERABILITY

We briefly consider findings of genetic, neuroimaging, and neurotransmitter research in BD, although the interested reader is referred to much more detailed reviews (Strakowski, 2012). Increasing evidence suggests that factors such as trauma (Burghy et al., 2011) and medication exposure (van Erp et al., 2012) have powerful influences on key brain regions and neurotransmitter systems. Given this evidence, we note studies of unaffected family members of those with BD when available.

Genetic Vulnerability

Genetic influences play an important role in the etiology of BD, with heritability estimates of .85–.93 in large-scale, community-based twin studies (Kieseppa, Partonen, Haukka, Kaprio, & Lonnqvist, 2004; McGuffin et al. 2003). The few available adoption studies in BD also are consistent with high heritability (Wender, 1986). Although genetic vulnerability for depression and mania are correlated, data from a large twin study suggest that these vulnerabilities should be considered as distinct (McGuffin et al. 2003).

A large body of research focuses on identifying genetic polymorphisms (variations in the DNA sequence that occur at a particular locus on the chromosome) associated with BD. Two major approaches dominate this research. Genomewide association studies (GWAS) examine a large array of the most common genetic loci. In contrast, candidate gene studies focus on a particular gene or smaller set of genes of interest. Although we provide examples of the findings of both, the reader should be aware that this literature is replete with nonreplications (Kato, 2007).

GWAS have been informative in highlighting that many psychiatric conditions overlap in the polymorphisms involved. For example, many of the polymorphisms that are associated with BD are also implicated in schizophrenia (Talkowski et al., 2012). Similarly, some polymorphisms involved in BD appear involved in depression as well as schizophrenia (Cross-Disorder Group of the Psychiatric Genomics Consortium, 2013).

Most candidate gene studies have examined polymorphisms related to serotonin and dopamine function. Meta-analyses of the serotonin transporter region in BD have yielded positive but small effects (Cho et al., 2005). One large-scale study identified 12 polymorphisms related to dopamine (DA) function that were related to BD (Talkowski et al., 2012).

Imaging Research

Here we consider both structural imaging, which focuses on whether there are changes in the volume of key regions or in the integrity of tracts linking these regions, and functional imaging, which focuses on patterns of activation. Structural and functional models of BD emphasize several strongly interconnected regions involved in emotion and emotion regulation, in reward, and in impulsivity and response inhibition (e.g., the inferior frontal gyrus [IFG]).

Multiple models have been developed of the networks involved in emotion. Some have differentiated neural responses to valenced stimuli as compared with "hotter" emotion-inducing paradigms (Strakowski, 2012). Others focus on emotion generation versus regulation. Regions such as the amygdala, ventral striatum, and thalamus are activated during early phases of processing emotion-relevant stimuli. Other regions, including the parahippocampal gyrus, hippocampus, subgenual anterior cingulate cortex, and ventromedial and orbitofrontal regions of the prefrontal cortex, are implicated in appraisal and encoding of emotional significance and regulation of responses to emotional stimuli (Phillips, Ladouceur, & Drevets, 2008).

Beyond emotion processing, many have hypothesized that the mesolimbic dopaminergic pathway from the ventral tegmental area to the nucleus accumbens is of particular importance in BD (Depue, Krauss, & Spoont, 1987). This pathway is believed to facilitate motivation and energy in the context of opportunities for reward (Salamone, Correa, Farrar, & Mingote, 2007). Activation of this pathway has consistently been shown to produce changes in many of the behaviors and experiences associated with mania, including energy, positive mood, and goal pursuit (Depue & Iacono, 1989; Fowles, 1993).

Structural Studies

Findings regarding the volume of key brain structures in BD have been mixed. In a meta-analysis of eight studies of voxel-based morphometry, right ventral prefrontal cortex, insula, temporal gyrus, and IFG were reduced among adults with BD compared with controls (Selvaraj et al., 2012). Caution is warranted, though, because mood state (Foland-Ross et al., 2012) and medication (Hafeman, Chang, Garrett, Sanders, & Phillips, 2012; van Erp et al., 2012) influence volumes of these regions. In light of these influences on structural deficits, studies of those at risk for BP are of particular interest. Among offspring of parents diagnosed with BD, no volume abnormalities have been observed consistently across studies (Singh, DelBello, & Chang, 2012).

A growing body of research has used diffusor tensor imaging (DTI) to evaluate white matter tracts connecting brain regions. In one review, BD appeared to be uniquely related to deficits in white matter connectivity of the orbitofrontal cortex with the amygdala and subgenual cingulate gyrus (Almeida & Phillips, 2013). Disruptions in white matter tracts from the prefrontal cortex have also been identified among youth who are in early stages of BD across three studies and among offspring of parents with BD in one study, although there has been some variability in the specific tracts implicated across studies (see Singh, et al., 2012, for a review).

Functional Studies

A burgeoning literature is available of functional imaging profiles in BD, using multiple paradigms across depression, hypomania, and well periods. Meta-analysis, though, is particularly helpful given that small sample sizes and heterogeneous approaches complicate interpretation of the substantial cross-study heterogeneity. Findings from multiple studies suggest that, compared with those without mood disorders, people with BD demonstrate increased activation of a range of limbic structures, including the hippocampus, parahippocampal gyrus, and ventral striatum and, to a smaller extent, the amygdala, when processing emotion-relevant stimuli as compared with neutral stimuli (Chen, Suckling, Lennox, Ooi, & Bullmore, 2011). Although this profile of limbic hyperactivation appears relatively consistent during manic and euthymic periods, findings do not seem to consistently generalize to depressive periods. Across studies, diminished activation of the orbitofrontal cortex has also been observed during emotion processing tasks, and this pattern is observed across euthymic, manic, and depressive states (Altshuler & Townsend, 2012). Despite some inconsistencies, this general profile of limbic hyperactivation and diminished activation of prefrontal regions has also been observed among youth diagnosed with BD (Singh et al., 2012). In a meta-analysis of BD as compared with major depressive disorder across 37 studies using facial affect processing paradigms (Delvecchio et al., 2012), both disorders were related to enhanced limbic activation and diminished cortical activation.

Some, but not all, research on reward processing has found that mania is associated with increased neural activation to cues of potential reward. For example, on a task with monetary incentives, individuals with current mania exhibited increased orbitofrontal activity when expecting reward gains and decreased activity when expecting losses as compared with neutral trials, a pattern that was opposite to that observed in healthy controls (Bermpohl et al., 2010). Increased orbitofrontal activity to gain cues has also been observed during remission (Nusslock et al., 2012). In the above-mentioned meta-analysis of emotion processing, BD was related to greater activation of the ventral striatum in response to happy faces than was major depressive disorder, consistent with the idea of increased reactivity to reward stimuli (Delvecchio et al., 2012). Some, but not all, studies, then, support the idea of increased neural response to reward in BD.

Across studies employing either emotion processing or cognitive tasks, people with BD demonstrate diminished activation of the IFG, a region that is central in the inhibition of prepotent responses (Chen et al., 2011; Delvecchio et al., 2012. The relatively diminished activation of the IFG may help explain some of the difficulties with inhibition of behavior and impulsivity that are associated with BD. Although consistently observed during depressed and well periods, IFG hypoactivation appears to be particularly pronounced during manic episodes.

Few studies have examined resting state functional connectivity in BD, and the available studies are limited by small sample sizes and the heterogeneous sample sizes. Nonetheless, two of three studies suggest diminished corticolimbic connectivity during resting states among persons diagnosed with BD (Altshuler & Townsend, 2012).

In research using emotion processing tasks, persons with BD demonstrated diminished connectivity of the amygdala with ventromedial prefrontal cortex, but this appeared to be specifically related to positive stimuli. The lack of connectivity in response to positive stimuli differentiated participants with BD from those with unipolar disorder (Almeida et al., 2009).

Neurotransmitter Research

Substantial research has focused on neurotransmitter irregularities associated with BD. Much of the historical research focused on the levels of neurotransmitter metabolites. Multiple studies of this form helped document that people with BD demonstrated deficits in levels of metabolites of serotonin and DA in cerebrospinal fluid (Yatham, Srisurapanont, Zis, & Kusumakar, 1997). Building from this work, newer paradigms have been applied to refine understanding of the nature of serotonin and DA neurotransmitter dysfunction in BD. We focus here on two such approaches. One approach is to "challenge" the system by changing levels of a given neurotransmitter and measuring neurological, behavioral, affective, or cognitive responses. In addition to challenge research, SPECT imaging provides data on specific neurotransmitter processes, such as reuptake of neurotransmitter from the synaptic cleft.

Serotonin Research

Several pharmacological challenges for studying serotonin system sensitivity are available. One approach is to increase serotonin availability by administering either *d*-fenfluramine (which triggers the release of serotonin and inhibits reuptake) or tryptophan (a precursor to serotonin). Serotonin neurons that project from the raphe to the hypothalamus trigger release of the hormone prolactin. Hence one way to measure the responsivity of the serotonin system to these challenges is to measure change in prolactin levels. Six out of nine studies suggest that people with unipolar and bipolar depression demonstrate similarly blunted hormonal responses to *d*-fenfluramine or tryptophan administration (Sher et al., 2003; see Sobczak, Honig, van Duinen, & Riedel, 2002, for a review), even during remission (Nurnberger, Berrettini, Simmons-Alling, Lawrence, & Brittain, 1990).

Beyond studies of serotonin augmentation, acute tryptophan depletion (ATD) is widely used. In ATD, persons are asked to drink a milk shake that is rich in 15 amino acids other than tryptophan, aspartic acid, and glutamic acid (Moore et al., 2000). As a result of the body's processing of the other amino acids, tryptophan is depleted within 4–12 hours, leading to an acute reduction in serotonin by 10–50% that is reversed within hours. ATD findings suggest that serotonergic deficits are not secondary to effects of previous episodes or treatments. That is, unaffected family members of persons with BD demonstrate atypical cognitive and emotional responses to ATD (Quintin et al., 2001;

Sobczak, Honig, Nicolson, & Riedel, 1999; Sobczak, Reidel, Booij, Het Rot, & Deutz, 2002), indicating that serotonergic dysfunction can be observed among persons at risk for the disorder who have not yet experienced symptoms.

Dopamine Research

Several researchers have experimentally manipulated DA levels. For example, multiple studies have suggested that DA agonists, such as bromocriptine, trigger manic symptoms (cf. McGrath, Quitkin, & Klein, 1995; Willner, 1995). Researchers have also compared responses to amphetamine, which releases catecholamines into the synaptic cleft, among persons with BD as compared with controls. Although most people with no diagnosis of BD develop mild manic symptoms, such as increases in thought speed and activity, after amphetamine administration, those with BD demonstrate much more pronounced increases in manic symptoms (Anand et al., 2000).

Across paradigms, there is also evidence for disruptions in DA receptor and reuptake function as correlates of BD. For example, behavioral sensitization paradigms have been used to study the mesolimbic DA reward pathway described earlier. Findings of this paradigm indicate that regions implicated in reward responsivity might already be sensitized among people with BD (Strakowski, Sax, Setters, Stanton, & Keck, 1997). SPECT imaging also suggests heightened DA transporter (DAT) binding (which would promote sustained DA release) among remitted patients with BD (Nikolaus, Antke, & Muller, 2009). Finally, findings of several studies suggest that aspects of second messenger systems related to dopamine are disrupted in BD (Cousins, Butts, & Young, 2009). Taken together, several findings indicate BD may relate to sustained release of DA.

PSYCHOSOCIAL ANTECEDENTS TO BIPOLAR DEPRESSION

In this section, we review the socioenvironmental variables that have the most evidence as predictors of bipolar depression. We focus on trauma, life events, social support, family functioning, and personality traits.

Trauma

There is a large literature documenting the relationship between childhood abuse and the onset and course of unipolar depression (see Hammen, Henry, & Daley, 2000). People with BD, though, have a higher incidence of childhood abuse than do those with unipolar depression (Hyun, Friedman, & Dunner, 2000). Childhood abuse is associated not only with a diagnosis of BD but also with a more pernicious course of the disorder. In a comprehensive review that weighted studies based on methodological rigor, Daruy-Filho, Brietzke, Lafer, and Grassi-Oliveira (2011) found that childhood abuse (particularly physical abuse) was related to earlier onset, rapid cycling, more hospitalizations, psychosis, suicidality, impulsivity, aggression, symptom severity, more mood episodes, and more comorbidity in BD. Early adversity can also amplify the effects of stressful life events on BD recurrence in adulthood (Dienes, Hammen, Henry, Cohen, & Daley, 2006; Gershon, Johnson, & Miller, 2013).

In one available prospective study, trauma history predicted greater chronic stressors, and the greater chronic stressors predicted greater symptoms of depression, but not mania (Gershon et al., 2013). More prospective research is needed on specific outcomes related to trauma.

Negative Life Events

Although many studies have focused on life events in BD, most rely on self-report scales, which have lower validity and reliability than interview measures (McQuaid et al., 1992). We focus on studies that use the Bedford College Life Event and Difficulty Schedule (LEDS; Brown & Harris, 1978) or other interview measures that rule out events caused by the disorder. The LEDS assessment begins with a semistructured interview covering life events and their context. Raters who are unaware of the participant's subjective appraisal of the event provide consensus ratings of event severity and whether the event was independent or dependent (caused by the disorder).

Prospective studies using such interviews have demonstrated that independent, stressful life events predict increases in bipolar depression (Johnson, 2005) and delay recovery from episodes of depression (Johnson & Miller, 1997), but not mania (Cohen, Hammen, Henry, & Daley, 2004; Johnson, Winett, Meyer, Greenhouse, & Miller, 1999; Johnson et al., 2008). Life events also were found to predict depression, but not mania, when examined conjointly with social support (Ellicott, Hammen, Gitlin, Brown, & Jamison, 1990). BD depressive symptoms appear particularly related to events related to loss and danger (Hosang, Uher, Maughan, McGuffin, & Farmer, 2012).

One study examined the role of life events, as measured using the adolescent version of the LEDS, in predicting the onset of mood disorders among 140 offspring of parents with BD (Hillegers et al., 2004). At 5-year follow-up, 34 of the children had developed depressive disorders and 4 had developed bipolar spectrum disorders. The onset of these mood disorders was clearly related to the cumulative number of severe negative life events over a 5-year period: Each severe life event increased risk of future onset by approximately 10%. Findings, however, were limited by the 5-year period covered by interviews. To address this, the authors examined severe life events that occurred within 14 months of the interview as predictors of mood episodes (either new onsets or recurrences; Wals et al., 2005). As with previous analyses, life events were clearly tied to mood disorders, and particularly to depression. Hence, negative life events appear to be important in understanding initial depression onset among those at risk for BD. Mood disorders appear particularly likely to develop in the context of life events for offspring who demonstrate high emotionality (Duffy et al., 2007). Despite theory (Post, 1992), there is no consistent finding that life events are more powerful at predicting earlier episodes than later ones in BD (Bender & Alloy, 2011).

Low Social Support

The deleterious effects of low social support on unipolar depression have been well documented (cf. Brown & Andrews, 1986). In parallel, with the exception of one study with low recurrence rates (Staner et al., 1997), social support has been found in numerous studies to be a significant predictor of mood episodes and episode severity in BD (cf. O'Connell, Mayo, Eng, Jones, & Gabel, 1985; Stefos, Bauwens, Staner, Pardoen, & Mendlewicz, 1996).

Low social support appears to predict increases in depressive, but not manic, symptoms (Cohen et al., 2004; Johnson et al., 1999; Johnson, Lundström, Åberg-Wistedt, &

Mathé, 2003; Johnson, Meyer, Winett, & Small, 2000; Weinstock & Miller, 2010). The mechanism for this effect does not appear to be due to buffering against life stress (Cohen et al., 2004; Johnson et al., 1999). Rather, social support has been found to bolster self-esteem (Johnson et al., 1999; Johnson, Meyer, et al., 2000) and to predict more positive minor events within BD (Havermans, Nicolson, & deVries, 2007).

Family Functioning

Expressed emotion (EE), defined as overinvolvement, hostility, or criticism by family members toward the patient, is a robust predictor of the course of BD (Butzlaff & Hooley, 1998; Miklowitz, Goldstein, Nuechterlein, Snyder, & Mintz, 1988). Among patients with BD, living with a high-EE family is related to a two- to threefold increase in the risk of relapse within 9 months (Barrowclough & Hooley, 2003). Poor outcome is especially linked to the criticism element of EE (Hooley, Rosen, & Richters, 1995; Rosenfarb et al., 2001). EE predicted more severe depressive, but not manic, symptoms of BD in two studies (Kim & Miklowitz, 2004; Yan, Hammen, Cohen, Daley, & Henry, 2004).

Aside from EE, more general family functioning has been studied as a psychosocial predictor of BD. Among adults, family impairment (Gitlin, Swendsen, Heller, & Hammen, 1995; Weinstock & Miller, 2010) and poor family problem-solving ability (Townsend, Demeter, Youngstrom, Drotar, & Findling, 2007) have been shown to predict depressive more than manic symptoms. Family functioning, though, did not predict depressive symptoms after controlling for social support (Weinstock & Miller, 2010).

Among adolescents with BD, family difficulties have been linked to suicidal ideation (Goldstein et al., 2009) and have been found to predict depressive symptoms (Sullivan, Judd, Axelson, & Miklowitz, 2012). In contrast to the adult literature, family characteristics also appear to predict mania. For example, low maternal warmth is associated with more rapid recurrence of mania among youth with BD (Geller et al., 2002; Geller, Tillman, Craney, & Bolhofner, 2004). Among adolescents with BD, baseline levels of family conflict predicted both the severity and duration of mania symptoms (Sullivan et al., 2012). Even prospective studies of family influences on adolescent outcomes, though, can be difficult to interpret, as family conflict may emerge as parents attempt to adjust to and control emergent manic symptoms of their children. Parental mood dysregulation or bipolar diagnoses, which are common among adolescents with BD, will also influence family function.

Personality Traits

Several prospective studies have considered neuroticism and extraversion in BD. As with unipolar depression (Gunderson, Triebwasser, Phillips, & Sullivan, 1999), neuroticism predicts increases in bipolar depressive but not manic symptoms (Heerlein, Richter, Gonzalez, & Santander, 1998; Lozano & Johnson, 2001). High neuroticism and low extraversion predicted an index of relative number of days of depression to manic symptoms across a 6-month follow-up of over 2,200 patients with BD (Barnett et al., 2011). In sum, neuroticism and low extraversion appear predictive of bipolar depression.

Negative Cognition

Comparable to major depressive disorder, BD depression is associated with negative cognitive styles (see Cuellar, Johnson, & Winters, 2005; Jones, Sellwood, & McGovern,

2005, for reviews). Also like major depression, many of the negative cognitive facets documented during bipolar depression diminish somewhat with recovery (Cuellar et al., 2005). During interepisode periods of BD, negative cognitive styles and rumination have been found to be correlated with depressive symptom severity (Green et al., 2011; Gruber, Eidelman, & Harvey, 2008; Rowland et al., 2013; Van der Gucht, Morriss, Lancaster, Kinderman, & Bentall, 2009).

When present, negative cognitive styles predict greater increases over time in depressive, but not manic, symptoms (Johnson et al., 1999; Johnson & Fingerhut, 2004). Given that statistical power is more limited for predicting dichotomous outcomes compared with symptoms, it is not surprising that some results have indicated only nonsignificant trends for negative cognition on relapse occurrence (Scott & Pope, 2003). One study of individuals with current BD depression found that extreme attributions (for positive or negative events) predicted slower recovery from depression, as well as a lower chance of recovery (Stange et al., 2013). Hence negative cognitive styles and extreme attributions, when present, may predict bipolar depression. Unfortunately, little is known about whether information-processing biases can predict the course of bipolar symptoms.

Predictors of Mania

Compared with BD depression, less is known about the psychosocial variables influencing mania. Here, we focus on a set of variables that have received support in prospective research: schedule and sleep dysregulation, personality (particularly positive affectivity), reward sensitivity, and cognitive variables.

Sleep and Schedule Disruption

Over 25 years ago, Wehr, Sack, and Rosenthal (1987) hypothesized that sleep disruption might trigger episodes of BD. Research within bipolar samples has shown that manic symptoms are predicted by sleep deprivation, whether measured using total sleep deprivation in a laboratory setting (Barbini et al., 1998) or more minor naturalistically occurring sleep loss (Leibenluft, Albert, Rosenthal, & Wehr, 1996). In contrast, sleep deprivation predicts remission of depressive symptoms in both BD and unipolar disorder (see Colombo, Benedetti, Barbini, Campori, & Smeraldi, 1999, for a review). Consistent with this profile, sleep has been found to directly affect many of the biological and emotional factors that are implicated in BD (Murray & Harvey, 2010).

Wehr and colleagues (1987) noted that episodes of BD often followed life events that would disrupt sleep, such as flights across time zones and childbirth. He hypothesized that this type of event might trigger symptoms as a result of sleep deprivation. This theory was expanded to suggest that social rhythm disruptions (e.g., to daily routines and social plans) might predict bipolar symptoms above and beyond the role of sleep (Ehlers, Frank, & Kupfer, 1988). Life events involving social rhythm disruption, as assessed using the LEDS, have been found to be more common in the 8 weeks before manic recurrences than before depressive recurrences (Malkoff-Schwartz et al., 2000). Such findings provide one more potential mechanism for understanding how life events affect manic recurrence. Hence research suggests that BD is characterized by biological and behavioral disruptions in the circadian rhythm and that sleep deprivation and life events involving schedule disruption can trigger manic symptoms.

Personality

In studies of personality as a predictor of mania, researchers have examined extraversion, positive affectivity, and the Hyperthymic Temperament Scale (TEMPS-A; Akiskal et al., 2005), a scale that covers activity levels, gregariousness, preference for social activities, and dominance.

High extraversion, but not neuroticism, was found to predict the first onset of mania (Lönnqvist et al., 2009), although these findings were not replicated in one small study of 26 participants who converted to BD (Clayton, Ernst, & Angst, 1994). Hyperthymic temperament also has been found to predict the initial onset of mania (Akiskal et al., 1995, 2005; Egeland, Hostetter, Pauls, & Sussex, 2000; Regeer et al., 2006).

Consistent with the findings regarding onset, extraversion was found to predict a relative tendency toward mania as compared with depression over time among patients already diagnosed with BD (Barnett et al., 2011). Elevations in trait-like positive affectivity have also been found to predict increases in mania after controlling for baseline manic symptoms (Gruber et al., 2009; Strakowski, Stoll, Tohen, Faedda, & Goodwin, 1993).

Other personality traits may amplify the effects of extraversion and positive affectivity. Among persons who endorse high levels of positive affectivity and extraversion, impulsivity has been shown to predict the first onset of hypomanic episodes in two studies (Alloy, Urošević, et al., 2012; Kwapil et al., 2000). Among those with high levels of depression, mood variability has been found to predict onset (Kochman et al., 2005). Hence multifactorial models of personality that conjointly consider extraversion and positive affectivity, along with traits such as impulsivity, may be more powerful in the prediction of mania.

Reward Sensitivity

Across multiple studies, researchers have assessed sensitivity to reward among those with BD, most typically using the Carver and White (1994) Behavioral Activation Scales (BAS). These scales measure self-rated tendencies to be highly reactive to cues of incentive and reward, as manifested in motivation, energy, and enthusiasm. People with remitted BD describe themselves as more reward sensitive, even after controlling for any subsyndromal symptoms (Johnson, Edge, Holmes, & Carver, 2013). Elevated reward sensitivity has been found to predict increases over time in mania symptoms among those diagnosed with BD (Meyer, Johnson, & Winters, 2001) and conversion from bipolar spectrum disorder to more severe forms of disorder (Alloy, Urošević, et al., 2012), controlling for baseline symptoms.

Johnson, Sandrow, and colleagues (2000) hypothesized that excess reward sensitivity would heighten reactivity to reward, such that manic symptoms would be more likely after life events involving goal attainment, such as getting married, having a child, or completing a degree. Goal-attainment life events, as measured using the LEDS, predicted increases in manic but not depressive symptoms after controlling for baseline symptoms among persons with BD. These findings have been replicated (Johnson et al., 2008).

A key question is how life events involving goal attainment become translated into symptoms. One daily monitoring study suggests that people with BD may become more active and energized than controls do after making initial progress toward a goal (Fulford, Johnson, Llabre, & Carver, 2010). Increases in goal engagement (setting new goals and spending time pursuing goals) predicted increases in manic symptoms over several months among those diagnosed with BD (Lozano & Johnson, 2001). Hence hyperactivation appears to be a critical component of reward responsivity in BD.

Perhaps related to reward sensitivity, people with BD have been found to endorse extremely high life ambitions, for example, becoming highly famous or wealthy. In one study, such elevated lifetime ambitions predicted increases in manic symptoms, controlling for baseline symptom level (Johnson, Carver, & Gotlib, 2012). Heightened ambitions have also been found to predict the onset of BD (Alloy, Bender, et al., 2012).

SUMMARY OF BIOLOGICAL VULNERABILITY AND PSYCHOSOCIAL TRIGGERS

Heritability estimates in BD are high, and a large volume of research is being conducted to identify specific genetic polymorphisms tied to the disorder. DTI analyses suggest that the white matter integrity of corticolimbic tracts may be disrupted in BD. Functional imaging studies suggest that BD is related to increases in limbic system hyperactivity and decreases in orbitofrontal activity during emotion processing tasks and diminished activation of the IFG across a range of tasks. Functional connectivity analyses also suggest diminished regulation of limbic system activity by cortical regions. Taken together, findings suggest that BD may relate to impaired function of regions involved in emotion regulation and impulsivity/motor inhibition. People with BD and their family members show hypersensitivity to serotonergic challenges. Multiple paradigms also indicate that BD may be related to prolonged release of dopamine.

Many of the psychosocial variables that contribute to the course of major depressive disorder also appear to contribute to the course of bipolar depression. That is, history of trauma, negative life events, low social support, expressed emotion, poor family functioning, neuroticism, and negative cognitive styles each may help predict depression within BD. Bipolar depression and major depressive disorder also appear to share remarkable overlap in neurobiology.

Most of the psychosocial variables that predict unipolar and bipolar depression appear less predictive of mania. Rather, in longitudinal research, mania appears to be predicted by a set of variables that seem related to positive affectivity, to impulsivity, to reward system activity, and to sleep and schedule dysregulation. Support for reward system activity as predictive of manic symptoms has emerged from studies of dopamine agonists, self-rated reward sensitivity, ambition, and life events. Support for sleep and schedule disruption also has been shown across a wide array of paradigms, including life event assessments, as well as experimental sleep deprivation.

The overall profile of separable manic and depressive triggers has implications for understanding psychotherapy. Given the applicability of psychosocial models from major depressive disorder to bipolar depression, it is not surprising that psychosocial treatments with strong effects on major depressive disorder have fared well in addressing bipolar depression (see Miklowitz, Chapter 28, this volume). Most of the therapies that have been studied address problems that are more broadly drawn from the psychopathology field, as opposed to this relatively narrow set of risk factors. Not surprisingly, therapies that address interpersonal and family problems, as well as negative cognitive styles, are less powerful in addressing mania as opposed to depression (Frank et al., 2005; Lam, Hayward, Watkins, Wright, & Sham, 2005; Miklowitz et al., 2000). Similarly, patients who achieve social rhythm stabilization within interpersonal and social rhythm therapy have been shown to experience diminished mania over time (Frank et al., 2005). Case studies support the idea that targeting sleep disruptions can effectively reduce manic symptoms (cf. Wehr et al., 1998). Taken together, the literature on psychosocial triggers suggests that comprehensive psychotherapy should include techniques to address mechanisms involved in both depression and mania.

FUTURE DIRECTIONS

Although the empirical literature has burgeoned, we highlight a few issues here. Methodologically, research in BD suffers in comparison with that conducted on many other disorders by virtue of the sheer complexity of this disorder. The complex medication regimens (see Gitlin, Chapter 26, this volume) and variability in the severity and form of manic and depressive symptoms (see Youngstrom & Algorta, Chapter 8, this volume) are all important for understanding vulnerability and merit further attention.

Comorbidity is also of extreme importance. Data from epidemiological research suggests that more than 95% of persons diagnosed with BD meet diagnostic criteria for comorbid conditions. Nine out of 10 individuals with BD experience anxiety disorders, and 6 out of 10 experience substance-related disorders during their lifetimes (Merikangas et al., 2007). Given this tendency toward multiple comorbid syndromes, one might expect that beyond variables that intensify risk for depression and those that intensify risk for mania, there must be variables that increase risk for a range of symptoms. Potential candidates include variables that have been documented as related to mania and a range of other psychiatric conditions, including diminished corticolimbic connectivity, impulsivity (Swann, 2009) emotion regulation (Gruber, Harvey, & Gross, 2012), and early trauma and family conflict.

One concern is that the predictors of mania overlap so substantially with the symptoms observed during episodes. Positive affect, impulsivity, increased engagement in goal pursuit, and decreased need for sleep are all key symptoms of mania. Of course, similar overlap can be observed in the literature on depression, in which negative thinking and negative emotionality are studied as predictors of the episode, but also are core symptoms evident during episodes. Others have written elegantly about how to conceptualize highly overlapping systems in the study of risk factors and psychopathology (cf. Klein, Kotov, & Bufferd, 2011). Although most studies control for baseline symptoms in examining these predictors, the substantial overlap suggests the need to consider variables that would allow these systems to become dysregulated. Understanding how baseline qualities unfold into more full-blown symptoms is likely to require dynamical modeling.

Despite gaps, empirical literature on BD has grown dramatically over the past 10 years. Researchers have provided evidence across a multitude of paradigms in support of a set of biological and psychosocial risk variables in BD. It is hoped that the next generation of research will help build integrative models of how the various risk variables implicated in BD interact to predict the complex array of outcomes of importance in this disorder.

REFERENCES

Akiskal, H. S., Maser, J. D., Zeller, P. J., Endicott, J., Coryell, W., Keller, M., et al. (1995). Switching from "unipolar" to bipolar II: An 11-year prospective study of clinical and temperamental predictors of 559 patients. *Archives of General Psychiatry, 52,* 114–128.

Akiskal, H. S., Medlowicz, M. V., Jean-Louis, G., Rapaport, M. H., Kelsoe, J. R., Gillin, J. C., et al. (2005). TEMPS-A: Validation of a short version of a self-rated instrument designed to measure variations in temperament. *Journal of Affective Disorders, 85*, 45–52.

Alloy, L. B., Bender, R. E., Whitehouse, W. G., Wagner, C. A., Liu, R. T., Grant, D. A., et al. (2012). High Behavioral Approach System (BAS) sensitivity, reward responsiveness, and goal-striving predict first onset of bipolar spectrum disorders: A prospective behavioral high-risk design. *Journal of Abnormal Psychology, 121*, 339–351.

Alloy, L. B., Urošević, S., Abramson, L. Y., Jager-Hyman, S., Nusslock, R., Whitehouse, W. G., et al. (2012). Progression along the bipolar spectrum: a longitudinal study of predictors of conversion from bipolar spectrum conditions to bipolar I and II disorders. *Journal of Abnormal Psychology, 121*, 16–27.

Almeida, J. R., & Phillips, M. L. (2013). Distinguishing between unipolar depression and bipolar depression: Current and future clinical and neuroimaging perspectives. *Biological Psychiatry, 73*, 111–118.

Almeida, J. R. C., Versace, A., Mechelli, A., Hassel, S., Quevedo, K., Kupfer, D. J., et al. (2009). Orbitomedial prefrontal cortical–amygdala effective connectivity during positive emotion processing discriminates bipolar from major depression. *Biological Psychiatry, 65*, 14.

Altshuler, L. L., & Townsend, J. D. (2012). Functional brain imaging in bipolar disorder. In S. M. Strakowski (Ed.), *The bipolar brain: Integrating neuroimaging and genetics* (pp. 53–77). Oxford, UK: Oxford University Press.

Anand, A., Verhoeff, P., Seneca, N., Zoghbi, S. S., Seibyl, J. P., Charney, D. S., et al. (2000). Brain SPECT imaging of amphetamine-induced dopamine release in euthymic bipolar disorder patients. *American Journal of Psychiatry, 157*, 1108–1114.

Angst, J., Angst, F., Gerber-Werder, R., & Gamma, A. (2005). Suicide in 406 mood-disorder patients with and without long-term medication: A 40 to 44 years' follow-up. *Archives of Suicide Research, 9*, 279–300.

Barbini, B., Colombo, C., Benedetti, F., Campori, E., Bellodi, L., & Smeraldi, E. (1998). The unipolar–bipolar dichotomy and the response to sleep deprivation. *Psychiatric Research, 79*, 43–50.

Barnett, J. H., Huang, J., Perlis, R. H., Young, M. M., Rosenbaum, J. F., Nierenberg, A. A., et al. (2011). Personality and bipolar disorder: Dissecting state and trait associations between mood and personality. *Psychological Medicine, 41*, 1593–1604.

Barrowclough, C., & Hooley, J. M. (2003). Attributions and expressed emotion: A review. *Clinical Psychology Review, 23*, 849–880.

Bender, R. E., & Alloy, L. B. (2011). Life stress and kindling in bipolar disorder: Review of the evidence and integration with emerging biopsychosocial theories. *Clinical Psychology Review, 31*, 383–398.

Bermpohl, F., Kahnt, T., Dalanay, U., Hägele, C., Sajonz, B., Wegner, T., et al. (2010). Altered representation of expected value in the orbitofrontal cortex in mania. *Human Brain Mapping, 31*, 958–969.

Brown, G. W., & Andrews, B. (1986). Social support and depression. In M. H. Appley & R. Trumbull (Eds.), *Dynamics of stress: Physiological, psychological, and social perspectives* (pp. 257–282). New York: Plenum Press.

Brown, G. W., & Harris, T. O. (1978). *The Bedford College Life Events and Difficulty Schedule: Directory of contextual threat ratings of events*. London: University of London, Bedford College.

Burghy, C. A., Stodola, D. E., Ruttle, P. L., Molloy, E. K., Armstrong, J. M., Oler, J. A., et al. (2012). Developmental pathways to amygdala–prefrontal function and internalizing symptoms in adolescence. *Nature Neuroscience, 15*, 1736–1741.

Butzlaff, R. L., & Hooley, J. M. (1998). Expressed emotion and psychiatric relapse: A meta-analysis. *Archives of General Psychiatry, 55*, 547–552.

Carver, C. S., & White, T. L. (1994). Behavioral inhibition, behavioral activation, and affective responses to impending reward and punishment: The BIS/BAS scales. *Journal of Personality and Social Psychology, 67*, 319–333.

Chen, C. H., Suckling, J., Lennox, B. R., Ooi, C., & Bullmore, E. T. (2011). A quantitative meta-analysis of fMRI studies in bipolar disorder. *Bipolar Disorders, 13*, 1–15.

Cho, H. J., Meira-Lima, I., Cordeiro, Q., Michelon, L., Sham, P., Vallada, H., et al. (2005). Population-based and family-based studies on the serotonin transporter gene polymorphisms and BD: A systematic review and meta-analysis. *Molecular Psychiatry, 10*, 771–781.

Clayton, P. J., Ernst, C., & Angst, J. (1994). Premorbid personality traits of men who develop unipolar or bipolar disorders. *European Archives of Psychiatry and Clinical Neuroscience, 243*, 340–346.

Cohen, A. N., Hammen, C., Henry, R. M., & Daley, S. E. (2004). Effects of stress and social support on recurrence in bipolar disorder. *Journal of Affective Disorders, 82*, 143–147.

Colombo, C., Benedetti, F., Barbini, B., Campori, E., & Smeraldi, E. (1999). Rate of switch from depression into mania after therapeutic sleep deprivation in bipolar depression. *Psychiatry Research, 86*, 267–270.

Cousins, D. A., Butts, K., & Young, A. H. (2009). The role of dopamine in bipolar disorder. *Bipolar Disorders, 11*, 787–806.

Cross-Disorder Group of the Psychiatric Genomics Consortium. (2013). Identification of risk loci with shared effects on five major psychiatric disorders: A genome-wide analysis. *Lancet, 381*, 1371–1379.

Cuellar, A. K., Johnson, S. L., & Winters, R. (2005). Distinctions between bipolar and unipolar depression. *Clinical Psychology Review, 25*, 307–339.

Daruy-Filho, L., Brietzke, E., Lafer, B., & Grassi-Oliveira, R. (2011). Childhood maltreatment and clinical outcomes of bipolar disorder. *Acta Psychiatrica Scandinavica, 124*, 427–434.

Delvecchio, G., Fossati, P., Boyer, P., Brambilla, P., Falkai, P., Gruber, O., et al.(2012). Common and distinct neural correlates of emotional processing in bipolar disorder and major depressive disorder: A voxel-based meta-analysis of functional magnetic resonance imaging studies. *European Neuropsychopharmacology, 22*, 100–113.

Depue, R. A., & Iacono, W. G. (1989). Neurobehavioral aspects of affective disorders. *Annual Review of Psychology, 40*, 457–492.

Depue, R. A., Krauss, S. P., & Spoont, M. R. (1987). A two-dimensional threshold model of seasonal bipolar affective disorder. In D. Magnuson & A. Ohman (Eds.), *Psychopathology: An interactional perspective* (pp. 95–123), San Diego, CA: Academic Press.

Depue, R. A., Slater, J. F., Wolfstetter-Kausch, H., Klein, D., Goplerud, E., & Farr, D. (1981). A behavioral paradigm for identifying persons at risk for bipolar depressive disorder: A conceptual framework and five validation studies. *Journal of Abnormal Psychology, 90*, 381–437.

Dienes, K. A., Hammen, C., Henry, R. M., Cohen, A. N., & Daley, S. E. (2006). The stress sensitization hypothesis: Understanding the course of bipolar disorder. *Journal of Affective Disorders, 95*, 43–49.

Duffy, A., Alda, M., Tinneer, A., Demidenko, N., Grof, P., & Goodyer, I. M. (2007). Temperament, life events, and psychopathology among the offspring of bipolar parents. *European Child and Adolescent Psychiatry, 16*, 222–228.

Egeland, J. A., Hostetter, A. M., Pauls, D. L., & Sussex, J. N. (2000). Prodromal symptoms before onset of manic-depressive disorder suggested by first hospital admission histories. *Journal of the American Academy of Child and Adolescent Psychiatry, 39*, 1245–1252.

Ehlers, C. L., Frank, E., & Kupfer, D. J. (1988). Social zeitgebers and biological rhythms: A unified approach to understanding the etiology of depression. *Archives of General Psychiatry, 45*, 948–952.

Ellicott, A., Hammen, C., Gitlin, M., Brown, G., & Jamison, K. (1990). Life events and the course of bipolar disorder. *American Journal of Psychiatry, 147*, 1194–1198.

Fagiolini, A., Kupfer, D. J., Masalehdan, A., Scott, J. A., Houck, P. R., & Frank, E. (2005). Functional impairment in the remission phase of bipolar disorder. *Bipolar Disorders, 7*, 281–285.

Foland-Ross, L. C., Brooks, J. O., Mintz, J., Bartzokis, G., Townsend, J., Thompson, P. M., et al. (2012). Mood-state effects on amygdala volume in bipolar disorder. *Journal of Affective Disorders, 139*, 298–301.

Fowles, D. C. (1993). Biological variables in psychopathology: A psychobiological perspective. In P. B. Sutker & H. E. Adams (Eds.), *Comprehensive handbook of psychopathology* (2nd ed., pp. 57–82). New York: Plenum Press.

Frank, E., Kupfer, D. J., Thase, M. E., Mallinger, A. G., Swartz, H. A., Fagiolini, A. M., et al. (2005). Two-year outcomes for interpersonal and social rhythm therapy in individuals with bipolar I disorder. *Archives of General Psychiatry, 62,* 996–1004.

Fulford, D., Johnson, S. L., Llabre, M. M., & Carver, C. S. (2010). Pushing and coasting in dynamic goal pursuit: Coasting is attenuated in bipolar disorder. *Psychological Science, 21,* 1021–1027.

Geller, B., Craney, J. L., Bolhofner, K., Nickelsburg, M. J., Williams, M., & Zimmerman, B. (2002). Two-year prospective follow-up of children with a prepubertal and early adolescent bipolar disorder phenotype. *American Journal of Psychiatry, 159,* 927–933.

Geller, B., Tillman, R., Craney, J. L., & Bolhofner, K. (2004). Four-year prospective outcome and natural history of mania in children with a prepubertal and early adolescent bipolar disorder phenotype. *Archives of General Psychiatry, 61,* 459–467.

Gershon, A., Johnson, S. L., & Miller, I. (2013). Chronic stressors and trauma: Prospective influences on the course of bipolar disorder. *Psychological Medicine, 43,* 2583–2592.

Gitlin, M. J., Swendsen, J., Heller, T. L., & Hammen, C. (1995). Relapse and impairment in bipolar disorder. *American Journal of Psychiatry, 152,* 1635–1640.

Goldstein, T. R., Birmaher, B., Axelson, D., Goldstein, B. I., Gill, M. K., Esposito-Smythers, C., et al. (2009). Family environment and suicidal ideation among bipolar youth. *Archives of Suicide Research, 13,* 378–388.

Green, M. J., Lino, B. J., Hwang, E.-J., Sparks, A., James, C., & Mitchell, P. B. (2011). Cognitive regulation of emotion in bipolar I disorder and unaffected biological relatives. *Acta Psychiatrica Scandinavica, 124,* 307–316.

Gruber, J., Culver, J. L., Johnson, S. L., Nam, J. Y., Keller, K. L., & Ketter, T. A. (2009). Do positive emotions predict symptomatic change in bipolar disorder? *Bipolar Disorders, 11,* 330–336.

Gruber, J., Eidelman, P., & Harvey, A. G. (2008). Transdiagnostic emotion regulation processes in bipolar disorder and insomnia. *Behaviour Research and Therapy, 46,* 1096–1100.

Gruber, J., Harvey, A. G., & Gross, J. J. (2012). When trying is not enough: Emotion regulation and the effort-success gap in bipolar disorder. *Emotion, 12,* 997–1003.

Gunderson, J. G., Triebwasser, J., Phillips, K. A., & Sullivan, C. N. (1999). Personality and vulnerability to affective disorders. In C. R. Cloninger (Ed.), *Personality and psychopathology* (pp. 2–32). Arlington, VA: American Psychiatric Association.

Hafeman, D. M., Chang, K. D., Garrett, A. S., Sanders, E. M., & Phillips, M. L. (2012). Effects of medication on neuroimaging findings in bipolar disorder: An updated review. *Bipolar Disorders, 14,* 375–410.

Hammen, C., Henry, R., & Daley, S. E. (2000). Depression and sensitization to stressors among young women as a function of childhood adversity. *Journal of Consulting and Clinical Psychology, 68,* 782–787.

Havermans, R., Nicolson, N. A., & deVries, M. W. (2007). Daily hassles, uplifts, and time use in individuals with bipolar disorder in remission. *Journal of Nervous and Mental Disease, 195,* 745–751.

Heerlein, A., Richter, P., Gonzalez, M., & Santander, J. (1998). Personality patterns and outcome in depressive and bipolar disorders. *Psychopathology, 31,* 15–22.

Hillegers, M. H. J., Burger, H., Wals, M., Reichart, C. G., Verhulst, F. C., Nolen, W. A., et al. (2004). Impact of stressful life events, familial loading and their interaction on the onset of mood disorders: Study in a high-risk cohort of adolescent offspring of parents with bipolar disorder. *British Journal of Psychiatry, 185,* 97–101.

Hooley, J. M., Rosen, L. R., & Richters, J. E. (1995). Expressed emotion: Toward clarification of a critical construct. In G. Miller (Ed.), *The behavioral high-risk paradigm in psychopathology* (pp. 88–120). New York: Springer.

Hosang, G. M., Uher, R., Maughan, B., McGuffin, P., & Farmer, A. E. (2012). The role of loss and danger events in symptom exacerbation in bipolar disorder. *Journal of Psychiatric Research, 46,* 1584–1589.

Hyun, M., Friedman, S. D., & Dunner, D. L. (2000). Relationship of childhood physical and sexual abuse to adult bipolar disorder. *Bipolar Disorders, 2,* 131–135.

Johnson, L., Lundström, O., Åberg-Wistedt, A., & Mathé, A. A. (2003). Social support in bipolar disorder: Its relevance to remission and relapse. *Bipolar Disorders, 5,* 129–137.

Johnson, S. L. (2005). Life events in bipolar disorder: Towards more specific models. *Clinical Psychology Review, 25,* 1008–1027.

Johnson, S. L., Carver, C. S., & Gotlib, I. H. (2012). Elevated ambitions for fame among persons diagnosed with bipolar I disorder. *Journal of Abnormal Psychology, 121,* 602–609.

Johnson, S. L., Cuellar, A. K., Ruggero, C., Winett-Perlman, C., Goodnick, P., White, R., et al. (2008). Life events as predictors of mania and depression in bipolar I disorder. *Journal of Abnormal Psychology, 117,* 268–277.

Johnson, S. L., Edge, M. D., Holmes, M. K., & Carver, C. S. (2012). The behavioral activation system and mania. *Annual Review of Clinical Psychology, 8,* 243–267.

Johnson, S. L., & Fingerhut, R. (2004). Negative cognitions predict the course of bipolar depression, not mania. *Journal of Cognitive Psychotherapy, 18,* 149–162.

Johnson, S. L., Meyer, B., Winett, C., & Small, J. (2000). Social support and self-esteem predict changes in bipolar depression but not mania. *Journal of Affective Disorders, 58,* 79–86.

Johnson, S. L., & Miller, I. (1997). Negative life events and time to recovery from episodes of bipolar disorder. *Journal of Abnormal Psychology, 106,* 449–457.

Johnson, S. L., Sandrow, D., Meyer, B., Winters, R., Miller, I., Solomon, D., et al. (2000). Increases in manic symptoms after life events involving goal attainment. *Journal of Abnormal Psychology, 109,* 721–727.

Johnson, S. L., Winett, C. A., Meyer, B., Greenhouse, W. J., & Miller, I. (1999). Social support and the course of bipolar disorder. *Journal of Abnormal Psychology, 108,* 558–566.

Jones, S. H., Sellwood, W., & McGovern, J. (2005). Psychological therapies for bipolar disorder: The role of model-driven approaches to therapy integration. *Bipolar Disorders, 7,* 22–32.

Judd, L. L., Akiskal, H. S., Schettler, P. J., Endicott, J., Maser, J., Solomon, D. J., et al. (2002). The long-term natural history of the weekly symptomatic status of bipolar I disorder. *Archives of General Psychiatry, 59,* 530–545.

Karkowski, L. M., & Kendler, K. S. (1997). An examination of the genetic relationship between bipolar and unipolar illness in an epidemiological sample. *Psychiatric Genetics, 7,* 159–163.

Kato, T. (2007). Molecular genetics of bipolar disorder and depression. *Psychiatry and Clinical Neurosciences, 61,* 3–19.

Kieseppa, T., Partonen, T., Haukka, J., Kaprio, J., & Lonnqvist, J. (2004). High concordance of bipolar I disorder in a nationwide sample of twins. *American Journal of Psychiatry, 161,* 1814–1821.

Kim, E. Y., & Miklowitz, D. J. (2004). Expressed emotion as a predictor of outcome among bipolar patients undergoing family therapy. *Journal of Affective Disorders, 82,* 343–352.

Klein, D. N., Kotov, R. &. Bufferd, S. J. (2011). Personality and depression: Explanatory models and review of the evidence. *Annual Review of Clinical Psychology, 7,* 269–295.

Kochman, F. J., Hantouche, E. G., Ferrari, P., Lancrenon, S., Bayart, D., & Akiskal, H. S. (2005). Cyclothymia temperament as a prospective predictor of bipolarity and suicidality in children and adolescents with major depressive disorder. *Journal of Affective Disorders, 85,* 181–189.

Kwapil, T. R., Miller, M. B., Zinser, M. C., Chapman, L. J., Chapman, J., & Eckblad, M. (2000). A longitudinal study of high scorers on the Hypomanic Personality Scale. *Journal of Abnormal Psychology, 109,* 222–226.

Lam, D. H., Hayward, P., Watkins, E. R., Wright, K., & Sham, P. (2005). Relapse prevention in patients with bipolar disorder: Cognitive therapy outcome after 2 years. *American Journal of Psychiatry, 162,* 324–329.

Leibenluft, E., Albert, P. S., Rosenthal, N. E., & Wehr, T. A. (1996). Relationship between sleep and mood in patients with rapid-cycling bipolar disorder. *Psychiatry Research, 63*, 161–168.

Lobban, F., Taylor, K., Murray, C., & Jones, S. (2012). Bipolar disorder is a two-edged sword: A qualitative study to understand the positive edge. *Journal of Affective Disorders, 141*, 204–212.

Lönnqvist, J. E., Verkasalo, M., Haukka, J., Nyman, K., Tiihonen, J., Laaksonen, I., et al. (2009). Premorbid personality factors in schizophrenia and bipolar disorder: Results from a large cohort study of male conscripts. *Journal of Abnormal Psychology, 118*, 418–423.

Lozano, B., & Johnson, S. L. (2001). Personality traits on the NEO-V as predictors of depression and mania. *Journal of Affective Disorders, 63*, 103–111.

Malkoff-Schwartz, S., Frank, E., Anderson, B., Hlastala, S. A., Luther, J. F., Sherrill, J. T., et al. (2000). Social rhythm disruption and stressful life events in the onset of bipolar and unipolar episodes. *Psychological Medicine, 30*, 1005–1016.

McGrath, P. J., Quitkin, F. M., & Klein, D. F. (1995). Bromocriptine treatment of relapses seen during selective serotonin re-uptake inhibitor treatment of depression. *Journal of Clinical Psychopharmacology, 15*, 289–291.

McGuffin, P., Rijsdijk, F., Andrew, M., Sham, P., Katz, R., & Cardno, A. (2003). The heritability of bipolar affective disorder and the genetic relationship to unipolar depression. *Archives of General Psychiatry, 6*, 497–502.

McQuaid, J. R., Monroe, S. M., Roberts, J. R., Johnson, S. L., Garamoni, G. L., Kupfer, D. J., et al. (1992). Toward the standardization of life stress assessment: Definitional discrepancies and inconsistencies in methods. *Stress Medicine, 8*, 47–56.

Merikangas, K. R., Akiskal, H. S., Angst, J., Greenberg, P. E., Hirschfeld, R. M. A., Petukhova, M., et al. (2007). Lifetime and 12-month prevalence of bipolar spectrum disorder in the national comorbidity survey replication. *Archives of General Psychiatry, 64*, 543–552.

Meyer, B., Johnson, S. L., & Winters, R. (2001). Responsiveness to threat and incentive in bipolar disorder: Relations of the BIS/BAS Scales with symptoms. *Journal of Psychopathology and Behavioral Assessment, 23*, 133–143.

Miklowitz, D. J., Goldstein, M. J., Nuechterlein, K. H., Snyder, K. S., & Mintz, J. (1988). Family factors and the course of bipolar affective disorder. *Archives of General Psychiatry, 45*, 225–231.

Miklowitz, D. J., Simoneau, T. L., George, E. L., Richards, J. A., Kalbag, A., Sachs-Ericsson, N. (2000). Family-focused treatment of bipolar disorder: 1-year effects of a psychoeducational program in conjunction with pharmacotherapy. *Biological Psychiatry, 48*, 582–592.

Moore, P., Landolt, H.-P., Seifritz, E., Clark, C., Bhatti, T., Kelsoe, J., et al. (2000). Clinical and physiological consequences of rapid tryptophan depletion. *Neuropsychopharmacology, 23*, 601–622.

Murray, G., & Harvey, A. (2010). Circadian rhythms and sleep in bipolar disorder. *Bipolar Disorders, 12*, 459–472.

Nikolaus, S., Antke, C., & Muller, H. W. (2009). In vivo imaging of synaptic function in the central nervous system: II. Mental and affective disorders. *Behavioural Brain Research, 204*, 32–66.

Nurnberger, J. I., Jr., Berrettini, W., Simmons-Alling, S., Lawrence, D., & Brittain, H. (1990). Blunted ACTH and cortisol response to afternoon tryptophan infusion in euthymic bipolar patients. *Psychiatry Research, 31*, 57–67.

Nusslock, R. R., Almeida, J. R. C., Forbes, E. E., Versace, A., Frank, E., Labarbara, E. J., et al. (2012). Waiting to win: Elevated striatal and orbitofrontal cortical activity during reward anticipation in euthymic bipolar disorder adults. *Bipolar Disorders, 14*, 249–260.

O'Connell, R. A., Mayo, J. A., Eng, L. K., Jones, J. S., & Gabel, R. H. (1985). Social support and long-term lithium outcome. *British Journal of Psychiatry, 147*, 272–275.

Phillips, M. L., Ladouceur, C. D., & Drevets, W. C. (2008). A neural model of voluntary and automatic emotion regulation: Implications for understanding the pathophysiology and neurodevelopment of bipolar disorder. *Molecular Psychiatry, 13*, 829, 833–857.

Post, R. M. (1992). Transduction of psychosocial stress into the neurobiology of recurrent affective disorder. *American Journal of Psychiatry, 149*, 999–1010.

Quintin, P., Benkelfat, C., Launay, J. M., Arnulf, I., Pointereau-Bellenger, A., Barbault, S., et al. (2001). Clinical and neurochemical effect of acute tryptophan depletion in unaffected relatives of patients with bipolar affective disorder. *Biological Psychiatry, 50*, 184–190.

Regeer, E. J., Krabbendam, L., De Graaf, R., Ten Have, M., Nolen, W. A., & Van Os, J. (2006). A prospective study of the transition rates of subthreshold (hypo)mania and depression in the general population. *Psychological Medicine, 36*, 619–627.

Rosenfarb, I. S., Miklowitz, D. J., Goldstein, M. J., Harmon, L., Nuechterlein, K. H., & Rea, M. M. (2001). Family transactions and relapse in bipolar disorder. *Family Process, 40*, 5–14.

Rowland, J. E., Hamilton, M. K., Lino, B. J., Ly, P., Denny, K., Hwang, E.-J., et al. (2013). Cognitive regulation of negative affect in schizophrenia and bipolar disorder. *Psychiatry Research, 208*, 21–28.

Salamone, J. D., Correa, M., Farrar, A., & Mingote, S. M. (2007). Effort-related functions of nucleus accumbens dopamine and associated forebrain circuits. *Psychopharmacology, 191*, 461–482.

Scott, J., & Pope, M. (2003). Cognitive styles in individuals with bipolar disorder. *Psychological Medicine, 33*, 1081–1088.

Selvaraj, S., Arnone, D., Job, D., Stanfield, A., Farrow, T. F., Nugent, A. C., et al. (2012). Grey matter differences in bipolar disorder: A meta-analysis of voxel-based morphometry studies. *Bipolar Disorders, 14*, 135–145.

Sher, L., Oquendo, M. A., Li, S., Ellis, S., Brodsky, B. S., Malone, K. M., et al. (2003). Prolactin response to fenfluramine administration in patients with unipolar and bipolar depression and healthy controls. *Psychoneuroendocrinology, 28*, 559–573.

Singh, M. K., DelBello, M. P., & Chang, K. (2012). Neuroimaging studies of bipolar disorder in youth. In S. M. Strakowski (Ed.), *The bipolar brain: Integrating neuroimaging and genetics*. Oxford, UK: Oxford University Press.

Sobczak, S., Honig, A., Nicolson, N. A., & Riedel, W. J. (1999). Effects of acute tryptophan depletion on mood and cortisol release in first-degree relatives of type I and type II bipolar patients and healthy matched controls. *Neuropsychopharmacology, 27*, 834–842.

Sobczak, S., Honig, A., van Duinen, M. A., & Riedel, W. J. (2002). Serotonergic dysregulation in bipolar disorders: A literature review of serotonergic challenge studies. *Bipolar Disorders, 4*, 347–356.

Sobczak, S., Riedel, W. J., Booij, I., Het Rot, A. M., & Deutz, N. E. P. (2002). Cognition following acute tryptophan depletion: Difference between first-degree relatives of bipolar disorder patients and matched healthy control volunteers. *Psychological Medicine, 32*, 503–512.

Staner, L., Tracy, A., Dramaix, M., Genevrois, C., Vanderelst, M., Vilane, A., et al. (1997). Clinical and psychosocial predictors of recurrence in recovered bipolar and unipolar depressives: A one-year controlled prospective study. *Psychiatry Research, 69*, 39–51.

Stange, J. P., Sylvia, L. G., da Silva Magalhães, P. V., Miklowitz, D. J., Otto, M. W., Frank, E., et al. (2013). Extreme attributions predict the course of bipolar depression. *Journal of Clinical Psychiatry, 74*, 249–255.

Stefos, G., Bauwens, F., Staner, L., Pardoen, D., & Mendlewicz, J. (1996). Psychosocial predictors of major affective recurrences in bipolar disorder: A 4-year longitudinal study of patients on prophylactic treatment. *Acta Psychiatrica Scandinavica, 93*, 420–426.

Strakowski, S. M. (2012). *The bipolar brain: Integrating neuroimaging and genetics*. Oxford, UK: Oxford University Press.

Strakowski, S. M., Sax, K. W., Setters, M. J., Stanton, S. P., & Keck, P. E., Jr. (1997). Lack of enhanced response to repeated *d*-amphetamine challenge in first-episode psychosis: Implications for sensitization model of psychosis in humans. *Biological Psychiatry, 42*, 749–755.

Strakowski, S. M., Stoll, A. L., Tohen, M., Faedda, G. L., & Goodwin, D. C. (1993). The Tridimensional Personality Questionnaire as a predictor of six-month outcome in first episode mania. *Psychiatry Research, 48*, 1–8.

Sullivan, A. E., Judd, C. M., Axelson, D. A., & Miklowitz, D. J. (2012). Family functioning and the course of adolescent bipolar disorder. *Behavior Therapy, 43,* 837–847.

Swann, A. C. (2009). Impulsivity in mania. *Current Psychiatry Reports, 11,* 481–487.

Talkowski, M. E., Chowdari, K. V., Mansour, H., Prasad, K. M., Wood, J., & Nimgaonkar, V. L. (2012). Genetics of bipolar disorder and schizophrenia. In S. M. Strakowski (Ed.), *The bipolar brain: Integrating neuroimaging and genetics* (pp. 203–214). Oxford, UK: Oxford University Press.

Townsend, L. D., Demeter, C. A., Youngstrom, E., Drotar, D., & Findling, R. L. (2007). Family conflict moderates response to pharmacological intervention in pediatric bipolar disorder. *Journal of Child and Adolescent Psychopharmacology, 17,* 843–851.

Van der Gucht, E., Morriss, R., Lancaster, G., Kinderman, P., & Bentall, R. P. (2009). Psychological processes in bipolar affective disorder: Negative cognitive style and reward processing. *British Journal of Psychiatry, 194,* 146–151.

van Erp, T. G. M., Thompson, P. M., Kieseppä, T., Bearden, C. E., Marino, A. C., Hoftman, G. D., et al. (2012). Hippocampal morphology in lithium and non-lithium-treated bipolar I disorder patients, non-bipolar co-twins, and control twins. *Human Brain Mapping, 33,* 501–510.

Wals, M., Hillegers, M. H. J., Reichart, C. G., Verhulst, F. C., Nolen, W. A., & Ormel, J. (2005). Stressful life events and onset of mood disorders in children of bipolar parents during 14-month follow-up. *Journal of Affective Disorders, 87,* 253–263.

Wehr, T. A., Sack, D. A., & Rosenthal, N. E. (1987). Sleep reduction as a final common pathway in the genesis of mania. *American Journal of Psychiatry, 144,* 201–204.

Wehr, T. A., Turner, E. H., Shimada, J. M., Lowe, C. H., Barker, C., & Leibenluft, E. (1998). Treatment of rapidly cycling bipolar patient by using extended bed rest and darkness to stabilize the timing and duration of sleep. *Biological Psychiatry, 43,* 822–828.

Weinstock, L. M., & Miller, I. W. (2010). Psychosocial predictors of mood symptoms 1 year after acute phase treatment of bipolar I disorder. *Comprehensive Psychiatry, 51,* 497–503.

Wender, P. H., Kety, S. S., Rosenthal, D., Schulsinger, F., Ortmann, J., & Lunde, I. (1986). Psychiatric disorders in the biological and adoptive families of adopted individuals with affective disorders. *Archives of General Psychiatry, 43,* 923–929.

Willner, P. (1995). Sensitization of the dopamine D-sub-2- or D-sub-3-type receptors as a common pathway in antidepressant drug action. *Clinical Neuropharmacology, 18,* 49–56.

Yan, L. J., Hammen, C., Cohen, A. N., Daley, S. E., & Henry, R. M. (2004). Expressed emotion versus relationship quality variables in the prediction of recurrence in bipolar patients. *Journal of Affective Disorders, 83,* 199–206.

Yatham, L. N., Srisurapanont, M., Zis, A. P., & Kusumakar, V. (1997). Comparative studies of the biological distinction between unipolar and bipolar depressions. *Life Sciences, 61,* 1445–1455.

PART III

DEPRESSION IN SPECIFIC POPULATIONS

Although depressive disorders occur in all demographic groups, cultures, and ages, their manifestations, meanings, treatments, and possible causes may differ importantly from one population to another. The seven chapters in this section detail considerations about the experience of depression in particular groups. Chentsova-Dutton, Ryder, and Tsai (Chapter 18) discuss a growing body of research on cultural differences in the expression and experience of depression. The topic of gender differences is perhaps the most extensive and developed theme among specific populations, and we note with sadness the untimely death of a pioneer and former contributor, Susan Nolen-Hoeksema. The topic is reviewed in a chapter by Hilt and Nolen-Hoeksema (Chapter 19), which continues to challenge simple unitary explanations of this disorder. Depression in children, discussed by Gibb (Chapter 20), and depression in adolescents, discussed by Rudolph and Flynn (Chapter 21), are presented as separate chapters in recognition of both the unique features of these groups and the enormous body of recent research on these topics. Davila, Stroud, and Starr (Chapter 22) provide an overview of the literature on depression in the context of couple and family relationships—including families with members who have bipolar disorder—and highlight conceptual themes in this area of research. Blazer and Hybels (Chapter 23) review the experience of depression in later life, a topic of increasing social concern. Finally, although suicide is not uniquely associated with depressive disorders, Nock, Millner, Deming, and Glenn (Chapter 24) address the relatively common experience of suicidality in depressed individuals and discuss its management.

CHAPTER 18

Understanding Depression across Cultural Contexts

YULIA E. CHENTSOVA-DUTTON, ANDREW G. RYDER,
and JEANNE TSAI

Yi, a young U.S.-born Hmong woman, is seriously distressed. She is having difficulty sleeping; she has lost her appetite; and she lacks interest in her studies. Yi also says that she has little energy and is having a difficult time balancing school and family obligations. Although she does not spontaneously use emotional terms to describe how she feels, when asked she agrees that she is unhappy and anxious. All these symptoms are consistent with DSM criteria for major depressive disorder (American Psychiatric Association, 2013). And yet Yi reports other symptoms that are not typically associated with major depression. She describes bodily aches and pains, especially in her stomach and liver. She has become particularly concerned about what other people think of her, making it hard for her to get along with her family. Finally, she reports that at night, the spirit of a disgruntled ancestor visits her, right before she is about to fall sleep. These encounters sap her energy. Although she says that she knows other people who have been visited by spirits, she is nonetheless concerned about experiencing these visits herself.

Cases like Yi's raise questions about how culture shapes the experience and expression of depression, with clear implications for assessment and treatment. On the one hand, diagnosable major depression is observed across cultural contexts, albeit with varying prevalence rates (Bromet et al., 2011). It disrupts lives worldwide, posing significant threats to people's productivity and well-being. Indeed, depression is projected to become a leading contributor to the global burden of disease by 2030 (Lopez & Mathers, 2006; see Kessler et al., Chapter 1, this volume). Given the costs of depression for individual sufferers and for society as a whole, it is tempting to rely on dominant Western[1] models of conceptualizing, assessing, and treating this disorder in cultural contexts that, like Hmong contexts, do not conceptualize its symptoms in the same way. Indeed, from this perspective,

---

[1] By "Western" we refer to a broad set of cultural contexts with historical ties to Western Europe, with majority populations of European origin (e.g., United States, Canada, Western Europe, Australia, and New Zealand).

a failure to diagnose Yi's symptoms as depression may delay treatment and prolong her suffering (Lee, Lytle, Yang, & Lum, 2010).

For this reason, it may not be surprising that much research and clinical work assumes that Western-based criteria for major depression reflect the underlying, culturally universal pathology of the disorder. In part, this is because this research has primarily taken place in the Western world. Therefore, much cross-cultural research on depression involves examining whether Western-defined depressive symptoms are recognized in non-Western cultural contexts (Jorm et al., 2005). This approach assumes that depression is similar to medical conditions that have a clear etiology and pathology leading to a specific set of symptoms that transcend culture.

In contrast, we argue that depression is distinct from many other medical conditions because it is not only a neurological phenomenon, but also a psychological and cultural one, and therefore cannot be explained without referencing all of these levels (Ryder, Ban, & Chentsova-Dutton, 2011). Take the case of gender differences in depression. Across many cultural contexts, women are more likely to develop depression than men. This pattern can be attributed to a set of biological vulnerabilities (e.g., stress reactivity, hormonal differences, genetic factors). Yet, one cannot fully explain it without considering psychological and cultural factors (e.g., increased likelihood of stress and victimization, body dissatisfaction, gender roles) (Hyde, Mezulis, & Abramson, 2008; Parker & Brotchie, 2010; see Hilt & Nolen-Hoeksema, Chapter 19, this volume). Indeed, exceptions to this pattern have been observed in some cultural groups, such as the Amish or Orthodox Jews (Egeland & Hostetter, 1983; Loewenthal et al., 1995). In these homogeneous and stable contexts that reinforce very clear gender roles, the prevalence rates of depression are similar for men and women. Such findings demonstrate how the study of culture and depression requires attention to the cultural context and to the interaction of biological and sociocultural factors.

In this chapter, we start by defining our terms before turning to the central concepts of normative and deviant cultural scripts and how they shape symptom presentation. We follow with two specific research examples, focusing on cultural scripts of somatization and positive emotions. Finally, we discuss future directions for research and conclude with some remarks on clinical implications of this work.

DEFINING DEPRESSION, OR SERIOUS DISTRESS

Evolutionary accounts postulate that depression represents a breakdown in an evolved and otherwise adaptive response to scarcity and loss (Nesse & Ellsworth, 2009). These explanations provide a plausible biological origin story for why it can emerge in many different cultural contexts. Indeed, research indicates that across cultural contexts, depression is reliably linked to environmental factors such as demanding climatic conditions, stress, unemployment and poverty, and lack of social support (for a more thorough review, see Chentsova-Dutton & Tsai, 2009), as well as to vulnerability factors such as high level of neuroticism or being female (Kuehner, 2003; Matsumoto, Nakagawa, & Estrada, 2009). How do we define responses to these stressors in ways that would allow us to capture cultural similarities and differences in depression?

Much research on depression across cultural contexts has relied on the *Diagnostic and Statistical Manual of Mental Disorders*, now in its fifth edition (DSM-5; American Psychiatric Association, 2013). In DSM-5, major depression is described as a period of prolonged dysfunction that is characterized by the key symptoms of depressed mood and anhedonia. As many anthropologists and cultural psychologists have argued, however, these criteria are not culture-free: the DSM definition of depression emerges from and is understood within a cultural context that emphasizes the uniqueness and autonomy of each person and the importance of personal experiences, goals, values, and preferences (Kirmayer, 2007). Key markers of healthy functioning in this context include promotion of the individual self, cultivation of positive feelings, and open expression of emotions to signal personal preferences (Heine, Lehman, Markus, & Kitayama, 1999). Accordingly, the DSM definition of major depression emphasizes deviations from these cultural norms and ideals. Furthermore, although the depression criteria include both psychological and somatic symptoms, the emotional symptoms of depressed mood and anhedonia are considered the "cardinal" symptoms, reflecting the Western emphasis on mental (vs. physical) states.

Finally, the DSM criteria describe depression as primarily intrapersonal. There is a striking absence of interpersonal symptoms, despite the fact that social deficits and dysfunctional communication patterns associated with depression are well documented in the literature (Hammen & Shih, Chapter 15, this volume; Joiner, Coyne, & Blalock, 1999). Indeed, in the opening case study, Yi's physical problems, like stomach and liver pains, and relational problems, like her inability to get along with her family, would not be counted toward a DSM diagnosis. All of these assumptions reflect a culturally specific set of values, norms, and ideals. Because the term *depression* carries this set of cultural assumptions, we prefer throughout this chapter to use a broader and less culture-specific term, *serious distress*, to describe a set of problematic and often prolonged responses to real or perceived failures or interpersonal losses (see Ryder & Chentsova-Dutton, 2012). Standard terminology (e.g., *major depressive disorder, levels of depressive symptoms*) is used when reviewing previous research based on systems such as the DSM.

Defining Culture

In defining culture, we begin with Kroeber and Kluckhohn's (1952) classic statement:

> patterns, explicit and implicit, of and for behavior acquired and transmitted by symbols . . . including their embodiment in artifacts; the essential core of culture consists of traditional . . . ideas and especially their attached values; culture systems may, on the one hand, be considered as products of action, on the other, as conditional elements of future action. (p. 181)

This definition emphasizes that culture exists "in the head" as ideas and "in the world" as institutions (e.g., family and legal systems), artifacts (e.g., advertisements, texts, songs), and practices (e.g., greetings, ceremonies). The idea of "cultural scripts" bridges these aspects of culture, describing specific sequenced patterns of meaningful ideas leading to observable actions in the world, which in turn reinforce the ideas held by the actor and observers. This approach to culture highlights the fact that people create cultural ideas and practices, and that these cultural ideas and practices in turn create people. Thus, culture and mind mutually constitute each other, or "make each other up" (Shweder, 1990).

Consider an example of this mutual constitution in the context of depression. One study showed that the editors and writers of popular Australian women's magazines promoted a way of coping with depression that reflected Australian individualistic values, specifically, the importance of "pulling oneself up by one's bootstraps" and managing one's own distress (e.g., Gattuso, Fullagar, & Young, 2006). Australians in turn endorsed this view of coping with depression (Kokanovic, Dowrick, Butler, Herrman, & Gunn, 2008). This example highlights the fact that people do not passively absorb culture but recreate it as observable scripts and, in doing so, reinforce or change the cultural contexts in which they live (Kashima, 2000).

Before turning to the literature on culture and depression, a brief comment on methodology is warranted. Cross-national differences in prevalence rates are one way of establishing at least the possibility of important cultural variation. A key conclusion of these studies is that prevalence rates of major depression vary dramatically across cultural contexts. A person in Korea or Japan has less than a 1-in-50 chance of meeting DSM criteria for major depression in the previous 12 months. In contrast, a person living in Brazil has a much higher risk, as high as one in ten (Andrade et al, 2003; Bromet et al., 2011; Chang et al., 2008). Most of these studies do not directly examine cultural variables; rather, one must infer them from country-level differences. Such studies are useful, as they may contain valuable clues about how culture shapes reactions to serious distress. Yet they are best understood as only the beginning of a sustained line of inquiry. Cross-national differences raise but do not answer questions about underlying processes, about *why* a difference is observed.

The ethnographic tradition with its "thick description" (Geertz, 1973) offers a contrasting approach to the study of culture and depression, focusing on the local cultural worlds in which serious distress is experienced and expressed. Many of the findings we present in this chapter are informed by this approach. The ethnographic method can help us determine whether a seemingly unusual symptom is normative, or is a recognized symptom of distress, in an informed, nuanced way. Yet this approach is also only the beginning. Research on culture and depression increasingly uses epidemiological studies *and* ethnographic data as dual starting points (e.g., De Jong & Van Ommeren, 2002; Guarnaccia, 2003). Such a multimethod approach depends on an informed model of the cultural scripts that shape how people experience and express distress.

NORMATIVE AND DEVIANT CULTURAL SCRIPTS

Experiences of serious distress are best understood in reference to two broad sets of cultural scripts. The first set, which we refer to as *normative cultural scripts*, comprises the full range of possibilities for a person in a given cultural milieu to perceive, think, feel, and act in ways that are experienced, and seen by others, as normal. Our understanding of these scripts is informed by research on the fundamental properties of scripts in cognitive psychology (Schank & Abelson, 1977), as well as by work in cultural psychology and psycholinguistics describing the role of scripts in understanding a given cultural context (DiMaggio, 1997; Lewis, 1989; Wierzbicka, 1999). Normative cultural scripts provide the background against which serious distress is understood, and can differ markedly depending on the cultural context. For example, parents of Chinese toddlers see shyness as developmentally appropriate and consistent with the normative script of how to behave with strangers (Chen et al., 1998). Any study of social anxiety among children in Chinese cultural contexts would need to take this into account. In other words, when studying distress in a given cultural context, one must start by learning more about local norms for thoughts, emotions, and behaviors.

The second set, which we refer to as *deviant cultural scripts*, comprises the various possibilities for a person in a given cultural milieu to deviate from these norms in ways that are nonetheless culturally comprehensible. These scripts describe unusual and/or undesirable perceptions, thoughts, feelings, and actions in ways that are familiar for people living in a given cultural context. Cultural scripts for serious distress comprise a subset of these scripts. Our conception of deviant cultural scripts draws on research conducted on a variety of interrelated constructs, including work on "illness schemas," "illness narratives," "illness representations," "explanatory models," and the "sick role" (e.g., Hagger & Orbell, 2003; Kleinman, 1988; Leventhal, Meyer, & Nerenz, 1980; Parsons, 1951; Shilling, 2002; Stern & Kirmayer, 2004; Weiss, 1997).

Deviant cultural scripts flag a person's experience as abnormal (i.e., pathologization) while also helping that person and those around him or her make sense of what is happening (Ban, Kashima, & Haslam, 2012). Research suggests that culture shapes the ways in which lines are drawn between normal and deviant reactions to the experience of living in an unpredictable world. Indeed, whereas serious distress is understood as a diagnosable medical problem in some cultural contexts, it is recognized as a normal part of being human in others. For instance, mild levels of depressive symptoms and heightened negative emotions are viewed as culturally normative in Eastern European contexts (Jurcik, Chentsova-Dutton, Solopieva-Jurcikova, & Ryder, 2013; Turvey, Jogerst, Kim, & Frolova, 2012). Eastern Europe is not unique in this respect: Germans report less desire to avoid negative emotions compared with European Americans (Koopmann-Holm & Tsai, 2014), and Spaniards tend not to view symptoms of depression that are triggered by external events (e.g., family member's illness) as pathological (Durà-Vilà, Littlewood, & Leavey, 2013). Indeed, some Iranians see "Western"-based symptoms of depression as consistent with the normal experience of falling in love (Dejman et al, 2010; Essau, Olaya, Pasha, Pauli, & Bray, 2013). These beliefs stand in contrast to North American views on serious distress. Over the course of the 20th century, North American cultural models have increasingly pathologized symptoms of distress and emphasized positive emotions as the norm (Horwitz & Wakefield, 2007). Given these differences, it is not surprising that the understanding of serious distress that prevails in one cultural context does not always translate easily to other contexts.

Once a person's symptoms cross the culturally shaped threshold for being seen as problematic or pathological, deviant cultural scripts help people identify and understand instances of serious distress and communicate them to others. Even within a single cultural context, descriptive studies of responses to serious distress reveal that its symptoms are very often numerous, confusing, and potentially overwhelming. They are known to span the range of bodily sensations, perceptions, attentional processes, thoughts, emotions, and social interactions. For example, studies examining Koreans and Korean American cultural contexts show that in the somatic realm alone, depression is associated with complaints of constipation, heartburn, loss of appetite, indigestion, abdominal cramps, numbness, weakness, dizziness, faintness, hot flashes, fatigue, tiredness, sore muscles, swollen ankles, stiff muscles, stiff joints, palpitation, heart racing, and chest pain (Saint Arnault & Kim, 2008). There is also the sense of an "aching heart" and feeling that one's "body is not listening" (Bernstein, Lee, Park, & Young, 2008), as well as the reports of emotional entrapment—the experience of having to hide negative emotions (Bernstein et al., 2008). It can be difficult for people to understand such a large and confusing set of distress-related changes and communicate them to others.

Deviant cultural scripts reduce this complexity by guiding attention toward some experiences that are considered important and worth attending to, and away from others (Ryder & Chentsova-Dutton, 2012). Korean cultural scripts of serious distress (e.g., *hwabyung, han*) emphasize feelings of anger and unfairness and somatic sensations of heat, dry mouth, and epigastric mass, and describe gradual progression from these symptoms to sorrow, self-blame, and acceptance (Choi & Kim, 1993; Min, Suh, & Song, 2009). In contrast, Puerto Rican scripts prioritize crying jags, difficulty sleeping, and visions (Koss-Chioino, 1999), whereas rural Nepalese scripts emphasize numbness and tingling (Kohrt et al., 2005). Returning to the example of Yi, a Hmong script for "soul loss" alerts her that something unusual, wrong, and possibly dangerous is happening. Although soul loss in Hmong contexts is uncommon and troubling (i.e., "deviant"), it is neither bizarre nor incomprehensible (Lee et al., 2010). Deviant cultural scripts of serious distress turn experiences that are alarming and confusing (e.g., "Something is profoundly wrong with me and I don't know what it is") into experiences that are troubling, but comprehensible and meaningful (e.g., "I am suffering from neurasthenia due to overwork"), with a label, acceptable explanations for the distress, and specific ways to address it.

Most cultural contexts foster a number of alternative scripts for serious distress that shift in their popularity over time (Gattuso et al., 2006; Pritzker, 2007). For example, Pritzker (2007) observed that Chinese people with depression often go back and forth in their use of bodily metaphors, locating depression sometimes in the heart and sometimes in the brain, each with different manifestations and implications. Karasz (2005), meanwhile, showed that European Americans can recruit depression scripts that include contradictory psychological and biological ideas about etiology. Furthermore, the relative availability of these scripts may vary over time. Particular deviant scripts, such as those for hysteria, neurasthenia, and chronic fatigue syndrome, emerge and disappear (Abbey & Garfinkel, 1991). For example, from 1996 to 2006, Americans became increasingly convinced that symptoms of depression represented effects of chemical imbalances and genetic characteristics rather than environmental factors (Pescosolido et al., 2010). This increase in the popularity of a biologically focused depression script is likely due to a number of factors, ranging from public education efforts (Regier et al., 1988) to the persuasive power of brain imaging (Dumit, 2003). These findings indicate that even within a single cultural context, researchers and clinicians need to attend to the range of scripts that are currently available in that context.

Although normative and deviant sets of cultural scripts inform one another (Rebhun, 1994; Tousignant & Maldonaldo, 1989), the relationship between them is not always straightforward. Sometimes, normative and deviant scripts describe contradictory patterns of emotions, thoughts, and behavior. For example, in European American cultural contexts, the deviant cultural script for depression emphasizes low arousal negative states (e.g., low energy) and emotional numbness. This pattern represents the reversal of a culturally normative script that places value on high-arousal positive states, such as excitement (Tsai, Knutson, & Fung, 2006) and on the open expression of emotions (Matsumoto et al., 2008). Indeed, depressed European Americans show blunted emotional response relative to nondepressed controls (Chentsova-Dutton et al., 2007; Chentsova-Dutton, Tsai, & Gotlib, 2010). This pattern of emotional reactivity, however, is not culturally universal. In contrast to European Americans, Asian Americans with major depression show normal or even intensified patterns of emotional reactivity. This pattern, in turn, violates Asian American normative cultural scripts that emphasize emotional moderation and control. In both cases, evidence is consistent with the idea that deviant cultural scripts of emotional reactivity violate normative cultural scripts of emotional reactivity.

Other aspects of deviant cultural scripts, however, represent exaggerations rather than reversals of what is culturally normal. For example, European American cultural contexts foster preference for monitoring and understanding internal psychological states and sharing them with others (Markus & Kitayama, 1991). Chinese cultural contexts, by contrast, discourage focus on internal emotional experiences and emphasize the monitoring and sharing of somatic symptoms and social references (Dere, Falk, & Ryder, 2012; Tsai, Simeonova, & Watanabe, 2004). The relative emphasis placed by depressed Chinese patients on somatic symptoms can be partially explained by endorsement of this normative cultural focus (Ryder et al., 2008). Moreover, this tendency is associated with traditional Chinese values in both students and patients, further supporting the interpretation that in this case, the deviant cultural script can best be described as an extension of the normative cultural script (Dere et al., 2012, 2013). Because deviant scripts can violate or exaggerate normative scripts, the two sets cannot be easily deduced from one another.

Further complicating the task of studying culture and serious distress, some people experience symptoms that fit neither normative nor deviant cultural scripts. For example, some patients with depression studied in England report very rare psychotic-like symptoms such as depersonalization or paranoid delusions (Hamilton, 1989). These people are distressed in ways that may be hard for others in their cultural context to recognize as depression (Rothschild et al., 2008; Schatzberg, 2003). Interestingly, the same symptoms are a prominent part of cultural scripts of depression in other cultural contexts, such as South Africa (Mosotho, Louw, Calitz, & Esterhuyse, 2008).

The degree of fit between the symptom presentation and available normative and deviant cultural scripts may affect the illness experience. We know that being identified as "mentally ill" can have stigmatizing effects but can also confer benefits. The label can enhance understanding and self-control and contribute to effective treatment seeking (Wright, Jorm, Harris, & McGorry, 2007; for a review, see Link & Phelan, 1999). In contrast, people whose symptoms cannot be easily identified or labeled within the realm of deviant scripts available in their cultural context may feel more frightened, experience frustration with ineffective treatments, and feel more misunderstood by health care providers, family, and friends. Thus, the study of cultural shaping of serious distress requires researchers to consider the culturally normative (i.e., normative scripts), the deviant-but-comprehensible (i.e., deviant scripts), and the bizarre-and-incomprehensible (i.e., unscripted) patterns of symptoms in a given cultural context.

In sum, cultural scripts of serious distress help people draw the lines between understandable responses to stressors and problematic distress. They also serve to emphasize and reinforce some symptoms over others, thereby reducing complexity and enabling people to understand symptoms or distress and communicate about them. Finally, like any aspect of culture, they compete for attention with other scripts and are a moving target due to historical change. How does understanding cultural scripts of normality and deviance advance research on culture and depression? Let us consider two of the best-studied scripts of serious distress, the somatization script of distress in Chinese cultural context and the script focusing on diminished positive emotions in North American cultural contexts.

TWO RESEARCH EXAMPLES

Somatic Symptoms in Chinese Cultural Contexts

One consistent pattern reported over the past thirty years is the emphasis placed on somatic symptoms in East Asian cultural contexts, most notably in China (Ryder & Chentsova-Dutton, 2012). Consider these symptoms of a Chinese patient described by

Lee, Kleinman, and Kleinman (2007): "head swelling, very distressed and painful in the heart, my heart felt pressed" (p. 4). These types of symptoms are recognized as deviant in Chinese cultural contexts. For decades, the predominant script used to describe this form of serious distress in China was "neurasthenia," a disorder characterized by overwhelming and persistent mental and physical fatigue (Lee, 1999). In Chinese samples, the affective and cognitive symptoms of depression that are so common in North American clinics were relatively deemphasized in favor of somatic symptoms such as chronic fatigue, weakness, sleeplessness, "heartache," and bodily aches and pains (Kleinman, 1982; Lee et al., 2007). Symptoms of neurasthenia tend to unfold according to a sequential script. The sufferer first complains of circadian dysfunction, in which she would be kept awake by "too many thoughts" during the night. She would then, not surprisingly, be exhausted during the day. Although emotional symptoms are not entirely absent from this script, they are described as consequences of the fatigue, rather than as the primary problem (Kleinman, 1982; Lee, 1998; Liu, 1989). The key symptom of low energy is alarming and explicable in Chinese contexts, fitting with traditional Chinese medicine's concerns with low *qi* (described as "life force" or "energy") and societal concerns with economic productivity. Proposed explanations for the emergence of this script include the idea that physical symptoms gain one better access to scarce health care resources (Yen, Robins, & Lin, 2000), the influence of traditional Chinese medicine (Cheung, 1995), and even political censure of symptoms such as "hopelessness" during the Cultural Revolution (Kleinman & Kleinman, 1995).

With recent historical changes, neurasthenia is receding in China while depression-like presentations are becoming increasingly common—perhaps due to globalization, increased competition in the marketplace of ideas, the passing of the Cultural Revolution, and/or changing roles in Chinese society (Lee, 1998; Lee & Wong, 1995; Ryder, Sun, Zhu, Yao, & Chentsova-Dutton, 2012). Similar moves away from the somatization script of serious distress have been observed among South Indians (Rao, Young & Raguram, 2007; for a popular treatment of this theme, see Watters, 2010). Knowing more about the ways in which cultural changes engender shifts away from bodily complaints and toward psychological distress can help researchers better understand relationships between these symptoms and advance our scientific and clinical understanding of serious distress.

On the other side of the globe, European American normative and deviant scripts that encourage reflection on emotion also beg for cultural analysis (Kirmayer, 2001; Ryder et al., 2008). Although these scripts may seem more natural than Chinese somatization scripts to researchers steeped in Western cultural contexts, they are also culturally shaped. A particularly interesting aspect of these scripts is the role of positive emotion, specifically, their presence in scripts of normality and their absence in scripts of serious distress.

Positive Emotions in European American versus East Asian Cultural Contexts

Although "depressed mood" has not been recognized as a key feature of depression across different times and places, research suggests that there is a shared understanding that negative experiences accompany serious distress across cultural contexts. An absence of *positive* emotions intuitively seems to go hand-in-hand with these negative experiences. Dampened levels of positive affect are posited to be central to phenomenology of depression, distinguishing it from many forms of anxiety (Watson, Clark, & Carey, 1988). After all, one might wonder, how can a person be happy, joyful, peaceful, or amused while depressed?

Indeed, studies conducted in North America and Western Europe show that people meeting diagnostic criteria for depression do experience and express diminished levels of positive emotion relative to those who do not meet these criteria (see Bylsma, Morris & Rottenberg, 2008; Rottenberg & Bylsma, Chapter 6, this volume). These deficits go beyond self-report: Psychophysiological research, along with animal work on reward responsiveness, dovetails with human behavioral studies in demonstrating that diminished anticipation and experience of pleasure in depression have neurobiological correlates (Treadway & Zald, 2011; see Pizzagalli & Treadway, Chapter 11, this volume). Dampening of positive emotions appears to be particularly pronounced for self-focused positive emotions, such as pride (Gruber, Oveis, Keltner, & Johnson, 2011), and for high-arousal positive states such as excitement and enthusiasm (Tellegen, 1985). Researchers have therefore suggested that cultivation of positive emotion may be key to reducing depression (Fredrickson, 2000).

Yet our understanding of the role of positive emotions in depression is incomplete without considering the cultural context in which they occur. In European American cultural contexts, positive emotions are considered functional and desirable (Bellah, Sullivan, Tipton, Swidler, & Madsen, 1985). These preferences are particularly pronounced for high-arousal positive states, such as euphoria or excitement, and self-focused positive emotions, such as pride (Eid & Diener, 2001; Tsai et al., 2006). Despite the documented psychological risks of valuing and pursuing high levels of positive emotions, such as disappointed expectations or neglect of social cues (Gruber, Mauss, & Tamir, 2011), European Americans rarely demonstrate awareness of the drawbacks (Uchida & Kitayama, 2009) and instead view positive emotions as central to optimal psychological functioning. The pervasive influence of these scripts is further illustrated by studies of emotional adjustments made by migrants and their descendants. One study suggests that acculturation to mainstream European American culture among Korean Americans is associated with increased willingness to endorse higher levels of happiness and hopefulness on depression inventories (Jang, Kim, & Chiriboga, 2005).

East Asian cultural contexts, in contrast, promote a more balanced perspective on positive emotions. Indeed, people in East Asian contexts are less likely to want to maximize positive emotions and minimize negative emotions than people in European American cultural contexts (Sims, Tsai, Wang, Fung, & Zhang, 2014). In part, the reason may be that East Asians recognize that feeling positive—especially self-focused and high arousal positive states—may invite jealousy from others or make a person less responsive to others' feelings (Uchida & Kitayama, 2009). As a result, people in East Asian contexts are more likely to experience negative feelings during positive situations (Leu et al., 2010; Miyamoto, Uchida, & Ellsworth, 2010; Sims et al., 2014) and to value low-arousal positive states, such as peacefulness and calm, which facilitate attending to others (Tsai et al., 2006; Tsai, Miao, Seppala, Fung, & Yeung, 2007) than are people in European American contexts.

How do these normative scripts regarding positive emotions affect experience and expression of serious distress? Studies conducted in East Asian cultural contexts or with Asian American samples suggest that a lack of positive emotions, particularly high-arousal positive emotions, is not an integral part of depression for these groups. For instance, discrepancies between how much people actually feel high-arousal positive states and how much they want to feel those states are associated with depressive symptoms (as measured by the Center for Epidemiologic Studies Depression [CES-D] Scale) for European American college students but not Hong Kong Chinese college students (Tsai et al., 2006). For the latter, discrepancies between the extent to which people actually feel low-arousal positive states and how much they want to feel those states are associated with depressive symptoms. These findings have been replicated with community samples of European American and Hong Kong Chinese adults (Tsai, Sims, Thomas, & Fung, 2014). These differences have implications for how depression is assessed across cultures. Widely used self-report measures of depressive symptoms typically include items that assess presence of positive affect, positive self-image, hopefulness, and life satisfaction. However, these items tend to emphasize high-arousal rather than low-arousal positive emotion and therefore miss the positive states that are valued in East Asian contexts (Hong & Tsai, 2012).

Indeed, research has demonstrated that positive items on depression inventories are less useful as markers of depression in East Asian contexts than in "Western" contexts (Iwata & Buka, 2002; Kanazawa, White, & Hampson, 2007; Yen et al., 2000). Intensity of trait positive emotions is negatively associated with levels of depression among students from European American cultural contexts; however, this relation does not hold for students from East Asian cultural contexts (Leu, Wang, & Koo, 2011). College students with clinical depression in China report higher levels of depressive symptoms (e.g., "I felt sad") but the same levels of happiness or hopefulness compared to their nondepressed counterparts (Yen et al., 2000). Similarly, when comparing their reports of positive emotion in response to the same stimuli in a laboratory setting, East Asians without depression are similar to their counterparts with depression (Chentsova-Dutton et al., 2010).

Taken together, these studies indicate that diminished positivity, particularly diminished high-arousal positive emotions, cannot be relied on as a core feature of depression in East Asian cultural contexts. Although lack of positive emotions such as pride and enthusiasm may signal an inability to conform to European American normative cultural scripts, they are not as relevant in East Asian cultural contexts. This suggests that preventive and clinical intervention aimed to cultivate self-focused, high-arousal positive emotions may be more likely to enhance the quality of life in European American than in East Asian contexts (Boehm, Lyubomirsky, & Sheldon, 2011).

FUTURE RESEARCH DIRECTIONS

Current research on the cultural shaping of depression points in many exciting directions for future research. First, researchers need to develop better ways of identifying and assessing normative and deviant cultural scripts as they are instantiated in the head and in the world. This process will depend in part on recognizing that serious distress is not only intrapersonal, but also interpersonal (see Hammen & Shih, Chapter 15, this volume). Although some researchers have acknowledged this emphasis by going beyond self-report methods to use daily diary or live observational methods to study the interactions of patients with depression with their partners (e.g., Papp, Kouros, & Cummings, 2010), much research still treats psychopathology as something that happens within an individual person. As more studies focus on the interpersonal impact of depression, it becomes apparent that cultural factors cannot be overlooked in this endeavor. We know that culture powerfully shapes interpersonal relationships; indeed, interpersonal relationships are one means by which cultural scripts are propagated. "Social support," "teasing," and other interpersonal phenomena carry culturally specific meanings and take place in culturally specific ways, reinforcing cultural norms via repeatedly evoking or enacting them (Campos, Keltner, Beck, Gonzaga, & John, 2007; Chen, Kim, Mojaverian, & Morling, 2012). Not only do individual people within a cultural context hold culturally salient beliefs and act on them, but they also tend to assume that other people hold these beliefs and enact them for broadly similar reasons. In other words, cultural meanings and practices, including those that are relevant to serious distress, are intersubjectively understood (Chiu, Gelfand, Yamagishi, Shteynberg, & Wan, 2010). Integration of cultural research with interpersonal research on depression is one example of a potentially rich landscape for future researchers to explore.

Future work should also aim to better understand the ways in which culture interacts with biological and psychological factors in shaping serious distress. We believe that an organizing principle for cultural-clinical psychology is the idea that culture–mind–brain can be understood as a single, mutually constitutive, multilevel system (Ryder et al., 2011; see also Kitayama & Uskul, 2011). Rather than privileging a single explanatory level, this approach conceptualizes key phenomena, such as expression of serious distress, vulnerability, or resilience, as system properties (Chentsova-Dutton & Ryder, 2013). Thus "depression" is not only a biological disease, nor is it only a set of cognitive distortions, nor is it only a culturally sanctioned way of communicating social suffering. Instead, "depression" is a profoundly distressing set of experiences involving disruptions within the single complex system that encompasses culture, mind, and brain. All levels are implicated in the maintenance of these disruptions—and all are ultimately implicated in their resolution (Ryder & Chentsova-Dutton, 2012).

For example, genetic sensitivity to environmental stressors has been linked to variation in the serotonin transporter gene. Such sensitivity is an individual-difference characteristic thought to be associated with increased vulnerability to depression (Caspi, Hariri, Holmes, Uher, & Moffitt, 2010; Uher & McGuffin, 2008). Indeed, in Western cultural contexts, this genetic sensitivity is associated with higher levels of depression in the presence of environmental stress (e.g., Zalsman et al, 2006). However, cultural contexts differ in the percentage of people who are genetically sensitive to environmental stressors (Way & Lieberman, 2010), and cultures with higher rates of genetic sensitivity actually show *lower* rates of depression. The reason for this reverse pattern may be due to how genetics interrelates with culture. Genetically similar populations tend to share broad similarities in cultural context; in this case, people from ethnic groups with a genetically higher likelihood of sensitivity to environmental stress tend to inhabit cultural contexts that foster collectivistic values (e.g., East Asian). Collectivism may serve to protect such genetically vulnerable groups against serious distress; in fact, some researchers have argued that it may even have evolved to do so (Chiao & Blizinsky, 2009). These findings suggest that the degree to which genetic sensitivity is linked to depression depends on the cultural context (Kim et al., 2010).

Thus, concern for the cultural does not mean bypassing the biological. Although we have emphasized culture in this chapter, we believe that some of the most exciting directions for research in this area require the contributions of genetics and neuroscience (see Lau et al., Chapter 9, and Pizzagalli & Treadway, Chapter 11, in this volume). To be transformative, however, researchers need to engage seriously with all levels, recognizing the evolved legacy of the human brain throughout culture while simultaneously acknowledging that the human brain is profoundly shaped by culture (Kirmayer, 2012). Future research should characterize ways in which genotypes interact with cultural models of emotions and social relationships in shaping how people respond to losses (see Sherman, Kim, & Taylor, 2009, for a model). It should also investigate the brain mechanisms responsible for shifting attention to culturally salient aspects of the phenomenal field, such as specific body parts, emotional responses, or social perceptions, to help gain a better understanding of the processes underpinning the ways in which deviant cultural scripts contribute to cultural variation in symptom presentation.

These are only a few of the many directions that cultural research on depression and serious distress might take. One final direction involves improving assessment and treatment. Cultural variation in symptom presentation has important implications for psychological assessment, but there is little work at present to guide us in thinking about, let alone addressing, these implications. We know that tailoring treatments to particular cultural contexts improves treatment outcomes (Griner & Smith, 2006), but we know little about what drives these effects. Preliminary evidence supports the roles of language match, inclusion of culturally relevant content, adaptation of clinician style to culturally normative communication patterns, and greater attention to family dynamics (Sue, Zane, Nagayama Hall, & Berger, 2009). There is also early evidence suggesting that a cultural consultation approach, bringing together health professionals, social scientists, and "culture brokers" to assess and discuss complex cases, is helpful in guiding clinicians working with patients of differing cultural backgrounds (Kirmayer, Groleau, & Rousseau, 2014). However, more research is needed to advance our understanding of how cultural ideas and practices play a role in the treatment process.

CONCLUDING REMARKS

We argued at the beginning of this chapter that we cannot simply deal with Yi's symptoms as her failure to understand "true"—meaning "Western"—depression. Indeed, we have reviewed the literature on culture and depression in order to argue for a more complex and, we believe, more compelling perspective. Culturally informed clinical research should concern itself with identifying the ways in which culturally normative and deviant scripts shape Yi's experience. We need to understand whether encounters with spirits are widely shared in Hmong culture and whether Yi's symptoms are consistent with Hmong and American scripts of normality and deviance. Understanding these scripts can help us better predict the ways in which Yi will cope with her symptoms and the consequences they will have for her psychological functioning. We believe that cases like Yi's present opportunities to bring a truly integrative and culturally informed perspective into the mainstream of clinical psychology. Moreover, this perspective goes far beyond the assumption that culture is only for minorities and migrants: Culture is an integral part of understanding any aspect of human behavior, including experiences of serious distress.

REFERENCES

Abbey, S. E., & Garfinkel, P. E. (1991). Neurasthenia and chronic fatigue syndrome. *American Journal of Psychiatry, 148*(12), 1638–1646.

American Psychiatric Association. (2013). *Diagnostic and statistical manual of mental disorders* (5th ed.). Washington, DC: Author.

Andrade, L., Caraveo-Anduaga, J. J., Berglund, P., Bijl, R. V., Graaf, R. D., Vollebergh, W., et al. (2003). The epidemiology of major depressive episodes: Results from the International Consortium of Psychiatric Epidemiology (ICPE) Surveys. *International Journal of Methods in Psychiatric Research, 12*(1), 3–21.

Ban, L. M., Kashima, Y., & Haslam, N. (2012). Does understanding behaviour make it seem normal?: Perceptions of abnormality among Euro-Australians and Chinese-Singaporeans. *Journal of Cross-Cultural Psychology, 43*(2), 286–298.

Bellah, R. N., Sullivan, W. M., Tipton, S. M., Swidler, A., & Madsen, R. P. (1985). *Habits of the heart.* Berkeley: University of California Press.

Bernstein, K. S., Lee, J. S., Park, S. Y., & Young, J. P. (2008). Symptom manifestations and expressions among Korean immigrant women suffering with depression. *Journal of Advanced Nursing, 61*(4), 393–402.

Boehm, J. K., Lyubomirsky, S., & Sheldon, K. M. (2011). A longitudinal experimental study comparing the effectiveness of happiness-enhancing strategies in Anglo Americans and Asian Americans. *Cognition and Emotion, 25*(7), 1263–1272.

Bromet, E., Andrade, L. H., Hwang, I., Sampson, N. A., Alonso, J., de Girolamo, G., et al. (2011). Cross-national epidemiology of DSM-IV major depressive episode. *BMC Medicine, 9*(1), 90.

Bylsma, L. M., Morris, B. H., & Rottenberg, J. (2008). A meta-analysis of emotional reactivity in major depressive disorder. *Clinical Psychology Review, 28*(4), 676–691.

Campos, B., Keltner, D., Beck, J. M., Gonzaga, G. C., & John, O. P. (2007). Culture and teasing: The relational benefits of reduced desire for positive self-differentiation. *Personality and Social Psychology Bulletin, 33*(1), 3–16.

Caspi, A., Hariri, A. R., Holmes, A., Uher, R., & Moffitt, T. E. (2010). Genetic sensitivity to the environment: The case of the serotonin transporter gene and its implications for studying complex diseases and traits. *American Journal of Psychiatry, 167*(5), 509–527.

Chang, S. M., Hahm, B. J., Lee, J. Y., Shin, M. S., Jeon, H. J., Hong, J. P., et al. (2008). Cross-national difference in the prevalence of depression caused by the diagnostic threshold. *Journal of Affective Disorders, 106*(1–2), 159–167.

Chen, J. M., Kim, H. S., Mojaverian, T., & Morling, B. (2012). Culture and social support provision: Who gives what and why. *Personality and Social Psychology Bulletin, 38*(1), 3–13.

Chen, X., Hastings, P. D., Rubin, K. H., Chen, H., Cen, G., & Stewart, S. L. (1998). Child-rearing attitudes and behavioral inhibition in Chinese and Canadian toddlers: A cross-cultural study. *Developmental Psychology, 34*(4), 677–686.

Chentsova-Dutton, Y. E., Chu, J. P., Tsai, J. L., Rottenberg, J., Gross, J., & Gotlib, I. H. (2007). Depression and emotional reactivity: Variation among Asian Americans and European Americans. *Journal of Abnormal Psychology, 116*(4), 776–785.

Chentsova-Dutton, Y. E., & Ryder, A. G. (2013). Vulnerability to depression in culture, mind, and brain. In M. Power (Ed.), *Handbook of mood disorders* (pp. 433–450). Chichester, UK: Wiley-Blackwell.

Chentsova-Dutton, Y. E., & Tsai, J. L. (2009). Understanding depression across cultures. In I. H. Gotlib & C. L. Hammen (Eds.), *Handbook of depression* (2nd ed., pp. 363–385). New York: Guilford Press.

Chentsova-Dutton, Y. E., Tsai, J. L., & Gotlib, I. H. (2010). Further evidence for the cultural norm hypothesis: Positive emotion in depressed and control European American and Asian American women. *Cultural Diversity and Ethnic Minority Psychology, 16*(2), 284–295.

Cheung, F. M. (1995). Facts and myths about somatization among the Chinese. In T.-Y. Lin, W. S. Tseng, & E. K. Yeh (Eds.), *Chinese societies and mental health* (pp. 156–180). Hong Kong: Oxford University Press.

Chiao, J. Y., & Blizinsky, K. D. (2009). Culture–gene coevolution of individualism–collectivism and the serotonin transporter gene. *Proceedings of the Royal Society B: Biological Sciences, 277*, 529–537.

Chiu, C.-Y., Gelfand, M. J., Yamagishi, T., Shteynberg, G., & Wan, C. (2010). Intersubjective culture: The role of intersubjective perceptions in cross-cultural research. *Perspectives on Psychological Science, 5*, 482–493.

Choi, S. C., & Kim, U. (1993). Indigenous form of lamentation in Korea. Han: Conceptual, philosophical, and empirical analyses. *Chung-Ang Journal of Social Science, 6*, 185–205.

De Jong, J. T., & Van Ommeren, M. (2002). Toward a culture-informed epidemiology: Combining qualitative and quantitative research in transcultural contexts. *Transcultural Psychiatry, 39*(4), 422–433.

Dejman, M., Setareh Forouzan, A., Assari, S., Rasoulian, M., Jazayery, A., Malekafzali, H., et al. (2010). How Iranian lay people in three ethnic groups conceptualize a case of a depressed woman: An explanatory model. *Ethnicity and Health, 15*(5), 475–493.

Dere, J., Falk, C. M., & Ryder, A. G. (2012). Unpacking cultural differences in alexithymia: The role of cultural values among Euro-Canadian and Chinese-Canadian students. *Journal of Cross-Cultural Psychology, 43*(8), 1297–1312.

Dere, J., Tang, Q., Zhu, X., Lin, C., Yao, S., & Ryder, A. G. (2013). The cultural shaping of alexithymia: Values and externally oriented thinking in a Chinese clinical sample. *Comprehensive Psychiatry, 54*(4), 362–368.

DiMaggio, P. (1997). Culture and cognition. *Annual Review of Sociology, 23*, 263–287.

Dumit, J. (2003). Is it me or my brain?: Depression and neuroscientific facts. *Journal of Medical Humanities, 24*(1–2), 35–47.

Durà-Vilà, G., Littlewood, R., & Leavey, G. (2013). Depression and the medicalization of sadness: Conceptualization and recommended help-seeking. *International Journal of Social Psychiatry, 59*(2), 165–175.

Egeland, J. A., & Hostetter, A. M. (1983). Amish Study: I. Affective disorders among the Amish, 1976–1980. *American Journal of Psychiatry, 140*(1), 56–61.

Eid, M., & Diener, E. (2001). Norms for experiencing emotions in different cultures: Inter-and intranational differences. *Journal of Personality and Social Psychology, 81*(5), 869–885.

Essau, C. A., Olaya, B., Pasha, G., Pauli, R., & Bray, D. (2013). Iranian adolescents' ability to recognize depression and beliefs about preventative strategies, treatments and causes of depression. *Journal of Affective Disorders, 149*(1–3), 152–159.

Fischer, R., & Van de Vliert, E. (2011). Does climate undermine subjective well-being?: A 58-nation study. *Personality and Social Psychology Bulletin, 37*(8), 1031–1041.

Fredrickson, B. L. (2000). Cultivating positive emotions to optimize health and well-being. *Prevention and Treatment, 3*(1). Retrieved from *www.unc.edu/peplab/publications/Fredrickson_2000_Prev&Trmt.pdf.*

Gattuso, S., Fullagar, S., & Young, I. (2006). Speaking of women's "nameless misery": The everyday construction of depression in Australian women's magazines. *Social Science and Medicine, 61*(8), 1640–1648.

Geertz, C. (1973). *The interpretation of cultures.* New York: Basic Books.

Griner, D., & Smith, T. B. (2006). Culturally adapted mental health intervention: A meta-analytic review. *Psychotherapy, 43*(4), 531–548.

Gruber, J., Mauss, I. B., & Tamir, M. (2011). A dark side of happiness?: How, when, and why happiness is not always good. *Perspectives on Psychological Science, 6*(3), 222–233.

Gruber, J., Oveis, C., Keltner, D., & Johnson, S. L. (2011). A discrete emotions approach to positive emotion disturbance in depression. *Cognition and Emotion, 25*(1), 40–52.

Guarnaccia, P. J. (2003). Editorial: Methodological advances in the cross-cultural study of mental health: Setting new standards. *Culture, Medicine and Psychiatry, 27*, 249–257.

Hagger, M. S., & Orbell, S. (2003). A meta-analytic review of the common-sense model of illness representations. *Psychology and Health, 18*(2), 141–184.

Hamilton, M. (1989). Frequency of symptoms in melancholia (depressive illness). *British Journal of Psychiatry, 154*, 201–206.

Heine, S. J., Lehman, D. R., Markus, H. R., & Kitayama, S. (1999). Is there a universal need for positive self-regard? *Psychological Review, 106*(4), 766–794.

Hong, J., & Tsai, J. L. (2012). *Cultural differences in ideal affect shape conceptions of happiness and depression.* Manuscript in preparation.

Horwitz, A. V., & Wakefield, J. C. (2007). *The loss of sadness: How psychiatry transformed normal sorrow into depressive disorder.* New York: Oxford University Press.

Hyde, J. S., Mezulis, A. H., & Abramson, L. Y. (2008). The ABCs of depression: Integrating affective, biological, and cognitive models to explain the emergence of the gender difference in depression. *Psychological Review, 115*(2), 291–313.

Iwata, N., & Buka, S. (2002). Race/ethnicity and depressive symptoms: A cross-cultural/ethnic comparison among university students in East Asia, North and South America. *Social Science and Medicine, 55*(12), 2243–2252.

Jang, Y., Kim, G., & Chiriboga, D. (2005). Acculturation and manifestation of depressive symptoms among Korean-American older adults. *Aging and Mental Health, 9*(6), 500–507.

Joiner, T. E., Coyne, J. C., & Blalock, J. (1999). Overview and synthesis. In T. E. Joiner & J. C. Coyne (Eds.), *The interactional nature of depression* (pp. 3–19). Washington, DC: American Psychological Association.

Jorm, A. F., Nakane, Y., Christensen, H., Yoshioka, K., Griffiths, K. M., & Wata, Y. (2005). Public beliefs about treatment and outcome of mental disorders: A comparison of Australia and Japan. *BMC Medicine, 3*(1), 12.

Jurcik, T., Chentsova-Dutton, Y. E., Solopieva-Jurcikova, L., & Ryder, A. G. (2013). Russians in treatment: The evidence base supporting cultural adaptations. *Journal of Clinical Psychology, 69*(7), 774–791.

Kanazawa, A., White, P. M., & Hampson, S. E. (2007). Ethnic variation in depressive symptoms in a community sample in Hawaii. *Cultural Diversity and Ethnic Minority Psychology, 13*(1), 35–44.

Karasz, A. (2005). Cultural differences in conceptual models of depression. *Social Science and Medicine, 60*(7), 1625–1635.

Kashima, Y. (2000). Conceptions of culture and person for psychology. *Journal of Cross-Cultural Psychology, 31*(1), 14–32.

Kim, H. S., Sherman, D. K., Sasaki, J. Y., Xu, J., Chu, T. Q., Ryu, C., et al. (2010). Culture, distress, and oxytocin receptor polymorphism (OXTR) interact to influence emotional support seeking. *Proceedings of the National Academy of Sciences of the USA, 107*, 15717–15721.

Kirmayer, L. J. (2001). Cultural variations in the clinical presentation of depression and anxiety: Implications for diagnosis and treatment. *Journal of Clinical Psychiatry, 62*(Suppl. 13), 22–28.

Kirmayer, L. J. (2007). Psychotherapy and the cultural concept of the person. *Transcultural Psychiatry, 44*, 232–257.

Kirmayer, L. J. (2012). The future of critical neuroscience. In S. Choudhury & J. Slaby (Eds.), *Critical neuroscience: A handbook of the social and cultural contexts of neuroscience* (pp. 367–383). Oxford, UK: Wiley-Blackwell.

Kirmayer, L. J., Groleau, D., & Rousseau, C. (2014). Development and evaluation of the cultural consultation service. In L. J. Kirmayer, J. Guzder, & C. Rousseau (Eds.), *Cultural consultation* (pp. 21–45). New York: Springer.

Kitayama, S., Mesquita, B., & Karasawa, M. (2006). Cultural affordances and emotional experience: Socially engaging and disengaging emotions in Japan and the United States. *Journal of Personality and Social Psychology, 91*(5), 890–903.

Kitayama, S., & Uskul, A. K. (2011). Culture, mind, and the brain: Current evidence and future directions. *Annual Review of Psychology, 62*, 419–449.

Kleinman, A. (1982). Neurasthenia and depression: A study of somatization and culture in China. *Culture, Medicine, and Psychiatry, 6*(2), 117–190.

Kleinman, A. (1988). *The illness narratives: Suffering, healing, and the human condition.* New York: Basic Books.

Kleinman, A., & Kleinman, J. (1995). Remembering the Cultural Revolution: Alienating pains and the pain of alienation/transformation. In T.-Y. Lin, W. S. Tseng, & E.-K. Yeh (Eds.). *Chinese societies and mental health* (pp. 141–155). Hong Kong: Oxford University Press.

Kohrt, B. A., Kunz, R. D., Baldwin, J. L., Koirala, N. R., Sharma, V. D., & Nepal, M. K. (2005). "Somatization" and "comorbidity": A study of *jhum-jhum* and depression in rural Nepal. *Ethos, 33*(1), 125–147.

Kokanovic, R., Dowrick, C., Butler, E., Herrman, H., & Gunn, J. (2008). Lay accounts of depression amongst Anglo-Australian residents and East African refugees. *Social Science and Medicine, 66*(2), 454–466.

Koopmann-Holm, B., & Tsai, J. L. (2014). *Focusing on the negative: Expressions of sympathy in American and German contexts.* Manuscript under review.

Koss-Chioino, J. D. (1999). Depression among Puerto Rican women: Culture, etiology and diagnosis. *Hispanic Journal of Behavioral Sciences, 21*(3), 330–350.

Kroeber, A. L., & Kluckhohn, C. (1952). Culture: A critical review of concepts and definitions. *Papers of the Peabody Museum of Archaeology and Ethnology, 47.*

Kuehner, C. (2003). Gender differences in unipolar depression: An update of epidemiological findings and possible explanations. *Acta Psychiatrica Scandinavica, 108*(3), 163–174.

Lee, D. T., Kleinman, J., & Kleinman, A. (2007). Rethinking depression: An ethnographic study of the experiences of depression among Chinese. *Harvard Review of Psychiatry, 15*(1), 1–8.

Lee, H. Y., Lytle, K., Yang, P. N., & Lum, T. (2010). Mental health literacy in Hmong and Cambodian elderly refugees: A barrier to understanding, recognizing, and responding to depression. *International Journal of Aging and Human Development, 71*(4), 323–344.

Lee, S. (1998). Estranged bodies, simulated harmony, and misplaced cultures: Neurasthenia in contemporary Chinese society. *Psychosomatic Medicine, 60*(4), 448–457.

Lee, S. (1999). Diagnosis postponed: Shenjing Shuairuo and the transformation of psychiatry in post-Mao China. *Culture, Medicine, and Psychiatry, 23*(3), 349–380.

Lee, S., & Wong, K. C. (1995). Rethinking neurasthenia: The illness concepts of shenjing shuairuo among Chinese undergraduates in Hong Kong. *Culture, Medicine, and Psychiatry, 19*(1), 91–111.

Leu, J., Mesquita, B., Ellsworth, P. C., ZhiYong, Z., Huijuan, Y., Buchtel, E., et al. (2010). Situational differences in dialectical emotions: Boundary conditions in a cultural comparison of North Americans and East Asians. *Cognition and Emotion, 24*(3), 419–435.

Leu, J., Wang, J., & Koo, K. (2011). Are positive emotions just as "positive" across cultures? *Emotion, 11*(4), 994–999.

Leventhal, H., Meyer, D., & Nerenz, D. (1980). The common sense representation of illness danger. In S. Rachman (Ed.), *Contributions to medical psychology* (Vol. 2, pp. 7–30). Oxford, UK: Pergamon Press.

Lewis, M. (1989). Cultural differences in children's knowledge of emotional scripts. In C. Saarni & P. L. Harris (Eds.), *Children's understanding of emotion* (pp. 350–357). Cambridge, UK: Cambridge University Press.

Link, B. G. & Phelan, J. C. (1999). The labeling theory of mental disorder: II. The consequences of labeling. In A. V. Horwitz & T. L. Scheid (Eds.), *A handbook for the study of mental health: Social contexts, theories, and systems* (pp. 361–376). New York: Cambridge University Press.

Liu, S. (1989). Neurasthenia in China: Modern and traditional criteria for its diagnosis. *Culture, Medicine, and Psychiatry, 13*(2), 163–186.

Loewenthal, K., Goldblatt, V., Gorton, T., Lubitsch, G., Bicknell, H., Fellowes, D., et al. (1995). Gender and depression in Anglo-Jewry. *Psychological Medicine, 25*(5), 1051–1064.

Lopez, A. D., & Mathers, C. D. (2006). Measuring the global burden of disease and epidemiological transitions: 2002–2030. *Annals of Tropical Medicine and Parasitology, 100*(5–6), 481–499.

Markus, H. R., & Kitayama, S. (1991). Culture and the self: Implications for cognition, emotion, and motivation. *Psychological Review, 98*(2), 224–253.

Matsumoto, D., Nakagawa, S., & Estrada, A. (2009). The role of dispositional traits in accounting for country and ethnic group differences on adjustment. *Journal of Personality, 77*(1), 177–212.

Matsumoto, D., Yoo, S. H., Fontaine, J. R. J., Anguas-Wong, A. M., Arriola, M., Ataca, B., et al. (2008). Mapping expressive differences around the world: The relationship between emotional display rules and individualism vs. collectivism. *Journal of Cross-Cultural Psychology, 39,* 55–74.

Min, S. K., Suh, S. Y., & Song, K. J. (2009). Symptoms to use for diagnostic criteria of hwa-byung, an anger syndrome. *Psychiatry investigation, 6,* 7–12.

Miyamoto, Y., Uchida, Y., & Ellsworth, P. C. (2010). Culture and mixed emotions: Co-occurrence of positive and negative emotions in Japan and the United States. *Emotion, 10*(3), 404–415.

Mosotho, N. L., Louw, D. A., Calitz, F. J. W., & Esterhuyse, K. G. F. (2008). Depression among Sesotho speakers in Mangaung, South Africa. *African Journal of Psychiatry, 11*(1), 35–43.

Nesse, R. M., & Ellsworth, P. C. (2009). Evolution, emotions, and emotional disorders. *American Psychologist, 64*(2), 129–139.

Papp, L. M., Kouros, C. D., & Cummings, E. M. (2010). Emotions in marital conflict interactions: Empathic accuracy, assumed similarity, and the moderating context of depressive symptoms. *Journal of Social and Personal Relationships, 27*(3), 367–387.

Parker, G., & Brotchie, H. (2010). Gender differences in depression. *International Review of Psychiatry, 22*(5), 429–436.

Parsons, T. (1951). *The social system*. London: Routledge.

Pescosolido, B. A., Martin, J. K., Long, J. S., Medina, T. R., Phelan, J. C., & Link, B. G. (2010). A disease like any other?: A decade of change in public reactions to schizophrenia, depression, and alcohol dependence. *American Journal of Psychiatry, 167*(11), 1321–1330.

Pritzker, S. (2007). Thinking hearts, feeling brains: Metaphor, culture, and the self in Chinese narratives of depression. *Metaphor and Symbol, 22*(3), 251–274.

Rao, D., Young, M., & Raguram, R. (2007). Culture, somatization, and psychological distress: Symptom presentation in South Indian patients from a public psychiatric hospital. *Psychopathology, 40*(5), 349–355.

Rebhun, L. A. (1994). Swallowing frogs: Anger and illness in Northeast Brazil. *Medical Anthropology Quarterly, 8*(4), 360–382.

Regier, D. A., Hirschfeld, R. M., Goodwin, F. K., Burke, J. D., Jr., Lazar, J. B., & Judd, L. L. (1988). The NIMH Depression Awareness, Recognition, and Treatment Program: Structure, aims, and scientific basis. *American Journal of Psychiatry, 145*(11), 1351–1357.

Rothschild, A. J., Winer, J., Flint, A. J., Mulsant, B. H., Whyte, E. M., Heo, M. et al. (2008). Missed diagnosis of psychotic depression at 4 academic medical centers. *Journal of Clinical Psychiatry, 69*(8), 1293–1296.

Ryder, A. G., Ban, L. M., & Chentsova-Dutton, Y. E. (2011). Towards a cultural-clinical psychology. *Social and Personality Psychology Compass, 5*(12), 960–975.

Ryder, A. G., & Chentsova-Dutton, Y. E. (2012). Depression in sociocultural context: "Chinese somatization," revisited. *Psychiatric Clinics of North America, 35*(1), 15–36.

Ryder, A. G., Sun, J., Zhu, X., Yao, S., & Chentsova-Dutton, Y. E. (2012). Depression in China: Integrating developmental psychopathology and cultural-clinical psychology. *Journal of Clinical Child and Adolescent Psychology, 41*(5), 682–694.

Ryder, A. G., Yang, J., Zhu, X., Yao, S., Yi, J., Heine, S. J., et al. (2008). The cultural shaping of depression: Somatic symptoms in China, psychological symptoms in North America? *Journal of Abnormal Psychology, 117*(2), 300–313.

Saint Arnault, D., & Kim, O. (2008). Is there an Asian idiom of distress?: Somatic symptoms in female Japanese and Korean students. *Archives of Psychiatric Nursing, 22*(1), 27–38.

Schank, R. C., & Abelson, R. P. (1977). *Scripts, plans, goals, and understanding: An inquiry into human knowledge structures*. Hillsdale, NJ: Erlbaum.

Schatzberg, A. F. (2003). New approaches to managing psychotic depression. *Journal of Clinical Psychiatry, 64*(Suppl. 1), 19–23.

Sherman, D. K., Kim, H. S., & Taylor, S. E. (2009). Culture and social support: Neural bases and biological impact. *Progress in Brain Research, 178*, 227–237.

Shilling, C. (2002). Culture, the "sick role" and the consumption of health. *British Journal of Sociology, 53*(4), 621–638.

Shweder, R. A. (1990). Cultural psychology: What is it? In J. W. Stigler, R. A. Shweder, & G. Herdt (Eds.), *Cultural psychology: Essays on comparative human development* (pp. 1–43). New York: Cambridge University Press.

Sims, T., Tsai, J. L., Wang, I., Fung, H. H., & Zhang, X. (2014). *Wanting to maximize the positive and minimize the negative: Implications for affective experience in American and Chinese contexts*. Manuscript under review.

Stern, L., & Kirmayer, L. (2004). Knowledge structures in illness narratives: Development and reliability of a coding scheme. *Transcultural Psychiatry, 41*(1), 130–142.

Sue, S., Zane, N., Nagayama Hall, G. C., & Berger, L. K. (2009). The case for cultural competency in psychotherapeutic interventions. *Annual Review of Psychology, 60,* 525–548.

Tellegen, A. (1985). Structures of mood and personality and their relevance to assessing anxiety, with an emphasis on self-report. In A. H. Tuma & J. D. Maser (Eds.), *Anxiety and the anxiety disorders* (pp. 681–706). Hillsdale, NJ: Erlbaum.

Tousignant, M., & Maldonaldo, M. (1989). Sadness, depression and social reciprocity in highland Ecuador. *Social Science and Medicine, 28*(9), 899–904.

Treadway, M. T., & Zald, D. H. (2011). Reconsidering anhedonia in depression: Lessons from translational neuroscience. *Neuroscience and Biobehavioral Reviews, 35*(3), 537–555.

Tsai, J. L., Knutson, B., & Fung, H. H. (2006). Cultural variation in affect valuation. *Journal of Personality and Social Psychology, 90*(2), 288–307.

Tsai, J. L., Miao, F. F., Seppala, E., Fung, H. H., & Yeung, D. Y. (2007). Influence and adjustment goals: Sources of cultural differences in ideal affect. *Journal of Personality and Social Psychology, 92*(6), 1102–1117.

Tsai, J. L., Simeonova, D. I., & Watanabe, J. T. (2004). Somatic and social: Chinese Americans talk about emotion. *Personality and Social Psychology Bulletin, 30*(9), 1226–1238.

Tsai, J. L., Sims, T., Thomas, E., & Fung, H. H. (2014). *Paths to increased well-being in older adulthood vary by culture: A comparison of European American, Chinese American, and Hong Kong Chinese adults.* Manuscript in preparation.

Turvey, C. L., Jogerst, G., Kim, M. Y., & Frolova, E. (2012). Cultural differences in depression-related stigma in late life: A comparison between the USA, Russia, and South Korea. *International Psychogeriatrics, 24*(10), 1642–1647.

Uher, R., & McGuffin, P. (2008). The moderation by the serotonin transporter gene of environmental adversity in the aetiology of mental illness: Review and methodological analysis. *Molecular Psychiatry, 13*(2), 131–146.

Uchida, Y., & Kitayama, S. (2009). Happiness and unhappiness in East and West: Themes and variations. *Emotion, 9*(4), 441–456.

Watson, D., Clark, L. A., & Carey, G. (1988). Positive and negative affectivity and their relations to anxiety and depressive disorders. *Journal of Abnormal Psychology, 97*(3), 346–353.

Watters, E. (2010). *Crazy like us: The globalization of the American psyche.* New York: Free Press.

Way, B. M., & Lieberman, M. D. (2010). Is there a genetic contribution to cultural differences?: Collectivism, individualism and genetic markers of social sensitivity. *Social Cognitive and Affective Neuroscience, 5*(2–3), 203–211.

Weiss, M. (1997). Explanatory Model Interview Catalogue (EMIC): Framework for comparative study of illness. *Transcultural Psychiatry, 34*(2), 235–263.

Wierzbicka, A. (1999). *Emotions across languages and cultures: Diversity and universals.* Cambridge, UK: Cambridge University Press.

Wright, A., Jorm, A. F., Harris, M. G., & McGorry, P. D. (2007). What's in a name?: Is accurate recognition and labeling of mental disorders by young people associated with better help-seeking and treatment preferences? *Social Psychiatry and Psychiatric Epidemiology, 42*(3), 244–250.

Yen, S., Robins, C. J., & Lin, N. (2000). A cross-cultural comparison of depressive symptom manifestation: China and the United States. *Journal of Consulting and Clinical Psychology, 68*(6), 993–999.

Zalsman, G., Huang, Y. Y., Oquendo, M., Burke, A., Hu, X. Z., Brent, D., et al. (2006). Association of a triallelic serotonin transporter gene promoter region (5-HTTLPR) polymorphism with stressful life events and severity of depression. *American Journal of Psychiatry, 163*(9), 1588–1593.

CHAPTER 19

Gender Differences in Depression

LORI M. HILT *and* SUSAN NOLEN-HOEKSEMA

O ne of the most striking demographic features of depression is that it affects about twice as many women as men. The National Comorbidity Survey (NCS) found a lifetime prevalence for major depressive disorder of 21.3% in women and 12.7% in men (Kessler, McGonagle, Swartz, Blazer, & Nelson, 1993). The absolute prevalence of depression varies substantially across cultures and nations, but the gender difference in depression remains significant across most demographic and cultural groups (Andrade et al., 2003; Bromet et al., 2011). The World Health Organization estimated that depression is the leading cause of disease-related disability for women in the world today (Murray & Lopez, 1996).

We review the epidemiology of gender differences in depression and describe research on the most prominent explanations for this difference, including biological, psychological, and social explanations. Finally, we suggest how these explanations may be integrated to best understand the gender difference in depression and provide suggestions for future research.

EPIDEMIOLOGICAL DATA

Patterns of Comorbidity

Depression is highly comorbid with many disorders, but patterns of comorbidity vary with gender. Women with depression are more likely than men with depression to have a history of anxiety disorders (Breslau, Schultz, & Peterson, 1995; Kessler, 2000). Furthermore, depression and generalized anxiety disorder are more strongly genetically related to each other in women than in men (Kendler, Gardner, Gatz, & Pedersen, 2007). Substance

Susan Nolen-Hoeksema passed away before this chapter was completed. She authored previous editions of this chapter and dedicated her career to understanding depression among women. She is greatly missed, and this chapter is dedicated to her memory.

abuse is also frequently comorbid with depression (Marcus et al., 2005), but women are more likely to report having developed depression before they developed an alcohol use disorder, whereas men are more likely to have developed an alcohol use disorder prior to depression (Kessler et al., 1997; Sannibale & Hall, 2001), suggesting that substance use is more often secondary to depression in women, whereas the reverse holds for men.

Suicidal behavior frequently occurs in the context of depression. For example, having a mood disorder increases the odds of a first suicide attempt by a factor of 5.2 (Nock, Hwang, Sampson, & Kessler, 2010). Suicide attempts and completions also show complex gender patterns. Women are much more likely than men to report suicide attempts (Brockington, 2001; Lewinsohn, Rohde, & Seeley, 1996). Men, however, are much more likely than women to die by suicide (Centers for Disease Control and Prevention, 2010). Men's greater rate of completed suicide may be due to the fact that they tend to choose more lethal means of suicide than do women (Canetto & Sakinofsky, 1998; Crosby, Cheltenham, & Sacks, 1999) and because of their higher rate of alcohol abuse (see Stack, 2000).

Gender Differences across the Lifespan

Whereas the prevalence of depression increases from childhood to adolescence and adulthood before leveling off and decreasing slightly later in life (Kessler et al., 2010), the gender difference in depression follows a slightly different pattern. Epidemiological studies of children often find no gender difference in depression or that boys have somewhat higher depressive symptoms than girls (Twenge & Nolen-Hoeksema, 2002). At about age 12 or 13 years, however, girls' rates of depression begin to increase, whereas boys' rates remain stable or increase much less. By mid- to late adolescence, girls are twice as likely as boys to be diagnosed with unipolar depression, and they score significantly higher on continuous measures of depressive symptoms (Galambos, Leadbeater, & Barker, 2004; Hankin et al., 1998). For example, the NCS Replication Study—Adolescent Supplement, which surveyed 13- to 17-year-olds, found rates of major depressive disorder (MDD) and dysthymia to be higher among older adolescents compared with younger ones, yet the 2:1 gender difference was found for the total sample (Merikangas et al., 2010). The absolute prevalence of diagnosable depression varies across the adult age span, but the gender difference remains significant and is especially strong among older adults (ages 65+; Kessler et al., 2010).

Gender Differences across Cultures

The gender difference in depression is found across racial/ethnic groups in the United States and appears to be even more pronounced among black and Hispanic adults than among white adults (Blazer, Kessler, McGonagle, & Swartz, 1994; Williams et al., 2007). Among adolescents, Hispanic girls appear to be at particularly high risk for depressive symptoms. In a study of more than 1,000 young adolescents from a low-income community, we found that Hispanic girls had significantly higher depressive symptoms than white or black girls or any group of boys (McLaughlin, Hilt, & Nolen-Hoeksema, 2007). Research has found that acculturation factors are more strongly linked to depression among Hispanic girls compared with boys. For example, one study of Hispanic adolescents found that girls (but not boys) experienced a loss of family cohesion as they moved away from traditional gender roles. This was associated with subsequent depressive symptoms, suggesting a possible mechanism of the gender difference in depression among Hispanic individuals (Lorenzo-Blanco, Unger, Baezconde-Garbanati, Ritt-Olson, & Soto, 2012).

Cross-national studies typically find a similar gender difference in depression. For example, one study of 25 European countries found evidence of cross-national variation, but women generally reported significantly more depression than men (Van de Velde, Bracke, Levecque, & Meuleman, 2010). Another study of 18 countries varying in geographic region and income found that the average ratio of depression in women compared with men was 2:1 (Bromet et al., 2011), paralleling findings from U.S. samples.

Understanding the Gender Difference in Depression

The rather stable 2:1 gender ratio across cultures might argue for a biological explanation of gender differences in depression; however, variation in cross-national data supports social explanations. For example, one country in the recent large European study did not show a gender difference in depression (Van de Velde et al., 2010). Another large, cross-national study found that the gender difference in depression was much smaller in more recent cohorts compared with earlier cohorts, and this narrowing of the gender difference in depression was associated with increases in gender equality (Seedat et al., 2009). Although data thus far are largely correlational, precluding testing of specific mechanisms, Seedat and colleagues' findings suggest that increases in opportunities for women may reduce exposure to stress and subsequent depression.

The observed greater prevalence of depression among women compared with men may be due to women having a greater number of first onsets, longer depressive episodes, a greater recurrence of depression than men, or all of these. Data from several studies of adults (Eaton et al., 1997; Kessler et al., 1993) and children or adolescents (Hankin et al., 1998; Kovacs, 2001) suggest that the gender difference is primarily due to a greater number of first onsets of depression and not to differences in the duration or recurrence of depression (for a review, see Kessler, 2003; for an exception, see Essau, Lewinsohn, Seeley, & Sasagawa, 2010). This suggests that factors associated with gender contribute to more women than men crossing the line from dysphoria into a major depressive episode, but once individuals are in an episode, factors unrelated to gender determine the duration of episodes. Next, we explore biological, psychological, and social explanations for the gender difference in depression.

BIOLOGICAL EXPLANATIONS

The relatively consistent cross-cultural and cross-national preponderance of depression among women suggests that biological factors may play a role in the gender difference in depression. Most biological explanations have focused on the effects of gonadal hormones on women's moods. Recently, several studies have investigated whether women may carry a greater genetic vulnerability to depression than men. Both of these biological explanations are reviewed in this section.

Hormonal Variation

Hormones have long been thought to play a role in women's depression because some women experience new onsets of depression, or significant exacerbation of existing depression, during periods when levels of their gonadal hormones are undergoing substantial change, specifically, puberty, the premenstrual phase of the menstrual cycle, the postpartum period, and menopause. The literature on hormones and moods among women is vast (for detailed reviews, see DeRose, Wright, & Brooks-Gunn, 2006;

Korszun, Altemus, & Young, 2006; Somerset, Newport, Ragan, & Stowe, 2007; Young & Korszun, 2010). We summarize the major trends in the literatures on each of the periods of the life cycle during which women are thought to be especially prone to depression.

Puberty

Because the gender difference in depression first emerges during puberty in mid-adolescence, some investigators have suggested that the activation of gonadal hormone systems plays a role in the increase in rates of depression in girls. The evidence that hormonal changes play a direct role in the emergence of gender differences in depression in early adolescence is inconsistent. In a report on more than 1,000 U.S. children ages 9–13 years, depression levels in girls rose significantly in mid-puberty, whereas boys' depression levels did not (Angold, Costello, & Worthman, 1998). In analyses of hormonal data, testosterone and estradiol levels better accounted for increases in depressive symptoms in the girls than did pubertal stage or age (Angold, Costello, Erklani, & Worthman, 1999). Several other studies have found no relationship between pubertal stage, or hormonal levels, and mood in girls or boys going through puberty (for reviews, see Buchanan, Eccles, & Becker, 1992; DeRose et al., 2006).

Several researchers have found that the *timing* of puberty (compared with that of a girl's or boy's peers) rather than a specific stage of puberty is associated with risk for psychopathology. Girls who go through the peak pubertal changes (e.g., menarche, weight gain, development of secondary sex characteristics) several months or more before their female peer group are more likely than girls who mature around the same time as their peer group to show depression, anxiety disorders, eating disorders, substance abuse, and delinquent symptoms (e.g., Graber, Lewinsohn, Seeley, & Brooks-Gunn, 1997; Kaltiala-Heino, Kosunen, & Rimpela, 2003; Rierdan & Koff, 1991; Siegel, Yancey, Aneshensel, & Schuler, 1999; Stice, Presnell, & Bearman, 2001), although other studies have found no effects of early maturation for girls (e.g., Angold et al., 1998; Paikoff, Brooks-Gunn, & Warren, 1991). For boys, it may be that late maturation is a risk factor for increases in depressive symptoms (e.g., Siegel et al., 1999), although two other studies found that both early and late perceived timing predicted higher depressive symptoms for boys (Graber et al., 1997; Kaltiala-Heino et al., 2003). The mixed findings on the effects of pubertal timing may be due to differences in measurement method (e.g., informant, retrospective recall, perceived vs. actual timing; see Dorn, Dahl, Woodward, & Biro, 2006).

The reasons for these differences in the impact of pubertal timing on girls' and boys' vulnerabilities are not entirely clear, but several investigators have suggested that the meanings associated with pubertal changes are very different for boys and girls (see Brooks-Gunn, 1988). Girls are much more likely than boys to dislike the physical changes that accompany puberty, particularly the weight gain in fat and the loss of the long, lithe, prepubescent look idealized in modern fashion (Siegel et al., 1999). Girls who reach menarche considerably earlier than their peers (e.g., in sixth grade) are more dissatisfied and unhappy with their bodies (Rierdan & Koff, 1991). In turn, several studies have shown that more negative body image is associated with increased levels of depressive symptoms in girls compared with boys (Allgood-Merten, Lewinsohn, & Hops, 1990).

Premenstrual Phase of the Menstrual Cycle

The luteal phase of the menstrual cycle has been associated with greater stress reactivity (Young & Korszun, 2010) and worsened symptoms of psychiatric disorders, including mood disorders (Kornstein et al., 2005). Researchers have advocated the inclusion of premenstrual dysphoric disorder (PMDD) in the *Diagnostic and Statistical Manual of Mental Disorders* (e.g., Kornstein, 2010), and the recently published fifth edition (DSM-5; American Psychiatric Association, 2013) provides a diagnosis of PMDD for the first time (PMDD was included in the appendix of the previous edition of the DSM). PMDD includes the presence, during most menstrual cycles in the preceding year, of five or more symptoms, representing a significant mood disturbance, which emerge during the last week of the luteal phase of the menstrual cycle and begin to remit a few days after the onset of menses. Although many women self-report that they have mild to moderate physical symptoms (e.g., bloating and breast tenderness) during the premenstrual phase of the menstrual cycle, many fewer women (approximately 3–8%) have symptoms meeting the criteria for PMDD (see Somerset et al., 2007).

Evidence that PMDD is heritable (Chang, Holroyd, & Chau, 1995) and that premenstrual complaints can be eliminated with suppression of ovarian activity or surgical menopause (Casper & Hearn, 1990) suggests that the disorder has biological roots. However, investigations of hormonal imbalances in women with PMDD have resulted in few consistently positive findings (Somerset et al., 2007; Steiner & Born, 2000). The current consensus in the field is that normal hormonal fluctuations trigger biochemical events within the central nervous system and other target tissues, resulting in premenstrual symptoms in vulnerable women (Steiner, Dunn, & Born, 2003). In particular, serotonin systems may be dysregulated by normal hormonal changes in biologically vulnerable women, leading to changes in their mood. The selective serotonin reuptake inhibitors (SSRIs) are effective in treating premenstrual symptoms, even when the drugs are taken only around the premenstrual phase (Steiner & Born, 2000).

Postpartum Phase

More than half of all women experience postpartum blues (dysphoria, mood lability, crying, anxiety, insomnia, poor appetite, and irritability) in the first few weeks after giving birth. Although upsetting, these symptoms are usually not debilitating and typically subside within 2–3 weeks' postpartum. *Postpartum depression* is the term used for an episode of major depression that occurs within the first several weeks after giving birth. Major depression with postpartum onset can be very debilitating and, if not treated, can linger for months or more (Flynn, 2005).

A meta-analysis of studies of postpartum depression found that 13% of women experience a depressive episode severe enough to qualify for a diagnosis of major depression in the first few weeks after giving birth, a rate not significantly higher than the approximately 12% of nonpostpartum women who are depressed in the same time period (O'Hara & Swain, 1996). A very large Danish study, however, found that women in the postpartum phase were at increased risk for depression compared with women who were not in the postpartum period (Munk-Olsen, Laursen, Pedersen, Mors, & Mortensen, 2006). The researchers compared more than 1 million adults who had become new parents during a designated period with adults who had not become parents during the same period on rates of hospital admissions or outpatient visits for mental disorders. New mothers had a much higher risk of unipolar depressive disorders in the first 5 months after birth and of any mental disorder in the first 3 months, compared with women who were not new mothers. Based on these findings, some researchers have argued that the postpartum specifier for MDD be extended from 4 weeks after giving birth to 3 months for the fifth edition of the DSM (e.g., Kornstein, 2010). The only change related to the postpartum specifier for DSM-5 is a name change to "peripartum onset" to reflect that many episodes of MDD related to childbirth actually begin during pregnancy (American Psychiatric Association, 2013).

Because the onset of major depression during the postpartum phase coincides with large changes in levels of estrogen, progesterone, and several other hormones, these changes have been thought to play a causal role (Steiner, Dunn, & Born, 2003). Studies comparing women with and without postpartum depression have failed to find consistent hormonal differences, however (Somerset et al., 2007). Also, studies show that women with postpartum depression often have family or personal histories of depression prior to becoming pregnant (O'Hara & Swain, 1996; Steiner & Tam, 1999). Thus it may be primarily women with an underlying vulnerability to depression who tend to develop postpartum depression.

Menopause

Perimenopause is the period immediately before menopause, from the time when the hormonal and clinical features of approaching menopause begin until the end of the first year after menopause. During menopause, estrogen levels decline gradually. Symptoms associated with this decline include hot flashes, night sweats, and vaginal dryness. The Harvard Study of Moods and Cycles followed a group of women ages 36–45 through the transition to menopause and found a twofold increase in new onsets of depression in those who entered perimenopause (Cohen, Soares, Vitonis, Otto, & Harlow, 2006). Some studies comparing women known to be in perimenopause or menopause with women who are not undergoing these biological changes have found that perimenopausal or menopausal women have higher levels of depressive symptoms or general negative mood (e.g., Bromberger et al., 2001; Freeman, Sammel, Lin, & Nelson, 2006; for exceptions, see Avis, 2003). Freeman and colleagues' (2006) longitudinal study of women also found that menopause was associated with a 2.5 times greater increase in risk for developing a first depressive episode. Interestingly, variable levels of estradiol (both low and high relative to each woman's mean level) predicted depression, suggesting that rapidly changing hormone levels may trigger depression.

Gonadal Hormone Effects on the Serotonin System and HPA Axis

There are multiple, complex relationships between gonadal hormones and the neurotransmitters that regulate mood, including serotonin. Estrogens, in particular, have profound effects on serotonergic function, from modulating pre- and postsynaptic serotonin receptors and serotonin reuptake to enhancing and diminishing serotonin synthesis and catabolism, respectively (Amin, Canli, & Epperson, 2005; Steiner et al., 2003). Interestingly, studies have found gender differences in response to pharmacological treatment of depression, with women responding better to SSRI antidepressants and men to tricyclic antidepressants (e.g., Kornstein et al., 2000).

There are also important interactions between ovarian hormones and the major stress-response system, the hypothalamic–pituitary–adrenal (HPA) axis. When the HPA axis is activated, a cascade of activity ends with cortisol output, which typically acts as a negative feedback loop to control the stress response. Depression has been associated with problems in this negative feedback, resulting in hypercortisolemia (see Gillespie & Nemeroff, 2005). Ovarian hormones help regulate the magnitude of the stress response, and they are associated with dysregulated HPA-axis functioning in women with depression (see Young & Korszun, 2010), suggesting a role of hormones in understanding the gender difference in depression.

In sum, though few studies have found linear associations between hormone levels and mood, women seem to be more susceptible to depression during times when hormone levels vary the most. Thus it appears that the rapidly changing hormone levels women experience may make them more vulnerable to depression (Young & Korszun, 2010).

Genetic Factors

In addition to hormones, genetic factors have been examined with respect to gender differences in depression. Family history studies show that depression runs in families, particularly among female members (MacKinnon, Jamison, & DePaulo, 1997). Several studies show greater genetic effects of major depression among females than among males (e.g., Bierut et al., 1999; Boomsma et al., 2000; Happonen et al., 2002; Jacobson & Rowe, 1999; Jansson et al., 2004; Kendler, Gatz, Gardner, & Pedersen, 2006; Silberg et al., 1999). Other studies find greater genetic effects in males than in females (Rice, Harold, & Thapar, 2002) or no gender differences in genetic effects (e.g., Kendler & Prescott, 1999; Rutter, Silberg, O'Connor, & Simonoff, 1999; Thapar & McGuffin, 1994). A recent review of studies on the heritability of depression suggests that there is greater evidence of genetic factors being associated with depression later in development, such that adult and adolescent studies find greater evidence of genetic effects than child studies; however, this same review, which focused on youth studies, suggested that the gender differences in genetic effects were small and mixed (Franic, Middledorp, Dolan, Ligthart, & Boomsma, 2010). Thus there is at best mixed evidence that women's greater vulnerability to depression is genetically based. It may be that women have a greater genetic vulnerability to certain risk factors for depression (e.g., affiliative needs or experiencing stressful life events, especially social stressors beginning in adolescence) rather than a greater genetic vulnerability to depression per se (see Rudolph & Flynn, Chapter 21, this volume; Silberg et al., 1999).

In addition to heritability studies, there have been several studies examining specific genotypes that predict depression, and some gender differences have emerged in this research. Although a thorough review of this literature is beyond the scope of this chapter, we provide an illustrative example involving the serotonin transporter gene (*5-HTTLPR*).

Variation in a polymorphism of the serotonin transporter gene (*5-HTTLPR*) has been associated with depression in a number of studies, especially in interaction with negative life stress (see Caspi, Hariri, Holmes, Uher, & Moffitt, 2010). Individuals with one or two copies of the short allele of the gene are thought to be more vulnerable to developing depression in the face of stress, perhaps because of heightened stress reactivity. A handful of studies have found that gender moderates this association such that the interaction between being an *s*-carrier and negative life stress predicting depression is only significant for females (e.g., Brummett et al., 2008; Hammen, Brennan, Keenan-Miller, Hazel, & Najman, 2010; Sjoberg et al., 2006). There are many possible explanations for the gender-specific findings, including the possibility of the serotonin system being more strongly related to depression in women, perhaps through the role of ovarian hormones in the serotonin system or the HPA axis.

Although association studies involving other genes related to depression have found gender differences (e.g., see Bradley et al., 2008, on the corticotropin-releasing hormone type 1 receptor gene), research has been rather limited. Additionally, although large genomewide association studies (GWAS) have found genetic variants associated with depression, they have not examined gender differences (e.g., Cross-Disorder Group of the Psychiatric Genomics Consortium, 2013; McMahon et al., 2010). In sum, there is mixed evidence regarding women's greater genetic vulnerability to depression. Future research may further explore gender as a moderator in association studies of gene–environment interactions predicting depression.

Psychological Explanations

Several psychological factors have been associated with depression, including various cognitive and interpersonal vulnerabilities. Because a review of this literature and associated gender differences would be beyond the scope of this chapter (for reviews, see Nolen-Hoeksema, 1990; Nolen-Hoeksema & Girgus, 1994), we focus on two psychological variables that have been studied extensively in relation to the gender difference in depression over the past several years: rumination and interpersonal orientation.

Rumination

Rumination is the tendency to focus on one's symptoms of distress and the possible causes and consequences of these symptoms in a repetitive and passive manner rather than in an active, problem-solving manner (Nolen-Hoeksema, 1991; Nolen-Hoeksema, Wisco, & Lyubomirsky, 2008). When people ruminate, they have thoughts such as "Why am I so unmotivated? I just can't get going. I'm never going to get my work done feeling this way." Although some rumination may be a natural response to distress and depression, there are stable individual differences in the tendency to ruminate (Nolen-Hoeksema & Davis, 1999). People who ruminate a great deal in response to sad moods have longer periods of depressive symptoms and are more likely to be diagnosed with MDD (Aldao, Nolen-Hoeksema, & Schweizer, 2010; Nolen-Hoeksema, 2000; Rood, Bogels, Nolen-Hoeksema, & Schouten, 2009). The effects of rumination on depression over time remain significant even after accounting for baseline levels of depression.

Women are more likely than men to ruminate in response to sad, depressed, or anxious moods (Nolen-Hoeksema & Jackson, 2001; Nolen-Hoeksema, Larson, & Grayson, 1999). The gender difference in rumination is found both in self-report survey and interview studies, as well as in laboratory studies in which women's and men's responses to sad moods are observed (Butler & Nolen-Hoeksema, 1994). In turn, when statistically controlling for gender differences in rumination, the gender difference in depression becomes nonsignificant, suggesting that rumination helps to account for the gender difference in depression (e.g., Nolen-Hoeksema et al., 1999). We found evidence for this same pattern among young adolescents in a prospective study: Adolescent girls reported ruminating more than boys, and the gender difference in rumination statistically accounted for the gender difference in depression (Hilt, McLaughlin, & Nolen-Hoeksema, 2010).

We noted earlier that the gender difference in depression is found for onsets but not for the duration of episodes. Interestingly, several researchers have found that rumination predicts new onsets of major depression but does not predict the duration of episodes of major depression (see Nolen-Hoeksema et al., 2008). Although this contradicts the original formulation of rumination (Nolen-Hoeksema, 1991), it parallels the findings that women have more onsets but not longer episodes of depression than men. Thus a greater tendency to ruminate may lead more women than men to transition from dysphoria to major depression, but once a woman (or a man) has crossed that line, other processes may influence the duration of episodes.

Interpersonal Orientation

One of the most consistent psychological differences between women and men is in interpersonal orientation (Feingold, 1994). Women are more likely than men to feel strong emotional ties with a wide range of people in their lives, to see their roles vis-à-vis others (i.e., mother, daughter, wife/partner) as central to their self-concepts, to care what others think of them, and to be emotionally affected by events in the lives of other people. An interpersonal orientation leads women to develop strong social support networks that can buffer them against adversity. For some women, however, this interpersonal orientation can develop into excessive concern about their relationships with others, which leads them to silence their own wants and needs in favor of maintaining a positive emotional tone in the relationships and to feel too responsible for the quality of the relationship (Helgeson, 1994; Jack, 1991). These characteristics lead these women to have less power in and to obtain less benefit from relationships. Women score higher than men on measures of excessive concern with relationships, and scores on these measures correlate with depression (Nolen-Hoeksema & Jackson, 2001). Similarly, studies of children and adolescents find that girls score higher than boys on need for social approval, reassurance seeking, and social-evaluative concerns, all of which are associated with proneness to depressive symptoms (Little & Garber, 2005; Prinstein, Borelli, Cheah, Simon, & Aikins, 2005; Rudolph, Caldwell, & Conley, 2005). For example, Rudolph and Conley (2005) found that social-evaluative concerns fully mediated the gender difference in depression in a group of adolescents.

Stress Reactivity and Stress Generation

Women's interpersonal orientation also appears to make them more emotionally reactive to interpersonal stress. Adult women, more than adult men, report that interpersonal stressors affect their well-being (Leadbeater, Blatt, & Quinlan, 1995). Similarly, in a study of pubertal girls and boys, Rudolph and Flynn (2007) found that interpersonal stressors were more likely to lead to depression in girls than boys (see also Ge, Lorenz, Conger, Elder, & Simons, 1994).

Some of the excess interpersonal stressors women experience may be created by themselves. Hammen's (1991) model of stress generation conceptualizes certain stressors as dependent (i.e., contributed to, in part or in whole, by the individual), and Hammen finds that women are more likely than men to experience dependent stressors. Women who overvalue relationships may seek reassurance to an extent that is excessive and annoys others (Joiner, Metalsky, Katz, & Beach, 1999). This can lead to interpersonal conflict or rejection, which then feeds a woman's concern regarding the relationship. Adolescent girls are more likely to report dependent stressors (especially within the interpersonal domain; e.g., peer conflict) compared with adolescent boys (Rudolph & Hammen, 1999; Shih, Eberhart, Hammen, & Brennan, 2006). Furthermore, Shih and colleagues (2006) found that dependent interpersonal stress mediated the gender difference in adolescent depression. There was also evidence in this study of higher stress reactivity among the adolescent girls, who were more likely than adolescent boys to become depressed when experiencing stressful life events.

Corumination

Additional research with adolescents has helped to elucidate the adjustment tradeoffs associated with an interpersonal association for girls. Work by Amanda Rose (2002) has found that adolescent girls are much more likely than boys to engage in the rumi-native process in a dyadic context by excessively discussing their problems in a passive manner, usually with a close girlfriend. This tendency to coruminate is simultaneously associated with high relationship quality (i.e., interpersonal closeness and support) and depressive symptoms, both concurrently and over time for girls (e.g., Rose, Carlson, & Waller, 2007). For boys, corumination predicted increases only in friendship quality, not in depressive symptoms, suggesting that corumination may be associated with poor adjustment only for girls.

In summary, the psychological factors reviewed in this section—rumination, stress generation, and corumination—are associated with depression concurrently and predict increases over time. Adolescent girls and adult women score higher than males on these constructs, which helps explain the gender difference in depression. Interestingly, all of these constructs have reciprocal relationships with depression, creating a vicious cycle that may be difficult to exit from once in motion.

SOCIAL EXPLANATIONS: STRESS EXPOSURE (VERSUS SENSITIVITY)

The biological and psychological factors reviewed so far are often viewed as vulnerability factors that increase the likelihood of depression, especially in the face of stress. Because the gender difference in depression appears to be related more to first onsets than to recurrence, we now turn to one of the major findings in this area—that first episodes of depression tend to be preceded by a negative life event more so than subsequent episodes (for reviews, see Mazure, 1998; Monroe & Harkness, 2005; Stroud, Davila, & Moyer, 2008). In this section, we review research on gender differences in stress exposure and sensitivity that might help to explain why more women than men develop depression.

Childhood Maltreatment and Other Adversities

A consistent predictor of both childhood- and adult-onset depression is the experience of childhood sexual abuse (e.g., Jaffee, Moffitt, Caspi, Fombonne, Poulton, & Martin, 2002). Other forms of childhood maltreatment, such as physical and emotional abuse and neglect, have also been associated with depression among both women and men (e.g., Arnow, Blasey, Hunkeler, Lee, & Hayward, 2011). It is possible that women's higher rate of depression could be partially explained by greater exposure to child maltreatment and/or greater sensitivity to it.

Girls are much more likely to be the victims of childhood sexual assault than boys. One review estimated that 35% of the gender difference in adult depression could be attributed to the higher rate of childhood sexual assault experienced by girls (Cutler & Nolen-Hoeksema, 1991). Two very large recent studies also showed that women are exposed to more childhood maltreatment than men and that this partially explained the gender difference in depression (Arnow et al., 2011; Dunn, Gilman, Willett, Slopen, & Molnar, 2012). Thus evidence for women's greater exposure to child maltreatment con-tributing to their higher rates of depression is strong.

Evidence regarding women's sensitivity to childhood stressors is more mixed. The two large studies just referenced did not find evidence that gender moderated the rela-tionship between childhood maltreatment and depression (Arnow et al., 2011; Dunn et al., 2012), suggesting that childhood maltreatment is equally detrimental for males and females. However, some research on other childhood adversities (e.g., parental separation or loss, poverty) has found that girls may be more sensitive to these stressors (Daley, Hammen, & Rao, 2000). For example, Rudolph and Flynn (2007) found that early childhood adversity sensitized pubertal girls, but not pubertal boys, to subsequent stress, increasing their risk for depressive symptoms. Additionally, girls appear to be more negatively affected than boys by maternal depression and, more generally, by family discord and disruption (Downey & Coyne, 1990; Goodman, Brogan, Lynch, & Fielding, 1993), perhaps because of their stronger interpersonal orientation.

Interpersonal Stress

Perhaps also because of their relatively strong interpersonal orientation, adolescent girls and women experience more interpersonal stress relative to males. Because women tend to have more people to whom they feel emotionally close, there is a higher chance that hardship will affect someone in their social circle, resulting in a negative emotional impact on their own well-being, a hypothesis that Kessler, McLeod, and Wethington (1985) term the *cost of caring*. Kessler and McLeod (1984) found that women reported a greater number of negative events occurring among people in their social networks than did men, presumably because these networks were larger for women than for men. Adolescent girls also report more interpersonal stressors than do boys (e.g., Ge et al., 1994; Hankin, Mermelstein, & Roesch, 2007; Rudolph & Hammen, 1999; Shih et al., 2006). In one daily diary study of adolescents, girls' higher rate of interpersonal stressors partially explained their higher rates of depressive symptoms (Hankin et al., 2007).

Chronic interpersonal stress often comes in the form of discord with one's partner. In intimate heterosexual relationships, some women face inequities in the distribution of power over making important decisions, such as the decision to move to a new city or how to spend the family's income (Nolen-Hoeksema et al., 1999). Even when they voice their opinions, women may feel these opinions are not taken seriously or that their viewpoints on important issues are not respected and affirmed by their partners. Nolen-Hoeksema and colleagues (1999) grouped inequities in workload and in heterosexual relationships under a variable labeled *chronic strain* and showed that chronic strain predicted increases in depression over time and partially mediated the gender difference in depression.

Hammen and colleagues (e.g., Daley et al., 2000) have differentiated between this type of chronic interpersonal strain and episodic interpersonal stress (e.g., the breakup of a relationship, a close friend moving away). In studies of young adult women, they found that whereas chronic interpersonal stress predicts first onsets but not recurrence of depression, episodic interpersonal stress predicts both first onsets and recurrence of depression.

In sum, there is evidence that women experience more childhood maltreatment and interpersonal stress, placing them at greater risk for depression. Additionally, women may be more sensitive to certain types of stress, such as childhood adversity, also contributing to their higher rates of depression.

INTEGRATIONS AND FUTURE DIRECTIONS

All of the factors reviewed in this chapter may independently contribute to women's higher rates of depression compared with men; however, complex interactions among these factors are likely to best explain the gender difference in depression. For example, the biological and psychological factors associated with depression may be detrimental only in the face of stress, that is, a diathesis–stress interaction.

The introduction of GWAS has made the search for main effects of gene associations with psychiatric disorders possible; however, this research has generally not succeeded in finding genetic main effects. For example, a recent GWAS of MDD did not find any common variants associated with depression (Wray et al., 2012). More fruitful avenues of research might involve examination of gene–environment interactions (or gene–gene interactions), intermediate phenotypes (such as rumination or stress reactivity), and gender differences in epigenetic mechanisms. We found evidence for the brain-derived neurotrophic factor (BDNF *Val66Met*) gene predicting rumination and subsequent depression in a sample of females (Hilt, Sander, Nolen-Hoeksema, & Simen, 2007). A study with mice found evidence of depression-like behavior in females with a simulated BDNF gene mutation but not in males (Monteggia et al., 2007), suggesting that this may be an interesting avenue for future research on gender differences in depression.

Interactions among multiple factors are possible both within and among different domains (i.e., biological, psychological, and social). Hormonal fluctuations and genetic risk for depression may interact with the stresses of puberty to put adolescent girls at greater risk for depression than boys. Additionally, early childhood adversities, which are more commonly experienced by girls, may sensitize their stress response systems to be overly reactive, putting them at greater risk for depression when experiencing stressful events. Women's greater likelihood of experiencing interpersonal stressors combined with the tendency to ruminate, which may amplify the negative mood associated with such stressors, may be more likely to contribute to depression than either factor alone. Women who face chronic stressors because of inequities in their heterosexual relationships become more ruminative over time (Nolen-Hoeksema et al., 1999). In turn, rumination impairs problem solving, increasing the likelihood of new stressors and subsequent depression. Complex models have been proposed that integrate multiple factors to help explain the gender difference in depression (e.g., Hankin & Abramson, 2001; Hyde, Mezulis, & Abramson, 2008), though aspects of these models have not been adequately tested, suggesting an important avenue for future research.

It is also important to note that many of these factors have reciprocal relationships with depression. For example, depression may result in increased rumination (see Nolen-Hoeksema et al., 2008), stress generation (Hammen, 1991), stress sensitization (Post, 1992), and interpersonal difficulties (Joiner & Coyne, 1999). Factors that predict a first onset may or may not be the same factors that maintain depression or cause recurrent episodes. Because epidemiological data suggest that the gender difference in depression is largely accounted for by first onsets of depression, future research should focus on understanding gender differences in predictors of onset.

Understanding the gender difference in depression may be best accomplished by focusing on its emergence in adolescence (see Hilt & Nolen-Hoeksema, 2009). For example, rumination predicts the gender difference in depressive symptoms by adolescence (Hilt et al., 2010); thus understanding the development of rumination may help to further elucidate the gender difference in depression. Limited longitudinal research on the development of rumination has not found gender differences in risk factors (Hilt, Armstrong, & Essex, 2012), but one retrospective study found that child sexual abuse predicted rumination in women but not men (Spasojevic & Alloy, 2002). Future research on the development of risk factors that mediate the gender difference in depression may clarify developmental trajectories and offer avenues for prevention.

What is clear from the existing literature on the gender differences in depression is that no single factor is likely to explain these differences. Instead, the differences may be overdetermined by a confluence of social, psychological, and biological differences between women and men.

REFERENCES

Aldao, A., Nolen-Hoeksema, S., & Schweizer, S. (2010). Emotion regulation strategies across psychopathology: A meta-analytic review. *Clinical Psychology Review, 30,* 217–237.

Allgood-Merten, B., Lewinsohn, P. M., & Hops, H. (1990). Sex differences and adolescent depression. *Journal of Abnormal Psychology, 99,* 55–63.

American Psychiatric Association. (2013). *Diagnostic and statistical manual of mental disorders* (5th ed.). Arlington, VA: Author.

Amin, Z., Canli, T., & Epperson, C. N. (2005). Effect of estrogen–serotonin interactions on mood and cognition. *Behavioral and Cognitive Neuroscience Reviews, 4,* 43–58.

Andrade, L., Caraveo-Anduaga, J. J., Berglund, P., Bijl, R. V., DeGraaf, R., Volbergh, W., et al. (2003). The epidemiology of major depressive episodes: Results from the International Consortium of Psychiatric Epidemiology (ICPE) surveys. *International Journal of Methods in Psychiatric Research, 12,* 3–21.

Angold, A., Costello, E. J., Erkanli, A., & Worthman, C. M. (1999). Pubertal changes in hormones of adolescent girls. *Psychological Medicine, 29,* 1043–1053.

Angold, A., Costello, E. J., & Worthman, C. M. (1998). Puberty and depression: The roles of age, pubertal status and pubertal timing. *Psychological Medicine, 28,* 51–61.

Arnow, B., Blasey, C. M., Hunkeler, E. M., Lee, J., & Hayward, C. (2011). Does gender moderate the relationship between childhood maltreatment and adult depression? *Child Maltreatment, 16,* 175–183.

Avis, N. E. (2003). Depression during the menopausal transition. *Psychology of Women Quarterly, 27,* 91–100.

Bierut, L. J., Heath, A. C., Bucholz, K. K., Dinwiddie, S. H., Madden, P. A. F., Statham, D. J., et al. (1999). Major depressive disorder in a community-based twin sample: Are there different genetic and environmental contributions for men and women? *Archives of General Psychiatry, 57,* 557–563.

Blazer, D. G., Kessler, R. C., McGonagle, K. A., & Swartz, M. S. (1994). The prevalence and distribution of major depression in a national community sample: The National Comorbidity Survey. *American Journal of Psychiatry, 151,* 979–986.

Boomsma, D. I., Beem, A. L., van den Berg, M., Dolan, C. V., Koopmans, J. R., Vink, J. M., et al. (2000). Netherlands twin family study of anxious depression (NETSAD). *Twin Research, 3,* 323–334.

Bradley, R. G., Binder, E. B., Epstein, M. P., Tang, Y., Nair, H. P., Liu, W., et al. (2008). Influence of child abuse on adult depression. *Archives of General Psychiatry, 65,* 190–200.

Breslau, N., Schultz, L., & Peterson, E. (1995). Sex differences in depression: A role for preexisting anxiety. *Psychiatry Research, 58,* 1–12.

Brockington, I. (2001). Suicide in women. *International Clinical Psychopharmacology, 16*(Suppl. 12), 7–19.

Bromberger, J. T., Meyer, P. M., Kravitz, H. M., Sommer, B., Cordal, A., Powell, L., et al. (2001). Dysphoric mood and natural menopause: A multi-ethnic community study. *American Journal of Public Health, 91,* 1435–1442.

Bromet, E., Andrade, L. H., Hwang, I., Sampson, N. A. Alonso, J., de Girolamo, G., et al. (2011). Cross-national epidemiology of DSM-IV major depressive episode. *BMC Medicine, 9,* 90.

Brooks-Gunn, J. (1988). Antecedents and consequences of variations in girls' maturational timing. *Journal of Adolescent Health Care, 9,* 365–373.

Brummett, B. H., Boyle, S. H., Siegler, I. C., Kuhn, C. M., Ashley-Koch, A., Jonassant, C. R., et al. (2008). Effects of environmental stress and gender on association among symptoms of depression and the serotonin transporter gene linked polymorphic region (*5-HTTLPR*). *Behavior Genetics, 38,* 34–43.

Buchanan, C. M., Eccles, J. S., & Becker, J. B. (1992). Are adolescents the victims of raging hormones: Evidence for activational effects of hormones on moods and behavior at adolescence. *Psychological Bulletin, 111,* 62–107.

Butler, L. D., & Nolen-Hoeksema, S. (1994). Gender differences in responses to a depressed mood in a college sample. *Sex Roles, 30,* 331–346.

Canetto, S. S., & Sakinofsky, I. (1998). The gender paradox in suicide. *Suicide and Life-Threatening Behavior, 28*, 1–23.

Casper, R. F., & Hearn, M. T. (1990). The effect of hysterectomy and bilateral oophorectomy in women with severe premenstrual syndrome. *American Journal of Obstetrics and Gynecology, 162*, 105–109.

Caspi, A., Hariri, A. R., Holmes, A., Uher, R., & Moffitt, T. E. (2010). Genetic sensitivity to the environment: The case of the serotonin transporter gene and its implications for studying complex diseases and traits. *American Journal of Psychiatry, 167*, 509–527.

Centers for Disease Control and Prevention. (2010). Fatal injury reports. Retrieved April 28, 2013, from *www.cdc.gov/injury/wisqars/fatal_injury_reports.html*.

Chang, A. M., Holroyd, E., & Chau, J. P. C. (1995). Premenstrual syndrome in employed Chinese women in Hong Kong. *Health Care for Women International, 16*, 551–561.

Cohen, L. S., Soares, C. N., Vitonis, A. F., Otto, M. W., & Harlow, B. L. (2006). Risk for new onset of depression during the menopausal transition: The Harvard study of moods and cycles. *Archives of General Psychiatry, 63*, 385–390.

Crosby, A. E., Cheltenham, M. P., & Sacks, J. J. (1999). Incidence of suicidal ideation and behavior in the United States, 1994. *Suicide and Life-Threatening Behavior, 29*, 131–140.

Cross-Disorder Group of the Psychiatric Genomics Consortium. (2013). Identification of risk loci with shared effects on five major psychiatric disorders: A genome-wide analysis. *Lancet, 381*, 1371–1379.

Cutler, S. E., & Nolen-Hoeksema, S. (1991). Accounting for sex differences in depression through female victimization: Childhood sexual abuse. *Sex Roles, 24*, 425–438.

Daley, S. E., Hammen, C., & Rao, U. (2000). Predictors of first onset and recurrence of major depression in young women during the 5 years following high school graduation. *Journal of Abnormal Psychology, 109*, 525–533.

DeRose, L. M., Wright, A. J., & Brooks-Gunn, J. (2006). Does puberty account for the gender differential in depression? In C. L. M. Keyes & S. H. Goodman (Eds.), *Women and depression* (pp. 89–128). New York: Cambridge University Press.

Dorn, L. D., Dahl, R. E., Woodward, H. R., & Biro, F. (2006). Defining the boundaries of early adolescence: A user's guide to assessing pubertal status and pubertal timing in research with adolescents. *Applied Developmental Science, 10*, 30–56.

Downey, G., & Coyne, J. C. (1990). Children of depressed parents: An integrative review. *Psychological Bulletin, 108*, 50–76.

Dunn, E. C., Gilman, S. E., Willett, J. B., Slopen, N. B., & Molnar, B. E. (2012). The impact of exposure to interpersonal violence on gender differences in adolescent-onset major depression: Results from the National Comorbidity Survey Replication (NCS-R). *Depression and Anxiety, 29*, 392–399.

Eaton, W., Anthony, J., Gallo, J., Cai, G., Tien, A., Romanoski, A., et al. (1997). Natural history of Diagnostic Interview Schedule/DSM-IV major depression. *Archives of General Psychiatry, 54*, 993–999.

Essau, C. A., Lewinsohn, P. M., Seeley, J. R., & Sasagawa, S. (2010). Gender differences in the developmental course of depression. *Journal of Affective Disorders, 127*, 185–190.

Feingold, A. (1994). Gender differences in personality: A meta-analysis. *Psychological Bulletin, 116*, 429–456.

Flynn, H. A. (2005). Epidemiology and phenomenology of postpartum mood disorders. *Psychiatric Annals, 35*, 522–551.

Franic, S., Middledorp, C. M., Dolan, C. V., Ligthart, L., & Boomsma, D. I. (2010). Childhood and adolescence anxiety and depression: Beyond heritability. *Journal of the American Academy of Child and Adolescent Psychiatry, 49*, 820–829.

Freeman, E. W., Sammel, M. D., Lin, H., & Nelson, D. B. (2006). Associations of hormones and menopausal status with depressed mood in women with no history of depression. *Archives of General Psychiatry, 63*, 375–382.

Galambos, N. L., Leadbeater, B. J., & Barker, E. T. (2004). Gender differences in and risk factors for depression in adolescence: A 4-year longitudinal study. *International Journal of Behavior Development, 28,* 16–25.

Ge, X., Lorenz, F. O., Conger, R. D., Elder, G. H., & Simons, R. L. (1994). Trajectories of stressful life events and depressive symptoms during adolescence. *Developmental Psychology, 30,* 467–483.

Gillespie, C. F., & Nemeroff, C. B. (2005). Hypercortisolemia and depression. *Psychosomatic Medicine, 67,* 26–28.

Goodman, S. H., Brogan, D., Lynch, M. E., & Fielding, B. (1993). Social and emotional competence in children of depressed mothers. *Child Development, 64,* 516–531.

Graber, J. A., Lewinsohn, P. M., Seeley, J. R., & Brooks-Gunn, J. (1997). Is psychopathology associated with the timing of pubertal development? *Journal of the American Academy of Child and Adolescent Psychiatry, 36,* 1768–1776.

Hammen, C., Brennan, P. A., Keenan-Miller, D., Hazel, M. A., & Najman, J. M. (2010). Chronic and acute stress, gender, and serotonin transporter gene–environment interactions predicting depression symptoms in youth. *Journal of Child Psychology and Psychiatry, 51,* 180–187.

Hammen, C. L. (1991). *Depression runs in families: The social context of risk and resilience in children of depressed mothers.* New York: Springer-Verlag.

Hankin, B. L., & Abramson, L. (2001). Development of gender differences in depression: An elaborated cognitive vulnerability–transactional stress theory. *Psychological Bulletin, 127,* 773–796.

Hankin, B. L., Abramson, L. Y., Moffitt, T. E., McGee, R., Silva, P., & Angell, K. E. (1998). Development of depression from preadolescence to young adulthood: Emerging gender differences in a 10-year longitudinal study. *Journal of Abnormal Psychology, 107,* 128–140.

Hankin, B. L., Mermelstein, R., & Roesch, L. (2007). Sex differences in adolescent depression: Stress exposure and reactivity models. *Child Development, 78,* 279–295.

Happonen, M., Pulkkinen, L., Kaprio, J., Van der Meere, M. J., Viken, R. J., & Rose, R. J. (2002). The heritability of depressive symptoms: Multiple informants and multiple measures. *Journal of Child Psychology and Psychiatry, 43,* 471–479.

Helgeson, V. (1994). Relation of agency and communion to well-being: Evidence and potential explanations. *Psychological Bulletin, 116,* 412–428.

Hilt, L. M., Armstrong, J. M., & Essex, M. J. (2012). Early family context and development of adolescent ruminative style: Moderation by temperament. *Cognition and Emotion, 26,* 916–926.

Hilt, L. M., McLaughlin, K. A., & Nolen-Hoeksema, S. (2010). Examination of the Response Styles Theory in a community sample of young adolescents. *Journal of Abnormal Child Psychology, 38,* 545–556.

Hilt, L. M., & Nolen-Hoeksema, S. (2009). The emergence of gender differences in depression in adolescence. In S. Nolen-Hoeksema & L. M. Hilt (Eds.), *Handbook of depression in adolescents* (pp. 111–135). New York: Routledge.

Hilt, L. M., Sander, L. C., Nolen-Hoeksema, S., & Simen, A. A. (2007). The BDNF Val66Met polymorphism predicts rumination and depression differently in young adolescent girls and their mothers. *Neuroscience Letters, 429,* 12–16.

Hyde, J. S., Mezulis, A. H., & Abramson, L. Y. (2008). The ABCs of depression: Integrating affective, biological, and cognitive models to explain the emergence of gender difference in depression. *Psychological Review, 115,* 291–313.

Jack, D. C. (1991). *Silencing the self: Women and depression.* New York: HarperPerennial.

Jacobson, K. C., & Rowe, D. C. (1999). Genetic and environmental influences on the relationships between family connectedness, school connectedness, and adolescent depressed mood: Sex differences. *Developmental Psychology, 35,* 926–939.

Jaffee, S. R., Moffitt, T. E., Caspi, A., Fombonne, E., Poulton, R., & Martin, J. (2002). Differences in early childhood risk factors for juvenile-onset and adult-onset depression. *Archives of General Psychiatry, 59,* 215–222.

Jansson, M., Gatz, M., Berg, S., Johansson, B., Malberg, B., McClearn, G. E., et al. (2004).

Gender differences in the heritability of depressive symptoms in the elderly. *Psychological Medicine, 34,* 471–479.

Joiner, T., & Coyne, J. C. (1999). *The interactional nature of depression: Advances in interpersonal approaches.* Washington, DC: American Psychological Association.

Joiner, T., Metalsky, G., Katz, J., & Beach, S. R. (1999). Depression and excessive reassurance-seeking. *Psychological Inquiry, 10,* 269–278.

Kaltiala-Heino, R., Kosunen, E., & Rimpela, M. (2003). Pubertal timing, sexual behaviour and self-reported depression in middle adolescence. *Journal of Adolescence, 26,* 531–545.

Kendler, K. S., Gardner, C. O., Gatz, M., & Pedersen, N. L. (2007). The sources of comorbidity between major depression and generalized anxiety disorder in a Swedish national twin sample. *Psychological Medicine, 37,* 453–462.

Kendler, K. S., Gatz, M., Gardner, C. O., & Pedersen, N. L. (2006). A Swedish national twin study of lifetime major depression. *American Journal of Psychiatry, 163,* 109–114.

Kendler, K. S., & Prescott, C. A. (1999). A population-based twin study of lifetime major depression in men and women. *Archives of General Psychiatry, 56,* 39–44.

Kessler, R. C. (2000). Gender differences in major depression: Epidemiological findings. In E. Frank (Ed.), *Gender and its effects on psychopathology* (pp. 61–84). Washington, DC: American Psychiatric.

Kessler, R. C. (2003). Epidemiology of women and depression. *Journal of Affective Disorders, 74,* 5–13.

Kessler, R. C., Birnbaum, H., Bromet, E., Hwang, I., Sampson, N., & Shahly, V. (2010). Age differences in major depression: Results from the National Comorbidity Surveys Replication (NCS-R). *Psychological Medicine, 40,* 225–237.

Kessler, R. C., Crum, R. M., Warner, L. A., Nelson, C. B., Schulenberg, J., & Anthony, J. C. (1997). Lifetime co-occurrence of DSM-III-R alcohol abuse and dependence with other psychiatric disorders in the National Comorbidity Survey. *Archives of General Psychiatry, 54,* 313–321.

Kessler, R. C., McGonagle, K. A., Swartz, M., Blazer, D. G., & Nelson, C. B. (1993). Sex and depression in the National Comorbidity Survey: I. Lifetime prevalence, chronicity, and recurrence. *Journal of Affective Disorders, 29,* 85–96.

Kessler, R. C., & McLeod, J. D. (1984). Sex differences in vulnerability to undesirable life events. *American Sociological Review, 49,* 620–631.

Kessler, R. C., McLeod, J., & Wethington, E. (1985). The costs of caring: A perspective on the relationship between sex and psychological distress. In I. G. Sarason & B. R. Sarason (Eds.), *Social support: Theory, research and applications* (pp. 491–506). Dordrecht, The Netherlands: Martinus Nijhoff.

Kornstein, S. G. (2010). Gender issues and DSM-V. *Archives of Women's Mental Health, 13,* 11–13.

Kornstein, S. G., Harvey, A. T., Rush, A. J., Wisniewski, S. R., Trivedi, M. H., Svikis, D. S., et al. (2005). Self-reported premenstrual exacerbation of depressive symptoms in patients seeking treatment for major depression. *Psychological Medicine, 35,* 1–10.

Kornstein, S. G., Schatzberg, A. F., Thase, M. T., Yonkers, K. A., McCullough, J. P., Keitner, G. I., et al. (2000). Gender differences in treatment response to sertraline versus imipramine in chronic depression. *American Journal of Psychiatry, 157,* 1445–1452.

Korszun, A., Altemus, M., & Young, E. A. (2006). The biological underpinnings of depression. In C. L. M. Keyes & S. H. Goodman (Eds.), *Women and depression* (pp. 41–61). New York: Cambridge University Press.

Kovacs, M. (2001). Gender and the course of major depressive disorder through adolescence in clinically referred youngsters. *Journal of the American Academy of Child and Adolescent Psychiatry, 40,* 1079–1085.

Leadbeater, B. J., Blatt, S. J., & Quinlan, D. M. (1995). Gender-linked vulnerabilities to depressive symptoms, stress, and problem behaviors in adolescents. *Journal of Research on Adolescence, 5,* 1–29.

Lewinsohn, P. M., Rohde, P., & Seeley, J. R. (1996). Adolescent suicidal ideation and attempts: Prevalence, risk factors, and clinical implications. *Clinical Psychology: Science and Practice, 3,* 25–46.

Little, S. A., & Garber, J. (2005). The role of social stressors and interpersonal orientation in explaining the longitudinal relation between externalizing and depressive symptoms. *Journal of Abnormal Psychology, 114,* 432–443.

Lorenzo-Blanco, E. I., Unger, J. B., Baezconde-Garbanati, L., Ritt-Olson, A., & Soto, D. (2012). Acculturation, enculturation, and symptoms of depression in Hispanic youth: The roles of gender, Hispanic cultural values, and family functioning. *Journal of Youth and Adolescence, 41,* 1350–1365.

MacKinnon, D., Jamison, K. R., & DePaulo, J. R. (1997). Genetics of manic depressive illness. *Annual Review of Neuroscience, 20,* 355–373.

Marcus, S. M., Young, E. A., Kerber, K. B., Kornstein, S., Farabaugh, A. H., Mitchell, J., et al. (2005). Gender differences in depression: Findings from the STAR*D study. *Journal of Affective Disorders, 87,* 141–150.

Mazure, C. M. (1998). Life stressors as risk factors in depression. *Clinical Psychology: Science and Practice, 5,* 291–313.

McLaughlin, K., Hilt, L., & Nolen-Hoeksema, S. (2007). Racial/ethic differences in internalizing and externalizing symptoms in adolescents. *Journal of Abnormal Child Psychology, 35,* 801–806.

McMahon, F. J., Akula, N., Schulze, T. G., Muglia, P., Tozzi, F., Detera-Wadleigh, S. D., et al. (2010). Meta-analysis of genome-wide association data detects a risk locus for major mood disorders on chromosome 3p21.1. *Nature Genetics, 42,* 128–131.

Merikangas, K. R., He, J., Burstein, M., Swanson, S. A., Avenevoli, S., Cui, L., et al. (2010). Lifetime prevalence of mental disorders in U. S. adolescents: Results from the National Comorbidity Survey Replication—Adolescent Supplement (NCS-A). *Journal of the American Academy of Child and Adolescent Psychiatry, 49,* 980–989.

Monroe, S. M., & Harkness, K. L. (2005). Life stress, the "kindling" hypothesis, and the recurrence of depression: Considerations from a life stress perspective. *Psychological Review, 112,* 417–445.

Monteggia, L. M., Luikart, B., Barrot, M., Theobold, D., Malkovska, I., Nef, S., et al. (2007). Brain-derived neurotrophic factor conditional knockouts show gender differences in depression-related behaviors. *Biological Psychiatry, 61,* 187–197.

Munk-Olsen, T., Laursen, T. M., Pedersen, C. B., Mors, O., & Mortensen, P. B. (2006). New parents and mental disorders: A population-based register study. *Journal of the American Medical Association, 296,* 2582–2589.

Murray, C., & Lopez, E. (Eds.). (1996). *The global burden of disease, injuries and risk factors in 1990 and projected to 2020.* Cambridge, MA: Harvard University Press.

Nock, M. K., Hwang, I., Sampson, N. A., & Kessler, R. C. (2010). Mental disorders, comorbidity, and suicidal behavior: Results from the National Comorbidity Survey Replication. *Molecular Psychiatry, 15,* 868–876.

Nolen-Hoeksema, S. (1990). *Sex differences in depression.* Stanford, CA: Stanford University Press.

Nolen-Hoeksema, S. (1991). Responses to depression and their effects on the duration of depressive episodes. *Journal of Abnormal Psychology, 100,* 569–582.

Nolen-Hoeksema, S. (2000). The role of rumination in depressive disorders and mixed anxiety/depressive symptoms. *Journal of Abnormal Psychology, 109,* 504–511.

Nolen-Hoeksema, S., & Davis, C. G. (1999). "Thanks for sharing that": Ruminators and their social support networks. *Journal of Personality and Social Psychology, 77,* 801–814.

Nolen-Hoeksema, S., & Girgus, J. S. (1994). The emergence of gender differences in depression in adolescence. *Psychological Bulletin, 115,* 424–443.

Nolen-Hoeksema, S., & Jackson, B. (2001). Mediators of the gender difference in rumination. *Psychology of Women Quarterly, 25,* 37–47.

Nolen-Hoeksema, S., Larson, J., & Grayson, C. (1999). Explaining the gender difference in depression. *Journal of Personality and Social Psychology, 77*, 1061–1072.

Nolen-Hoeksema, S., Wisco, B., & Lyubomirsky, S. (2008). Rethinking rumination. *Perspectives on Psychological Science, 3*, 400–424.

O'Hara, M. W., & Swain, A. M. (1996). Rates and risk of postpartum depression: A meta-analysis. *International Review of Psychiatry, 8*, 37–54.

Paikoff, R. L., Brooks-Gunn, J., & Warren, M. P. (1991). Effects of girls' hormonal status on depressive and aggressive symptoms over the course of one year. *Journal of Youth and Adolescence, 20*, 191–215.

Post, R. M. (1992). Transduction of psychosocial stress into the neurobiology of recurrent affective disorder. *American Journal of Psychiatry, 149*, 999–1010.

Prinstein, M. J., Borelli, J. L., Cheah, C. S. L., Simon, V. A., & Aikins, J. W. (2005). Adolescent girls' interpersonal vulnerability to depressive symptoms: A longitudinal examination of reassurance-seeking and peer relationships. *Journal of Abnormal Psychology, 114*, 676–688.

Rice, F., Harold, G. T., & Thapar, A. (2002). Assessing the effects of age, sex, and shared environment on the genetic aetiology of depression in childhood and adolescence. *Journal of Child Psychology and Psychiatry, 43*, 1039–1051.

Rierdan, J., & Koff, E. (1991). Depressive symptomatology among very early maturing girls. *Journal of Youth and Adolescence, 20*, 415–425.

Rood, L. R., Bogels, S. J., Nolen-Hoeksema, S., & Schouten, E. (2009). The influence of emotion-focused rumination and distraction on depressive symptoms in non-clinical youth: A meta-analytic review. *Clinical Psychology Review, 29*, 607–616.

Rose, A. J. (2002). Co-rumination in the friendships of girls and boys. *Child Development, 73*, 1830–1843.

Rose, A. J., Carlson, W., & Waller, E. M. (2007). Prospective associations of co-rumination with friendship and emotional adjustment: Considering the socioeconomical trade-offs of co-rumination. *Developmental Psychology, 43*, 1019–1031.

Rudolph, K. D., Caldwell, M. S., & Conley, C. S. (2005). Need for approval and children's well-being. *Child Development, 76*, 309–323.

Rudolph, K. D., & Conley, C. S. (2005). The socioemotional costs and benefits of social-evaluative concerns: Do girls care too much? *Journal of Personality, 73*, 115–137.

Rudolph, K. D., & Flynn, M. (2007). Childhood adversity and youth depression: Influence of gender and pubertal status. *Development and Psychopathology, 19*, 497–521.

Rudolph, K. D., & Hammen, C. (1999). Age and gender as determinants of stress exposure, generation, and reactions in youngsters: A transactional perspective. *Child Development, 70*, 660–677.

Rutter, M., Silberg, J., O'Connor, T., & Simonoff, E. (1999). Genetics and child psychiatry: II. Empirical research findings. *Journal of Child Psychology and Psychiatry, 40*, 19–55.

Sannibale, C., & Hall, W. (2001). Gender-related symptoms and correlates of alcohol dependence among men and women with a lifetime diagnosis of alcohol use disorders. *Drug and Alcohol Review, 20*, 369–383.

Seedat, S., Scott, K. M., Angermeyer, M. C., Berglund, P., Bromet, E. J., Brugha, T. S., et al. (2009). Cross-national associations between gender and mental disorders in the WHO World Mental Health Surveys. *Archives of General Psychiatry, 66*, 785–795.

Shih, J. H., Eberhart, N. K., Hammen, C. L., & Brennan, P. A. (2006). Differential exposure and reactivity to interpersonal stress predict sex differences in adolescent depression. *Journal of Clinical Child and Adolescent Psychology, 35*, 103–115.

Siegel, J. M., Yancey, A. K., Aneshensel, C. S., & Schuler, R. (1999). Body image, perceived pubertal timing, and adolescent mental health. *Journal of Adolescent Health, 25*, 155–165.

Silberg, J., Pickles, A., Rutter, M., Hewitt, J., Simonoff, E., Maes, H., et al. (1999). The influence of genetic factors and life stress on depression among adolescent girls. *Archives of General Psychiatry, 56*, 225–232.

Sjoberg, R. L., Nilsson, K. W., Nordquist, M., Phrik, J., Leppert, J., Lindstrom, L., et al. (2006).

Development of depression: Sex and the interaction between environment and a promoter polymorphism of the serotonin transporter gene. *International Journal of Neuropsychopharmacology, 9,* 443–449.

Somerset, W., Newport, D. J., Ragan, K., & Stowe, Z. N. (2007). Depressive disorders in women: From menarche to beyond the menopause. In C. L. M. Keyes & S. H. Goodman (Eds.), *Women and depression* (pp. 62–88). New York: Cambridge University Press.

Spasojevic, J., & Alloy, L. B. (2002). Who becomes a depressive ruminator?: Developmental antecedents of ruminative response style. *Journal of Cognitive Psychotherapy, 16,* 405–419.

Stack, S. (2000). Suicide: A 15-year review of the sociological literature: Part I. Cultural and economic factors. *Suicide and Life-Threatening Behavior, 30,* 145–162.

Steiner, M., & Born, L. (2000). Advances in the treatment of premenstrual dysphoria. *CNS Drugs, 13,* 286–304.

Steiner, M., Dunn, E., & Born, L. (2003). Hormones and mood: From menarche to menopause and beyond. *Journal of Affective Disorders, 74,* 67–83.

Steiner, M., & Tam, W. Y. K. (1999). Postpartum depression in relation to other psychiatric disorders. In L. Miller (Ed.), *Postpartum mood disorders* (pp. 47–63). Washington, DC: American Psychiatric Press.

Stice, E., Presnell, K., & Bearman, S. K. (2001). Relation of early menarche to depression, eating disorders, substance abuse, and comorbid psychopathology among adolescent girls. *Developmental Psychology, 37,* 608–619.

Stroud, C. B., Davila, J., & Moyer, A. (2008). The relationship between stress and depression in first onsets versus recurrences: A meta-analytic review. *Journal of Abnormal Psychology, 117,* 206–213.

Thapar, A., & McGuffin, P. (1994). A twin study of depressive symptoms in childhood. *British Journal of Psychiatry, 165,* 259–265.

Twenge, J. M., & Nolen-Hoeksema, S. (2002). Age, gender, race, SES, and birth cohort differences on the Children's Depression Inventory: A meta-analysis. *Journal of Abnormal Psychology, 111,* 578–588.

Van de Velde, S., Bracke, P., Levecque, K., & Meuleman, B. (2010). Gender differences in depression in 25 European countries after eliminating measurement bias in the CES-D 8. *Social Science Research, 39,* 396–404.

Williams, D. R., Gonzalez, H. M., Neighbors, H., Nesse, R., Abelson, J. M., Sweetman, J., et al. (2007). Prevalence and distribution of major depressive disorder in African Americans, Caribbean blacks, and non-Hispanic whites. *Archives of General Psychiatry, 64,* 305–315.

Wray, N. R., Pergadia, M. L., Blackwood, D. H., Penninx, B. W., Gordon, S. D., Nyholt, D. R., et al. (2012). Genome-wide association study of major depressive disorder: New results, meta-analysis, and lessons learned. *Molecular Psychiatry, 17,* 36–48.

Young, E., & Korszun, A. (2010). Sex, trauma, stress hormones and depression. *Molecular Psychiatry, 15,* 23–28.

CHAPTER 20

Depression in Children

BRANDON E. GIBB

The goal of this chapter is to give a general overview of the characteristics and risk factors for depression in prepubertal children. At the outset, it should be noted that there is significantly less research in child populations than in adolescents and adults. In addition, research with youth samples typically combine children and adolescents, rarely examining child versus adolescent participants separately. As much as possible, the current chapter focuses on research with children specifically, and age ranges are noted when adolescents are also included in the study.

PREVALENCE

In the late 1970s and early 1980s, theorists and researchers still debated whether children were capable of experiencing clinical levels of depression (e.g., Lefkowitz & Burton, 1978). We now recognize that children not only do experience clinical depression, including major depressive disorder (MDD), but also that they do so at alarming rates. Results of the National Health and Nutrition Examination Survey (NHANES) indicate that the 12-month prevalence of mood disorders in children ages 8–11 years old is approximately 2.5% (MDD: 1.6%; dysthymia: 0.8%; Merikangas et al., 2010). Similar estimates have been observed in other studies suggesting that approximately 2% of 6- to 11-year-olds have a history of depressive diagnoses (for a review, see Centers for Disease Control and Prevention [CDC], 2013a. There is also growing recognition that major depression can occur even earlier in life, including in preschool-age children (Domènech-Llaberia et al., 2009; Luby et al., 2002, 2006). Although few epidemiological studies have been conducted with children this young, it is estimated that 0.5–2% of children ages 3–6 years old experience major depression (CDC, 2013a; Domènech-Llaberia et al., 2009; Egger & Angold, 2006; Wichstrøm et al., 2012). In addition, although the occurrence of documented suicide is rare in children younger than age 8, suicide is the seventh leading cause of death among 8- to 12-year-olds and the third leading cause of death when focused specifically on 11- to 12-year-olds. This rate continues into adolescence, with suicide being the second leading cause of death among 13- to 18-year-olds (CDC, 2013b). Clearly, then, clinically significant episodes of depression not only occur during childhood, but they are also far too frequent and are sometimes fatal.

There is a well-known sex difference in rates of major depression among adolescents and adults, with the gender gap starting around age 13 and reaching the 2:1 female:male ratio observed in adults by age 18 (Hankin et al., 1998). In contrast, among children, studies have either found no evidence for gender differences in depressive symptoms or diagnoses (Domènech-Llaberia et al., 2009; Egger & Angold, 2006; Twenge & Nolen-Hoeksema, 2002) or have suggested that boys have higher rates of depression than girls (Angold, Costello, & Worthman, 1998; McGee & Williams, 1988; Wichstrøm et al., 2012).

PHENOMENOLOGY

The DSM criteria for diagnosing MDD in children are identical to those used for adults, with the exception that the Criterion A symptom of sadness may be exhibited as irritability. In addition, the criteria for diagnosing dysthymia (DSM-IV)/persistent depressive disorder (DSM-5) require only 1 year of illness rather than 2 years. However, there have been questions about whether there may be other developmental differences in the expression of depression in children.

For example, some have suggested that certain cognitive symptoms, such as low self-esteem, hopelessness, and depressive guilt, may not be apparent in children with depression because of developmental differences in cognitive development (i.e., prior to the development of abstract thought; Weiss & Garber, 2003). However, findings from studies testing this hypothesis are mixed. Partially supporting theories of developmental differences in cognitive development on symptom expression, concerns about the future (e.g., hopelessness) loaded more strongly onto a depression latent variable in adolescents than in children; however, guilt loaded more strongly onto depression for children than for adolescents (Weiss & Garber, 2003). In addition, other studies have found no difference in factor structure or patterns of item-total correlations for measures of depressive symptoms in children versus adolescents (e.g., Mitchell, McCauley, Burke, & Moss, 1988; Ryan et al., 1987; Smucker, Craighead, Craighead, & Green, 1986). Currently, therefore, there is no clear evidence for developmental differences in the relevance of cognitive symptoms of depression in children versus adolescents or adults. This said, there is evidence for age-related increases in cognitive (and other) symptoms of depression (i.e., hopelessness, as well as anhedonia, hypersomnia, weight gain, decreased energy, and social withdrawal; for a review, see Weiss & Garber, 2003). However, this may speak more to developmental differences in *rates* of depression than to developmental differences in the *expression* of depression.

More recently, theorists and researchers have suggested that appetite and weight symptoms of depression utilized in DSM may need to be modified for pediatric samples. According to current DSM criteria, appetite/weight disturbance can be exhibited by either an increase or a decrease from usual. However, there are normative increases in appetite and weight as children age, calling into question the utility of increases in appetite or weight as a clear feature of depression in youth. Indeed, there is growing evidence that, although decreases in appetite and weight are associated with depression in children and adolescents, increases are not (e.g., Cole et al., 2012).

Finally, there is some evidence that the duration criteria for MDD could be reduced, at least for very young children (Luby et al., 2002). As noted earlier, the duration criteria for dysthymia/persistent depressive disorder in children and adolescents is currently 1 year rather than the 2 years required for the diagnosis in adults. However, the duration criterion for MDD is 2 weeks, regardless of the age of the person. There is evidence, however, that when diagnosing MDD in preschoolers, those children who do versus do not meet the 2-week duration criterion but who meet all of the other diagnostic criteria exhibit greater depression severity and functional impairment than healthy controls at a baseline assessment and 2 years later (Gaffrey, Belden, & Luby, 2011). In addition, both depression groups, regardless of whether they met the 2-week duration criteria, exhibit similar levels of depression and functional impairment, as well as risk for full MDD at 2-year follow-up (Gaffrey et al., 2011). Furthermore, preschoolers who meet all symptom and impairment criteria for MDD, whether or not they meet the duration criteria, exhibit higher levels of each of the typical MDD symptoms than children with externalizing disorders (attention-deficit/hyperactivity disorder [ADHD] and/or oppositional defiant disorder [ODD]) and nonclinical controls and greater levels of functional impairment than controls (Luby et al., 2002). Finally, the 6-month stability of MDD diagnoses is similar whether the 2-week duration criteria was met (ϕ = .81) or not (ϕ = .71; Luby et al., 2002). This suggests that all the hallmarks of a clinically significant major depressive episode may be present in preschool children even if the episode lasts less than 2 weeks.

COURSE AND OUTCOME

Depression in childhood, as in older samples, is a chronic and recurrent disorder. Research suggests that the median episode length of MDD in childhood is 9 months, with a mean of 11 months, suggesting that a significant minority of children have episodes of MDD lasting over a year (for a review, see Kovacs, 1996). However, almost all children do achieve full remission eventually, with 99% remitting within 6 years of disorder onset (Kovacs, 1996). For dysthymia, the median duration is 4 years, with 91% of children experiencing a full remission within 9 years (Kovacs, 1996).

Childhood depression also shows substantial homotypic continuity over time. For example, preschoolers (ages 3–6 years) diagnosed with MDD were at elevated risk for MDD at 12-month and 24-month follow-up and were more likely to meet criteria for MDD than for other disorders at follow-up (Luby, Si, Belden, Tandon, & Spitznagel, 2009). Of those meeting criteria for MDD at the baseline assessment, 46% recovered and stayed depression-free at 24 months, 35% recovered but then had a recurrence of MDD, and the remaining 19% experienced chronic MDD over the follow-up. In addition, 40% of children (ages 8–13 years) who had initially recovered from MDD relapsed within 2 years (Kovacs et al., 1984). Similarly, 35% of child psychiatric inpatients with depression were rehospitalized within a year of discharge, and 45% were rehospitalized by the end of the 2nd year (Asarnow et al., 1988). Furthermore, in a sample of children recruited from the community, those exhibiting elevated depressive symptoms at age 9 continued to show these elevations at ages 11 and 13 (McGee & Williams, 1988). There is also evidence that children diagnosed with MDD are at increased risk for suicide attempts in adolescence and young adulthood compared with children with anxiety disorders or individuals with no psychiatric diagnoses in childhood, though in this study there was no difference in risk for future MDD (Weissman et al., 1999). Finally, in a study that focused on youth psychiatric inpatients and outpatients, children with a history of MDD were more likely to meet criteria for MDD in adulthood than were psychiatric controls without depression, though there was some evidence that the reoccurrence of MDD in adulthood was more likely among youth diagnosed with MDD occurring during adolescence than during childhood (Harrington, 1996).

COMORBIDITY

As in older samples, diagnostic comorbidity is common in children with depression, with the highest rates of comorbidity observed for anxiety and disruptive behavior disorders (Copeland, Shanahan, Costello, & Angold, 2009; Kovacs, Gatsonia, Paulauskas, & Richards, 1989; Kovacs, Paulauskas, Gatsonis, & Richards, 1988; McGee & Williams, 1988; Merikangas et al., 2010). This outcome appears to be due at least in part to shared genetic influences between depression and these other disorders (Eley & Stevenson, 1999; Rice, van den Bree, & Thapar, 2004; Subbarao et al., 2008; Thapar & McGuffin, 1997). There is some evidence of sex differences in patterns of comorbidity, with antisocial behavior more common in boys than in girls diagnosed with depression (McGee & Williams, 1988; but see Kovacs et al., 1988). With regard to temporal ordering, behavior disorders (e.g., conduct disorder) are more likely to develop subsequent to depression in children than prior to it (Kovacs et al., 1988). In contrast, anxiety disorders are more likely to precede the development of depression than to follow it (Kovacs et al., 1989) though there is also evidence of bidirectional influences, particularly for generalized anxiety disorder (GAD; Copeland et al., 2009). In terms of sequential comorbidity, there is evidence that youth with childhood-onset MDD are also at increased risk for substance abuse later in life (Weissman et al., 1999; but see also Copeland et al., 2009).

ETIOLOGY

Depression is a stress-related disorder that is often preceded by the occurrence of negative life events. However, there is also considerable individual variability in reactions to negative events, and models of depression risk focus on factors thought to increase stress reactivity, often within a vulnerability–stress or stress–diathesis framework. In this section, research on neurobiological, genetic, and cognitive models of risk is reviewed, as is research on specific types of environmental influences.

Neurobiology

Neural Circuits

Neural models of depression, developed largely from structural and functional neuroimaging studies of adults, emphasize disruption in corticolimbic circuits, with heightened activity in limbic regions such as the amygdala that is not effectively down-regulated by prefrontal cortical regions (e.g., dorsolateral prefrontal cortex; for reviews, see Cusi, Nazarov, Holshausen, MacQueen, & McKinnon, 2012; Hamilton et al., 2012). For example, a recent meta-analysis of neuroimaging data in adults with MDD showed that, compared with adults with no history of MDD, adults with MDD exhibited greater reactivity to negative stimuli (e.g., sad faces) in the amygdala, dorsal anterior cingulate, and insula and lower reactivity in the dorsolateral prefrontal cortex and dorsal striatum (Hamilton et al., 2012). The results of this meta-analysis also suggested that individuals with depression exhibit higher resting activity than controls in the pulvinar nucleus.

Findings in child samples are largely consistent with the adult literature (for a review, see Hulvershorn, Cullen, & Anand, 2011). For example, severity of MDD in preschool children is associated with greater amygdala activation when viewing sad, but not happy or neutral, faces (Gaffrey, Luby, et al., 2011). In addition, among 7- to 11-year-olds without current depression, severity of prior preschool-onset MDD (PO-MDD) was associated with increased reactivity to sad faces in various regions of the corticolimbic circuit including amygdala, hippocampus, parietal regions, and orbital frontal cortex (Barch, Gaffrey, Botteron, Belden, & Luby, 2012), which suggests that disruptions in this circuit are not simply correlates of current depression. Furthermore, these differences in reactivity were largely specific to sad faces rather than angry or happy faces. There is also evidence for a link between functional and structural differences in PO-MDD. For example, one study found that 7- to 12-year-old children with a history of PO-MDD have significantly smaller hippocampal volumes than children with no depression history (Suzuki et al., 2013). Furthermore, smaller right hippocampal volume in children with a history of PO-MDD was associated with greater putamen activation to sad faces and greater amygdala activation to negative faces generally (sad, angry, fearful), with the link between hippocampal volume and amygdala activation being significantly stronger in children with a history of PO-MDD than in controls (Suzuki et al., 2013). Finally, there is evidence for differences in functional connectivity between limbic regions and both prefrontal and striatal regions among children with a history of PO-MDD compared with children with no history of depression. For example, children with a history of PO-MDD, compared with children with no history of depression, exhibited reduced connectivity between the amygdala and regions of dorsal prefrontal and parietal cortex (Luking et al., 2011).

Hypothalamic–Pituitary–Adrenal Axis

Limbic areas directly influence activity in the hypothalamic–pituitary–adrenal (HPA) axis, the body's stress-response system, via projections to the thalamus (Guerry & Hastings, 2011; Gunnar & Quevedo, 2007). In normal functioning, a perceived stressor triggers the release of corticotropin-releasing hormone (CRH) from the hypothalamus, which causes adrenocorticotropic hormone (ACTH) to be released by the pituitary, causing glucocorticoids, including cortisol, to be synthesized and released by the adrenal cortex. HPA-axis reactivity to acute stressors is typically self-limiting, with cortisol downregulating production of CRH through a negative feedback loop. In nonclinical samples, preschool and school-age children exhibit hyporesponsiveness of the HPA axis such that they exhibit lower cortisol response to stressors than do infants, adolescents, and adults (Guerry & Hastings, 2011; Gunnar & Quevedo, 2007; Lupien, McEwen, Gunnar, & Heim, 2009). The results of one study suggest that this may be particularly true among children with depression. Specifically, one study found that preschool and prepubertal children with dysphoria exhibited significantly lower cortisol reactivity to a laboratory-based stressor (for preschoolers, exposure to a scary robot and a frustration task; for older children, the Trier Social Stress Test) than did children without dysphoria, whereas adolescents with dysphoria exhibited the expected greater cortisol reactivity compared with adolescents without dysphoria (Hankin, Badanes, Abela, & Watamura, 2010). In contrast, however, a second study of preschool-age children found that children with MDD exhibited greater cortisol increases following a stressor (separation from mothers) than children with ADHD or ODD or children with no history of psychopathology (Luby et al., 2003), differences that appear to have been due to the inclusion of children with anhedonic depression (Luby et al., 2003; Luby, Mrakotsky, Heffelfinger, Brown, & Spitznagel, 2004).

The reasons for the differences in reactivity findings across studies are unclear. It may be due to the difference in severity of depression examined (elevated symptoms vs. diagnoses of MDD) or differences in the types of stress tasks used. Or it may be that heightened cortisol reactivity characterizes only a subset of children with depression. Consistent with this latter possibility, approximately 45% of children with depression exhibit cortisol nonsuppression following the dexamethasone suppression test (for a review, see Guerry & Hastings, 2011), suggesting the role of altered HPA-axis activity in at least a subset of children with depression. Also similar to adults, rates of nonsuppression among child inpatients were approximate those seen in outpatients (Guerry & Hastings, 2011), suggesting that rates of dexamethasone nonsuppression track severity of disease. There is also evidence from a meta-analysis that children with depression exhibit slightly, but significantly, higher basal cortisol levels than children without depression (Hankin et al., 2010; Lopez-Duran, Kovacs, & George, 2009). Similar results have been observed among infants exposed to prenatal or postnatal depression in their mothers (for a review, see Guerry & Hastings, 2011).

Genetic Influences

There are clear genetic influences on depression risk, with heritability estimates suggesting that approximately 40% of the variance in depression risk is due to genetic factors (Eley, 1997; Sullivan, Neale, & Kendler, 2000). There are also developmental changes in the strength of genetic influences that increase as children age into adolescence (Eley & Stevenson, 1999; Rice, Harold, & Thapar, 2003; Silberg et al., 1999; Thapar & McGuffin, 1996). These changes are attributed to an increased role for gene–environment correlations, reflecting adolescents' greater control over their environments, which can lead to an increase in negative life events (Eley & Stevenson, 1999; Rice et al., 2003; Silberg et al., 1999). Twin studies have also noted clear evidence for genetic moderation of the impact of negative life events on depression risk (Silberg, Rutter, Neale, & Eaves, 2001; Wilkinson, Trzaskowski, Haworth, & Eley, 2013) in addition to gene–environment correlation effects.

Although twin and adoption studies can tell us what proportion of variance in depression risk is attributed to genetic influences, they do not tell us which specific genes or genetic pathways may be implicated. More recently, therefore, there has been increasing emphasis on examining specific genes that may increase risk for depression. Researchers have taken two approaches to identifying specific genes: genomewide association studies (GWAS) and candidate gene studies. GWAS are largely atheoretical investigations requiring extremely large sample sizes in which hundreds of thousands of single nucleotide polymorphisms (SNPs) are compared between individuals with current or past MDD versus those with no depression history. Despite the strengths of GWAS, they have revealed few replicable genetic loci for depression risk thus far (Cohen-Woods, Craig, & McGuffin, 2013; Major Depressive Disorder Working Group of the Psychiatric GWAS Consortium et al., 2013).

In contrast, candidate gene studies are theory-driven investigations and typically include much smaller sample sizes. In these studies, candidate genes are chosen because of their known or hypothesized influence on neural or physiological mechanisms underlying depression risk. The first of these studies was conducted by Caspi and colleagues (2003) and focused on a functional polymorphism (5-HTTLPR) in the serotonin transporter gene (*SLC6A4*). In this study, adults who carried one or two copies of the 5-HTTLPR short allele, which is associated with less transcriptional efficiency of *SLC6A4* compared with the long allele, were at greater risk for developing MDD in the context of negative life events than were adults homozygous for the long allele. Intriguingly, similar results were observed when focusing on adults' histories of childhood abuse, suggesting that early life stress could increase lifelong risk for depression among carriers of specific genetic polymorphisms. In the years following the publication of this study, there has been considerable debate about the influence of 5-HTTLPR on depression risk (Karg, Burmeister, Shedden, & Sen, 2011; Risch et al., 2009). However, consistent with neural models of depression risk, there is evidence from meta-analyses that the presence of the 5-HTTLPR short allele is associated with increased amygdala activation to emotional stimuli (Munafò, Brown, & Hariri, 2008), as well as greater cortisol reactivity in youth (Dougherty, Klein, Congdon, Canli, & Hayden, 2010; Gotlib, Joormann, Minor, & Hallmayer, 2008; Mueller, Brocke, Fries, Lesch, & Kirschbaum, 2010). In addition, there is growing evidence for its role in moderating the impact of negative life events on depression risk in youth (for a review, see Dunn et al., 2011).

It is clear, however, that genetic risk for depression is not limited to any single gene, and a number of studies have focused on other candidate polymorphisms, primarily those thought to influence disruptions in corticolimbic areas (e.g., the Val158Met polymorphism in the catechol-*O*-methyl transferase [*COMT*] gene) or HPA-axis functioning (e.g., the protective TAT haplotype in the corticotropin-releasing hormone receptor 1 [*CRHR1*] gene). Although few studies have examined these polymorphisms in childhood depression, there is preliminary support for their role in moderating the impact of environmental stress (Cicchetti, Rogosch, & Oshri, 2011; Conway, Hammen, Brennan, Lind, & Najman, 2010). This said, depression risk is likely to be influenced by variation in a number of genes acting together, and future research is needed to examine aggregate levels of influence across a number of genes. In addition, research is needed that moves beyond a simple examination of genotypes to explore methylation and gene expression to gain a more detailed understanding of the actual activity of specific genes within an individual.

Information-Processing Biases

Cognitive models of depression focus on biases in the processing of information. Specifically, biases in attention to, interpretation of, and memory for depression-relevant information are thought to contribute to the development and maintenance of depression. These information-processing biases are driven by altered neural reactivity in the same regions reviewed earlier as underlying depression risk (i.e., corticolimbic circuits and hypothalamus; Disner, Beevers, Haigh, & Beck, 2011). The biases are hypothesized to develop during childhood and then stabilize during adolescence, increasing risk for depression across the lifespan.

The majority of research on cognitive vulnerability to depression in children has focused on cognitive vulnerability as defined in the reformulated theory of learned helplessness (Abramson, Seligman, & Teasdale, 1978) or the hopelessness theory of depression (Abramson, Metalsky, & Alloy, 1989). In the reformulated theory of learned helplessness, cognitive vulnerability is defined as the tendency to attribute the occurrence of negative events to internal, stable, and global causes. In revising the theory as the hopelessness theory, the internality dimension of causal attributions was deemphasized, and the authors added two new domains of inferences—the tendency to infer negative consequences and the tendency to infer negative self-characteristics following the occurrence of negative events. Consistent with a vulnerability–stress model of risk, negative attributional or inferential styles are hypothesized to increase risk for depression in the presence, but not absence, of negative life events. There is consistent evidence for the impact of children's attributional and inferential styles on prospective increases in depression, as well as growing evidence that these styles moderate the impact of negative life events on future depression (Abela & Hankin, 2008; Cohen, Young, & Abela, 2012).

There is also growing support for the role of rumination in contributing to the development of depression in children. According to the response-styles theory (Nolen-Hoeksema, Wisco, & Lyubomirsky, 2008), the tendency to ruminate, or passively reflect on one's thoughts and feelings of sadness, contributes to the development and maintenance of depression. Although the response-styles theory was originally developed to help explain the gender difference in depression, with studies of adults consistently showing that women exhibit higher levels of rumination than men (Nolen-Hoeksema et al., 2008), there is little evidence for a gender difference in rumination in children (for a review, see Abela & Hankin, 2008). This said, a number of studies have now shown that rumination, perhaps specifically brooding rumination, contributes to prospective changes in depressive symptoms and to the development of depressive disorders in both girls and boys (Abela & Hankin, 2008; Gibb, Grassia, Stone, Uhrlass, & McGeary, 2012; Rood, Roelofs, Bögels, Nolen-Hoeksema, & Schouten, 2009).

In contrast to hopelessness theory and response-styles theory, which were developed in adults and later extended to explain depression risk in children, Cole's (1991) competency-based model of depression was developed specifically for children. According to this theory, children's levels of self-perceived competence in various domains (e.g., scholastic competence or social acceptance) increase risk for depression. A number of studies have now found that children's levels of self-perceived competence (particularly perceived levels of academic competence and social acceptance) increase risk for depression, though it remains unclear whether self-perceived competence mediates or moderates the influence of negative events on children's levels of depressive symptoms, nor whether there is a transition from mediation to moderation as children age into adolescence (Cole et al., 2011; Jacquez, Cole, & Searle, 2004; Uhrlass, Crossett, & Gibb, 2008).

Despite the strengths of each of these studies, the majority focus on children's self-report of their cognitions, which may be subject to response bias and may inflate relations with children's self-reported depressive symptoms. More recently, therefore, researchers have focused on computer-based assessments of information-processing biases in children. For example, there is growing evidence that children with depression or at risk for depression due to a positive family history of MDD exhibit attentional biases for depression-relevant stimuli (i.e., sad face) and, consistent with cognitive models' specificity hypothesis, these biases appear to be specific sad, rather than angry or happy, faces (e.g., Gibb, Benas, Grassia, & McGeary, 2009; Joormann, Talbot, & Gotlib, 2007; Kujawa et al., 2011; but see Johnson & Gibb, in press). In addition, attentional biases for sad faces predict prospective increases in children's depressive symptoms (Gibb et al., 2009). However, although there is clear evidence for the presence of attentional biases to sad faces, evidence is mixed with regard to the direction of the bias, with some studies finding evidence for preferential attention to sad faces (Joormann et al., 2007; Kujawa et al., 2011) and others finding evidence for attentional avoidance (Gibb et al., 2009; Johnson & Gibb, in press). Future research is needed to clarify this discrepancy in findings.

Finally, there is evidence for memory biases in children with depression, particularly overgeneral autobiographical memory biases. For example, children with a lifetime history of depressive disorders report fewer specific autobiographical memories than children with other forms of psychopathology (e.g., anxiety or behavior disorders) or nonclinical controls (Vrielynck, Deplus, & Philippot, 2007). Similar results have been observed in nonclinical samples of children, with higher levels of depressive symptoms associated with less specific autobiographical memories (Drummond, Dritschel, Astell, O'Carroll, & Dalgleish, 2006; Raes, Verstraeten, Bijttebier, Vasey, & Dalgleish, 2010). Despite the strengths of these studies, longitudinal research is needed to determine whether memory biases are simply a correlate or a consequence of depression in children or whether they predict the onset of depressive disorders.

Environmental Influences

As noted earlier, depression is considered a stress-related disorder, and the majority of episodes are preceded by some type of negative life event. As also noted earlier, there is considerable individual variability in reactivity to environmental stressors based on neurobiological, cognitive, and genetic influences. In this section, specific types of environmental influences are reviewed with a focus on those that are most strongly linked to depression risk in children.

Parents and Parenting

One of the strongest risk factors for depression in childhood is having a parent with depression (for reviews, see Goodman, 2007; Gotlib & Colich, Chapter 13, this volume). This risk is conveyed by both genetic and environmental influences. There is evidence that specific parenting styles and behaviors, even in the absence of parental depression, increase risk for depression in children. For example, parenting styles that are characterized by low levels of warmth and high levels of psychological control, referred to as "affectionless control," are associated with depression risk in children (Alloy, Abramson, Smith, Gibb, & Neeren, 2006). In terms of specific parenting behavior, one of the strongest risk factors identified for childhood depression is maternal criticism. Mothers of children with depression are rated as more critical than are mothers of children without depression (Asarnow, Tompson, Woo, & Cantwell, 2001; Silk et al., 2009). In addition, children exposed to heightened levels of maternal criticism over time are at increased risk for developing depressive disorders in the future (Burkhouse, Uhrlass, Stone, Knopik, & Gibb, 2012). There is evidence that maternal criticism mediates the link between maternal and child depression and also that it contributes to the development of cognitive vulnerabilities to depression in children (Goodman, 2007; Gotlib & Colich, Chapter 13, this volume).

Peer Influences

In addition to parents, peers also have a strong influence on a child's functioning. Of the various forms of peer influences, the one most consistently linked to risk for depression is peer victimization. Researchers have focused on two forms of peer victimization—overt victimization and relational victimization. Overt victimization includes behaviors designed to directly hurt someone (e.g., hitting, pushing, or kicking), whereas relational victimization is more indirect and includes behaviors designed to reduce someone's standing within a social group (e.g., spreading rumors, purposefully excluding someone; Crick, Casas, & Nelson, 2002). Although there are consistent gender differences in overt victimization, with boys reporting higher levels than girls, research suggests that girls and boys experience equivalent amounts of relational victimization (Crick et al., 2002). Both forms of victimization are associated with prospective increases in levels of depression among both boys and girls (for a meta-analytic review, see Reijntjes, Kamphuis, Prinzie, & Telch, 2010). As with criticism from parents, there is growing evidence that peer victimization also contributes to the development of various cognitive vulnerabilities to depression in children (Gibb, Stone, & Crossett, 2012; Sinclair et al., 2012).

Stress Generation

In addition to the well-known impact of negative life events on depression, there is growing evidence that individuals with depression contribute to the generation of additional negative events in their lives (Hammen, 2006). Although the stress-generation model was originally developed to explain the cyclic nature of depression risk in adults, there has been growing support for stress-generation models in children (Cole, Nolen-Hoeksema, Girgus, & Paul, 2006; Gibb & Alloy, 2006; Gibb & Hanley, 2010). These studies help to explain one mechanism by which early experiences with depression may lead to additional stressors in the child's life, setting in motion a vicious cycle of risk.

CONCLUSIONS AND FUTURE DIRECTIONS

Research on childhood depression has come quite a long way since the early 1980s. No longer questioning whether children can experience clinically significant episodes of depression, we now have reliable estimates of its prevalence in children and a better understanding of its presentation and course. Significant strides have also been made in understanding the neural and physiological underpinnings of depression in children, as well as cognitive, genetic, and environmental risk factors.

A key direction for future research, which is already beginning to happen, is to develop more integrated models of depression risk at multiple levels of analysis to understand how these various factors operate together to increase risk for depression in children. For example, researchers are now seeking to integrate cognitive and genetic models of risk (cf. Gibb, Beevers, & McGeary, 2013) by examining whether the information-processing biases featured in cognitive theories of depression may represent endophenotypes for specific genetic influences. One promising aspect of this approach is that genetic effects (main effects or genetic moderation of environmental influences) should be stronger for more basic processes, such as attentional biases, than for heterogeneous constructs such as MDD. A number of studies have now supported the link between specific candidate genes and various information-processing biases in children, adolescents, and adults (for a review, see Gibb et al., 2013). Another way in which these models may be integrated is by examining the combined impact of cognitive and genetic factors that increase reactivity to environmental influences within a gene × cognition × environment model of risk. These models also have garnered initial support. For example, in one study, the relation between mothers' and children's depressive symptom levels over time was strongest among children carrying the 5-HTTLR short or L_G allele who also exhibited attentional avoidance of sad faces (Gibb et al., 2009). In another study, children with negative inferential styles were at increased risk for depression in response to maternal criticism, but again only if they also carried at least one copy of the 5-HTTLR short or L_G allele (Gibb, Uhrlass, Grassia, Benas, & McGeary, 2009).

A related area for future research is to gain a better understanding of factors underlying diagnostic comorbidity in children. For example, results from twin studies suggest that depression and anxiety share common genetic influences (Eley & Stevenson, 1999; Rice et al., 2004; Subbarao et al., 2008). Also, the neural circuitry underlying depression and anxiety are similar (disruption in corticolimbic pathways), suggesting shared influence. In addition, cognitive models of psychopathology suggest that both disorders are characterized by the same types of information-processing biases—biases in attention, interpretation, and memory—and differ only in the content or focus of these biases (loss and threat for depression and anxiety, respectively; for a review, see Gibb & Coles, 2005). Recognizing the need to better understand the core mechanisms underlying disorders that may contribute to comorbidity using current diagnostic systems, the National Institute of Mental Health has begun its Research Domain Criteria (RDoC) initiative, the specific focus of which is to define mechanisms that cut across current diagnostic categories and to describe those mechanisms at the levels of genes, molecules, cells, neural circuits, physiology, and behavior (see *www.nimh.nih.gov/research-priorities/rdoc/index.shtml*). Explicit in this initiative is also gaining a better understanding of environmental influences, as well as the developmental context in which these processes occur.

Advances in both of these areas will help to integrate previously separate lines of research and will contribute to a fuller, more detailed understanding of depression risk in children. It is hoped that these advances will also pave the way for the development of novel intervention and prevention programs (cf. Hamilton, Glover, Hsu, Johnson, & Gotlib, 2011; Rozenman, Weersing, & Amir, 2011) that can alter the developmental trajectory of depressed and at-risk youth so that they can escape the vicious cycle of risk that often accompanies childhood depression.

ACKNOWLEDGMENT

This project was supported by grants from the National Institute of Child Health and Human Development (R01 HD057066) and the National Institute of Mental Health (R01 MH098060).

REFERENCES

Abela, J. R. Z., & Hankin, B. L. (2008). Cognitive vulnerability to depression in children and adolescents: A developmental psychopathology perspective. In J. R. Z. Abela & B. L. Hankin (Eds.), *Handbook of depression in children and adolescents* (pp. 35–78). New York: Guilford Press.

Abramson, L. Y., Metalsky, G. I., & Alloy, L. B. (1989). Hopelessness depression: A theory-based subtype of depression. *Psychological Review, 96*(2), 358–372.

Abramson, L. Y., Seligman, M. E., & Teasdale, J. D. (1978). Learned helplessness in humans: Critique and reformulation. *Journal of Abnormal Psychology, 87*(1), 49–74.

Alloy, L. B., Abramson, L. Y., Smith, J. M., Gibb, B. E., & Neeren, A. M. (2006). Role of parenting and maltreatment histories in unipolar and bipolar mood disorders: Mediation by cognitive vulnerability to depression. *Clinical Child and Family Psychology Review, 9*(1), 23–64.

Angold, A., Costello, E. J., & Worthman, C. M. (1998). Puberty and depression: The roles of age, pubertal status and pubertal timing. *Psychological Medicine, 28*(1), 51–61.

Asarnow, J. R., Goldstein, M. J., Carlson, G. A., Perdue, S., Bates, S., & Keller, J. (1988). Childhood-onset depressive disorders: A follow-up study of rates of rehospitalization and out-of-home placement among child psychiatric inpatients. *Journal of Affective Disorders, 15*(3), 245–253.

Asarnow, J. R., Tompson, M., Woo, S., & Cantwell, D. P. (2001). Is expressed emotion a specific risk factor for depression or a nonspecific correlate of psychopathology? *Journal of Abnormal Child Psychology, 29*(6), 573–583.

Barch, D. M., Gaffrey, M. S., Botteron, K. N., Belden, A. C., & Luby, J. L. (2012). Functional brain activation to emotionally valenced faces in school-aged children with a history of preschool-onset major depression. *Biological Psychiatry, 72*(12), 1035–1042.

Burkhouse, K., Uhrlass, D., Stone, L., Knopik, V., & Gibb, B. (2012). Expressed emotion–criticism and risk of depression onset in children. *Journal of Clinical Child and Adolescent Psychology, 41*(6), 771–777.

Caspi, A., Sugden, K., Moffitt, T. E., Taylor, A., Craig, I. W., Harrington, H., et al. (2003). Influence of life stress on depression: Moderation by a polymorphism in the *5-HTT* gene. *Science, 301,* 386–389.

Centers for Disease Control and Prevention. (2013a). Mental health surveillance among children—United States, 2005–2011. *Morbidity and Mortality Weekly Report, 62*(Suppl. 2), 1–35.

Centers for Disease Control and Prevention (2013b). Web-based Injury Statistics Query and Reporting System (WISQARS). Retrieved May 17, 2013, from *http://webappa.cdc.gov/sasweb/ncipc/leadcaus10_us.htm.*

Cicchetti, D., Rogosch, F. A., & Oshri, A. (2011). Interactive effects of corticotropin releasing hormone receptor 1, serotonin transporter linked polymorphic region, and child maltreatment on diurnal cortisol regulation and internalizing symptomatology. *Development and Psychopathology, 23*(4), 1125–1138.

Cohen, J. R., Young, J. F., & Abela, J. R. Z. (2012). Cognitive vulnerability to depression in children: An idiographic, longitudinal examination of inferential styles. *Cognitive Therapy and Research, 36*(6), 643–654.

Cohen-Woods, S., Craig, I. W., & McGuffin, P. (2013). The current state of play on the molecular genetics of depression. *Psychological Medicine, 43*(4), 673–687.

Cole, D. A. (1991). Preliminary support for a competency-based model of depression in children. *Journal of Abnormal Psychology, 100*(2), 181–190.

Cole, D. A., Cho, S., Martin, N. C., Youngstrom, E. A., March, J. S., Findling, R. L., et al. (2012). Are increased weight and appetite useful indicators of depression in children and adolescents? *Journal of Abnormal Psychology, 121*(4), 838–851.

Cole, D. A., Jacquez, F. M., LaGrange, B., Pineda, A. Q., Truss, A. E., Weitlauf, A. S., et al. (2011). A longitudinal study of cognitive risks for depressive symptoms in children and young adolescents. *Journal of Early Adolescence, 31*(6), 782–816.

Cole, D. A., Nolen-Hoeksema, S., Girgus, J., & Paul, G. (2006). Stress exposure and stress generation in child and adolescent depression: A latent trait–state–error approach to longitudinal analyses. *Journal of Abnormal Psychology, 115*(1), 40–51.

Conway, C. C., Hammen, C., Brennan, P. A., Lind, P. A., & Najman, J. M. (2010). Interaction of chronic stress with serotonin transporter and catechol-O-methyltransferase polymorphisms in predicting youth depression. *Depression and Anxiety, 27*(8), 737–745.

Copeland, W. E., Shanahan, L., Costello, J., & Angold, A. (2009). Childhood and adolescent psychiatric disorders as predictors of young adult disorders. *Archives of General Psychiatry, 66*(7), 764–772.

Crick, N. R., Casas, J. F., & Nelson, D. A. (2002). Toward a more comprehensive understanding of peer maltreatment: Studies of relational victimization. *Current Directions in Psychological Science, 11*(3), 98–101.

Cusi, A. M., Nazarov, A., Holshausen, K., MacQueen, G. M., & McKinnon, M. C. (2012). Systematic review of the neural basis of social cognition in patients with mood disorders. *Journal of Psychiatry and Neuroscience, 37*(3), 154–169.

Disner, S. G., Beevers, C. G., Haigh, E. A. P., & Beck, A. T. (2011). Neural mechanisms of the cognitive model of depression. *Nature Reviews Neuroscience, 12*(8), 467–477.

Domènech-Llaberia, E., Viñas, F., Pla, E., Jané, M. C., Mitjavila, M., Corbella, T., et al. (2009). Prevalence of major depression in preschool children. *European Child and Adolescent Psychiatry, 18*(10), 597–604.

Dougherty, L. R., Klein, D. N., Congdon, E., Canli, T., & Hayden, E. P. (2010). Interaction between *5-HTTLPR* and BDNF *Val66Met* polymorphisms on HPA-axis reactivity in preschoolers. *Biological Psychology, 83*(2), 93–100.

Drummond, L. E., Dritschel, B., Astell, A., O'Carroll, R. E., & Dalgleish, T. (2006). Effects of age, dysphoria, and emotion focusing on autobiographical memory specificity in children. *Cognition and Emotion, 20*(3–4), 488–505.

Dunn, E. C., Uddin, M., Subramanian, S. V., Smoller, J. W., Galea, S., & Koenen, K. C. (2011). Research review: Gene–environment interaction research in youth depression: A systematic review with recommendations for future research. *Journal of Child Psychology and Psychiatry, 52*(12), 1223–1238.

Egger, H. L., & Angold, A. (2006). Common emotional and behavioral disorders in preschool children: Presentation, nosology, and epidemiology. *Journal of Child Psychology and Psychiatry, 47*(3–4), 313–337.

Eley, T. C. (1997). Depressive symptoms in children and adolescents: Etiological links between normality and abnormality: A research note. *Child Psychology and Psychiatry and Allied Disciplines, 38*(7), 861–865.

Eley, T. C., & Stevenson, J. (1999). Exploring the covariation between anxiety and depression symptoms: A genetic analysis of the effects of age and sex. *Journal of Child Psychology and Psychiatry, 40*(8), 1273–1282.

Gaffrey, M. S., Belden, A. C., & Luby, J. L. (2011). The 2-week duration criterion and severity and course of early childhood depression: Implications for nosology. *Journal of Affective Disorders, 133*(3), 537–545.

Gaffrey, M. S., Luby, J. L., Belden, A. C., Hirshberg, J. S., Volsch, J., & Barch, D. M. (2011). Association between depression severity and amygdala reactivity during sad face viewing in depressed preschoolers: An fMRI study. *Journal of Affective Disorders, 129*(1–3), 364–370.

Gibb, B. E., & Alloy, L. B. (2006). A prospective test of the hopelessness theory of depression in children. *Journal of Clinical Child and Adolescent Psychology, 35*(2), 264–274.

Gibb, B. E., Beevers, C. G., & McGeary, J. E. (2013). Toward an integration of cognitive and genetic models of risk for depression. *Cognition and Emotion, 27*(2), 193–216.

Gibb, B. E., Benas, J. S., Grassia, M., & McGeary, J. (2009). Children's attentional biases and *5-HTTLPR* genotype: Potential mechanisms linking mother and child depression. *Journal of Clinical Child and Adolescent Psychology, 38*(3), 415–426.

Gibb, B. E., & Coles, M. E. (2005). *Cognitive vulnerability–stress models of psychopathology: A developmental perspective.* Thousand Oaks, CA: Sage.

Gibb, B. E., Grassia, M., Stone, L. B., Uhrlass, D. J., & McGeary, J. E. (2012). Brooding rumination and risk for depressive disorders in children of depressed mothers. *Journal of Abnormal Child Psychology, 40*(2), 317–326.

Gibb, B. E., & Hanley, A. J. (2010). Depression and interpersonal stress generation in children: Prospective impact on relational versus overt victimization. *International Journal of Cognitive Therapy, 3*(4), 358–367.

Gibb, B. E., Stone, L. B., & Crossett, S. E. (2012). Peer victimization and prospective changes in children's inferential styles. *Journal of Clinical Child and Adolescent Psychology, 41*(5), 561–569.

Gibb, B. E., Uhrlass, D. J., Grassia, M., Benas, J. S., & McGeary, J. (2009). Children's inferential styles, 5-HTTLPR genotype, and maternal expressed emotion–criticism: An integrated model for the intergenerational transmission of depression. *Journal of Abnormal Psychology, 118*(4), 734–745.

Goodman, S. H. (2007). Depression in mothers. *Annual Review of Clinical Psychology, 3*, 107–135.

Gotlib, I. H., Joormann, J., Minor, K. L., & Hallmayer, J. (2008). HPA-axis reactivity: A mechanism underlying the associations among 5-HTTLPR, stress, and depression. *Biological Psychiatry, 63*(9), 847–851.

Guerry, J. D., & Hastings, P. D. (2011). In search of HPA-axis dysregulation in child and adolescent depression. *Clinical Child and Family Psychology Review, 14*(2), 135–160.

Gunnar, M., & Quevedo, K. (2007). The neurobiology of stress and development. *Annual Review of Psychology, 58*, 145–173.

Hamilton, J. P., Etkin, A., Furman, D. J., Lemus, M. G., Johnson, R. F., & Gotlib, I. H. (2012). Functional neuroimaging of major depressive disorder: A meta-analysis and new integration of baseline activation and neural response data. *American Journal of Psychiatry, 169*(7), 693–703.

Hamilton, J. P., Glover, G. H., Hsu, J., Johnson, R. F., & Gotlib, I. H. (2011). Modulation of subgenual anterior cingulate cortex activity with real-time neurofeedback. *Human Brain Mapping, 32*(1), 22–31.

Hammen, C. (2006). Stress generation in depression: Reflections on origins, research, and future directions. *Journal of Clinical Psychology, 62*(9), 1065–1082.

Hankin, B. L., Abramson, L. Y., Moffitt, T. E., Silva, P. A., McGee, R., & Angell, K. E. (1998). Development of depression from preadolescence to young adulthood: Emerging gender differences in a 10-year longitudinal study. *Journal of Abnormal Psychology, 107*(1), 128–140.

Hankin, B. L., Badanes, L. S., Abela, J. R. Z., & Watamura, S. E. (2010). Hypothalamic–pituitary–adrenal axis dysregulation in dysphoric children and adolescents: Cortisol reactivity to psychosocial stress from preschool through middle adolescence. *Biological Psychiatry, 68*(5), 484–490.

Harrington, R. C. (1996). Adult outcomes of childhood and adolescent depression: Influences on the risk for adult depression. *Psychiatric Annals, 26*(6), 320–325.

Hulvershorn, L. A., Cullen, K., & Anand, A. (2011). Toward dysfunctional connectivity: A review of neuroimaging findings in pediatric major depressive disorder. *Brain Imaging and Behavior, 5*(4), 307–328.

Jacquez, F., Cole, D. A., & Searle, B. (2004). Self-perceived competence as a mediator between maternal feedback and depressive symptoms in adolescents. *Journal of Abnormal Child Psychology, 32*(4), 355–367.

Johnson, A. L., & Gibb, B. E. (in press). Attentional biases in currently depressed children: An eye-tracking study of biases in sustained attention to emotional stimuli. *Journal of Child and Adolescent Psychology.*

Joormann, J., Talbot, L., & Gotlib, I. H. (2007). Biased processing of emotional information in girls at risk for depression. *Journal of Abnormal Psychology, 116*(1), 135–143.

Karg, K., Burmeister, M., Shedden, K., & Sen, S. (2011). The serotonin transporter promoter variant (5-HTTLPR), stress, and depression meta-analysis revisited: Evidence of genetic moderation. *Archives of General Psychiatry, 68*(5), 444–454.

Kovacs, M. (1996). The course of childhood-onset depressive disorders. *Psychiatric Annals, 26*(6), 326–330.

Kovacs, M., Feinberg, T. L., Crouse-Novak, M., Paulauskas, S. L., Pollock, M., Finkelstein, R. (1984). Depressive disorders in childhood: II. A longitudinal study of the risk for a subsequent major depression. *Archives of General Psychiatry, 41*(7), 643–649.

Kovacs, M., Gatsonia, C., Paulauskas, S. L., & Richards, C. (1989). Depressive disorders in childhood: IV. A longitudinal study of comorbidity with and risk for anxiety disorders. *Archives of General Psychiatry, 46*(9), 776–782.

Kovacs, M., Paulauskas, S., Gatsonis, C., & Richards, C. (1988). Depressive disorders in childhood: III. A longitudinal study of comorbidity with and risk for conduct disorders. *Journal of Affective Disorders, 15*(3), 205–217.

Kujawa, A. J., Torpey, D., Kim, J., Hajcak, G., Rose, S., Gotlib, I. H., et al. (2011). Attentional biases for emotional faces in young children of mothers with chronic or recurrent depression. *Journal of Abnormal Child Psychology, 39*(1), 125–135.

Lefkowitz, M. M., & Burton, N. (1978). Childhood depression: A critique of the concept. *Psychological Bulletin, 85*, 716–726.

Lopez-Duran, N. L., Kovacs, M., & George, C. J. (2009). Hypothalamic–pituitary–adrenal axis dysregulation in depressed children and adolescents: A meta-analysis. *Psychoneuroendocrinology, 34*(9), 1272–1283.

Luby, J. L., Heffelfinger, A., Mrakotsky, C., Brown, K., Hessler, M., & Spitznagel, E. (2003). Alterations in stress cortisol reactivity in depressed preschoolers relative to psychiatric and no-disorder comparison groups. *Archives of General Psychiatry, 60*(12), 1248–1255.

Luby, J. L., Heffelfinger, A. K., Mrakotsky, C., Hessler, M. J., Brown, K. M., & Hildebrand, T. (2002). Preschool major depressive disorder: Preliminary validation for developmentally modified DSM-IV criteria. *Journal of the American Academy of Child and Adolescent Psychiatry, 41*(8), 928–937.

Luby, J. L., Mrakotsky, C., Heffelfinger, A., Brown, K., & Spitznagel, E. (2004). Characteristics of depressed preschoolers with and without anhedonia: Evidence for a melancholic depressive subtype in young children. *American Journal of Psychiatry, 161*(11), 1998–2004.

Luby, J. L., Si, X., Belden, A. C., Tandon, M., & Spitznagel, E. (2009). Preschool depression: Homotypic continuity and course over 24 months. *Archives of General Psychiatry, 66*(8), 897–905.

Luby, J. L., Sullivan, J., Belden, A., Stalets, M., Blankenship, S., & Spitznagel, E. (2006). An observational analysis of behavior in depressed preschoolers: Further validation of early-onset depression. *Journal of the American Academy of Child and Adolescent Psychiatry, 45*(2), 203–212.

Luking, K. R., Repovs, G., Belden, A. C., Gaffrey, M. S., Botteron, K. N., Luby, J. L., et al. (2011). Functional connectivity of the amygdala in early-childhood-onset depression. *Journal of the American Academy of Child and Adolescent Psychiatry, 50*(10), 1027–1041.e3.

Lupien, S. J., McEwen, B. S., Gunnar, M. R., & Heim, C. (2009). Effects of stress throughout the lifespan on the brain, behaviour and cognition. *Nature Reviews Neuroscience, 10*(6), 434–445.

Major Depressive Disorder Working Group of the Psychiatric GWAS Consortium, Ripke, S., Wray, N. R., Lewis, C. M., Hamilton, S. P., Weissman, M. M., et al. (2013). A mega-analysis of genome-wide association studies for major depressive disorder. *Molecular Psychiatry, 18*(4), 497–511.

McGee, R., & Williams, S. (1988). A longitudinal study of depression in nine-year-old children. *Journal of the American Academy of Child and Adolescent Psychiatry, 27*(3), 342–348.

Merikangas, K. R., He, J., Brody, D., Fisher, P. W., Bourdon, K., & Koretz, D. S. (2010). Prevalence and treatment of mental disorders among U.S. children in the 2001–2004 NHANES. *Pediatrics, 125*(1), 75–81.

Mitchell, J. R., McCauley, E., Burke, P. M., & Moss, S. J. (1988). Phenomenology of depression in children and adolescents. *Journal of the American Academy of Child and Adolescent Psychiatry, 27*(1), 12–20.

Mueller, A., Brocke, B., Fries, E., Lesch, K., & Kirschbaum, C. (2010). The role of the serotonin transporter polymorphism for the endocrine stress response in newborns. *Psychoneuroendocrinology, 35*(2), 289–296.

Munafò, M. R., Brown, S. M., & Hariri, A. R. (2008). Serotonin transporter (*5-HTTLPR*) genotype and amygdala activation: A meta-analysis. *Biological Psychiatry, 63*(9), 852–857.

Nolen-Hoeksema, S., Wisco, B. E., & Lyubomirsky, S. (2008). Rethinking rumination. *Perspectives on Psychological Science, 3*(5), 400–424.

Raes, F., Verstraeten, K., Bijttebier, P., Vasey, M. W., & Dalgleish, T. (2010). Inhibitory control mediates the relationship between depressed mood and overgeneral memory recall in children. *Journal of Clinical Child and Adolescent Psychology, 39*(2), 276–281.

Reijntjes, A., Kamphuis, J. H., Prinzie, P., & Telch, M. J. (2010). Peer victimization and internalizing problems in children: A meta-analysis of longitudinal studies. *Child Abuse and Neglect, 34*(4), 244–252.

Rice, F., Harold, G. T., & Thapar, A. (2003). Negative life events as an account of age-related differences in the genetic aetiology of depression in childhood and adolescence. *Journal of Child Psychology and Psychiatry, 44*(7), 977–987.

Rice, F., van den Bree, M. B. M., & Thapar, A. (2004). A population-based study of anxiety as a precursor for depression in childhood and adolescence. *BMC Psychiatry, 4*, 43.

Risch, N., Herrell, R., Lehner, T., Liang, K., Eaves, L., Hoh, J., et al. (2009). Interaction between the serotonin transporter gene (*5-HTTLPR*), stressful life events, and risk of depression: A meta-analysis. *Journal of the American Medical Association, 301*, 2462–2471.

Rood, L., Roelofs, J., Bögels, S. M., Nolen-Hoeksema, S., & Schouten, E. (2009). The influence of emotion-focused rumination and distraction on depressive symptoms in non-clinical youth: A meta-analytic review. *Clinical Psychology Review, 29*(7), 607–616.

Rozenman, M., Weersing, V. R., & Amir, N. (2011). A case series of attention modification in clinically anxious youths. *Behaviour Research and Therapy, 49*(5), 324–330.

Ryan, N. D., Puig-Antich, J., Ambrosini, P., Rabinovich, H., Robinson, D., Nelson, B., et al. (1987). The clinical picture of major depression in children and adolescents. *Archives of General Psychiatry, 44*(10), 854–861.

Silberg, J., Rutter, M., Neale, M., & Eaves, L. (2001). Genetic moderation of environmental risk for depression and anxiety in adolescent girls. *British Journal of Psychiatry, 179*, 116–121.

Silberg, J. L., Pickles, A., Rutter, M., Hewitt, J., Simonoff, E., Maes, H., et al. (1999). The influence of genetic factors and life stress on depression among adolescent girls. *Archives of General Psychiatry, 56*(3), 225–232.

Silk, J. S., Ziegler, M. L., Whalen, D. J., Dahl, R. E., Ryan, N. D., Dietz, L. J., et al. (2009). Expressed emotion in mothers of currently depressed, remitted, high-risk, and low-risk youth: Links to child depression status and longitudinal course. *Journal of Clinical Child and Adolescent Psychology, 38*(1), 36–47.

Sinclair, K. R., Cole, D. A., Dukewich, T., Felton, J., Weitlauf, A. S., Maxwell, M. A., et al. (2012). Impact of physical and relational peer victimization on depressive cognitions in children and adolescents. *Journal of Clinical Child and Adolescent Psychology, 41*(5), 570–583.

Smucker, M. R., Craighead, W. E., Craighead, L. W., & Green, B. J. (1986). Normative and reliability data for the Children's Depression Inventory. *Journal of Abnormal Child Psychology, 14*(1), 25–39.

Subbarao, A., Rhee, S. H., Young, S. E., Ehringer, M. A., Corley, R. P., & Hewitt, J. K. (2008). Common genetic and environmental influences on major depressive disorder and conduct disorder. *Journal of Abnormal Child Psychology, 36*(3), 433–444.

Sullivan, P. F., Neale, M. C., & Kendler, K. S. (2000). Genetic epidemiology of major depression: Review and meta-analysis. *American Journal of Psychiatry, 157*(10), 1552–1562.

Suzuki, H., Botteron, K. N., Luby, J. L., Belden, A. C., Gaffrey, M. S., Babb, C. M., et al. (2013). Structural–functional correlations between hippocampal volume and cortico–limbic emotional responses in depressed children. *Cognitive, Affective, and Behavioral Neuroscience, 13*(1), 135–151.

Thapar, A., & McGuffin, P. (1996). The genetic etiology of childhood depressive symptoms: A developmental perspective. *Development and Psychopathology, 8*(4), 751–760.

Thapar, A., & McGuffin, P. (1997). Anxiety and depressive symptoms in childhood: A genetic study of comorbidity. *Child Psychology and Psychiatry and Allied Disciplines, 38*(6), 651–656.

Twenge, J. M., & Nolen-Hoeksema, S. (2002). Age, gender, race, socioeconomic status, and birth cohort difference on the children's depression inventory: A meta-analysis. *Journal of Abnormal Psychology, 111*(4), 578–588.

Uhrlass, D. J., Crossett, S. E., & Gibb, B. E. (2008). Self-perceived competence, relational victimization, and children's depressive symptoms: Evidence for a sex-specific vulnerability–stress model. *International Journal of Cognitive Therapy, 1*(4), 284–297.

Vrielynck, N., Deplus, S., & Philippot, P. (2007). Overgeneral autobiographical memory and depressive disorder in children. *Journal of Clinical Child and Adolescent Psychology, 36*(1), 95–105.

Weiss, B., & Garber, J. (2003). Developmental differences in the phenomenology of depression. *Development and Psychopathology, 15*(2), 403–430.

Weissman, M. M., Wolk, S., Wickramaratne, P., Goldstein, R. B., Adams, P., Greenwald, S., et al.(1999). Children with prepubertal-onset major depressive disorder and anxiety grown up. *Archives of General Psychiatry, 56*(9), 794–801.

Wichstrøm, L., Berg-Nielsen, T. S., Angold, A., Egger, H. L., Solheim, E., & Sveen, T. H. (2012). Prevalence of psychiatric disorders in preschoolers. *Journal of Child Psychology and Psychiatry, 53*(6), 695–705.

Wilkinson, P. O., Trzaskowski, M., Haworth, C. M. A., & Eley, T. C. (2013). The role of gene–environment correlations and interactions in middle childhood depressive symptoms. *Development and Psychopathology, 25*(1), 93–104.

CHAPTER 21

Depression in Adolescents

KAREN D. RUDOLPH *and* MEGAN FLYNN

Depression is a serious mental health problem that carries significant personal and societal costs. Contemporary perspectives highlight adolescence as a high-risk period for the emergence of depression. No longer viewed as reflecting normative storm and stress, depression in adolescents is recognized as a pernicious and recurrent disorder that creates significant impairment across development. Understanding depression in adolescents can therefore inform theories of the etiology, course, and consequences of depression, as well as interventions to alleviate current suffering and prevent lifelong impairment.

Several characteristics of adolescence are particularly relevant to understanding how this period creates a context of risk for depression. Major transformations in brain structure and function and related biological processes heighten vulnerability to emotion dysregulation, cognitive dysfunction, and stress sensitivity (Ladouceur, 2012). Normative changes in social systems intensify stress, with accompanying implications for depression (Rudolph, 2009). These normative biological, psychological, and social challenges may tip the scale from mental health to psychopathology in vulnerable youth or those who progress through puberty earlier than their peers (Rudolph, 2014). Thus understanding depression in adolescents requires considering the unique features of this developmental stage.

DESCRIPTION OF DEPRESSION IN ADOLESCENTS

Epidemiology

Epidemiological research reveals a marked increase in depression during adolescence. By mid- to late adolescence, rates of diagnosable depression are comparable to those in adults (prevalence rates of 15–25%; Kaminski & Garber, 2002). Prospective community studies similarly reveal a sharp rise in rates of clinical depression from childhood through late adolescence (Rohde, Beevers, Stice, & O'Neil, 2009). Subclinical depression affects a large minority of adolescents. Using diagnostic criteria, approximately 20% of youth experience subsyndromal or minor depression (Van Voorhees, Melkonian, Marko, Humensky, & Fogel, 2010). Using conventional cutoffs on self-report measures, an even greater percentage of youth (20–50%) experience significant symptoms (Kessler, Avenevoli, & Merikangas, 2001). Moreover, research tracking depressive symptoms over time indicates rising rates during adolescence (Dekker et al., 2007). These elevated and persistent levels of symptoms are associated with comorbidity (Van Voorhees et al., 2010) and herald the onset of depressive disorders (Klein, Shankman, Lewinsohn, & Seeley, 2009).

Prospective research indicates that the peak age of onset for depression occurs during mid-adolescence, at approximately 13–15 years. In the Oregon Adolescent Depression Project, the mean age of onset of major depressive disorder (MDD) was about age 15 (Lewinsohn & Essau, 2002). In a sample of females, the 1-year prevalence for depression diagnoses peaked at age 16 (Rohde et al., 2009). The length of major depressive episodes (MDEs) during adolescence varies across studies, with longer durations in clinical (mean duration of 7–9 months; Birmaher, Arbeleaz, & Brent, 2002; Rao et al., 1995) than community (mean duration of 5.3–6.5 months; Kaminski & Garber, 2002; Rohde et al., 2009) samples. Most MDEs remit within 2 years, whereas persistent depressive disorder (formerly dysthymia; American Psychiatric Association, 2013) has a mean duration of 2.4–4 years (Birmaher et al., 1996; Kaminski & Garber, 2002).

Depression carries a strong risk for recurrence, with as many as 40–70% of adolescents experiencing another MDE within 2–5 years after recovery (Birmaher et al., 1996; Pettit, Hartley, Lewinsohn, Seeley, & Klein, 2013). Predictors of chronicity and recurrence include symptom severity, personal or family MDD history, comorbidity, suicidality, negative beliefs, and family adversity (Birmaher et al., 2002; Pettit et al., 2013).

Less clarity exists about the continuity of depression across developmental periods. Evidence from both community (Copeland et al., 2013) and clinical (Rao et al., 1995) studies attests that adolescent depression portends depression in adulthood. However, there is a possible discontinuity between pre- versus postadolescence onset depression, as reflected in differing course, correlates, and etiology (Hill, Pickles, Rollinson, Davies, & Byatt, 2004). These findings indicate the need to identify factors that distinguish between depressive disorders with differing periods of onset and to elucidate processes that underlie continuity versus discontinuity over time.

Phenomenology and Developmental Features

In the most recent *Diagnostic and Statistical Manual of Mental Disorders* (DSM-5; APA, 2013), the same criteria are used to diagnose depression across development, with only small differences (in adolescents, irritability can be one of the mood changes, and there is a 1-year duration criteria for persistent depressive disorder). However, there may be developmental changes in the experience and expression of symptoms. In a meta-analysis comparing *rates* of symptoms across age groups, Weiss and Garber (2003) found differences in many of the core (e.g., agitation, retardation, fatigue, guilt, and sadness) and associated (e.g., anxiety, somatic complaints) symptoms. Evidence is mixed regarding whether a similar *structure* underlies the depressive syndrome across age (Weiss & Garber, 2003). Thus, although depression shows some homotypic continuity, there are phenomenological differences. These differences may reflect developmentally specific manifestations of the same syndrome or the possibility that childhood- versus adolescence- or adult-onset depression are distinct disorders.

Comorbidity

Comorbidity between adolescent depression and other disorders is common (Rohde, 2009). Community research reveals that adolescent depression highly co-occurs with anxiety disorders (odds ratios of 11.0–13.2) and conduct/oppositional defiant disorders (odds ratio of 3.5–8.6; Romano, Tremblay, Vitaro, Zoccolillo, & Pagani, 2005). A recent analysis of three large-scale prospective studies revealed that depression in adolescence is preceded by anxiety and conduct disorders in childhood and predicts anxiety and substance use disorders in adulthood (Copeland et al., 2013).

Comorbidity may reflect inadequate diagnostic systems or assessment instruments. Alternatively, comorbidity may stem from common etiologies (e.g., shared genetic liability for depression and conduct disorder; Tackett, Waldman, Van Hulle, & Lahey, 2011) or co-occurring risk factors (e.g., family psychiatric history and childhood adversity create a risk for depression and anxiety; Moffitt et al., 2007). Given the sequential association between depression and other disorders, comorbidity also may be explained by the progression of one disorder into another.

Illustrating the significance of depression comorbidity, it is associated with more severe and recurrent depression (Karlsson et al., 2008), as well as more life stress (Rudolph et al., 2000) and substance use (Evans & Frank, 2004). Comorbidity also might obscure certain correlates of depression, such as atypical patterns of brain functioning (Kentgen et al., 2000). Thus future research must consider how comorbidity influences the nature, course, etiology, consequences, and treatment of depression.

Sex Differences

One of the most robust features of depression is the emerging sex difference during adolescence, with girls beginning to show more depressive symptoms and disorders by early to mid-adolescence (12–14 years); this difference increases through adolescence until it reaches a 2:1 ratio, which persists through the life span (Hankin, Wetter, & Cheely, 2008). Adolescent girls with depression experience more weight and appetite disturbances, feelings of worthlessness and guilt (Lewinsohn, Rohde, & Seeley, 1998), sadness and loneliness (Abdel-Khalek & Soliman, 2002), and suicidality (Yorbik, Birmaher, Axelson, Williamson, & Ryan, 2004), as well as more comorbid depression and anxiety disorders (Romano et al., 2005). Theoretical models attempt to account for the rising rates and the emerging sex difference in depression during adolescence (Rudolph, 2009). These models focus on the interactive contributions of biological, psychological, and contextual changes associated with the adolescent transition, often with a focus on sex-linked roles, beliefs, and experiences within interpersonal relationships (see later sections).

ORIGINS AND DEVELOPMENT OF DEPRESSION IN ADOLESCENTS

Understanding the origins of depression in adolescents requires a developmental, multilevel conceptualization that integrates multiple domains of personal and contextual risk. Moreover, an integrative framework must consider how adolescent transitions serve as a backdrop for increasing depression, particularly in girls.

Genetic Vulnerability

Behavior genetic research reveals moderate heritability of depressive disorders, with significant variability depending on age, sex, informant, and operationalization of depression. A recent review (Rice, 2010) concluded that heritability is nonsignificant in child samples but increases during adolescence, with estimates (around 40%) similar to those in adults. These findings indicate different origins of childhood and adolescent depression, suggesting age of onset might be a marker for distinct subtypes. When tracked over time, some new genetic influences emerge and others are attenuated (Kendler, Gardner, & Lichtenstein, 2008; Lau & Eley, 2006), suggesting that heritability is dynamic and may be expressed through transactions and interactions with novel developmental and environmental experiences. Indeed, genes can affect the likelihood that individuals are exposed to depressogenic environments through passive or evocative gene–environment correlations or can increase sensitivity to stressors (Lau & Eley, 2008), thereby resulting in changing associations between genes and depression across development. Although behavior genetic research indicates small to negligible sex differences in heritability (Franić, Middeldorp, Dolan, Ligthart, & Boomsma, 2010), one twin study revealed significant heritability that was specific to pubertal girls. Moreover, in another study, genetic liability to life events accounted in part for higher rates of depression in girls after puberty (Silberg et al., 1999).

Molecular genetic research has identified candidate genes for depression vulnerability, with a particular focus on those involved in emotion regulation and stress reactivity. Research suggests that adolescents with the short allele variant of the serotonin transporter gene (*5-HTTLPR*) are at greater risk for depression when faced with life stress (Hankin, Jenness, Abela, & Smolen, 2011) or elevated morning cortisol (Goodyer, Croudace, Dudbridge, Ban, & Herbert, 2010), with some studies yielding effects in adolescent girls but not boys (Hammen, Brennan, Keenan-Miller, Hazel, & Najman, 2010). Research also documents gene–gene–environment (Kaufman et al., 2006) and gene–cortisol (Goodyer et al., 2010) interactions for brain-derived neurotropic factor (*BDNF*). However, significant debate exists concerning the robustness of gene × environment interactions for depression (e.g., Karg, Burmeister, Shedden, & Sen, 2011; Risch et al., 2009).

Scientists now are seeking to identify endophenotypes, or processes through which genes create a liability to stress reactivity and depression. Research supports a genetic liability to cognitive vulnerability (Beevers, Wells, Ellis, & McGeary, 2009; Lau, Rijsdijk, & Eley, 2006). Variants of the *5-HT* and *BDNF* genes linked with depression also are associated with relevant biological risks, such as amygdala activation to negative emotional stimuli (Furman, Hamilton, Joormann, & Gotlib, 2011; Lau et al., 2010), as well as heightened basal cortisol and cortisol reactivity (Chen, Joormann, Hallmayer, & Gotlib, 2009; Gotlib, Joormann, Minor, & Hallmayer, 2008), implicating neural and hormonal pathways through which genetic risk is expressed.

In sum, research implicates gene–environment interactions and transactions as risks for adolescent depression. Genetic liability seems to be activated during adolescence, particularly in girls. This developmental expression of liability may be triggered by biological changes, as well as increasing psychological and social challenges during puberty that create an opportunity for genetically mediated exposure or reactivity to stress. However, given inconsistencies in candidate gene research, continued research is needed to elucidate the precise nature and limits of genetic liability and to determine the specific biological, psychological, and social mechanisms (e.g., temperamental characteristics, neurobiological dysfunction, cognitive vulnerability, stress exposure or reactivity) through which this liability is translated into depression. Exciting advances are likely to emerge as the field of epigenetics continues to unravel how social experiences guide individual differences in the biological and phenotypic expression (or silencing) of genes (Meaney, 2010).

Biological Vulnerability

Recent efforts to understand the unique biological substrates of depression in adolescents have yielded several compelling models. Despite diversity across the models, they converge on the idea that biological transformations of puberty, reflected in changes in brain structure and function and downstream consequences, can help account for the dramatic rise and, to some extent, the emerging sex difference in depression during adolescence.

Progress in uncovering clues regarding risk for depression has been spurred by emerging models of adolescent brain development (Dahl, 2004), which focus on a maturational imbalance between neural regions involved in cognitive control (prefrontal cortex; PFC) and socioaffective circuitry involved in emotional reactivity and motivation (amygdala, ventral striatum). According to these models, increasing neural and hormonal sensitivity to emotionally salient or stressful stimuli during puberty overwhelms cognitive regulation systems, which mature more gradually. These changes, driven in part by increases in puberty-related sex hormones and their influences on neurotransmitter systems, are presumed to heighten emotion dysregulation and risk for affective disorders, particularly in vulnerable youth (Ladouceur, 2012).

Pubertal changes occur across multiple neurobiological systems, with converging evidence for heightened emotional and stress reactivity as instantiated in sensitivity of the hypothalamic–pituitary–adrenal (HPA) axis and sympathetic nervous system (SNS; Gunnar, Wewerka, Frenn, Long, & Griggs, 2009; Stroud et al., 2009). During puberty, surges in sex hormones along with psychosocial changes may have a particularly strong influence on youths' social orientation, triggering a unique attunement to social rewards (status, dominance) and punishment (negative evaluation, rejection) (Forbes & Dahl, 2010). This reorientation, or social sensitivity (Somerville, 2013), is thought to amplify the emotional salience of social cues in ways that influence affective reactivity and regulation (Ladouceur, 2012). Relative to younger children, adolescents show elevated amygdala activation to fearful faces (Hare et al., 2008), potentiation of physiological indexes of approach and avoidance (Quevedo, Benning, Gunnar, & Dahl, 2009), and heightened neural reactivity to rejection versus acceptance (Silk et al., 2012). Suggesting an association with hormonal changes, Forbes, Phillips, Ryan, and Dahl (2011) found that pubertal maturation rather than age predicts more reactivity to unambiguous (relative to ambiguous) social threat. Along with heightened reactivity, adolescents show poorer neural regulation. Relative to adults, adolescents more strongly recruit the medial PFC (part of the socioaffective circuitry) and less strongly recruit regulatory regions of the lateral PFC while processing social exclusion (Sebastian et al., 2011).

Theory and research thus implicate adolescence as a stage during which normative changes create difficulties integrating processes that regulate arousal, attention, motivation, and emotion with those that regulate cognitive control; this lack of coordination may pose particular challenges for youth who enter adolescence with prior vulnerabilities, creating a context of risk for depression. Indeed, hormonal and neural reactivity to emotional stimuli and stress plays an important role in adolescent depression. HPA sensitivity—reflected in basal cortisol (Adam et al., 2010; Mathew et al., 2003) and cortisol reactivity to social challenge (Giletta et al., in press)—predicts future depression and suicidality in adolescents (for a review, see Guerry & Hastings, 2011); this link may be specific to girls (Gunnar et al., 2009). Neural sensitivity to emotion, such as heightened ventromedial PFC and dorsal anterior cingulate cortex (dACC) activity when processing fearful faces (Killgore & Yurgelun-Todd, 2006) and heightened amydala reactivity when processing angry faces (Forbes et al., 2011), also is linked with adolescent depression. Reflecting impairments in regulation, youth with affective disorders show less effective attentional control over emotionally salient distractors (e.g., negative emotional faces) than healthy adolescents (for a review, see Ladouceur, 2012), suggesting dampened functional connectivity between prefrontal cortical regions and the subcortical regions they modulate. One study using resting-state fMRI confirmed compromised functional connectivity within neural circuits involved in emotion processing (Cullen et al., 2009). This compromised connectivity is likely due in part to observed structural differences in limbic (amygdala, hippocampus, and pituitary) and cortical (PFC, orbifrontal cortext, and ACC) circuitry involved in emotion regulation, although findings vary across samples (Hulvershorn, Cullen, & Anand, 2011).

Dysregulation of motivation systems—both heightened neural sensitivity to punishment and dampened neural sensitivity to reward—also serves as a risk for depression. Neural sensitivity (subgenual ACC activation) to social exclusion—so-called "social pain"—predicts adolescent depression (Masten et al., 2011). Consistent with behavioral indicators of low approach motivation (e.g., anhedonia), blunted neural sensitivity to reward predicts subsequent symptoms and first onset of an MDE (Bress, Foti, Kotov, Klein, & Hajcak, 2013; for a review, see Forbes & Dahl, 2012). This pattern is consistent with psychophysiological models of depression suggesting that left-sided hypoactivation of prefrontal cortical regions reflects an underactivation of the approach system, leading to withdrawal and depression (Davidson, Pizzagalli, Nitschke, & Putnam, 2002).

Given that adolescence is marked by normative biological changes in reactivity and regulation, why are some youth particularly vulnerable, such that puberty triggers depression during this stage? The origin of this vulnerability likely lies in a combination of genetic liability and early social adversity. Consistent with both explanations, compared with youth not at risk, the offspring of parents with depression show HPA dysregulation (for a review, see Guerry & Hastings, 2011), greater amygdala and nucleus accumbens activation to fearful faces (Monk et al., 2008), atypical neural processing of reward and punishment (Gotlib et al., 2010), and dampened neural activation during mood regulation (Joormann, Cooney, Henry, & Gotlib, 2012). A small body of research also implicates structural differences in adolescents with a family history of depression (Hulvershorn et al., 2011). This research supports the idea that heightened reactivity and poorer regulation may be risk markers, but more research is needed to determine whether these patterns predict subsequent depression in youth.

Vulnerability in the face of normative biological changes of adolescence also may emerge from early social adversity, which can create permanent changes in brain structure and function, thereby sensitizing the stress-response system (Post, 1992) in ways that heighten risk for emotion dysregulation and subsequent depression. This biological embedding of experience has the potential to explain why youth exposed to early adversity show increasing depression during adolescence. "Social pain" theory (Eisenberger, 2012) suggests that threats to human needs for social belonging trigger activation in the same neural circuitry as that underlying physical pain. Indeed, experimental exposure to social injury activates brain regions (dACC and anterior insula) implicated in the affective component of physical pain. These effects are heightened for individuals with traits or experiences indicative of social sensitivity (Eisenberger, 2012). Social adversity also can lead to activation of stress-response systems and a pattern of proinflammatory processes that heighten risk for depression (Slavich, O'Donovan, Epel, & Kemeny, 2010). Thus it is plausible that early experiences are instantiated in anomalous patterns of biological function, which then confer risk for depression.

Still to be determined is how early-developing biological vulnerabilities intersect with hormonal changes during puberty to account for emerging depression. It is well established that advancing puberty represents a context of risk for depression (Rudolph, 2014). Pubertal changes may have a direct effect on depression through proximal modulatory effects of sex steroids and interactions with other neurotransmitter and hormonal systems involved in central nervous system reactivity and stress regulation, as well as through organizational effects of hormones on neural development (Ladouceur, 2012; Rudolph, 2014). These structural and functional changes may set the stage for problems (e.g., emotion dysregulation, avoidance) that trigger depression. Yet research also documents unique effects of the timing, or even perceived timing, of puberty, particularly early maturation in girls, on depression and the sex difference therein, suggesting that psychological and social aspects of puberty may contribute to risk beyond hormones (Rudolph, 2014).

In sum, adolescence represents a period of rapid brain development during which preexisting vulnerability may be expressed in the form of heightened sensitivity and compromised regulation in emotion and stress-response systems. However, ideas about the biological origins of risk are mainly speculative. Moreover, research has not yet directly examined theoretical assumptions that biological processes mediate the interactive contribution of early risk and proximal social stressors to adolescent depression. Also awaiting investigation is the intriguing idea that adolescence can serve as a period of developmental plasticity, allowing for recalibration of biological systems and potential reversal of early risk along with resilience against depression (Esposito & Gunnar, 2014).

Emotional Vulnerability

Difficulty processing and regulating emotions is a core feature of depression. Converging lines of research identify developmental origins, correlates, and proximal predictors of these core emotional deficits. Conceptualizations of emotional vulnerability to depression consider individual differences in temperament, emotional awareness, emotion processing, and emotional reactivity.

Theoretical models of temperament implicate trait-like differences in positive emotionality (PE; activity, sociability) and negative emotionality (NE; fear, sadness, anger) in depression (Clark & Watson, 1991). Indeed, low PE and high NE predict subsequent adolescent depression (Davies & Windle, 2001). Related aspects of temperament are reflected in approach (sensitivity to reward and positive stimuli) and avoidance (sensitivity to punishment and negative stimuli; Gray, 1994). Compared with youth without depression, mixed-age youth with depression exhibit reduced reward anticipation following positive outcomes (Olino et al., 2011); adolescents with depression also report fewer approach goals/plans and more avoidance plans (Dickson & MacLeod, 2004).

Deficits in emotional awareness and processing also serve as risks for depression. In terms of affective experience, compromised emotional understanding predicts adolescent depressive symptoms over time (Flynn & Rudolph, in press). Using neuropsychological methods (assessment of perceptual asymmetry) to assess the processing of emotional expressions, one study found that a reduced posterior right hemisphere bias was associated with depressive symptoms in youth exposed to high levels of interpersonal stress (Flynn & Rudolph, 2007). Two recent studies identified maladaptive interpersonal stress responses as a mechanism accounting for the effects of compromised emotional understanding (Flynn & Rudolph, in press) and atypical regional brain activity (Flynn & Rudolph, 2010) on adolescent depression.

Depression-linked emotional dysfunction likely emerges from both personal (discussed earlier; e.g., genetic and biological contributions to atypical emotional reactivity and regulation; puberty-driven developmental changes in emotion) and environmental factors. Both distal (e.g. parental depression, maltreatment) and proximal (e.g. maladaptive parent socialization) environmental influences contribute to depression-linked emotional dysfunction (Abaied & Rudolph, 2014). Deviant processing of facial emotions (selective attention to sadness) occurs in the never-depressed daughters of mothers with depression, implicating this pattern as a possible marker of vulnerability (Joormann, Talbot, & Gotlib, 2007). Parents also can contribute directly to poor regulatory abilities through caregiving behaviors that disrupt the development of emotional competence (Denham, Bassett, & Wyatt, 2007) and effective responses to stress (Abaied & Rudolph, 2010). A recent review of observational research indicates that youth depression is associated with parental behaviors that reinforce dysphoria, reciprocate anger and aggression, and fail to reinforce positive emotions (Schwartz, Sheeber, Dudgeon, & Allen, 2012). Moreover, parental encouragement to disengage from rather than engage with stress predicts depression in youth experiencing high levels of interpersonal stress (Abaied & Rudolph, 2010).

Thus several lines of research implicate emotional dysfunction in adolescent depression. Although illuminating, future research will benefit from prospective investigations examining integrated biological, cognitive, and interpersonal mediators and moderators of the links between emotional vulnerabilities and adolescent depression. Continued investigation into how adolescence, particularly the pubertal transition, serves to heighten emotional vulnerability also may help explain increasing rates of depression during this stage.

Cognitive Vulnerability

Cognitive vulnerability–stress models of depression assert that negative belief systems and maladaptive information processing serve as diatheses for depression, which are activated in the context of stress. Three prominent theories identify negative cognitive schemas and core dysfunctional attitudes (Beck, 1967), negative inferences and hopelessness (Abramson, Metalsky, & Alloy, 1989), and ruminative response style (Nolen-Hoeksema, 1991) as cognitive vulnerabilities that confer vulnerability to depression during stressful circumstances.

Contemporary research using prospective designs and evaluating cognitive vulnerability–stress interactions supports the basic tenets of cognitive models (Abela & Hankin, 2008). In adolescents, dysfunctional attitudes (Hankin, Abramson, Miller, & Haeffel, 2004), depressive attributions (Carter & Garber, 2011), and rumination (Abela & Hankin, 2011) interact with stress to predict depressive symptoms and episodes. However, studies revealing partial or even no support for cognitive models have led to refinements of these theories. The "weakest link hypothesis" (Abela & Sarin, 2002) proposes that identifying youths' most negative inferential style may maximize predictive validity (for supportive evidence in adolescents, see Morris, Ciesla, & Garber, 2008).

Less well studied is the role of implicit information-processing biases in depression in adolescents. One study of mixed-age youth revealed that youth with pure depression show an attentional bias toward sad faces (Hankin, Gibb, Abela, & Flory, 2010). Although research in this area is limited by its concurrent design, research also reveals attentional (Joormann et al., 2007) and memory (Flynn & Rudolph, 2012) biases associated with maternal depression, implicating these biases as potential markers of vulnerability. Finally, exposure to peer stress during mid- to late childhood predicts depression in adolescent girls, but not boys, with shifting deficits (inability to refocus attention, rigid thinking; Agoston & Rudolph, 2014). Such deficits may create cognitive inflexibility that sets the stage for rumination and eventual depression. Collectively, these studies suggest that information-processing biases and associated cognitive control deficits predict subsequent depression; however, more prospective research is needed.

Recent efforts focus on understanding the development of cognitive vulnerability. Research identifies its early roots in individual differences in genes, temperament, neural activation, and self-regulation, as well as social-contextual adversity (Abela & Hankin, 2008). Proximal stressors (Tram & Cole, 2000) and depressive symptoms (LaGrange et al., 2011) also leave a cognitive scar reflected in maladaptive attributions and appraisals. Despite its origins in early-emerging traits and experiences, cognitive vulnerability may amplify across adolescence, perhaps helping to explain the concomitant rise in depression. During this stage, changes in the capacity for abstract reasoning, generalization, and self-consciousness, along with the growing disjuncture between cognitive control and emotional reactivity, may intensify risk for stable negative cognitions and unchecked cognitive activity (attentional biases, rumination, maladaptive inferences). Indeed, a quantitative review (Lakdawalla, Hankin, & Mermelstein, 2007) revealed that the cognitive vulnerability–depression link strengthens with age, indicating the importance of understanding changes in the stability, consolidation, and predictive power of cognitive vulnerability across development.

Interpersonal Vulnerability

According to interpersonal theories, individuals with depression and those prone to depression engage in maladaptive behaviors that elicit negative responses and generate stress in their relationships. These relationship difficulties perpetuate symptoms and promote recurrence (Hammen, 2006). Although originally developed to explain adult depression, more recent perspectives emphasize how normative personal and social challenges of adolescence interact with prior interpersonal vulnerability, anchored in exposure to early adversity, to heighten risk for depression and the sex difference therein during this stage (Cyranowski, Frank, Young, & Shear, 2000; Rudolph, 2009).

Developmental theories implicate early family adversity (parental depression, insecure parent–child attachment, maltreatment) as a significant risk factor for interpersonal vulnerability and consequent depression. Family adversity sensitizes youth to subsequent stress, such that adolescents with, compared to without, a history of adversity are more likely to become depressed when faced with mild stress (Hammen, Henry, & Daley, 2000; Rudolph & Flynn, 2007). This sensitization may occur via multiple pathways. Family adversity may heighten maladaptive appraisals of relationships (e.g., interpersonal sensitivity; negative self-appraisals) by conveying messages that youth are unworthy and relationships are unpredictable or unrewarding, as well as by sensitizing youth to imagined or actual evaluation and social stress (Rudolph, 2009). Exposure to early adversity also may undermine youths' social prowess by fostering difficulties in self-regulation, social disengagement, and an interpersonal style characterized by a negative self-focus (Rudolph, 2009). In turn, maladaptive relationship appraisals (Hammen et al., 1995) and social-behavioral deficits (Flynn & Rudolph, 2011; Prinstein, Borelli, Cheah, Simon, & Aikins, 2005) heighten risk for adolescent depressive symptoms, particularly in the face of interpersonal stress.

Maladaptive relationship appraisals and social-behavioral deficits also may generate stress in adolescents' relationships, causing them to act in ways that trigger aversive reactions from others. Youth who feel insecure or who are highly sensitive to evaluation and approval may disengage from relationships or overreact to perceived slights, leaving them socially isolated. Alternatively, seeking excessive reassurance or engaging in negative self-focused exchanges with peers may elicit overt rejection, victimization, or conflict (Rudolph, 2009). Consistent with these ideas, maladaptive relationship schemas (Eberhart, Auerbach, Bigda-Peyton, & Abela, 2011) and excessive reassurance seeking (Shih, Abela, & Starrs, 2009) contribute to interpersonal stress. Dysregulated stress responses then exacerbate relationship disturbances (Flynn & Rudolph, 2011), creating a self-perpetuating cycle of dysfunction. Interpersonal stressors, in turn, play a key role in the emergence of depression, particularly in girls (Rudolph, Flynn, Abaied, Groot, & Thompson, 2009), and help account for the sex difference in depression in adolescents (Shih, Eberhart, Hammen, & Brennan, 2006).

Early adversity also may heighten risk for depression in adolescents by creating proximal family disturbances. Family adversities, such as depression in parents and maltreatment, often are reflected in disrupted parenting and stressful family contexts (Abaied & Rudolph, 2014). Proximal family stressors predict depression in adolescents (Auerbach & Ho, 2012) and help account for the contribution of depression in mothers to depression in adolescents (Hammen, Brennan, & Keenan-Miller, 2008). Parenting and family disturbances also may exacerbate the effects of other interpersonal stressors (DeLay, Hafen, Cunha, Weber, & Laursen, 2013) or contribute to self-generated stress (Auerbach & Ho, 2012). Thus early adversity may serve as a marker of continued vulnerability within relationships during adolescence.

Early and ongoing interpersonal vulnerability is likely to be amplified during the adolescent transition as a result of normative social-contextual, physical-maturational, and cognitive-developmental changes accompanying this stage (Rudolph, 2009). This intensification process is particularly salient in girls due to their increased exposure and susceptibility to social challenges (Mazza et al., 2009; Rudolph, 2002; Shih et al., 2006). Moreover, preexisting vulnerabilities associated with early family adversity may be activated by challenges that accompany the adolescent transition, such as emerging adolescent autonomy and peer reliance, along with heightened parental expectations and concerns (Rudolph, 2014). Indeed, stress sensitization occurs in pubertal but not prepubertal girls, suggesting that this transition heightens susceptibility to ongoing interpersonal stressors in girls with a history of adversity (Rudolph & Flynn, 2007).

Consistent with transactional models, depression may exacerbate prior interpersonal vulnerability by creating stress in adolescents' relationships. Depression in adolescents predicts poorer communication and more conflict with parents (Brière, Archambault, & Janosz, 2013). In the peer group, depressive symptoms contribute to victimization (Tran, Cole, & Weiss, 2012), more negative and less positive relationship qualities (Oppenheimer & Hankin, 2011), and lower social status (Agoston & Rudolph, 2013). In romantic relationships, depression predicts more conflict (Vujeva & Furman, 2011) and the use of more negative, and fewer positive, conflict resolution strategies (Ha, Overbeek, Cillessen, & Engles, 2012).

Depression also may shape adolescents' interpersonal worlds through peer selection, deselection, and influence processes, which result in homophily in symptoms within peer networks (Rudolph, Lansford, & Rodkin, in press; Schaefer, Kornienko, & Fox, 2011). Active selection into social groups with other youth with depression could operate through preference effects, whereby adolescents with depression seek out peers with similar characteristics; unfortunately, relationships among friends with depression may exacerbate dysfunction. Default selection also may occur, whereby aversive characteristics of youth with depression constrain their friendship options or social withdrawal causes them to detach from mainstream peer groups, resulting in social isolation or affiliation with other marginalized peers. Consistent with these ideas, youth with depression are less likely to be selected, and more likely to be deselected, as friends over time and are more likely themselves to deselect friends over time (Van Zalk, Kerr, Branje, Stattin, & Meeus, 2010). Of course, homophily also can result from peer influence, through either contagion effects (transmission of negative cognitions; corumination) or active socialization effects (Van Zalk et al., 2010). Overall, research confirms that peer selection, deselection, and influence all contribute to depression homophily within friendship networks, with particularly strong effects for girls (Rudolph et al., in press; Schaefer et al., 2011).

In sum, research supports interpersonal theories of depression in adolescents, suggesting that relationship dysfunction operates as both an antecedent and a consequence of depression. These processes may be particularly salient during the adolescent transition, especially in girls, when prior individual differences in interpersonal vulnerability interact with normative developmental challenges to contribute to rising rates of depression. During this stage, relationships undergo significant change (disruptions in peer groups, formation of new networks, entrance into heterosexual relationships); these changes seem to create particular difficulties for girls. Thus increasing interpersonal challenges likely contribute to the emerging sex difference in depression across the adolescent transition (Rudolph, 2009).

Integrating Domains of Risk

Considerable advances in the use of rigorous, prospective designs and sophisticated assessment and analytical methods have prompted a rapid progression in the field's understanding of depression in adolescents. Perhaps most notable is the push toward developing multilevel models that consider synergistic and transactional contributions across domains of risk. Although thorough validation of these models awaits the test of time, major inroads have been made in linking domains, as well as providing insight into how genetic and early environmental risks are reflected in endophenotypes (biological, cognitive, and emotional processes) that heighten risk for psychopathology across development.

Depression risk begins with heritable or early-acquired temperamental vulnerabilities (NE, avoidance motivation), cognitive biases (inferential biases, difficulty disengaging from negative stimuli), and heightened stress reactivity (poor regulatory skills, dysregulated stress-response systems), which serve as diatheses that increase susceptibility to proximal stressors and foster the generation of stress, particularly within the interpersonal domain. The adolescent transition, including the timing of puberty, creates a developmental context of risk in light of accompanying brain reorganization (imbalance between maturation of reactive and regulatory processes), thereby increasing stress sensitivity, psychological and cognitive challenges, and social disruptions. Early stress and depressive episodes can then result in a scarring or kindling (Post, 1992) effect, thereby sensitizing adolescents to recurrent or persistent symptoms across development.

CONCLUSIONS AND FUTURE DIRECTIONS

Depression often emerges during adolescence and follows a chronic or recurring course, often generating significant psychosocial impairment. For the most part, the depressive syndrome shows significant continuity across developmental stages. However, unique age-linked characteristics indicate the need to explore differences in the nature, etiology, course, and consequences of disorders during different stages. It is possible that the syndrome is essentially comparable across the life span but that some vulnerability factors do not become active contributors until later in development, when biological, emotional, and cognitive capabilities and social experiences coalesce into more stable and organized systems. Many questions remain concerning how these risks work together to predict adolescent depression.

First, research needs to investigate whether the multiple contributors to depression reflect distinct or overlapping risks, as well as to identify the complex mechanisms that link these risks. For example, are compromised emotion regulation and cognitive biases the expression of joint genetic liability, or do they represent independent pathways to depression? Is early adversity translated into vulnerability through the sensitization of biological, emotional, and cognitive pathways? What are the unique genetic versus environmental contributions to depression arising from depression in parents? How and when is biological dysregulation in high-risk youth translated into emotional or psychological processes that create a vulnerability to depression? What are the processes through which youth with depression create and select stressful environments? Answering these questions has implications for theory, as well as efforts to identify high-risk youth and prevent the expression of future liability for depression.

Another critical direction is continued investigation of the specificity of particular risk factors to depression in adolescents. Significant efforts also are needed to investigate alternative explanations for depression comorbidity. Clues may stem from the temporal sequencing of disorders, but more research is needed to determine whether this sequence reflects the developmental unfolding of a generalized vulnerability to negative affect and stress reactivity, a functional association between earlier and later disorders, or some combination of the two.

A third avenue for exploration is to elucidate why depression increases during adolescence and why girls are particularly susceptible at this time. A growing number of developmentally informed theories addressing these questions, along with advances in the field's understanding of adolescent brain development, provide insight into why risk is amplified during the adolescent transition. However, relatively little is known about how biological, psychological, and social challenges of adolescence interact to predict depression. It also is unclear whether the adolescent transition creates new vulnerabilities to depression in previously healthy youth or merely exacerbates risk in youth with preexisting liabilities.

Finally, transitions can represent turning points at which some youth progress down a deviant trajectory toward increasing impairment, whereas others move toward a more adaptive trajectory. Understanding the factors that determine trajectories across the adolescent transition would shed considerable light on characteristics or experiences that amplify or protect youth from depression through adolescence and adulthood.

REFERENCES

Abaied, J. L., & Rudolph, K. D. (2010). Mothers as a resource in times of stress: Interactive contributions of socialization of coping and stress to youth psychopathology. *Journal of Abnormal Child Psychology, 38*, 273–289.

Abaied, J. L., & Rudolph, K. D. (2014). Family relationships, emotional processes, and adolescent depression. In C. S. Richards & M. W. O'Hara (Eds.), *Oxford handbook of depression and comorbidity* (pp. 460–475). Oxford, UK: Oxford University Press.

Abdel-Khalek, A. M., & Soliman, H. H. (2002). Sex differences in symptoms of depression among American children and adolescents. *Psychological Reports, 90*, 185–188.

Abela, J. R. Z., & Hankin, B. L. (2008). Cognitive vulnerability to depression in children and adolescents: A developmental psychopathology approach. In J. R. Z. Abela & B. L. Hankin (Eds.), *Handbook of child and adolescent depression* (pp. 35–78). New York: Guilford Press.

Abela, J. R. Z., & Hankin, B. L. (2011). Rumination as a vulnerability factor to depression during the transition from early to middle adolescence: A multi-wave longitudinal study. *Journal of Abnormal Psychology, 120*, 259–271.

Abela, J. R. Z., & Sarin, S. (2002). Cognitive vulnerability to hopelessness depression: A chain is only as strong as its weakest link. *Cognitive Therapy and Research, 26*, 811–829.

Abramson, L. Y., Metalsky, G. I., & Alloy, L. B. (1989). Hopelessness depression: A theory-based subtype of depression. *Psychological Review, 96*, 358–372.

Adam, E. K., Doane, L. D., Zinbarg, R. E., Mineka, S., Craske, M. G., & Griffith, J. W. (2010). Prospective prediction of major depressive disorder from cortisol awakening responses in adolescence. *Psychoneuroendocrinology, 35*, 921–931.

Agoston, A. M., & Rudolph, K. D. (2013). Pathways from depressive symptoms to low social status. *Journal of Abnormal Child Psychology, 41*, 295–308.

Agoston, A. M., & Rudolph, K. D. (2014). *Interactive contributions of peer stress and executive function deficits to adolescent depression.* Manuscript in preparation.

American Psychiatric Association. (2013). *Diagnostic and statistical manual of mental disorders* (5th ed.). Arlington, VA: Author.

Auerbach, R. P., & Ho, M. (2012). A cognitive-interpersonal model of adolescent depression: The impact of family conflict and depressogenic cognitive styles. *Journal of Clinical Child and Adolescent Psychology, 41*, 792–802.

Beck, A. T. (1967). *Depression: Clinical, experimental, and theoretical aspects.* New York: Harper & Row.

Beevers, C. G., Wells, T. T., Ellis, A. J., & McGeary, J. E. (2009). Association of the serotonin transporter gene promoter region (*5-HTTLPR*) polymorphism with biased attention for emotional stimuli. *Journal of Abnormal Psychology, 118*, 670–681.

Birmaher, B., Arbelaez, C., & Brent, D. (2002). Course and outcome of child and adolescent major depressive disorder. *Child and Adolescent Psychiatric Clinics of North America, 11*, 619–638.

Birmaher, B., Ryan, N. D., Williamson, D. E., Brent, D. A., Kaufman, J., Dahl, R. E., et al. (1996). Childhood and adolescent depression: A review of the past 10 years: Part I. *Journal of the American Academy of Child and Adolescent Psychiatry, 35*, 1427–1439.

Bress, J. N., Foti, D., Kotov, R., Klein, D. N., & Hajcak, G. (2013). Blunted neural response to rewards prospectively predicts depression in adolescent girls. *Psychophysiology, 50*, 74–81.

Brière, F. N., Archambault, K., & Janosz, M. (2013). Reciprocal prospective associations between depressive symptoms and perceived relationship with parents in early adolescence. *Canadian Journal of Psychiatry, 58*, 169–176.

Carter, J., & Garber, J. (2011). Predictors of the first onset of a major depressive episode and changes in depressive symptoms across adolescence: Stress and negative cognitions. *Journal of Abnormal Psychology, 120*, 779–796.

Chen, M. C., Joormann, J., Hallmayer, J., & Gotlib, I. H. (2009). Serotonin transporter polymorphism predicts waking cortisol in young girls. *Psychoneuroendocrinology, 34*, 681–686.

Clark, L. A., & Watson, D. (1991). A tripartite model of anxiety and depression: Psychometric evidence and taxonomic implications. *Journal of Abnormal Psychology, 100*, 316–336.

Copeland, W. E., Adair, C. E., Smetanin, P., Stiff, D., Briante, C., Colman, I., et al. (2013). Diagnostic transitions from childhood to adolescence to early adulthood. *Journal of Child Psychology and Psychiatry, 54*, 791–799.

Cullen, K. R., Gee, D. G., Klimes-Dougan, B., Gabbay, V., Hulvershorn, L., Mueller, B. A., et al. (2009). A preliminary study of functional connectivity in comorbid adolescent depression. *Neuroscience Letters, 460*, 227–231.

Cyranowski, J. M., Frank, E., Young, E., & Shear, K. (2000). Adolescent onset of the gender difference in lifetime rates of depression. *Archives of General Psychiatry, 57*, 21–27.

Dahl, R. E. (2004). Adolescent brain development: A period of vulnerabilities and opportunities. *Annals of the New York Academy of Sciences, 1021*, 1–22.

Davidson, R., Pizzagalli, D., Nitschke, J., & Putnam, K. (2002). Depression: Perspectives from affective neuroscience. *Annual Review of Psychology, 53*, 545–574.

Davies, P. T., & Windle, M. (2001). Interparental discord and adolescent adjustment trajectories: The potentiating and protective role of intrapersonal attributes. *Child Development, 74*, 1163–1178.

Dekker, M. C., Ferdinand, R. F., van Lang, N. J., Bongers, I. L., van der Ende, J., & Verhulst, F. C. (2007). Developmental trajectories of depressive symptoms from early childhood to late adolescence: Gender differences and adult outcome. *Journal of Child Psychology and Psychiatry, 48*, 657–666.

DeLay, D., Hafen, C. A., Cunha, J. M., Weber, L. D., & Laursen, B. (2013). Perceptions of parental support buffer against depression for Brazilian youth with interpersonal difficulties. *International Journal of Behavioral Development, 37*, 29–34.

Denham, S. A., Bassett, H. H., & Wyatt, T. (2007). The socialization of emotional competence. In J. E. Grusec & P. D. Hastings (Eds.), *Handbook of socialization: Theory and research* (pp. 614–637). New York: Guilford Press.

Dickson, J. M., & MacLeod, A. K. (2004). Approach and avoidance goals and plans: Their relationship to anxiety and depression. *Cognitive Therapy and Research, 28*, 415–432.

Eberhart, N. K., Auerbach, R. P., Bigda-Peyton, J., & Abela, J. Z. (2011). Maladaptive schemas and depression: Tests of stress generation and diathesis–stress models. *Journal of Social and Clinical Psychology, 30*, 75–104.

Eisenberger, N. I. (2012). Broken hearts and broken bones: A neural perspective on the similarities between social and physical pain. *Current Directions in Psychological Science, 21*, 42–47.

Esposito, E., & Gunnar, M. R. (2014). Early deprivation and developmental psychopathology. In M. Lewis & K. D. Rudolph (Eds.), *Handbook of developmental psychopathology* (3rd ed., pp. 371–388). New York: Plenum Press.

Evans, A., & Frank, S. J. (2004). Adolescent depression and externalizing problems: Testing two models of comorbidity in an inpatient sample. *Adolescence, 39*, 1–18.

Flynn, M., & Rudolph, K. D. (2007). Perceptual asymmetry and youths' responses to stress: Understanding vulnerability to depression. *Cognition and Emotion, 21*, 773–788.

Flynn, M., & Rudolph, K. D. (2010). Neuropsychological and interpersonal antecedents of youth depression. *Cognition and Emotion, 24*, 94–110.

Flynn, M., & Rudolph, K. D. (2011). Stress generation and adolescent depression: Contribution of interpersonal stress responses. *Journal of Abnormal Child Psychology, 39*, 1187–1198.

Flynn, M., & Rudolph, K. D. (2012). The trade-offs of emotional reactivity for youths' social information processing in the context of maternal depression. *Frontiers in Integrative Neuroscience, 6*, 43.

Flynn, M., & Rudolph, K. D. (in press). A prospective examination of emotional clarity, stress responses, and depressive symptoms during early adolescence. *Journal of Early Adolescence.*

Forbes, E. E., & Dahl, R. E. (2010). Pubertal development and behavior: Hormonal activation of social and motivational tendencies. *Brain and Cognition, 72*, 66–72.

Forbes, E. E., & Dahl, R. E. (2012). Research review: Altered reward function in adolescent depression: What, when, and how? *Journal of Child Psychology and Psychiatry, 53,* 3–15.

Forbes, E. E., Phillips, M. L., Ryan, N. D., & Dahl, R. E. (2011). Neural systems of threat processing in adolescents: Role of pubertal maturation and relation to measures of negative affect. *Developmental Neuropsychology, 36,* 429–452.

Franić, S., Middeldorp, C. M., Dolan, C. V., Ligthart, L., & Boomsma, D. I. (2010). Childhood and adolescent anxiety and depression: Beyond heritability. *Journal of the American Academy of Child and Adolescent Psychiatry, 49,* 820–829.

Furman, D., Hamilton, J. P., Joormann, J., & Gotlib, I. H. (2011). Altered timing of limbic system activation during elaboration of sad mood as a function of serotonin transporter polymorphism. *Social Cognitive and Affective Neuroscience, 6,* 270–276.

Giletta, M., Calhoun, C. D., Hastings, P. D., Rudolph, K. D., Nock, M. K., & Prinstein, M. J. (in press). Multi-level risk factors for suicidal ideation among at-risk adolescent females: The role of hypothalamic–pituitary–adrenal axis responses to stress. *Journal of Abnormal Child Psychology.*

Goodyer, I. M., Croudace, T., Dudbridge, F., Ban, M., & Herbert, J. (2010). Polymorphisms in BDNF (*Val66Met*) and *5-HTTLPR*, morning cortisol and subsequent depression in at-risk adolescents. *British Journal of Psychiatry, 197,* 365–371.

Gotlib, I., Hamilton, J. P., Cooney, R., Singh, M., Henry, M., & Joormann, J. (2010). Neural processing of reward and loss in girls at risk for major depression. *Archives of General Psychiatry, 67,* 380–387.

Gotlib, I. H., Joormann, J., Minor, K. L., & Hallmayer, J. (2008). HPA axis reactivity: A mechanism underlying the associations among *5-HTTLPR*, stress, and depression. *Biological Psychiatry, 63,* 847–851.

Gray, J. A. (1994). Three fundamental emotion systems. In P. Ekman & R. J. Davidson (Eds.), *The nature of emotion: Fundamental questions* (pp. 243–247). New York: Oxford University Press.

Guerry, J. D., & Hastings, P. D. (2011). In search of HPA axis dysregulation in child and adolescent depression. *Clinical Child and Family Psychology Review, 14,* 135–160.

Gunnar, M. R., Wewerka, S., Frenn, K., Long, J. D., & Griggs, C. (2009). Developmental changes in HPA activity over the transition to adolescence: Normative changes and associations with puberty. *Development and Psychopathology, 21,* 69–85.

Ha, T., Overbeek, G., Cillessen, A. N., & Engels, R. E. (2012). A longitudinal study of the associations among adolescent conflict resolution styles, depressive symptoms, and romantic relationship longevity. *Journal of Adolescence, 35,* 1247–1254.

Hammen, C. (2006). Stress generation in depression: Reflections on origins, research, and future directions. *Journal of Clinical Psychology, 62,* 69–82.

Hammen, C., Brennan, P. A., & Keenan-Miller, D. (2008). Patterns of adolescent depression to age 20: The role of maternal depression and youth interpersonal dysfunction. *Journal of Abnormal Child Psychology, 36,* 1189–1198.

Hammen, C., Brennan, P. A., Keenan-Miller, D., Hazel, N. A., & Najman, J. M. (2010). Chronic and acute stress, gender, and serotonin transporter gene–environment interactions predicting depression symptoms in youth. *Journal of Child Psychology and Psychiatry, 51,* 180–187.

Hammen, C., Burge, D., Daley, S. E., Davila, J., Paley, B., & Rudolph, K. D. (1995). Interpersonal attachment cognitions and prediction of symptomatic responses to interpersonal stress. *Journal of Abnormal Psychology, 104,* 436–443.

Hammen, C., Henry, R., & Daley, S. E. (2000). Depression and sensitization to stressors among young women as a function of childhood adversity. *Journal of Consulting and Clinical Psychology, 68,* 782–787.

Hankin, B. L., Abramson, L. Y., Miller, N., & Haeffel, G. J. (2004). Cognitive vulnerability–stress theories of depression: Examining affective specificity in the prediction of depression versus anxiety in three prospective studies. *Cognitive Therapy and Research, 28,* 309–345.

Hankin, B. L., Gibb, B. E., Abela, J. R. Z., & Flory, K. (2010). Selective attention to affective stimuli and clinical depression among youths: Role of anxiety and specificity of emotion. *Journal of Abnormal Psychology, 119,* 491–501.

Hankin, B. L., Jenness, J., Abela, J. R. Z., & Smolen, A. (2011). Interaction of *5-HTTLPR* and idiographic stressors predicts prospective depressive symptoms specifically among youth in a multiwave design. *Journal of Clinical Child and Adolescent Psychology, 40,* 572–585.

Hankin, B. L., Wetter, E., & Cheely, C. (2008). Sex differences in child and adolescent depression: A developmental psychopathological approach. In J. R. Z. Abela & B. L. Hankin (Eds.), *Handbook of depression in children and adolescents* (pp. 377–414). New York: Guilford Press.

Hare, T. A., Tottenham, N., Galvan, A., Voss, H. U., Glover, G. H., & Casey, B. J. (2008). Biological substrates of emotional reactivity and regulation in adolescence during an emotional go-nogo task. *Biological Psychiatry, 63,* 927–934.

Hill, J., Pickles, A., Rollinson, L., Davies, R., & Byatt, M. (2004). Juvenile- versus adult-onset depression: Multiple differences imply different pathways. *Psychological Medicine, 34,* 1483–1493.

Hulvershorn, L., Cullen, K., & Anand, A. (2011). Toward dysfunctional connectivity: A review of neuroimaging findings in pediatric major depressive disorder. *Brain Imaging and Behavior, 5,* 307–328.

Joormann, J., Cooney, R., Henry, M., & Gotlib, I. (2012). Neural correlates of automatic mood regulation in girls at high risk for depression. *Journal of Abnormal Psychology, 121,* 61–72.

Joormann, J., Talbot, L., & Gotlib, I. H. (2007). Biased processing of emotional information in girls at risk for depression. *Journal of Abnormal Psychology, 116,* 135–143.

Kaminski, K. M., & Garber, J. (2002). Depressive spectrum disorders in high-risk adolescents: Episode duration and predictors of time to recovery. *Journal of the American Academy of Child and Adolescent Psychiatry, 41,* 410–418.

Karg, K., Burmeister, M., Shedden, K., & Sen, S. (2011). The serotonin transporter promoter variant (5-HTTLPR), stress and depression meta-analysis revisited: Evidence of genetic moderation. *Archives of General Psychiatry, 68,* 444–454.

Karlsson, L., Kiviruusu, O., Miettunen, J., Heilä, H., Holi, M., Ruuttu, T., et al. (2008). One-year course and predictors of outcome of adolescent depression: A case-control study in Finland. *Journal of Clinical Psychiatry, 69,* 844–853.

Kaufman, J., Yang, B., Douglas-Palumberi, H., Grasso, D., Lipschitz, D., Houshyar, S., et al. (2006). Brain-derived neurotrophic factor–*5-HTTLPR* gene interactions and environmental modifiers of depression in children. *Biological Psychiatry, 59,* 673–680.

Kendler, K. S., Gardner, C. O., & Lichtenstein, P. (2008). A developmental twin study of symptoms of anxiety and depression: Evidence for genetic innovation and attenuation. *Psychological Medicine, 38,* 1567–1575.

Kentgen, L. M., Tenke, C. E., Pine, D. S., Fong, R., Klein, R. G., & Bruder, G. E. (2000). Electroencephalographic asymmetries in adolescents with major depression: Influence of comorbidity with anxiety disorders. *Journal of Abnormal Psychology, 109,* 797–802.

Kessler, R. C., Avenevoli, S., & Merikangas, K. R. (2001). Mood disorders in children and adolescents: An epidemiologic perspective. *Biological Psychiatry, 49,* 1002–1014.

Killgore, W. D. S., & Yurgelun-Todd, D. A. (2006). Ventromedial prefrontal activity correlates with depressed mood in adolescent children. *NeuroReport, 17,* 167–171.

Klein, D. N., Shankman, S. A., Lewinsohn, P. M., & Seeley, J. R. (2009). Subthreshold depressive disorder in adolescents: Predictors of escalation to full-syndrome depressive disorders. *Journal of the American Academy of Child and Adolescent Psychiatry, 48,* 703–710.

Ladouceur, C. D. (2012). Neural systems supporting cognitive–affective interactions in adolescence: The role of puberty and implications for affective disorders. *Frontiers in Integrative Neuroscience, 6,* 65.

LaGrange, B., Cole, D. A., Jacquez, F., Ciesla, J., Dallaire, D., Pineda, A., et al. (2011). Disentangling the prospective relations between maladaptive cognitions and depressive symptoms. *Journal of Abnormal Psychology, 120,* 511–527.

Lakdawalla, Z., Hankin, B. L., & Mermelstein, R. (2007). Cognitive theories of depression in children and adolescents: A conceptual and quantitative review. *Clinical Child and Family Psychology Review, 10,* 1–24.

Lau, J. Y., & Eley, T. C., (2006). Changes in genetic and environmental influences on depressive symptoms across adolescence and young adulthood. *British Journal of Psychiatry, 189,* 422–427.

Lau, J. Y., & Eley, T. C. (2008). Disentangling gene–environment correlations and interactions on adolescent depressive symptoms. *Journal of Child Psychology and Psychiatry, 49,* 142–150.

Lau, J. Y., Goldman, D., Buzas, B., Hodgkinson, C., Leibenluft, E., Nelson, E., et al. (2010). BDNF gene polymorphism (*Val66Met*) predicts amygdala and anterior hippocampus responses to emotional faces in anxious and depressed adolescents. *Neuroimage, 53,* 952–961.

Lau, Y. F., Rijsdijk, F., & Eley, T. C. (2006). I think, therefore I am: A twin study of attributional style in adolescents. *Journal of Child Psychology and Psychiatry, 47,* 696–703.

Lewinsohn, P. M., & Essau, C. A. (2002). Depression in adolescents. In I. H. Gotlib & C. L. Hammen (Eds.), *Handbook of depression* (pp. 541–559). New York: Guilford Press.

Lewinsohn, P. M., Rohde, P., & Seeley, J. R. (1998). Major depressive disorder in older adolescents: Prevalence, risk factors, and clinical implications. *Clinical Psychology Review, 18,* 765–794.

Masten, C. L., Eisenberger, N. I., Borofsky, L. A., McNealy, K., Pfeifer, J. H., & Dapretto, M. (2011). Subgenual anterior cingulate responses to peer rejection: A marker of adolescents' risk for depression. *Development and Psychopathology, 23,* 283–292.

Mathew, S. J., Coplan, J. D., Goetz, R. R., Feder, A., Greenwald, S., Dahl, R. E., et al. (2003). Differentiating depressed adolescent 24h cortisol secretion in light of their adult clinical outcome. *Neuropsychopharmacology, 28,* 1336–1343.

Mazza, J. J., Abbott, R. D., Fleming, C. B., Harachi, T. W., Cortes, R. C., Park, J., et al. (2009). Early predictors of adolescent depression: A 7-year longitudinal study. *Journal of Early Adolescence, 29,* 664–692.

Meaney, M. J. (2010). Epigenetics and the biological definition of gene × environment interactions. *Child Development, 81,* 41–79.

Moffitt, T. E., Caspi, A., Harrington, H., Milne, B. J., Melchior, M., Goldberg, D., et al. (2007). Generalized anxiety disorder and depression: Childhood risk factors in a birth cohort followed to age 32. *Psychological Medicine, 37,* 441–452.

Monk, C. S., Klein, R. G., Telzer, E. H., Schroth, E. A., Mannuzza, S., Moulton, J. L., et al. (2008). Amygdala and nucleus accumbens activation to emotional facial expressions in children and adolescents at risk for major depression. *American Journal of Psychiatry, 165,* 90–98.

Morris, M. C., Ciesla, J. A., & Garber, J. (2008). A prospective study of the cognitive-stress model of depressive symptoms in adolescents. *Journal of Abnormal Psychology, 117,* 719–734.

Nolen-Hoeksema, S. (1991). Responses to depression and their effects on the duration of depressive episodes. *Journal of Abnormal Psychology, 100,* 569–582.

Olino, T. M., McMakin, D. L., Dahl, R. E., Ryan, N. D., Silk, J. S., Birmaher, B., et al. (2011). "I won, but I'm not getting my hopes up": Depression moderates the relationship of outcomes and reward anticipation. *Psychiatry Research: Neuroimaging, 194,* 393–395.

Oppenheimer, C. W., & Hankin, B. L. (2011). Relationship quality and depressive symptoms among adolescents: A short-term multiwave investigation of longitudinal, reciprocal associations. *Journal of Clinical Child and Adolescent Psychology, 40,* 486–493.

Pettit, J. W., Hartley, C., Lewinsohn, P. M., Seeley, J. R., & Klein, D. N. (2013). Is liability to recurrent major depressive disorder present before first episode onset in adolescence or acquired after the initial episode? *Journal of Abnormal Psychology, 122,* 353–358.

Post, R. M. (1992). Transduction of psychosocial stress into the neurobiology of recurrent affective disorder. *American Journal of Psychiatry, 149,* 999–1010.

Prinstein, M. J., Borelli, J. L., Cheah, C. S. L., Simon, V. A., & Aikins, J. W. (2005). Adolescent girls' interpersonal vulnerability to depressive symptoms: A longitudinal examination of reassurance-seeking and peer relationships. *Journal of Abnormal Psychology, 114,* 676–688.

Quevedo, K. M., Benning, S. D., Gunnar, M. R., & Dahl, R. E. (2009). The onset of puberty: Effects on the psychophysiology of defensive and appetitive motivation. *Development and Psychopathology, 21,* 27–45.

Rao, U., Ryan, N. D., Birmaher, B., Dahl, R. E., Williamson, D. E., Kaufman, J., et al. (1995). Unipolar depression in adolescents: Clinical outcomes in adulthood. *Journal of the American Academy of Child and Adolescent Psychiatry, 34,* 566–578.

Rice, F. (2010). Genetics of childhood and adolescent depression: Insights into etiological heterogeneity and challenges for future genomic research. *Genome Medicine, 2,* 68–73.

Risch, N., Herrell, R., Lehner, T., Liang, K.-Y., Eaves, L., Hoh, J., et al. (2009). Interaction between the serotonin transporter gene (5-HTTLPR), stressful life events, and risk of depression: A meta-analysis. *Journal of the American Medical Association, 301,* 2462–2471.

Rohde, P. (2009). Comorbidities with adolescent depression. In S. Nolen-Hoeksema & L. M. Hilt (Eds.), *Handbook of depression in adolescents* (pp. 139–177). New York: Routledge/Taylor & Francis.

Rohde, P., Beevers, C. G., Stice, E., & O'Neil, K. (2009). Major and minor depression in female adolescents: Onset, course, symptom presentation, and demographic associations. *Journal of Clinical Psychology, 65,* 1339–1349.

Romano, E., Tremblay, R. E., Vitaro, F., Zoccolillo, M., & Pagani, L. (2005). Sex and informant effects on diagnostic comorbidity in an adolescent community sample. *Canadian Journal of Psychiatry, 50,* 479–489.

Rudolph, K. D. (2002). Gender differences in emotional responses to interpersonal stress during adolescence. *Journal of Adolescent Health, 30,* 3–13.

Rudolph, K. D. (2009). The interpersonal context of adolescent depression. In S. Nolen-Hoeksema & L. M. Hilt (Eds.), *Handbook of depression in adolescents* (pp. 377–418). New York: Routledge.

Rudolph, K. D. (2014). Puberty and the development of psychopathology. In M. Lewis & K. D. Rudolph (Eds.), *Handbook of developmental psychopathology* (3rd ed., pp. 331–356). New York: Plenum Press.

Rudolph, K. D., & Flynn, M. (2007). Childhood adversity and youth depression: The role of gender and pubertal status. *Development and Psychopathology, 19,* 497–521.

Rudolph, K. D., Flynn, M., Abaied, J. L., Groot, A., & Thompson, R. (2009). Why is past depression the best predictor of future depression?: Stress generation as a mechanism of depression continuity in girls. *Journal of Clinical Child and Adolescent Psychology, 38,* 473–485.

Rudolph, K. D., Hammen, C., Burge, D., Lindberg, N., Herzberg, D., & Daley, S. (2000). Toward an interpersonal life-stress model of depression: The developmental context of stress generation. *Development and Psychopathology, 12,* 215–234.

Rudolph, K. D., Lansford, J. E., & Rodkin, P. (in press). Interpersonal theories of psychopathology. In D. Cicchetti (Ed.), *Developmental psychopathology* (3rd ed.). London: Wiley.

Schaefer, D. R., Kornienko, O., & Fox, A. M. (2011). Misery does not love company: Network selection mechanisms and depression homophily. *American Sociological Review, 76,* 764–785.

Schwartz, O. S., Sheeber, L. B., Dudgeon, P., & Allen, N. B. (2012). Emotion socialization within the family environment and adolescent depression. *Clinical Psychology Review, 32,* 447–453.

Sebastian, C., Tan, G. C. Y., Roiser, J. P., Viding, E., Dumontheil, I., & Blakemore, S. J. (2011). Developmental influences on the neural bases of responses to social rejection: Implications of social neuroscience for education. *NeuroImage, 57,* 686–694.

Shih, J. H., Abela, J. Z., & Starrs, C. (2009). Cognitive and interpersonal predictors of stress generation in children of affectively ill parents. *Journal of Abnormal Child Psychology, 37,* 195–208.

Shih, J. H., Eberhart, N. K., Hammen, C. L., & Brennan, P. A. (2006). Differential exposure and reactivity to interpersonal stress predict sex differences in adolescent depression. *Journal of Clinical Child and Adolescent Psychology, 35*, 103–115.

Silberg, J. L., Pickles, A., Rutter, M., Hewitt, J., Simonoff, E., Maes, H., et al. (1999). The influence of genetic factors and life stress on depression among adolescent girls. *Archives of General Psychiatry, 56*, 225–232.

Silk, J. S., Stroud, L. R., Siegle, G. J., Dahl, R. E., Lee, K. H., & Nelson, E. E. (2012). Peer acceptance and rejection through the eyes of youth: Pupillary, eyetracking and ecological data from the Chatroom Interact task. *Social Cognitive and Affective Neuroscience, 7*, 93–105.

Slavich, G. M., O'Donovan, A., Epel, E. S., & Kemeny, M. E. (2010). Black sheep get the blues: A psychobiological model of social rejection and depression. *Neuroscience and Biobehavioral Reviews, 35*, 39–45.

Somerville, L. H. (2013). The teenage brain: Sensitivity to social evaluation. *Current Directions in Psychological Science, 22*, 121–127.

Stroud, L. R., Foster, E., Papandonatos, G., Handwerger, K., Granger, D. A., Kivlighan, K. T., et al. (2009). Stress response and the adolescent transition: Performance versus social rejection stress. *Development and Psychopathology, 21*, 47–68.

Tackett, J. L., Waldman, I. D., Van Hulle, C. A., & Lahey, B. B. (2011). Shared genetic influences on negative emotionality and major depression/conduct disorder comorbidity. *Journal of the American Academy of Child and Adolescent Psychiatry, 50*, 818–827.

Tram, J. M., & Cole, D. A. (2000). Self-perceived competence and the relation between life events and depressive symptoms in adolescence: Mediator or moderator? *Journal of Abnormal Psychology, 109*, 753–760.

Tran, C. V., Cole, D. A., & Weiss, B. (2012). Testing reciprocal longitudinal relations between peer victimization and depressive symptoms in young adolescents. *Journal of Clinical Child and Adolescent Psychology, 41*, 353–360.

Van Voorhees, B. W., Melkonian, S., Marko, M., Humensky, J., & Fogel, J. (2010). Adolescents in primary care with sub-threshold depressed mood screened for participation in a depression prevention study: Co-morbidity and factors associated with depressive symptoms. *Open Psychiatry Journal, 4*, 10–18.

Van Zalk, M. H. W., Kerr, M., Branje, S. J. T., Stattin, H., & Meeus, W. H. J. (2010). It takes three: Selection, influence, and de-selection processes of depression in adolescent friendship networks. *Developmental Psychology, 46*, 927–938.

Vujeva, H. M., & Furman, W. (2011). Depressive symptoms and romantic relationship qualities from adolescence through emerging adulthood: A longitudinal examination of influences. *Journal of Clinical Child and Adolescent Psychology, 40*, 123–135.

Weiss, B., & Garber, J. (2003). Developmental differences in the phenomenology of depression. *Development and Psychopathology, 15*, 403–430.

Yorbik, O., Birmaher, B., Axelson, D., Williamson, D. E., & Ryan, N. D. (2004). Clinical characteristics of depressive symptoms in children and adolescents with major depressive disorder. *Journal of Clinical Psychiatry, 65*, 1654–1659.

CHAPTER 22

Depression in Couples and Families

JOANNE DAVILA, CATHERINE B. STROUD, *and* LISA R. STARR

As other chapters in this book also attest, depression is associated with significant interpersonal impairment, both as a cause and as a consequence of the disorder (see Hammen & Shih, Chapter 15, this volume). This is particularly evident in the context of couple and family relationships. This chapter provides an overview of the literature on depression in these contexts and provides directions for future research.

DEPRESSION IN THE CONTEXT OF COUPLE RELATIONSHIPS

In this section, we focus on the main processes and components of couple relationships, including how they start, function, and end, and discuss their association with depression. Although research in this area has largely focused on adults, there is a growing literature on adolescents. Because depression rates increase markedly from childhood into adolescence, depression has the potential to impair interpersonal functioning early on. Adolescent interpersonal experiences, especially romantic ones, may serve important socialization functions and result in learning that guides later relational ability. Therefore, the association between depression and poor romantic functioning may begin early and set the stage for continued impairment across the lifespan.

Relationship Formation

A recent cross-national study of adults found that depression was associated with a lower likelihood of on-time or late marriage (Breslau et al., 2011), suggesting that depression decreases the odds of marrying in adulthood. Marriage, however, decreases the odds of depression. Although some studies comparing married and never-married people show no differences in depression (e.g., Kessler et al., 2003) or find that the never married are less depressed (Romanoski et al., 1992), the majority indicate that being married or in a relationship in adulthood is associated with less depression (e.g., Gutiérrez-Lobos, Wölfl,

Scherer, Anderer, & Schmidl-Mohl, 2000; Inaba, Thoits, & Ueno, 2005). Perhaps the clearest evidence to date comes from a twin study comparing married or cohabiting individuals with those not in a relationship, excluding individuals with a history of divorce. Horn, Xu, Beam, Turkheimer, and Emery (2013) found that, compared with being single, being coupled remained significantly associated with fewer depressive symptoms after controlling for genetic and shared environmental factors. This suggests that being coupled, on average, has a quasi-causal positive effect on depressive symptoms, that is, that relationships may be protective for adults.

However, there is growing evidence that involvement in dating activities and romantic relationships during adolescence, particularly if frequent or steady, is associated with depressive symptoms, particularly for girls (see Davila, 2008). Indeed, a number of studies suggest that early-onset depression is associated with early marriage (e.g., Gotlib, Lewinsohn, & Seeley, 1998; Kessler, Walters, & Forthofer, 1998) and that depressive symptoms in adolescence are associated with entry into romantic relationships (Davila et al., 2009). Though the reasons for this are unclear, one possibility is that depressed or dysphoric youth may seek out romantic experiences to meet dependence needs, compensate for poor family or peer relations, or in search of mood-regulating experiences (Davila, 2008). These ideas are speculative (see also Gotlib et al., 1998) and important targets for research. It also is possible that adolescent romantic experiences are inherently challenging. As such, they may put youth at risk for depression, particularly youth with poor coping, support, or personal resources that impair their ability to manage such challenges. In line with this idea, the association between romantic experiences and depressive symptoms among early adolescent girls has been found to be strongest among those with emotionally unavailable parents (Steinberg & Davila, 2008), those who engage in corumination (a maladaptive emotion regulation strategy; Starr & Davila, 2009), and those with a more preoccupied attachment style (i.e., who are needy and fearful of rejection; Davila, Steinberg, Kachadourian, Cobb, & Fincham, 2004).

Relationship Satisfaction and Functioning

Research consistently documents that, among adult couples of various ages, depression and depressive symptoms are associated with less relationship satisfaction and that these associations are bidirectional (e.g., Davila, Karney, Hall, & Bradbury, 2003; Whisman, 2001; Whisman & Uebelacker, 2009). Furthermore, this association is strengthened in a variety of contexts, including among partners with high levels of neuroticism (Davila et al., 2003), avoidant attachment (Smith, Breiding, & Papp, 2012), and hostile communication (Kouros, Papp, & Cummings, 2008) and among those who face greater chronic stress (Poyner-del Vento & Cobb, 2011) and who make blame-oriented attributions about partners' negative behavior (Gordon, Friedman, & Miller, 2005). Mediators of the relationship satisfaction–depression association also have been identified, including self-silencing (i.e., not voicing one's thoughts, feelings, and needs out of fear of how the other person will respond; Uebelacker, Courtnage, & Whisman, 2003) and maladaptive conflict styles (DuRocher Schudlich, Papp, & Cummings, 2011).

In line with these findings, there is ample evidence that depression and depressive symptoms are associated with a variety of maladaptive relational processes, including poor problem solving (e.g., Jackman-Cram, Dobson, & Martin, 2006; see Rehman, Gollan, & Mortimer, 2008, for a review), negative reactions to problem solving (e.g., Whisman, Weinstock, & Uebelacker, 2002), low levels of support (e.g., Monroe, Bromet, Connell, & Steiner, 1986), poor support skills (e.g., Davila, Bradbury, Cohan, & Tochluk, 1997), criticism and hostility (e.g., Hooley & Teasdale, 1989; Proulx, Buehler, & Helms, 2009), low empathic accuracy (e.g., Papp, Kouros, & Cummings, 2010), relational insecurity (e.g., Whiffen, Kallos-Lilly, & MacDonald, 2001), poor romantic competence (Rehman, Beausoleil, & Karimiha, 2013), and negative relationship events (e.g., Christian-Herman, O'Leary, & Avery-Leaf, 2001). Individual factors that play a role in these associations have begun to be examined. For example, anxiety about abandonment and excessive reassurance seeking predict romantic conflict, which then predicts increases in depressive symptoms (Eberhart & Hammen, 2010).

Though less well studied, the adolescent relationship literature mirrors these findings. For example, among adolescent girls, depressive symptoms and depressed mood are associated with less intimacy (Williams, Connolly, & Segal, 2001), lower support and higher relationship stress (Daley & Hammen, 2002), and more negative interactions, as well as inequality in the contribution of emotional resources and in decision making (Galliher, Rostosky, Welsh, & Kawaguchi, 1999; La Greca & Harrison, 2005). Depressive symptoms also are associated with more negative conflict resolution styles (Ha, Overbeek, Cillessen, & Engels, 2012), as well as increases in conflict and poor problem solving over time (Vujeva & Furman, 2011). Adolescent girls' depressive symptoms also are associated with romantic partners' ratings of them as less interpersonally competent (Daley & Hammen, 2002).

Relationship Dissolution

Loss of a relationship confers significant risk for depression. Divorced, separated, and widowed individuals show higher rates of depressive symptoms, are more likely to meet criteria for major depression, and are at higher risk for developing depression than are married individuals (e.g., Kessler et al., 2003; Osler, McGue, Lund, & Christensen, 2008). In line with this, in adolescence, relationship breakups are associated with first onset of depression (Monroe, Rohde, Seeley, & Lewinsohn, 1999).

Depression also is associated with subsequent divorce (e.g., Breslau et al., 2011; Kessler et al., 1998), suggesting that depression (or its consequences) might impair relationships to the point of dissolution. However, in some cases, depression may be associated with staying in an unhappy marriage (Davila & Bradbury, 2001). The circumstances under which depression leads to divorce versus staying in an unhappy marriage would be an important target for research.

DEPRESSION IN THE CONTEXT OF FAMILY RELATIONSHIPS

Youth Depression and Family Functioning

Parent–Child and Family Environment Factors

A number of factors distinguish the rearing behaviors of parents of youth who have or do not have depression, with research suggesting that parents of youth with depression are more controlling and less supportive and warm and that they exhibit higher levels of criticism, use more coercion, and communicate less effectively (for reviews, see Kaslow, Jones, & Palin, 2005; McLeod, Weisz, & Wood, 2007). A recent meta-analysis of the cross-sectional association between parenting and childhood depression indicated that, as compared with parental control, parental rejection (i.e., low warmth, hostility, and overinvolvement) was more strongly associated with childhood depression, with parental hostility toward the child yielding the strongest association (McLeod et al., 2007).

Importantly, there also is evidence that parenting behaviors prospectively predict increases in depressive symptoms (e.g., Branje, Hale, Frijns, & Meeus, 2010; Schwartz, Dudgeon, et al., 2012) and future onsets of depression (Burkhouse, Uhrlass, Stone, Knopik, & Gibb, 2012; Silk et al., 2009). In turn, greater depressive symptoms prospectively predict changes in parenting behaviors and lower quality parent–child relationships (Branje et al., 2010; Manongdo & Ramirez Garcia, 2011). Thus youth depression and parenting reciprocally influence one another over time.

Research has identified key moderators of the association between parenting and youth depression. For instance, larger bilateral hippocampal volumes may render girls more susceptible to the negative influence of maternal aggressive behavior (Whittle et al., 2011). Associations may also differ as a function of ethnicity. For example, the associations between caregiver conflict, openness, warmth, and internalizing symptoms were reduced in African American compared with European American children (Vendlinski, Silk, Shaw, & Lane, 2006).

More work is needed to elucidate the mechanisms underlying associations between parenting and youth depression. Initial work suggests that parenting practices may contribute to youth depression via reducing children's self-esteem (e.g., Soenens et al., 2008) and increasing parent–child conflict (e.g., Bámaca-Colbert, Umaña-Taylor, & Gayles, 2012), highlighting the role that both parents and children play in these associations. In line with this, an emerging body of research has utilized sequential analyses of observed mother–adolescent interactions to elucidate the ways in which parents' and adolescents' responses to each other's emotional expression engender risk for depression. Overall, this work suggests that maternal responses that reinforce adolescents' dysphoric behavior, reciprocate adolescents' aggressive behavior, or invalidate or dampen adolescents' positive emotions are associated with depression in adolescents (for a review, see Schwartz, Sheeber, Dudgeon, & Allen, 2012). Greater maternal negativity may contribute to adolescents' depressive symptoms by increasing adolescents' use of maladaptive emotion regulation strategies (e.g., Yap, Schwartz, Byrne, Simmons, & Allen, 2010). In turn, consistent with the bidirectional, transactional nature of the association between parent and child behavior, girls with high depressive symptoms are more likely to reciprocate their mothers' negative affective behavior (Yap et al., 2010).

In terms of the family environment, research shows that high conflict and low cohesiveness prospectively predict the development of depression in children and adolescents (Kaslow et al., 2005; Sheeber, Hops, & Davis, 2001). The influence of family conflict on depression varies. For example, the association between family conflict and depression was found to be greater in children and adolescents who were at high genetic risk for depression (Rice, Harold, Shelton, & Thapar, 2006). In addition, the importance of family conflict and family cohesion may vary by ethnicity, with low cohesion uniquely linked to depression for African American adolescents and high family conflict uniquely linked to depression for European American adolescents (Herman, Ostrander, & Tucker, 2007). Moreover, greater acculturation-based conflict, but not levels of everyday conflict (Juang, Syed, & Cookston, 2012), predicted *lower* levels of depressive symptoms in Chinese American adolescents, further highlighting the ways in which aspects of family environment that are associated with depression vary according to cultural background.

Parental Marital Factors

In addition to parenting and family environment variables, support for the association between interparental conflict and depression in youth is robust (see Kaslow et al., 2005). Consistent with the emotional security hypothesis (Davies & Cummings, 1994) and the cognitive-contextual perspective (Grych & Fincham, 1993), research has documented how children's cognitive, emotional, and behavioral responses to interparental conflict may underlie the link between interparental conflict and depressive symptoms (e.g., Buehler, Lange, & Franck, 2007; Cummings, George, McCoy, & Davies, 2012). Investigators have also explored aspects of the parent–child relationship, including parental acceptance and harshness (e.g., Benson, Buehler, & Gerard, 2008), as well as aspects of the family system, including youth-perceived triangulation (e.g., Franck & Buehler, 2007), as mechanisms of this association. Further study of the moderators of this association is warranted, such as biological factors (e.g., El-Sheikh, Keiley, Erath, & Dyer, 2013) and other aspects of the family environment (e.g., Kennedy, Bybee, Sullivan, & Greeson, 2010) that may buffer the impact of parental conflict.

Given the links between depression and interparental and family conflict, it is not surprising that children from divorced families are more likely to experience depression (e.g., Ge, Natsuaki, & Conger, 2006). Stressful events around the time of divorce may be one avenue by which divorce influences future depression (Ge et al., 2006). Consistent with this, some evidence suggests that environmental factors surrounding the divorce may account for most of the relation between divorce and depression (e.g., D'Onofrio et al., 2006); however, other work suggests the relation may be due to children's and parent's shared genetic vulnerability to internalizing disorders (e.g., D'Onofrio et al., 2007). Notably, the impact of childhood divorce appears to vary according to race/ethnicity (Van Voorhees, Paunesku, Fogel, & Bell, 2009).

Parental Depression and Family Functioning

Effects on Children of Parents with Depression

The impact of parental depression predates even birth. Maternal prenatal depression is associated with placental abnormalities, elevated fetal heart rate, increased fetal physiological activity, birth complications, low birthweight, and lower positive affect at birth (Field, Diego, & Hernandez-Reif, 2006). From these beginnings, parental depression continues to predict impairments in offspring functioning throughout the lifespan. Infants more often have difficult temperaments, lower social engagement, and impaired mental and motor development. Toddlers have trouble with emotion regulation and self-soothing. Older children and adolescents have greater emotional distress, more school problems and peer difficulties, and poor self-esteem, and young adults have lower life satisfaction, greater mental health service utilization, and poorer romantic functioning (Feldman et al., 2009; Goodman & Gotlib, 1999; Katz, Hammen, & Brennan, 2013; Lewinsohn, Olino, & Klein, 2005). Furthermore, children of parents with depression are, not surprisingly, at heightened risk for depression and other forms of psychopathology themselves, propagating the scourge of depression across generations (Goodman et al., 2011), as discussed in detail by Gotlib and Colich (Chapter 13, this volume). Here, we focus specifically on the effects of parental depression on relationships, behaviors, and functioning within the family system.

Parental depression puts tension on the entire family system. Families in which either the mother or the father has depression are less cohesive and more conflictual (reviewed in Hughes & Gullone, 2008). Family functioning may be especially poor among families in which both a parent and a child have depression (Hammen & Brennan, 2001; Shiner & Marmorstein, 1998). Within the spousal subsystem, as we discussed earlier, depression is strongly linked to marital distress, which in turn directly affects child adjustment. As such, marital discord may partially mediate or moderate the association between parental depression and negative offspring outcomes (Cummings, Keller, & Davies, 2005; Fendrich, Warner, & Weissman, 1990).

Parental depression strains parent–child relationships beginning early in the life of the offspring; in fact, researchers have even speculated that depression during pregnancy impedes prenatal mother–child bonding (Pearson et al., 2012). During infancy, parents with depression speak to their babies using more negative content and focusing less on the infant's experience and more on the parents themselves (Murray, Kempton, Woolgar, & Hooper, 1993; Sethna, Murray, & Ramchandani, 2012). Mothers with depression are less responsive to their infants' cries (Donovan, Leavitt, & Walsh, 1998), touch their babies less frequently (Herrera, Reissland, & Shepherd, 2004), and interpret infant facial expressions less accurately (Arteche et al., 2011). These factors likely disrupt parent–child bonding. As such, maternal depression predicts problems in offspring attachment security (Atkinson et al., 2000). On the positive side, children who do build positive relationships with one of their parents are more resilient to the effects of parental depression (Brennan, Le Brocque, & Hammen, 2003; Pargas, Brennan, Hammen, & Le Brocque, 2010; Tannenbaum & Forehand, 1994).

Depression influences parenting behaviors in multiple ways, although specific patterns may vary by individual. Some parents with depression may adopt ineffective and nonauthoritarian parenting behaviors, including inconsistency, poor monitoring, and confrontation avoidance (Arellano, Harvey, & Thakar, 2012; Elgar, Mills, McGrath, Waschbusch, & Brownridge, 2007; Kochanska, Kuczynski, Radke-Yarrow, & Welsh, 1987), whereas others employ harsh, intrusive, and rejecting parenting styles (Lovejoy, Graczyk, O'Hare, & Neuman, 2000). Parents with depression generally are less warm and nurturing toward their children (Arellano et al., 2012; Elgar et al., 2007) and report more negativity and lower confidence about parenthood (Elgar et al., 2007; Lovejoy et al., 2000; Teti & Gelfand, 1991). Although much research has focused on mothers, studies examining fathers have found comparable parenting impairments (Elgar et al., 2007; Wilson & Durbin, 2010). Not surprisingly, parenting deficits accompanied by depression in turn predict negative outcomes in children (Hammen, Shih, & Brennan, 2004).

Some evidence suggests that treating parental depression improves youth outcomes (Foster et al., 2008; Shaw, Connell, Dishion, Wilson, & Gardner, 2009). Other interventions directed at mothers with depression have shown success in improving the mother–child relationship and increasing attachment security (Goodman, Broth, Hall, & Stowe, 2008; Toth, Rogosch, Manly, & Cicchetti, 2006). Although these findings offer promising evidence that the negative impact of parental depression may be reparable, other studies suggest that effective treatments for maternal depression will not completely eliminate maladaptive effects on the mother–child relationship and child outcomes (Forman et al., 2007; Murray, Cooper, Wilson, & Romaniuk, 2003). Similarly, after remission of maternal depression, negative parenting behaviors are reduced but not abolished (Lovejoy et al., 2000). Perhaps some of depression's impact on the family system is not a consequence of depression per se but rather of stable risk factors (e.g., personality traits, stressful context) that conjointly contribute to risk of depression and family dysfunction; these features may not be traditional targets of treatment. Although further research should determine how to best reduce the residual effects of parental depression, it is heartening that treatment has at least some potential to lessen the burden on the family system.

Effects of Children on Depression in Parents

Much research on parental depression has operated under the implicit assumption that effects are unidirectional, with parents molding offspring. The notion that children are passive recipients of their parents' behaviors (consistent with the outdated "mal-de-mère" model, in which mothers were saddled with sole culpability for their children's misbehaviors) has long been criticized as oversimplified (e.g., Belsky, 1984). Nonetheless, to date, relatively few studies have explored the nature of child effects on parents, or the extent to which child behaviors or characteristics influence parental symptomatology.

Existing studies offer some support for child effects on parental depression. Offspring behavior affects maternal depression beginning in infancy (Murray, Stanley, Hooper, King, & Fiori-Cowley, 1996). Furthermore, parental and offspring psychopathology appear to be reciprocally related (Ge, Conger, Lorenz, Shanahan, & Elder, 1995; Hammen, Burge, & Stansbury, 1990), in part because child psychopathology increases the parent's exposure to stressors (Raposa, Hammen, & Brennan, 2011). A growing number of studies suggest that child externalizing symptoms influence parental depression (Allen, Manning, & Meyer, 2010; Gartstein & Sheeber, 2004; Gross, Shaw, Burwell, & Nagin, 2009; Gross, Shaw, & Moilanen, 2008). For example, Gross and colleagues (2009) found that toddler noncompliance predicted higher severity and chronicity of maternal depression trajectories. A few studies also support the impact of child internalizing symptoms on maternal depression. For example, Hughes and Gullone (2010) showed reciprocal prospective associations between the internalizing symptoms of adolescents and those of their mothers.

However, other research has been less supportive of child effects on parental depression. Hanington, Ramchandani, and Stein (2010) found little evidence that child temperament influenced parental depression. In one diary study, daily maternal depressed mood preceded child externalizing symptoms, and not vice versa (Elgar, Waschbusch, McGrath, Stewart, & Curtis, 2004). Other studies offer mixed support for child effects. In a multiwave cross-lagged study, Elgar, Curtis, McGrath, Waschbush, and Stewart (2003) found that maternal depression preceded child externalizing symptoms but followed child internalizing problems. Nicholson, Deboeck, Farris, Boker, and Borkowski (2011) used dynamical systems analysis to test bidirectional transactional coupling between maternal and offspring symptoms. This technique fits a coupled damped linear oscillator model to time-series data to examine complex, bidirectional associations over time. Offspring internalizing and externalizing symptoms fluctuated in concert with maternal depressive symptoms, supporting reciprocity, but effects of mothers' symptoms on offspring were stronger than offspring effects on mothers. Several mechanisms of transmission apply only from parent to child. Aside from genetic transmission, parental depression has unique potential to disrupt the child's development during critical time periods. In sum, children's functioning may have an impact on parental depression, but effects may depend on how offspring functioning is defined, and parents may more powerfully influence their children than vice versa.

BIPOLAR DISORDER

Couple Relationships

Although limited, research suggests that individuals with bipolar disorder are less likely to be married, but this varies as a function of gender, age of onset, and disorder subtype (Lieberman, Massey, & Goodwin, 2010). When individuals with bipolar disorder do marry, they are more likely to marry someone with a psychiatric illness, compared with unipolar patients and healthy controls (for a review, see Mathews & Reus, 2001).

However, marriage may benefit the treatment and course of bipolar disorder. For example, those with a partner at onset of the disorder are more likely to achieve full interepisodic remission (Johnson, Lundstrom, Aberg-Wistedt, & Mathe, 2003), and, among women with bipolar disorder (but not men), marriage predicts fewer and less severe depressive episodes (Lieberman et al., 2010).

Regarding marital distress, individuals with bipolar disorder, like those with unipolar depression, report higher levels of marital distress than controls (Radke-Yarrow, 1998), even in remission (Bauwens, Tracy, Pardoen, Vander Elst, & Mandlewicz, 1991), and particularly when their partners without bipolar disorder also show higher levels of depression (Rowe & Morris, 2012). In fact, bipolar disorder had the strongest association with marital distress among the psychiatric disorders examined in the National Comorbidity Study replication (Whisman, 2007). In addition, a consistent finding is that spouses of individuals with bipolar disorder report less satisfaction than do their partners, even when their partners are in remission (e.g., Levkovitz, Fennig, Horesh, Barak, & Treves, 2000). Depressive symptoms appear to be particularly toxic to spouses' level of satisfaction (e.g., Lam, Donaldson, Brown, & Malliaris, 2005; Rowe & Morris, 2012; cf., Sheets & Miller, 2010) and level of caregiver burden (Ostacher et al., 2008). In contrast, partners report lower levels of burden and dissatisfaction when they believe their spouses have lower levels of control over their illness (e.g., Lam et al., 2005).

Similar to unipolar depression, the relationships of those with bipolar disorder are characterized by impairments in social support (e.g., Levkovitz et al., 2000), high levels of conflict (Hoover & Fitzgerald, 1981), low levels of partner warmth, and high levels of partner hostility (Rowe & Morris, 2012). Partners' (and other caregivers') expressed emotion (EE; levels of criticism, hostility, emotional overinvolvement; Leff & Vaughn, 1985) predicts relapse in treated patients over time (for a review, see Miklowitz, 2004), although this may be specific to depressive episodes (Yan, Hammen, Cohen, Daley, & Henry, 2004). Similarly, greater levels of romantic impairment predict greater levels of depressive, but not manic, symptoms over time (Weinstock & Miller, 2008). Finally, rates of divorce are elevated among individuals with bipolar disorder (Walid & Zaytseva, 2011), and it is likely that relationship dissolution is a stressor that triggers an episode.

Family Functioning

The families of youth with bipolar disorder are characterized by lower levels of warmth, adaptability, and cohesion, as well as higher levels of conflict (for a review, see Keenan-Miller & Miklowitz, 2011). Although most research is cross-sectional, the relationship between childhood bipolar disorder and family functioning is likely bidirectional, with both parent and child contributing to the family environment. For example, among youth with bipolar disorder, earlier age of onset, greater duration of illness, elevated manic symptoms, comorbid attention-deficit/hyperactivity disorder (ADHD) and oppositional defiant disorder (ODD), and presence of parental psychopathology are associated with greater levels of family dysfunction (Belardinelli et al., 2008; Schenkel, West, Harral, Patel, & Pavuluri, 2008; Sullivan & Miklowitz, 2010). In turn, family environment factors, such as parental warmth, EE, and family conflict, affect course (Geller, Tillman, Bolhofner, & Zimmerman, 2008; Miklowitz, Biuckians, & Richards, 2006) and treatment (e.g., Sullivan, Judd, Axelson, & Miklowitz, 2012). The limited research on interparental conflict suggests that living with biological parents in an intact marriage predicts stabilization among youth with bipolar disorder (Geller et al., 2002), but the influence of youth bipolar disorder on parent's marital functioning remains to be investigated.

Similarly, offspring of parents with bipolar disorder show impairments, including increased rates of psychopathology (particularly affective disorders) and cognitive deficits (Klimes-Dougan, Ronsaville, Wiggs, & Martinez, 2006; Lapalme, Hodgins, & LaRoche, 1997). This is likely in part explained by the shared genetic vulnerability, given the pronounced genetic component in bipolar disorder (McGuffin et al., 2003). However, a few studies suggest that bipolar disorder also has negative impacts on qualitative aspects of the family. Family functioning is typically impaired among families with a parent with bipolar disorder (Du Rocher Schudlich, Youngstrom, Calabrese, & Findling, 2008; Weinstock, Keitner, Ryan, Solomon, & Miller, 2006), especially during acute mood episodes (Uebelacker et al., 2006). Compared with normative data, families with a parent with bipolar disorder report less cohesion, independence, and achievement orientation and more conflict (Chang, Blasey, Ketter, & Steiner, 2001). However, other studies suggest that family functioning is comparable to that in major depression, making it unclear whether manic episodes confer unique risk (Weinstock et al., 2006). Substantially more research is needed.

CONCLUSIONS AND FUTURE DIRECTIONS

Despite the large and consistent literature on associations between depression and relationship processes, there are important gaps in knowledge. For example, taxometric research suggests that change in marital discord may show its strongest connection to depression only at high levels and may show less powerful connections at other points (Beach, Fincham, & Leonard, 2006). Taxonomy has not been examined in other types of relationships or at other ages, making it unclear whether the emergence of taxonic associations may be a developmental process that emerges over time or a marriage-specific process. Future research should similarly examine whether depression needs to reach a critical severity level to trigger family discord. In addition, most adolescent research has focused on subclinical depressive symptoms, but depression severity may be important. The adolescents with the most severe depression may not have romantic experiences, which may result in a different type of impairment than that resulting from involvement in dysfunctional relationships.

Questions of gender differences remain unresolved. Although some research suggests that associations are stronger for women, this is not a consistent finding (see Brock & Lawrence, 2011; Simon & Barrett, 2010), nor have gender effects been adequately examined, as research has tended to focus on females (for a review, see Whisman, Weinstock, & Tolejko, 2006). This is particularly true in the adolescent literature, as virtually no research has examined males. In addition, conceptual models of the association between depression and romantic dysfunction largely have not focused on gender differences, leaving the field to proceed without the benefit of a theoretical framework from which to explore them. Within the family literature, the overall association between childhood depression and parenting is not moderated by parent or child gender (McLeod et al., 2007). However, other work suggests that boys and girls may be differentially sensitive to certain aspects of the family system (e.g., Harkness & Lumley, 2008; Yap et al., 2010). Although research on the impact of paternal depression is limited, one meta-analysis suggests that paternal depression affects parenting behaviors in a manner comparable to maternal depression (Wilson & Durbin, 2010). To further our understanding of gender differences, future work should continue to include both mothers and fathers, to explore whether gender differences emerge during certain developmental periods, and to investigate whether the mechanisms underlying associations differ according to parent and child gender.

Questions of specificity of marital and family quality to depression also exist. Although associations between marital discord and depression remain after controlling for personality pathology and for what were termed Axis I disorders prior to DSM-5 (Whisman, 1999; Whisman, Uebelacker, Tolejko, Chatav, & McKelvie, 2006), other research supports a model that includes internalizing symptoms more broadly defined (Brock & Lawrence, 2011). Further research should consider implementing advanced statistical methods, such as latent variable modeling, to differentiate between broad internalizing pathology versus depression-specific components in examining the reciprocal effects of depression on family functioning (South, Krueger, & Iacono, 2011; Starr, Conway, Hammen, & Brennan, 2014). Finally, as noted earlier, far more research is needed to understand the unique challenges that bipolar disorder, with both mania and depression, presents to couples and families.

Another issue is that the literatures on children, adolescents, and adults are quite separate from one another. Given the field's emphasis on viewing psychopathology developmentally and the evidence for links between adolescent and adult relational functioning (Madsen & Collins, 2011), it would behoove researchers to adopt a developmental focus toward understanding associations between depression and romantic and family functioning over the life course.

Finally, continued research is needed on diverse groups with regard to relationship type, ethnic/cultural differences, and age. The literature has focused on heterosexual relationships more than on gay, lesbian, and bisexual relationships and rarely incorporates same-sex-parented families. With the growing number and recognition of these relationships, as well as recognition of unique stressors associated with sexual minority status, it will be important to examine associations with depression. The couples literature also has neglected examination of ethnic/cultural differences that may moderate associations between depression and relationship dysfunction. As noted, an emerging body of work indicates that such associations vary in the context of childhood depression and family relationships. For example, the importance of family, parent–child conflict, and family cohesion differs according to cultural factors (e.g., Herman et al., 2007; Kim, Chen, Li, Huang, & Moon, 2009). Whether they do so also in romantic relationships is largely unknown. And, although there are growing data on relationships and depression at diverse ages, including adolescence and older adulthood, understanding associations at different ages and adopting a developmental focus may be a useful next step.

REFERENCES

Allen, J. P., Manning, N., & Meyer, J. (2010). Tightly linked systems: Reciprocal relations between maternal depressive symptoms and maternal reports of adolescent externalizing behavior. *Journal of Abnormal Psychology, 119*, 825–835.

Arellano, P. A. E., Harvey, E. A., & Thakar, D. A. (2012). A longitudinal study of the relation between depressive symptomatology and parenting practices. *Family Relations: An Interdisciplinary Journal of Applied Family Studies, 61*, 271–282.

Arteche, A., Joormann, J., Harvey, A., Craske, M., Gotlib, I. H., Lehtonen, A., et al. (2011). The effects of postnatal maternal depression and anxiety on the processing of infant faces. *Journal of Affective Disorders, 133*, 197–203.

Atkinson, L., Paglia, A., Coolbear, J., Niccols, A., Parker, K. C. H., & Guger, S. (2000). Attachment security: A meta-analysis of maternal mental health correlates. *Clinical Psychology Review, 20,* 1019–1040.

Bámaca-Colbert, M. Y., Umaña-Taylor, A. J., & Gayles, J. G. (2012). A developmental-contextual model of depressive symptoms in Mexican-origin female adolescents. *Developmental Psychology, 48*(2), 406–421.

Bauwens, F., Tracy, A., Pardoen, D., Vander Elst, M., & Mandlewicz, J. (1991). Social adjustment of remitted bipolar and unipolar out-patients. *British Journal of Psychiatry, 159,* 239–244.

Beach, S. R. H., Fincham, F. D., & Leonard, K. E. (2006, November). *Nuances in the connection between marriage and depression.* Paper presented at the annual convention of the Association for Behavioral and Cognitive Therapies, Chicago.

Belardinelli, C., Hatch, J. P., Olvera, R. L., Fonseca, M., Caetano, S. C., Nicoletti, M., et al. (2008). Family environment patterns in families with bipolar children. *Journal of Affective Disorders, 107*(1–3), 299–305.

Belsky, J. (1984). The determinants of parenting: A process model. *Child Development, 55,* 83–96.

Benson, M. J., Buehler, C., & Gerard, J. M. (2008). Interparental hostility and early adolescent problem behavior: Spillover via maternal acceptance, harshness, inconsistency, and intrusiveness. *Journal of Early Adolescence, 28*(3), 428–454.

Branje, S. J. T., Hale, W. W., III, Frijns, T., & Meeus, W. H. J. (2010). Longitudinal associations between perceived parent–child relationship quality and depressive symptoms in adolescence. *Journal of Abnormal Child Psychology, 38*(6), 751–763.

Brennan, P. A., Le Brocque, R., & Hammen, C. (2003). Maternal depression, parent–child relationships, and resilient outcomes in adolescence. *Journal of the American Academy of Child and Adolescent Psychiatry, 42,* 1469–1477.

Breslau, J., Miller, E., Jin, R., Sampson, N. A., Alonso, J., Andrade, L. H., et al. (2011). A multinational study of mental disorders, marriage, and divorce. *Acta Psychiatrica Scandinavica, 124,* 474–486.

Brock, R. L. & Lawrence, E. (2011). Marriage as a risk factor for internalizing disorders: Clarifying scope and specificity. *Journal of Consulting and Clinical Psychology, 79,* 577–589.

Buehler, C., Lange, G., & Franck, K. L. (2007). Adolescents' cognitive and emotional responses to marital hostility. *Child Development, 78*(3), 775–789.

Burkhouse, K., Uhrlass, D., Stone, L., Knopik, V., & Gibb, B. (2012). Expressed emotion–criticism and risk of depression onset in children. *Journal of Clinical Child and Adolescent Psychology, 41*(6), 771–777.

Chang, K. D., Blasey, C., Ketter, T. A., & Steiner, H. (2001). Family environment of children and adolescents with bipolar parents. *Bipolar Disorders, 3,* 73–78.

Christian-Herman, J. L., O'Leary, K. D., & Avery-Leaf, S. (2001). The impact of severe negative events in marriage on depression. *Journal of Social and Clinical Psychology, 20,* 25–44.

Cummings, E. M., George, M. R. W., McCoy, K. P., & Davies, P. T. (2012). Interparental conflict in kindergarten and adolescent adjustment: Prospective investigation of emotional security as an explanatory mechanism. *Child Development, 83*(5), 1703–1715.

Cummings, E. M., Keller, P. S., & Davies, P. T. (2005). Towards a family process model of maternal and paternal depressive symptoms: Exploring multiple relations with child and family functioning. *Journal of Child Psychology and Psychiatry, 46,* 479–489.

Daley, S. E., & Hammen, C. (2002). Depressive symptoms and close relationships during the transition to adulthood: Perspectives from dysphoric women, their best friends, and their romantic partners. *Journal of Consulting and Clinical Psychology, 70,* 129–141.

Davies, P. T., & Cummings, E. M. (1994). Marital conflict and child adjustment: An emotional security hypothesis. *Psychological Bulletin, 116*(3), 387–411.

Davila, J. (2008). Depressive symptoms and adolescent romance: Theory, research, and implications. *Child Development Perspectives, 2,* 26–31.

Davila, J., & Bradbury, T. N. (2001). Attachment insecurity and the distinction between unhappy spouses who do and do not divorce. *Journal of Family Psychology, 15,* 371–393.

Davila, J., Bradbury, T. N., Cohan, C. L., & Tochluk, S. (1997). Marital functioning and depressive symptoms: Evidence for a stress generation model. *Journal of Personality and Social Psychology, 73,* 849–861.

Davila, J., Karney, B. R., Hall, T., & Bradbury, T. N. (2003). Depressive symptoms and marital satisfaction: Within-subject associations and the moderating effects of gender and neuroticism. *Journal of Family Psychology, 17,* 557–570.

Davila, J., Steinberg, S., Kachadourian, L., Cobb, R., & Fincham, F. (2004). Romantic involvement and depressive symptoms in early and late adolescence: The role of a preoccupied relational style. *Personal Relationships, 11,* 161–178.

Davila, J., Stroud, C. B., Starr, L. R., Ramsay Miller, M., Yoneda, A., & Hershenberg, R. (2009). Romantic and sexual activities, parent–adolescent stress, and depressive symptoms among early adolescent girls. *Journal of Adolescence, 32,* 909–924.

D'Onofrio, B. M., Turkheimer, E., Emery, R. E., Maes, H. H., Silberg, J., & Eaves, L. J. (2007). A Children of Twins study of parental divorce and offspring psychopathology. *Journal of Child Psychology and Psychiatry, 48*(7), 667–675.

D'Onofrio, B. M., Turkheimer, E., Emery, R. E., Slutske, W. S., Heath, A. C., Madden, P. A., et al. (2006). A genetically informed study of the processes underlying the association between parental marital instability and offspring adjustment. *Developmental Psychology, 42*(3), 486–499.

Donovan, W. L., Leavitt, L. A., & Walsh, R. O. (1998). Conflict and depression predict maternal sensitivity to infant cries. *Infant Behavior and Development, 21,* 505–517.

Du Rocher Schudlich, T. D., Papp, L. M., & Cummings, E. M. (2011). Relations between spouses' depressive symptoms and marital conflict: A longitudinal investigation of the role of conflict resolution styles. *Journal of Family Psychology, 25,* 531–540.

Du Rocher Schudlich, T. D., Youngstrom, E. A., Calabrese, J. R., & Findling, R. L. (2008). The role of family functioning in bipolar disorder in families. *Journal of Abnormal Child Psychology, 36,* 849–863.

Eberhart, N. K., & Hammen, C. L. (2010). Interpersonal style, stress, and depression: An examination of transactional and diathesis–stress models. *Journal of Social and Clinical Psychology, 29,* 23–38.

Elgar, F. J., Curtis, L. J., McGrath, P. J., Waschbusch, D. A., & Stewart, S. H. (2003). Antecedent–consequence conditions in maternal mood and child adjustment: A four-year cross-lagged study. *Journal of Clinical Child and Adolescent Psychology, 32,* 362–374.

Elgar, F. J., Mills, R. S. L., McGrath, P. J., Waschbusch, D. A., & Brownridge, D. A. (2007). Maternal and paternal depressive symptoms and child maladjustment: The mediating role of parental behavior. *Journal of Abnormal Child Psychology, 35,* 943–955.

Elgar, F. J., Waschbusch, D. A., McGrath, P. J., Stewart, S. H., & Curtis, L. J. (2004). Temporal relations in daily-reported maternal mood and disruptive child behavior. *Journal of Abnormal Child Psychology, 32,* 237–247.

El-Sheikh, M., Keiley, M., Erath, S., & Dyer, W. J. (2013). Marital conflict and growth in children's internalizing symptoms: The role of autonomic nervous system activity. *Developmental Psychology, 49*(1), 92–108.

Feldman, R., Granat, A., Pariente, C., Kanety, H., Kuint, J., & Gilboa-Schechtman, E. (2009). Maternal depression and anxiety across the postpartum year and infant social engagement, fear regulation, and stress reactivity. *Journal of the American Academy of Child and Adolescent Psychiatry, 48,* 919–927.

Fendrich, M., Warner, V., & Weissman, M. M. (1990). Family risk factors, parental depression, and psychopathology in offspring. *Developmental Psychology, 26,* 40–50.

Field, T., Diego, M., & Hernandez-Reif, M. (2006). Prenatal depression effects on the fetus and newborn: A review. *Infant Behavior and Development, 29,* 445–455.

Forman, D. R., O'Hara, M. W., Stuart, S., Gorman, L. L., Larsen, K. E., & Coy, K. C. (2007). Effective treatment for postpartum depression is not sufficient to improve the developing mother–child relationship. *Development and Psychopathology, 19,* 585–602.

Foster, C. E., Webster, M. C., Weissman, M. M., Pilowsky, D. J., Wickramaratne, P. J., Talati, A., et al. (2008). Remission of maternal depression: Relations to family functioning and youth internalizing and externalizing symptoms. *Journal of Clinical Child and Adolescent Psychology, 37*, 714–724.

Franck, K. L., & Buehler, C. (2007). A family process model of marital hostility, parental depressive affect, and early adolescent problem behavior: The roles of triangulation and parental warmth. *Journal of Family Psychology, 21*(4), 614–625.

Galliher, R. V., Rostosky, S. S., Welsh, D. P., & Kawaguchi, M. C. (1999). Power and psychological well-being in late adolescent romantic relationships. *Sex Roles, 40*, 689–710.

Gartstein, M. A., & Sheeber, L. (2004). Child behavior problems and maternal symptoms of depression: A mediational model. *Journal of Child and Adolescent Psychiatric Nursing, 17*, 141–150.

Ge, X., Conger, R. D., Lorenz, F. O., Shanahan, M., & Elder, G. H. (1995). Mutual influences in parent and adolescent psychological distress. *Developmental Psychology, 31*, 406–419.

Ge, X., Natsuaki, M. N., & Conger, R. D. (2006). Trajectories of depressive symptoms and stressful life events among male and female adolescents in divorced and nondivorced families. *Development and Psychopathology, 18*, 253–273.

Geller, B., Craney, J. L., Bolhofner, K., Nickelsburg, M. J., Williams, M., & Zimerman, B. (2002). Two-year prospective follow-up of children with prepubertal and early onset bipolar disorder phenotype. *American Journal of Psychiatry, 159*, 927–933.

Geller, B., Tillman, R., Bolhofner, K., & Zimerman, B. (2008). Child bipolar I disorder: Prospective continuity with adult bipolar I disorder; characteristics of second and third episodes; predictors of 8-year outcome. *Archives of General Psychiatry, 65*(10), 1125–1133.

Goodman, S. H., Broth, M. R., Hall, C. M., & Stowe, Z. N. (2008). Treatment of postpartum depression in mothers: Secondary benefits to the infants. *Infant Mental Health Journal, 29*, 492–513.

Goodman, S. H., & Gotlib, I. H. (1999). Risk for psychopathology in the children of depressed mothers: A developmental model for understanding mechanisms of transmission. *Psychological Review, 106*, 458–490.

Goodman, S. H., Rouse, M. H., Connell, A. M., Broth, M. R., Hall, C. M., & Heyward, D. (2011). Maternal depression and child psychopathology: A meta-analytic review. *Clinical Child and Family Psychology Review, 14*, 1–27.

Gordon, K. C., Friedman, M. A., & Miller, I. W. (2005). Marital attributions as moderators of the marital discord–depression link. *Journal of Social and Clinical Psychology, 24*, 876–893.

Gotlib, I. H., Lewinsohn, P. M., & Seeley, J. R. (1998). Consequences of depression during adolescence: Marital status and marital functioning in early adulthood. *Journal of Abnormal Psychology, 107*, 686–690.

Gross, H. E., Shaw, D. S., Burwell, R. A., & Nagin, D. S. (2009). Transactional processes in child disruptive behavior and maternal depression: A longitudinal study from early childhood to adolescence. *Development and Psychopathology, 21*, 139–156.

Gross, H. E., Shaw, D. S., & Moilanen, K. L. (2008). Reciprocal associations between boys' externalizing problems and mothers' depressive symptoms. *Journal of Abnormal Child Psychology, 36*, 693–709.

Grych, J. H., & Fincham, F. D. (1993). Children's appraisals of marital conflict: Initial investigations of the cognitive-contextual framework. *Child Development, 64*, 215–230.

Gutiérrez-Lobos, K., Wölfl, G., Scherer, M., Anderer, P., & Schmidl-Mohl, B. (2000). The gender gap in depression reconsidered: The influence of marital and employment status on the female/male ratio of treated incidence rates. *Social Psychiatry and Psychiatric Epidemiology, 35*, 202–210.

Ha, T., Overbeek, G., Cillessen, A. H. N., & Engels, R. C. M. E., (2012). A longitudinal study of the associations among adolescent conflict resolution styles, depressive symptoms, and romantic relationship longevity. *Journal of Adolescence, 35*, 1247–1254.

Hammen, C., & Brennan, P. A. (2001). Depressed adolescents of depressed and nondepressed mothers: Tests of an interpersonal impairment hypothesis. *Journal of Consulting and Clinical Psychology, 69,* 284–294.

Hammen, C., Burge, D., & Stansbury, K. (1990). Relationship of mother and child variables to child outcomes in a high-risk sample: A causal modeling analysis. *Developmental Psychology, 26,* 24–30.

Hammen, C., Shih, J. H., & Brennan, P. A. (2004). Intergenerational transmission of depression: Test of an interpersonal stress model in a community sample. *Journal of Consulting and Clinical Psychology, 72,* 511–522.

Hanington, L., Ramchandani, P., & Stein, A. (2010). Parental depression and child temperament: Assessing child to parent effects in a longitudinal population study. *Infant Behavior and Development, 33,* 88–95.

Harkness, K. L., & Lumley, M. N. (2008). Child abuse and neglect and the development of depression in children and adolescents. In J. R. Z. Abela & B. L. Hankin (Eds.), *Handbook of depression in children and adolescents* (pp. 466–488). New York: Guilford Press.

Herman, K. C., Ostrander, R., & Tucker, C. M. (2007). Do family environments and negative cognitions of adolescents with depressive symptoms vary by ethnic group? *Journal of Family Psychology, 21*(2), 325–330.

Herrera, E., Reissland, N., & Shepherd, J. (2004). Maternal touch and maternal child-directed speech: Effects of depressed mood in the postnatal period. *Journal of Affective Disorders, 81,* 29–23.

Hooley, J. M., & Teasdale, J. D. (1989). Predictors of relapse in unipolar depressives: Expressed emotion, marital distress, and perceived criticism. *Journal of Abnormal Psychology, 98,* 229–235.

Hoover, C. F., & Fitzgerald, G. (1981). Marital conflict of manic–depressive patients. *Archives of General Psychiatry, 38,* 65–67.

Horn, E. E., Xu, Y., Beam, C., Turkheimer, E., & Emery, R. E. (2013). Accounting for the physical and mental health benefits of entry into marriage: A genetically informed study of selection and causation. *Journal of Family Psychology, 27,* 30–41.

Hughes, E. K., & Gullone, E. (2008). Internalizing symptoms and disorders in families of adolescents: A review of family systems literature. *Clinical Psychology Review, 28,* 92–117.

Hughes, E. K., & Gullone, E. (2010). Reciprocal relationships between parent and adolescent internalizing symptoms. *Journal of Family Psychology, 24,* 115–124.

Inaba, A., Thoits, P. A., & Ueno, K. (2005). Depression in the United States and Japan: Gender, marital status, and SES patterns. *Social Science and Medicine, 61,* 2280–2292.

Jackman-Cram, S., Dobson, K. S., & Martin, R. (2006). Marital problem-solving behavior in depression and marital distress. *Journal of Abnormal Psychology, 115,* 380–384.

Johnson, L., Lundstrom, O., Aberg-Wistedt, A., & Mathe, A. A. (2003). Social support in bipolar disorder: Its relevance to remission and relapse. *Bipolar Disorders, 5,* 129–137.

Juang, L. P., Syed, M., & Cookston, J. T. (2012). Acculturation-based and everyday parent–adolescent conflict among Chinese American adolescents: Longitudinal trajectories and implications for mental health. *Journal of Family Psychology, 26*(6), 916–926.

Kaslow, N. J., Jones, C. A., & Palin, F. (2005). A relational perspective on depressed children: Family patterns and interventions. In W. M. Pinsof & J. L. Lebow (Eds.), *Family psychology: The art of the science* (pp. 215–242). New York: Oxford University Press.

Katz, S. J., Hammen, C. L., & Brennan, P. A. (2013). Maternal depression and the intergenerational transmission of relational impairment. *Journal of Family Psychology, 27,* 86–95.

Keenan-Miller, D., & Miklowitz, D. J. (2011). Interpersonal functioning in pediatric bipolar disorder. *Clinical Psychology: Science and Practice, 18*(4), 342–356.

Kennedy, A. C., Bybee, D., Sullivan, C. M., & Greeson, M. (2010). The impact of family and community violence on children's depression trajectories: Examining the interactions of violence exposure, family social support, and gender. *Journal of Family Psychology, 24*(2), 197–207.

Kessler, R. C., Berglund, P., Demler, O., Jin, R., Koretz, D., Merikangas, K. R., et al. (2003). The epidemiology of major depressive disorder: Results for the National Comorbidity Survey Replication (NCS-R). *Journal of the American Medical Association, 289*, 3095–3105.

Kessler, R. C., Walters, E. E., & Forthofer, M. S. (1998). The social consequences of psychiatric disorders: III. Probability of marital stability. *American Journal of Psychiatry, 155*, 1092–1096.

Kim, S. Y., Chen, Q., Li, J., Huang, X., & Moon, U. J. (2009). Parent–child acculturation, parenting, and adolescent depressive symptoms in Chinese immigrant families. *Journal of Family Psychology, 23*(3), 426–437.

Klimes-Dougan, B., Ronsaville, D., Wiggs, E. A., & Martinez, P. E. (2006). Neuropsychological functioning in adolescent children of mothers with a history of bipolar or major depressive disorders. *Biological Psychiatry, 60*, 957–965.

Kochanska, G., Kuczynski, L., Radke-Yarrow, M., & Welsh, J. D. (1987). Resolutions of control episodes between well and affectively ill mothers and their young children. *Journal of Abnormal Child Psychology, 15*, 441–456.

Kouros, C. D., Papp, L. M., & Cummings, E. M. (2008). Interrelations and moderators of longitudinal links between marital satisfaction and depressive symptoms among couples in established relationships. *Journal of Family Psychology, 22*, 667–677.

La Greca, A. M., & Harrison, H. M. (2005). Adolescent peer relations, friendships, and romantic relationships: Do they predict social anxiety and depression? *Journal of Clinical Child and Adolescent Psychology, 34*, 49–61.

Lam, D., Donaldson, C., Brown, Y., & Malliaris, Y. (2005). Burden and marital and sexual satisfaction in partners of bipolar patients. *Bipolar Disorders, 7*, 431–440.

Lapalme, M., Hodgins, S., & LaRoche, C. (1997). Children of parents with bipolar disorder: A meta-analysis of risk for mental disorders. *Canadian Journal of Psychiatry, 42*, 623–631.

Leff, J., & Vaughn, C. (1985). *Expressed emotion in families.* New York: Guilford Press

Levkovitz, V., Fennig, S., Horesh, N., Barak, V., & Treves, I. (2000). Perception of ill spouse and dyadic relationship in couples with affective disorder and those without. *Journal of Affective Disorders, 58*, 237–240.

Lewinsohn, P. M., Olino, T. M., & Klein, D. N. (2005). Psychosocial impairment in offspring of depressed parents. *Psychological Medicine, 35*, 1493–1503.

Lieberman, D. Z., Massey, S. H., & Goodwin, F. K. (2010). The role of gender in single vs. married individuals with bipolar disorder. *Comprehensive Psychiatry, 51*(4), 380–385.

Lovejoy, M. C., Graczyk, P. A., O'Hare, E., & Neuman, G. (2000). Maternal depression and parenting behavior: A meta-analytic review. *Clinical Psychology Review, 20*, 561–592.

Madsen, S. D., & Collins, W. A. (2011). The salience of adolescent romantic experiences for romantic relationship qualities in young adulthood. *Journal of Research on Adolescence, 21*, 789–801.

Manongdo, J. A., & Ramirez Garcia, J. I. (2011). Maternal parenting and mental health of Mexican American youth: A bidirectional and prospective approach. *Journal of Family Psychology, 25*(2), 261–270.

Mathews, C., & Reus, V. (2001). Assortative mating in the affective disorders: A systematic review and meta-analysis. *Comprehensive Psychiatry, 42*, 257–262.

McGuffin, P., Rijsdijk, F., Andrew, M., Sham, P., Katz, R., & Cardno, A. (2003). The heritability of bipolar affective disorder and the genetic relationship to unipolar depression. *Archives of General Psychiatry, 60*, 497–502.

McLeod, B. D., Weisz, J. R., & Wood, J. J. (2007). Examining the association between parenting and childhood depression: A meta-analysis. *Clinical Psychology Review, 27*, 986–1003.

Miklowitz, D. J. (2004). The role of family systems in severe and recurrent psychiatric disorders: A developmental psychopathology view. *Development and Psychopathology, 16*, 667–688.

Miklowitz, D. J., Biuckians, A., & Richards, J. A. (2006). Early-onset bipolar disorder: A family treatment perspective. *Development and Psychopathology, 18*, 1247–1265.

Monroe, S. M., Bromet, E. J., Connell, M. M., & Steiner, S. C. (1986). Social support, life events, and depressive symptoms: A 1-year prospective study. *Journal of Consulting and Clinical Psychology, 54,* 424–431.

Monroe, S. M., Rohde, P., Seeley, J. R., & Lewinsohn, P. M. (1999). Life events and depression in adolescence: Relationship loss as a prospective risk factor for first onset of major depressive disorder. *Journal of Abnormal Psychology, 108,* 606–614.

Murray, L., Cooper, P. J., Wilson, A., & Romaniuk, H. (2003). Controlled trial of the short- and long-term effect of psychological treatment of post-partum depressio:. 2. Impact on the mother–child relationship and child outcome. *British Journal of Psychiatry, 182,* 420–427.

Murray, L., Kempton, C., Woolgar, M., & Hooper, R. (1993). Depressed mothers' speech to their infants and its relation to infant gender and cognitive development. *Journal of Child Psychology and Psychiatry, 34,* 1083–1101.

Murray, L., Stanley, C., Hooper, R., King, F., & Fiori-Cowley, A. (1996). The role of infant factors in postnatal depression and mother–infant interactions. *Developmental Medicine and Child Neurology, 38,* 109–119.

Nicholson, J. S., Deboeck, P. R., Farris, J. R., Boker, S. M., & Borkowski, J. G. (2011). Maternal depressive symptomatology and child behavior: Transactional relationship with simultaneous bidirectional coupling. *Developmental Psychology, 47,* 1312–1323.

Osler, M., McGue, M., Lund, R., & Christensen, K. (2008). Marital status and twins' health and behavior: An analysis of middle-aged Danish twins. *Psychosomatic Medicine, 70,* 482–487.

Ostacher, M. J., Nierenberg, A. A., Iosifescu, D. V., Eidelman, P., Lund, H. G., Ametrano, R. M., et al. (2008). Correlates of subjective and objective burden among caregivers of patients with bipolar disorder. *Acta Psychiatrica Scandinavica, 118,* 49–56.

Papp, L. M., Kouros, C. D., & Cummings, E. M., (2010) Emotions in marital conflict interactions: Empathic accuracy, assumed similarity, and the moderating context of depressive symptoms. *Journal of Social and Personal Relationships, 27,* 367–387.

Pargas, R. C. M., Brennan, P. A., Hammen, C., & Le Brocque, R. (2010). Resilience to maternal depression in young adulthood. *Developmental Psychology, 46,* 805–814.

Pearson, R. M., Melotti, R., Heron, J., Joinson, C., Stein, A., Ramchandani, P. G., et al. (2012). Disruption to the development of maternal responsiveness?: The impact of prenatal depression on mother–infant interactions. *Infant Behavior and Development, 35,* 613–626.

Poyner-Del Vento, P. W., & Cobb, R. J. (2011). Chronic stress as a moderator of the association between depressive symptoms and marital satisfaction. *Journal of Social and Clinical Psychology, 30,* 905–936.

Proulx, C. M., Buehler, C., & Helms, H. (2009). Moderators of the link between marital hostility and change in spouses' depressive symptoms. *Journal of Family Psychology, 23,* 540–550.

Radke-Yarrow, M. (1998). *Children of depressed mothers: From early childhood to maturity.* Cambridge, UK: Cambridge University Press.

Raposa, E., Hammen, C., & Brennan, P. (2011). Effects of child psychopathology on maternal depression: The mediating role of child-related acute and chronic stressors. *Journal of Abnormal Child Psychology, 39,* 1177–1186.

Rehman, U. S., Beausoleil, A., & Karimiha, G. (2013). Competency lies in the eye of the beholder?: Comparing the interpersonal skills of currently, formerly and never depressed females using self and partner reports. *Cognitive Therapy and Research, 37,* 43–50.

Rehman, U. S., Gollan, J., & Mortimer, A. R. (2008). The marital context of depression: Research, limitations, and new directions. *Clinical Psychology Review, 28,* 179–198.

Rice, F., Harold, G. T., Shelton, K. H., & Thapar, A. (2006). Family conflict interacts with genetic liability in predicting childhood and adolescent depression. *Journal of the American Academy of Child and Adolescent Psychiatry, 45,* 841–848.

Romanoski, A. J., Folstein, M. F., Nestadt, G., Chahal, R., Merchant, A., Brown, C. H., et al. (1992). The epidemiology of psychiatrist-ascertained depression and DSM-III depressive disorders: Results from the Eastern Baltimore Mental Health Survey clinical reappraisal. *Psychological Medicine, 22,* 629–655.

Rowe, L. S., & Morris, A. M. (2012). Patient and partner correlates of couple relationship functioning in bipolar disorder. *Journal of Family Psychology, 26*(3), 328–337.

Schenkel, L. S., West, A. E., Harral, E. M., Patel, N. B., & Pavuluri, M. N. (2008). Parent–child interactions in pediatric bipolar disorder. *Journal of Clinical Psychology, 64*(4), 422–437.

Schwartz, O. S., Dudgeon, P., Sheeber, L. B., Yap, M. B. H., Simmons, J. G., & Allen, N. B. (2012). Parental behaviors during family interactions predict changes in depression and anxiety symptoms during adolescence. *Journal of Abnormal Child Psychology, 40*(1), 59–71.

Schwartz, O. S., Sheeber, L. B., Dudgeon, P., & Allen, N. B. (2012). Emotion socialization within the family environment and adolescent depression. *Clinical Psychology Review, 32*(6), 447–453.

Sethna, V., Murray, L., & Ramchandani, P. G. (2012). Depressed fathers' speech to their 3-month-old infants: A study of cognitive and mentalizing features in paternal speech. *Psychological Medicine, 42,* 2361–2371.

Shaw, D. S., Connell, A., Dishion, T. J., Wilson, M. N., & Gardner, F. (2009). Improvements in maternal depression as a mediator of intervention effects on early childhood problem behavior. *Development and Psychopathology, 21,* 417–439.

Sheeber, L., Hops, H., & Davis, B. (2001). Family processes in adolescent depression. *Clinical Child and Family Psychology Review, 4,* 19–35.

Sheets, E. S., & Miller, I. W. (2010). Predictors of relationship functioning for patients with bipolar disorder and their partners. *Journal of Family Psychology, 24,* 371–379.

Shiner, R. L., & Marmorstein, N. R. (1998). Family environments of adolescents with lifetime depression: Associations with maternal depression history. *Journal of the American Academy of Child and Adolescent Psychiatry, 37,* 1152–1160.

Silk, J. S., Ziegler, M. L., Whalen, D. J., Dahl, R. E., Ryan, N. D., Dietz, L. J., et al. (2009). Expressed emotion in mothers of currently depressed, remitted, high-risk, and low-risk youth: Links to child depression status and longitudinal course. *Journal of Clinical Child and Adolescent Psychology, 38*(1), 36–47.

Simon, R. W., & Barrett, A. E. (2010). Nonmarital romantic relationships and mental health in early adulthood: Does the association differ for women and men? *Journal of Health and Social Behavior, 51,* 168–182.

Smith, D. A., Breiding, M. J., & Papp, L. M. (2012). Depressive moods and marital happiness: Within-person synchrony, moderators, and meaning. *Journal of Family Psychology, 26,* 338–347.

Soenens, B., Luyckx, K., Vansteenkiste, M., Duriez, B., & Goossens, L. (2008). Clarifying the link between parental psychological control and adolescents' depressive symptoms: Reciprocal versus unidirectional models. *Merrill-Palmer Quarterly, 54*(4), 411–444.

South, S. C., Krueger, R. F., & Iacono, W. G. (2011). Understanding general and specific connections between psychopathology and marital distress: A model-based approach. *Journal of Abnormal Psychology, 120,* 935.

Starr, L. R., Conway, C. C., Hammen, C. L., & Brennan, P. A. (2014). Transdiagnostic and disorderspecific models of intergenerational transmission of internalizing pathology. *Psychological Medicine, 44*(1), 161–172.

Starr, L. R., & Davila, J. (2009). Clarifying co-rumination: Associations with internalizing symptoms and romantic involvement among adolescent girls. *Journal of Adolescence, 32*(1), 19–37.

Steinberg, S. J., & Davila, J. (2008). Romantic functioning and depressive symptoms among early adolescent girls: The moderating role of parental emotional availability. *Journal of Clinical Child and Adolescent Psychology, 37*(2), 350–362.

Sullivan, A. E., Judd, C. M., Axelson, D. A., & Miklowitz, D. J. (2012). Family functioning and the course of adolescent bipolar disorder. *Behavior Therapy, 43*(4), 837–847.

Sullivan, A. E., & Miklowitz, D. J. (2010). Family functioning among adolescents with bipolar disorder. *Journal of Family Psychology, 24*(1), 60–67.

Tannenbaum, L., & Forehand, R. (1994). Maternal depressive mood: The role of the father in preventing adolescent problem behaviors. *Behaviour Research and Therapy, 32,* 321–325.

Teti, D. M., & Gelfand, D. M. (1991). Behavioral competence among mothers of infants in the first year: The mediational role of maternal self-efficacy. *Child Development, 62,* 918–929.

Toth, S. L., Rogosch, F. A., Manly, J. T., & Cicchetti, D. (2006). The efficacy of toddler–parent psychotherapy to reorganize attachment in the young offspring of mothers with major depressive disorder: A randomized preventive trial. *Journal of Consulting and Clinical Psychology, 74,* 1006–1016.

Uebelacker, L. A., Beevers, C. G., Battle, C. L., Strong, D., Keitner, G. I., Ryan, C. E., et al. (2006). Family functioning in bipolar I disorder. *Journal of Family Psychology, 20,* 701–704.

Uebelacker, L. A., Courtnage, E. S., & Whisman, M. A. (2003). Correlates of depression and marital dissatisfaction: Perceptions of marital communication style. *Journal of Social and Personal Relationships, 20,* 757–769.

Van Voorhees, B. W., Paunesku, D., Fogel, J., & Bell, C. C. (2009). Differences in vulnerability factors for depressive episodes in African American and European American adolescents. *Journal of the National Medical Association, 101*(12), 1255–1267.

Vendlinski, M., Silk, J. S., Shaw, D. S., & Lane, T. J. (2006). Ethnic differences in relations between family process and child internalizing problems. *Journal of Child Psychology and Psychiatry, 47,* 960–969.

Vujeva, H. M., & Furman, W. (2011). Depressive symptoms and romantic relationship qualities from adolescence through emerging adulthood: A longitudinal examination of influences. *Journal of Clinical Child and Adolescent Psychology, 40,* 123–135.

Walid, M. S., & Zaytseva, N. V. (2011). Which neuropsychiatric disorder is more associated with divorce? *Journal of Divorce and Remarriage, 52*(4), 220–224.

Weinstock, L. M., Keitner, G. I., Ryan, C. E., Solomon, D. A., & Miller, I. W. (2006). Family functioning and mood disorders: A comparison between patients with major depressive disorder and bipolar I disorder. *Journal of Consulting and Clinical Psychology, 74,* 1192–1202.

Weinstock, L. M., & Miller, I. W. (2008). Functional impairment as a predictor of short-term symptom course in bipolar I disorder. *Bipolar Disorders, 10*(3), 437–442.

Whiffen, V. E., Kallos-Lilly, V., & MacDonald, B. J. (2001). Depression and attachment in couples. *Cognitive Therapy and Research, 25,* 421–434.

Whisman, M. A. (1999). Marital dissatisfaction and psychiatric disorders: Results from the national comorbidity survey. *Journal of Abnormal Psychology, 108,* 701–706.

Whisman, M. A. (2001). The association between depression and marital dissatisfaction. In S. R. H. Beach (Ed.), *Marital and family processes in depression: A scientific foundation for clinical practice* (pp. 3–24). Washington, DC: American Psychological Association.

Whisman, M. A. (2007). Marital distress and DSM-IV psychiatric disorders in a population-based national survey. *Journal of Abnormal Psychology, 116,* 638–643.

Whisman, M. A., & Uebelacker, L. A. (2009). Prospective associations between marital discord and depressive symptoms in middle-aged and older adults. *Psychology and Aging, 24,* 184–189.

Whisman, M. A., Uebelacker, L. A., Tolejko, N., Chatav, Y., & McKelvie, M. (2006, November). *Marital dissatisfaction and depression in older adults: Is the association confounded by personality?* Paper presented at the annual convention of the Association for Behavioral and Cognitive Therapies, Chicago.

Whisman, M. A., Weinstock, L. M., & Tolejko, N. (2006). Marriage and depression. In C. L. M. Keyes & S. H. Goodman (Eds.), *Women and depression: A handbook for the social, behavioral, and biomedical sciences* (pp. 219–240). New York: Cambridge University Press.

Whisman, M. A., Weinstock, L. M., & Uebelacker, L. A. (2002). Mood reactivity to marital conflict: The influence of marital dissatisfaction and depression. *Behavior Therapy, 33,* 299–314.

Whittle, S., Yap, M. B. H., Sheeber, L., Dudgeon, P., Yücel, M., Pantelis, C., et al. (2011). Hippocampal volume and sensitivity to maternal aggressive behavior: A prospective study of adolescent depressive symptoms. *Development and Psychopathology, 23*(1), 115–129.

Williams, S., Connolly, J., & Segal, Z. V. (2001). Intimacy in relationships and cognitive vulnerability to depression in adolescent girls. *Cognitive Therapy and Research, 25,* 477–496.

Wilson, S., & Durbin, C. E. (2010). Effects of paternal depression on fathers' parenting behaviors: A meta-analytic review. *Clinical Psychology Review, 30,* 167–180.

Yan, L. J., Hammen, C., Cohen, A. N., Daley, S. E., & Henry, R. M. (2004). Expressed emotion versus relationship quality variables in the prediction of recurrence in bipolar patients. *Journal of Affective Disorders, 83,* 199–206.

Yap, M. B. H., Schwartz, O. S., Byrne, M. L., Simmons, J. G., & Allen, N. B. (2010). Maternal positive and negative interaction behaviors and early adolescents' depressive symptoms: Adolescent emotion regulation as a mediator. *Journal of Research on Adolescence, 20*(4), 1014–1043.

CHAPTER 23

Depression in Later Life
Epidemiology, Assessment, Impact, and Treatment

DAN G. BLAZER *and* CELIA F. HYBELS

Depression, hopelessness, helplessness, uselessness, and loneliness are considered ubiquitous as people become older. The Buddha said, upon encountering an older person, "It's the world's pity, that weak and ignorant beings, drunk with the vanity of youth, do not behold old age. . . . What is the use of pleasures and delights in life, since I myself am the future dwelling-place of old-age?" (in de Beauvoir, 1973, p. 7).

Despite this discouraging perception of old age, most older adults experience good life satisfaction, especially if they are not plagued by excessive physical illness and functional incapacity (Gatz & Zarit, 1999). Even so, depression is the most frequent cause of emotional suffering in later life, and, when present, it significantly reduces the quality of life among older adults (Berkman et al., 1986; Blazer, 2002a). Interest in late-life depression has increased considerably among investigators over the past 25 years. Many gaps in our understanding of the phenomenology, diagnosis, and prognosis have been filled (Beekman et al., 2002; Schulz, Drayer, & Rollman, 2002). We have learned much about the etiology of depression in older adults (Blazer & Hybels, 2005). Finally, the evidence base for therapies used to treat late-life depression has increased dramatically (Reynolds, 2006; Reynolds et al., 1999; Tedeschini et al, 2011; Unutzer et al., 2002).

In this chapter, we explore late-life depression from a clinical and investigative perspective, identifying the significant increase in our knowledge and the gaps that remain. We first address case definitions of late-life depression and then review the epidemiology of mood disorders, both studies of symptom frequency and those that use diagnostic categories, such as those found in the fourth, text revision edition of the *Diagnostic and Statistical Manual of Mental Disorders* (DSM-IV-TR; American Psychiatric Association, 2000). We follow this discussion with a review of the longitudinal course and outcomes of late-life depressive disorders, then review the biological, psychological, and social origins of late-life depression. We next review the elements of a thorough diagnostic workup, the diagnostic interview, and treatment approaches, with a brief section on bipolar disorder. Finally, we review future directions for research into late-life mood disorders.

CASE DEFINITIONS OF LATE-LIFE DEPRESSION

The diagnosis for late-life depression is neither simple nor straightforward. First, investigators to date have found no biological markers for the most common depressive syndromes in later life (though many biological correlates have been identified). In addition, symptoms do not easily cluster into mutually exclusive categories that permit easy classification. Finally, neither clinicians nor clinical investigators agree as to what constitutes a clinically significant episode of depression (regardless of age). Therefore, we present some clinically useful case definitions of late-life depression. *Major depression* is the core diagnosis for clinical depression. To meet criteria for a diagnosis, the older adult must exhibit at least one of two basic symptoms (depressed mood and/or lack of interest) for 2 weeks or more. Older adults are more likely to complain of a loss of interest than to present with an overt expression of a depressed mood. In addition, to be diagnosed with major depression, the older adult must exhibit at least four or more of the following symptoms for at least 2 weeks. Older adults tend to differ somewhat from middle-aged adults in the presentation of these criteria symptoms (Blazer, Bachar, & Hughes, 1987):

- Feelings of worthlessness or inappropriate guilt (guilt is less frequent among older adults than among younger adults as a symptom of depression).
- Diminished ability to concentrate or to make decisions (older adults are no more likely than younger adults to complain of difficulty with concentration and memory, but they are more likely than younger adults to exhibit positive findings on psychological testing in the midst of an episode of depression).
- Fatigue (a common symptom regardless of age in the moderate to severely depressed).
- Psychomotor agitation or retardation (either can be seen in late life).
- Increase or decrease in weight or appetite (older adults rarely gain weight in the midst of a depression, whereas even a weight loss of 5 pounds is a cardinal symptom of late-life depression if no other explanation can be found for the weight loss).
- Recurrent thoughts of death or suicide (older adults are less likely to express suicidal ideation, though they may frequently ruminate about death in the midst of an episode of depression; American Psychiatric Association, 2013).

Older adults with major depression are less likely to have comorbid anxiety, and they report fewer lifetime episodes of depression than middle-aged adults (Hybels, Landerman, & Blazer, 2012). Even so, making the diagnosis of major depression in an older adult without comorbid physical illness or cognitive impairment should be no more difficult than it is in a younger adult.

The diagnosis of *minor, subsyndromal, or subthreshold depression* is made when the core symptoms are present, along with one to three additional symptoms, usually assessed by symptom scales. In epidemiological studies, the most common definition is a score of 16 or greater on the Center for Epidemiologic Studies Depression Scale (CES-D; Radloff, 1977), while not meeting criteria for major depression. Still others have suggested a diagnosis of subthreshold depression below the usual cutoff point on the CES-D (Hybels, Blazer, & Pieper, 2001). *Dysthymic disorder* is a less severe but more chronic variant of depression. To meet criteria, the older adult must experience symptoms most of the time for at least 2 years (American Psychiatric Association, 2013). This disorder does not usually begin in late life, but it can persist from midlife into late life (Blazer, 1994; Devenand et al., 1994).

Some differences between *early*-onset (a first episode prior to the age of 60) and *late*-onset (first episode at age 60 years or later) depression have been reported in addition to symptom presentation. For example, personality problems, a family history of psychiatric disorder, and stressful ongoing events, such as a dysfunctional marriage, are more common in early- than in late-onset depression. Interest in differentiating an early- versus late-onset episode of depression derives in part from recent interest in the etiology of first-onset depressions in late life.

Vascular depression, a depression proposed to be secondary to vascular lesions in the brain, appears to present with slightly different symptoms than typical episodes of major depression in late life. For example, these older adults experience problems with executive cognitive function, such as verbal fluency, recognition memory, and forward planning (Krishnan, Hays, & Blazer, 1997). Some investigators have proposed criteria for a *depression of Alzheimer's disease*. In persons who meet criteria for a dementing disorder of the Alzheimer's type, the appearance of three symptoms, such as depressed mood, anhedonia, social isolation (not a symptom criterion for major depression), poor appetite, poor sleep, psychomotor changes, irritability (not a symptom of major depression), fatigue and loss of energy, feelings of worthlessness, and suicidal thoughts, would qualify for the diagnosis (Olin et al., 2002). Finally, *psychotic depression* (in contrast to nonpsychotic depression) may occur in as many as 20–45% of hospitalized older adult patients but is much less frequent in the community (Meyers, 1992).

EPIDEMIOLOGY OF LATE-LIFE DEPRESSION

Table 23.1 lists the prevalence of depression reported in selected studies of older adults in community populations. The lifetime prevalence of major depression in these studies ranges from 2.6 to 10.6% (Hasin, Goodwin, Stinson, & Grant, 2005; Kessler et al., 2005; Lee et al., 2007), whereas the lifetime prevalence of dysthymia may be only 1.3% (see Kessler et al., Chapter 1, this volume). Current or 1-month prevalence of major depression in this age group may be less than 1% (Patten, Wang, & Williams, 2006; Regier et al., 1988). Among community-dwelling older adults, the prevalence of clinically significant depressive symptoms or minor depression is much higher than that of major depression (Blazer, Hughes, & George, 1987) and may range to 9% (Blazer, Burchett, Service, & George, 1991) or more in selected population subgroups, such as Hispanic older adults (Black, Goodwin, & Markides, 1998). Both major depression and depressive symptoms are more common in older adult females than in males (Black et al., 1998) and may be lower in African Americans than in European Americans and higher among some Asian Americans (Gonzalez, Tarraf, Whitfield, & Vega, 2010).

The prevalence of major and minor depression is generally higher in clinical than in community populations. Lyness, King, Cox, Yoediono, and Caine (1999) reported that the current prevalence of subsyndromal depression in a primary care sample was 9.9% compared with a prevalence of 6.5% for major depression, 5.2% for minor depression, and 0.9% for dysthymia. Among hospitalized patients, the prevalence of major or minor depression ranges from 11 to 23% (Koenig, Meador, Cohen, & Blazer, 1988). Finally, 12.4% of institutionalized older adults met criteria for major depression, and 30.5% had minor depression or clinically significant depressive symptomatology (Parmelee, Katz, & Lawton, 1989).

TABLE 23.1. Prevalence of Depression in Older Adults Reported from Selected Community Studies

Authors	Study	Location	n	Age	Instrument	Period	Outcome	Prevalence
Regier et al. (1988)	ECA	5 U.S. cities	5,702 (18,571)	65+	DIS	1 month	Major depression Dysthymia	0.7% 1.8%
Hasin et al. (2005)	NESARC	U.S.	(43,093)	65+	AUDADIS-IV	12 months Lifetime	Major depression Major depression	2.69% 8.19%
Kessler et al. (2005)	NCS-R	U.S.	(9,282)	60+	WMH–CIDI	Lifetime Lifetime	Major depression Dysthymia	10.6% 1.3%
Gum, King-Kallimanis, & Kohn (2009)	NCS-R	U.S.	(9,282)	65+	WMH–CIDI	12 months	Major depression Dysthymia Bipolar I and II	2.3% 0.5% 0.2%
Patten et al. (2006)	CCHS	Canada	(36,984)	65+	CIDI	12 months Current	Major depression Major depression	1.9% 0.9%
Lee et al. (2007)	WMH–China	Beijing and Shanghai	(5,201)	65+	WMH–CIDI	Lifetime	Major depression	2.6%
Gonzalez et al. (2010)	CPES	U.S.		65–74	CIDI	12 months	Major depression	7.8% Chinese 1.3% Vietnamese 6.5% Cubans 3.9% MAs 5.0% PRs 4.7% CBs 2.3% AAs 3.6% whites
Blazer et al. (1991)	EPESE	North Carolina	3,998	65+	CES-D		Depressive symptoms	9.0%
Black et al. (1998)	Hispanic EPESE	5 states	2,823	65+	CES-D		Depressive symptoms	17.3% males; 31.9% females

Note. Number of age eligible with (total sample size) provided, if available. ECA, Epidemiologic Catchment Area; DIS, Diagnostic Interview Schedule (Robins et al, 1981); NESARC, National Epidemiologic Survey on Alcoholism and Related Conditions; AUDADIS-IV, Alcohol Use Disorder and Associated Disabilities Interview Schedule–DSM-IV Version (Grant et al., 2001); NCS-R, National Comorbidity Study—Replication; CIDI, Composite International Diagnostic Interview (Kessler & Ustun, 2004); WMH, World Mental Health Survey; CCHS, Canadian Community Health Survey: Mental Health and Well-Being; CPES, Collaborative Psychiatric Epidemiologic Surveys; MAs, Mexican Americans; PRs, Puerto Ricans; AAs, African Americans; CBs, Caribbean blacks; EPESE, Established populations for epidemiologic studies of the elderly; CES-D, Center for Epidemiologic Studies Depression Scale (Radloff, 1977).

The annual incidence of major depressive disorder (MDD) per 100 person-years of risk reported from the Epidemiologic Catchment Area (ECA) study was 1.25 among those 65 or older (0.90 for males and 1.48 for females; Eaton et al., 1989), a lower incidence than that observed in younger adults. The incidence of depression follows the same female–male ratio in the very old, and the incidence of first-onset depression may increase with age among persons ages 70–85 (Palsson, Ostling, & Skoog, 2001).

OUTCOME OF LATE-LIFE DEPRESSION

Though episodes of depression across the life cycle, especially episodes of more severe depression, almost always remit, or at least partially remit, depression is a chronic and recurrent illness. Data from a community study of older adults from the Netherlands illustrate this chronicity. Among participants with clinically significant depressive symptoms, 23% improved, 44% experienced an unfavorable but fluctuating course, and 33% experienced a severe and chronic course over a 6-year period (Beekman et al., 2002).

Studies that have focused on older adults in clinic settings reveal similar chronicity (Alexopoulos et al., 1996). Brodaty, Luscombe, Peisah, Anstey, and Andrews (2001) found that only 12% of a group of older adult patients experiencing depression, who had been followed for 25 years and had experienced severe depression earlier in life, remained continuously well over the follow-up period (Brodaty et al., 2001). The prognosis from clinical studies of older adults with late-life depression, however, is similar to that of younger adults when the older adults are not plagued with comorbid medical illness, functional impairment, or cognitive impairment (Keller, Shapiro, Lavori, & Wolfe, 1982a, 1982b). Comorbid depression is associated with a less favorable prognosis. Factors predicting partial remission were similar to those predicting no remission, and poor social support and functional limitations increased the risk for poor outcomes in these individuals (Hybels, Blazer, & Steffens, 2005).

More severe depression in late life is often associated with cognitive impairment. When the depression improves, the cognitive impairment often improves as well. Nevertheless, the interaction of comorbid depression and cognitive impairment is a risk for the later emergence of Alzheimer's disease (Alexopoulos, Meyers, Young, Mattis, & Kakuma, 1993; van den Kommer et al., 2013). Therefore, early depressive symptoms associated with mild cognitive impairment may represent a preclinical sign and should be considered a risk for impending Alzheimer's disease or vascular dementia. Depression can further complicate Alzheimer's disease over time by increasing disability and physical aggression, thereby contributing to depression among caregivers (Gonzales-Salvador, Aragano, Lyketsos, & Barba, 1999). Depressive symptoms in patients with Alzheimer's disease resolve spontaneously at a greater frequency, without requiring intensive therapy (e.g., medication therapy), than those among older adults with depression and vascular dementia, in whom depressive symptoms tend to be persistent and refractory to drug treatment (Li, Meyer, & Thornby, 2001).

Depression and medical problems often coexist, and the causal pathway is bidirectional. For example, depression is a frequent and important contributing cause of weight loss in late life (Morley & Kraenzle, 1994). Frailty, leading to profound weight loss, can in turn contribute to clinically important depressive symptoms (Fried, 1994). Depression is also associated with many chronic medical illnesses, including cardiovascular disease and diabetes (Blazer, Moody-Ayers, Craft-Morgan, & Burchett, 2002; Williams et al., 2002; see Freedland & Carney, Chapter 7, this volume). The mechanisms that underlie the association between depression and physical illness in older adults are not well understood. Perhaps the best established association between depression and physical problems is that between depression and functional impairment (Blazer et al., 1991; Bruce, 2001). For example, in one study, older adults with depression were 67% more likely to experience impairment in activities of daily living and 73% more likely to experience mobility restrictions 6 years after initial evaluation than were those without depression (Penninx, Leveille, Ferrucci, van Eijk, & Guralnik, 1999). Disability, in turn, can increase the risk for depressive symptoms (Kennedy, Kelman, & Thomas, 1990). Explanations for this bidirectional association include the propensity for physical disability to lead to a higher frequency of negative life events, which in turn increases the risk for depression; restricted social and leisure activities secondary to physical disability; and the isolation and reduced quality of social support often inherent in physical disability (Blazer, 1983).

Suicide is the most tragic consequence of late-life depression. The association of depression and suicide across the life cycle has been well documented (Conwell, Duberstein, & Caine, 2002). Late-life suicide rates declined during much of the 20th century. From World War II until about 1980, suicide rates declined among older adults, especially among white males (who have a much higher suicide rate than do other age, sex, and racial/ethnic groups; National Center for Health Statistics, 2001). From 1991 to 2003, suicide rates were consistently higher among those 65 years and older compared with the younger age groups. The suicide rates in this age group declined from 19.70 suicides per 100,000 in 1991 to 14.78 suicides per 100,000 in 2009, and since 2005 rates have been lower for the 65+ age group compared with the 25–64 age group (see *www. cdc.gov/violenceprevention/suicide/statistics/trends02.html*). Despite their confined environment, hospitalized patients with mood disorders are also at risk for suicide. In a study of older inpatients hospitalized for psychiatric disorders in Denmark, those with mood disorders were twice as likely to commit suicide. More than one-half of the suicides occurred within the first week either after admission or after discharge (Erlangsen, Zarit, Tu, & Conwell, 2006). Despite the potential for widespread use of antidepressant medication in older adults to reduce the burden of depression (and therefore suicide), one group found a fivefold higher risk of completed suicide during the first month in older adults treated with selective serotonin reuptake inhibitors (SSRIs) compared with other antidepressants, independent of a recent diagnosis of depression or the receipt of psychiatric care, and suicide of a violent nature was clearly more frequent (Juurlink, Mamdani, Kopp, & Redelmeier, 2006).

ORIGINS OF LATE-LIFE DEPRESSION

Older adults present a paradox to clinicians and investigators who seek to understand the origins of depression (Blazer & Hybels, 2005). On the one hand, older adults appear to be at greater biological vulnerability than are people in midlife. As documented earlier, however, the frequency of severe depression (except in institutional settings) is lower in late life than in midlife, suggesting that psychological and social factors may offer protection.

Biological Origins

Twin studies of older adults in Scandinavia document the relative contribution of hereditary and environmental factors to self-reported depressive symptoms. In one study from Sweden, genetic influences accounted for 16% of the variance in depressive symptoms and 19% in symptoms specific to biological factors, such as sleep. On the other hand, genetic influences contributed only minimally to expressions of depressed mood and positive affect (Gatz, Pedersen, Plomin, Nesselroade, & McClearn, 1992). Therefore, not all depressive symptoms are equally influenced by heredity. Virtually every study of major depression has documented a relatively greater frequency among women than among men (Krause, 1986; see Hilt & Nolen-Hoeksema, Chapter 19, this volume), potentially due to selective survival (men die earlier than women do) or to a greater likelihood that women report symptoms more frequently than men do (Hinton, Zweifach, Oishi, Tang, & Unutzer, 2006); it is uncertain whether genetic factors contribute to this sex difference.

Though no single genetic marker has yet been identified for depression at any age, two markers are of some interest and represent the types of findings that may lead to significant changes in the way depression is conceptualized and treated in the future. In one study, older adults with late-onset depression presented a higher frequency of the *C677T* mutation of the *MTHFR* (methylenetetrahydrofolate reductase) enzyme than did patients with early-onset depression (Hickie et al., 2001). In a second study, investigators found that older adults with a homozygous short allele polymorphism in the serotonin transporter gene (*5-HTT*) were less likely to respond to SSRI treatment than were their counterparts with long alleles (Zhang et al., 2005). Other transporter genes appear to have only a minor association with late-life depression (Seripa et al, 2013).

In studies of depression across the life span, underactivity of serotonin neurotransmission has been a key focus of research into the pathophysiology of depression. Although serotonin activity, namely, 5-HT_{2A} receptor binding, decreases in a variety of brain regions throughout the lifespan, there is less decrease from midlife to late life than from young adulthood to midlife (Sheline, Mintun, Moerlein, & Snyder, 2002).

Another biological correlate of depression across the lifespan is hypersecretion of corticotropin-releasing factor (CRF). CRF, however, also declines as age advances (Gottfries, 1990). Other endocrine abnormalities have been associated with late-life depression, including high levels of cortisol (Yaffe, Ettinger, & Pressman, 1998), which may be associated with anatomical changes, specifically, atrophy of the hippocampus (Sapolsky, 2001). In a vicious cycle, depressive symptoms can lead to increased cortisol secretion, which inhibits neurogenesis, leading to hippocampal volume loss that may in turn mediate symptoms of depression.

Investigators have long noted the association of depressive symptoms and vascular risk factors. Hypertension has also been associated with an increased risk of depression, although results of studies have been inconsistent (Lyness, King, Conwell, Cox, & Caine, 2000). Brain scans, especially those using magnetic resonance imaging (MRI), have revealed white matter hyperintensities in the subcortical region, suggesting disruption of neural circuits associated with depression (Taylor et al., 2003; see Pizzagalli & Treadway, Chapter 11, this volume). As we noted earlier, these findings indicate depressive symptoms in concert with reduced executive cognitive function.

Many studies have been conducted over the past three decades documenting the association of late-life depression and changes in brain structure. In a recent meta-analysis, reduction in volume in the hippocampus was the most obvious correlate with depression, accompanied with similar but significant reductions in the orbitofrontal cortex, putamen, and thalamus (Sexton, Mackey, & Ebmeier, 2013).

Psychological Origins

Many different psychological theories have been postulated to explain depression across the lifespan. Older individuals with depression and with a personality disorder are much more likely than those without a personality disorder to experience reemergence of depressive symptoms, hopelessness, and ambivalence regarding emotional expression (Morse & Lynch, 2004). Personality may also interact with factors such as life events to increase risk for depression, for example, adjusting to physical illness or reduced physical function (Mazure, Maciejewski, Jacobs, & Bruce, 2002). In several studies, late-life depression has also been associated with neuroticism (Henderson, Jorm, & MacKinnon, 1993).

By far the most frequent psychological construct applied to depressive disorders across the lifespan is cognitive distortion (Beck, 1987; see Joormann & Arditte, Chapter 14, this volume). In a study of the experience and impact of adverse life events, older patients with dysthymia were more likely to report recent life events with greater negative impact, particularly interpersonal conflicts (Devenand, Kim, Paykina, & Sackeim, 2002). In a community-based study, older adult participants who endorsed more depressive symptoms used rumination and catastrophizing more frequently, and positive reappraisal less frequently, than did those with fewer symptoms (Kraaij & de Wilde, 2001). Perceived loss of internal locus of control has also been found to be associated with both the onset and the persistence of depressive symptoms in a community sample (Beekman, Deeg, & Geerlings, 2001).

Two factors are worth considering in understanding the psychological (as well as social and biological) risk for depression in late life (Blazer & Hybels, 2005). The first is socioemotional selectivity theory (Carstensen, Mayr, Pasupathi, & Nesselroade, 2000). According to this theory, older persons perceive time and past experience differently than do younger persons. Specifically, younger adults prioritize the pursuit of knowledge, recognizing that they have much to learn and relatively long futures, even if this requires suppressing emotional well-being. In contrast, older adults perceive time as relatively limited, leading them to deemphasize negative experiences and to prioritize emotionally meaningful goals. Older adults selectively recall and attend to positive information, termed the *positivity effect*, which may confer benefits to well-being.

Second, adults are postulated to acquire more wisdom as they grow older. Although wisdom can be a nebulous concept, investigators in Germany have operationalized this construct in community samples (Baltes & Staudinger, 2000). These investigators identified five criteria associated with wisdom: rich factual knowledge; rich procedural knowledge (i.e., knowing how to develop strategies for addressing problems); relativism of values and life priorities (e.g., developing tolerances for differences in society); lifespan contextualization (i.e., integrating life experiences that are seemingly conflicting); and the recognition and management of uncertainty (recognizing that the future cannot be known with certainty). Individuals who possess wisdom, therefore, can more easily address problems and respond to life stresses, reducing the risk of depression.

Social Origins

Many social factors have been associated with the onset and persistence of late-life depression. There is a strong association between severe stressful events, such as bereavement and life-threatening illnesses, and the onset of major depression in later life (Murphy, 1982). Older adults who lack a confidant are especially vulnerable to life stressors. Given that certain devastating life events are more common in late life, it is tempting to assume that older adults are at increased risk for experiencing stressful events that may be associated with depression. Yet most stressful events that lead to depression are predictable, that is, "on time," events. For example, the death of a sibling is a severe and perhaps catastrophic event that can frequently lead to depression. During midlife, such a death is unexpected, and the adjustment is more difficult. In contrast, although a loss in late life may be severe, the death is usually not unexpected. In addition, many events that lead to depression actually occur more frequently earlier than later in life, such as divorce and difficulties with the law (Hughes, Blazer, & George, 1988).

DIAGNOSTIC WORKUP

Older adults are much less likely than younger adults to use mental health services when they are depressed (Unutzer et al., 1997). Most older adults who do see a clinician for their late-life depression usually are seen in a primary care physician's office (Gallo & Coyne, 2000). Therefore, the diagnostic workup and initiation of therapy usually begins in this setting. Although many psychological tests are available to screen for and identify cases of late-life mood disorders, such as major depression and dysthymia, the diagnosis ultimately derives from a careful history. In obtaining information necessary to make a diagnosis, the clinician should focus on present symptoms, past history (especially a history of previous episodic symptoms similar to those presenting at the time of the interview), family history, recent life events, changes in social and economic status, recent medical problems, and family history. In the absence of comorbid disorders, such as Alzheimer's disease or significant physical dysfunction, the diagnostic criteria for major depression are applicable, as described earlier (Hinton et al., 2006).

A number of available scales have been used to screen for late-life depression in both clinical and community settings. These include the Geriatric Depression Scale (GDS; Yesavage, Brink, & Rose, 1983) and the CES-D (Radloff, 1977). A screen for depressive symptoms should be augmented with a screen for cognitive functioning, with a scale such as the Mini-Mental State Examination (MMSE; Folstein, Folstein, & McHugh, 1975). Investigators have reported sex differences in symptoms in the presentation of depression in late life. Specifically, older men are not only less likely than older women to be referred for depressive symptoms but also less likely to endorse core depressive symptoms and to have received treatment for depression (Blazer et al., 1991). Diagnostic instruments used for case finding in clinical settings include the Structured Clinical Interview for DSM (SCID; Robins, Helzer, & Croughan, 1981) and the Diagnostic Interview Schedule (DIS; Spitzer, Williams, Gibbon, & First, 1990; see Nezu et al., Chapter 2, this volume). In addition, the clinician should screen for suicidal thoughts or behaviors. The older adult can be asked a series of questions to determine progressive potential risk. As is the case with younger individuals, if the older patient with depression has considered a specific means for harming him- or herself (e.g., taking pills or hanging oneself), then the risk for suicide is increased. These questions are probably of less value in evaluating risk for suicide than is an assessment of known risk factors, such as being of white race or male sex; having lower income; being socially isolated, divorced, widowed, or bereaved; suffering from comorbid medical illness; having been diagnosed with depression in the past; abusing alcohol or other substances; and having a history of previous suicide attempts (Blazer, 2002a).

TREATMENT OF LATE-LIFE DEPRESSION

There are no true biological markers for any of the subtypes of late-life depression; therefore, no definitive laboratory tests assist the clinician in designing therapies for older patients with depression. The one exception is brain scanning in vascular depression, in which the presence of subcortical white matter hyperintensities can assist in the diagnosis. Routine laboratory tests, such as a chemistry screen or an electrocardiogram, are employed as a baseline for determining the biological effects of biological therapies. If a medical illness is suspected to contribute to the depressive disorder, a number of elective laboratory tests can be ordered, including a thyroid screen for undiagnosed thyroid dysfunction, vitamin B_{12} and folate assays, as well as polysomnography, if sleep abnormalities cannot be explained.

Biological Therapies

The foundation for the treatment of moderate to severe depression in late life is antidepressant medication (Jacobson, Pies, & Katz, 2007; Nezu, 1987). All of the currently available antidepressant medications are virtually equal in efficacy (see Gitlin, Chapter 26, this volume). Therefore, clinicians usually choose an antidepressant based on the side effects that they hope to avoid. Selective serotonin reuptake inhibitors (SSRIs) have become the preferred antidepressant medication of most clinicians. Side effects from earlier generations of antidepressants (specifically the tricyclic antidepressants), such as dry mouth, constipation, occasional confusion, postural hypotension, and urinary retention, are avoided with the SSRIs. Even so, the SSRIs can lead to side effects such as weight loss, agitation, sleep loss, and, in some rare situations, a potential increased risk for suicidal behavior. Currently available SSRI medications include citalopram, paroxetine, fluoxetine, fluvoxamine, and escitalopram. Other "new generation" antidepressants with both serotonergic and norepinergic effects include mirtazapine, venlafaxine, bupropion, and duloxetine. Duloxetine has also been approved for use in the treatment of fibromyalgia, yet the studies of its use in older adults are limited. Clinicians who treat older adults with medication (whether alone or in combination with current psychotherapeutic approaches) must be realistic regarding the prognosis for recovery from a moderate to severe episode of depression. African American men and women have significantly lower adherence to using antidepressant medications (Kales et al., 2013).

Most antidepressants exhibit efficacy within 4–6 weeks. Yet the actual time from the initiation of therapy to a subjective report that the older adult truly feels "like my old self" may take months and even up to a year for those experiencing a severe depressive episode. Biological symptoms, such as sleep difficulties, may improve more quickly with antidepressant therapy; subjective well-being and an interest in life requires a much longer time to reemerge. One reason is that older adults who recover from a moderate to severe episode of depression require time to reintegrate into their usual life activities because they often hesitate to return to past social activities for fear of embarrassment after a prolonged episode of depression.

When antidepressant therapy is not effective, change to another agent is usually the next step. However, in one large study, the success in attaining remission following a switch from one antidepressant to another was not dramatic and often unsuccessful (Gaynes et al., 2009). If a person did not respond to two different antidepressants, the likelihood of remission decreased dramatically. A more aggressive approach pharmacologically, one that is even less successful, is augmenting antidepressant therapy with a neuroleptic medication such as quetiapine or risperidone (Wright, Eiland, & Lorenz, 2013). When this augmentation strategy is implemented, side effects often become a major problem.

Some depressive episodes do not respond to antidepressant medication and are severe enough to require electroconvulsive therapy (ECT; Flint & Rifat, 1998). Severe depressive symptoms, psychotic symptoms, a potential for suicide, and a history of responding to ECT in the past are indications for ECT. The primary adverse reaction to ECT in late life is memory problems during the few weeks during and following treatment, and though this symptom almost always remits with time, it can be very disturbing to older adults. The ability to administer ECT to older adults as outpatients has greatly reduced both the cost and the inconvenience and stigma of receiving the treatment. Transcranial magnetic stimulation is yet another therapy that has been studied and is now approved by the Food and Drug Administration (FDA) for restricted conditions. In one study, however, the treatment was not effective in older (> 45 years of age) compared with younger (Aquirre et al., 2011) adults.

Psychological Therapies

Many different psychotherapies have been used with older adults with depression. An increasing body of literature supports the value of psychotherapy in the treatment of mild to moderate depressive disorders. Cognitive-behavioral therapies (CBTs) have been studied most frequently (Arean & Cook, 2002) and address problematic thoughts that initiate and perpetuate depressive symptoms. The goal of therapy is to change the thoughts and dysfunctional attitudes that initiate symptoms and may lead to a relapse. The process by which cognitive therapy works is not entirely clear (see Hollon & Dimidjian, Chapter 27, this volume). For example, some data suggest that the most important mechanism of change in cognitive therapy is altered thought attribution, such as reevaluation of events. Another aspect of CBT that is thought to be effective is actual change of behavior itself. Depressive symptoms lead to activities that in turn perpetuate the depression. The goal of therapy, therefore, is to change behaviors through, for example, skills training (problem solving and interpersonal skills) and even exercise. Older people with lifelong habits may be less inclined to change behavior, but this type of therapy can be effective.

A variant of CBT is social problem-solving therapy (PST). Ineffective coping in stressful situations is thought to lead to a breakdown of problem-solving abilities and, consequently, to an increase in the propensity to become depressed in late life (Nezu, 1987). The therapist teaches the patient a structured format for solving problems that includes problem details, goals, solutions, specific solution advantages, and an assessment of the final solution within context. In other words, PST refines and augments the usual strategies employed by older adults to handle day-to-day problems.

Interpersonal psychotherapy (IPT), a popular manualized treatment, focuses on four factors that are thought to initiate and perpetuate depressive symptoms (Frank, Frank, & Cornes, 1993; see Beach, Whisman, & Bodenmann, Chapter 29, this volume). Similar to CBT, IPT focuses on social context. Grief, interpersonal disputes, role transitions, and interpersonal deficits (e.g., the lack of ability to assert oneself in social situations) constitute the treatment focus. IPT utilizes role playing, communication analysis, clarification of the patient's wants and needs, and connections between the affect of the patient and environmental events. IPT has been found to be effective in preventing short-term relapse of major depression but not long-term outcome. One advantage of IPT is that older patients are less likely to drop out of treatment than is the case with many other psychotherapeutic approaches (Reynolds et al., 1999, 2006).

Older psychiatric patients are generally receptive to psychotherapy; the most commonly noted causes for seeking treatment were depression related to interpersonal problems, health conditions, grief/loss, finances, housing, and challenges due to executive dysfunction. They found support, problem-solving strategies, and a focus on interpersonal relationships to be most helpful in psychotherapy (Dakin & Arean, 2013). Predicting who will respond to psychotherapy, however, is not an easy task. In one small study, psychotherapy nonresponders demonstrated that reduced bilateral cortical thickness on MRI may be an important marker of individuals at higher risk for poor response to psychotherapy (Mackin et al., 2012).

Family Intervention

A clinician can rarely treat older adults without some interaction with family members, whether spouses, children, or siblings. Family members almost always accompany the older patient with depression to the office for an initial evaluation, and the patient rarely prohibits the clinician to discuss the depression with a family member. Clinicians should take advantage of this opportunity. Family members can provide valuable information to complement the interview with the older adult about the duration and severity of symptoms, about differences they witness in the older adult during the depression compared with his or her usual state, and about information concerning life events that may have contributed to the depressive episode. In addition, the clinician should address concerns of the family (whether these concerns are verbalized or not). Family members often benefit from an explanation by the clinician of the symptoms of depression (e.g., addressing the question, "Why does Mom sit in the chair all day?"). They also benefit from guidance about addressing disturbing behaviors, such as inactivity and negative ruminations. Finally, families should be warned of the risk for suicide (despite the best efforts of families and clinicians, suicide cannot be absolutely prevented) and instructed about means for reducing the risk of suicide, such as removing weapons from the house.

PREVENTION

Can late-life depression be prevented? From the perspective of public health, both secondary prevention (early detection and treatment) and tertiary prevention (rehabilitation) are the heart and soul of our current therapeutic approach. Yet this leaves unanswered the question of whether the onset of an episode of major depression in late life can be prevented in the first place. Blazer (2002b) proposed that targeting symptoms of sadness and loneliness through an enhancement of self-efficacy may prevent depressive symptoms from evolving into a full-blown episode of major depression. *Self-efficacy* is the belief that one can organize and execute the courses of action required to develop and enhance a person's belief that he or she can act in ways that lead to a desired goal.

Self-efficacy is strengthened not by some general or abstract instruction but by the experience of successfully dealing with and overcoming specific problems. A number of skills appear to increase self-efficacy: maintaining and promoting physical health (e.g., controlling blood glucose levels in borderline diabetes); enhancing cognitive performance (e.g., through the creative use of life review); enhancing physical functioning (e.g., age-appropriate exercise); developing a greater sense of personal control and mastery (e.g., developing coping strategies); improving social skills (e.g., through social skills training); and enhancing a sense of personal and existential integrity (e.g., working through past traumatic events).

There are few empirical studies to inform the clinician and investigator of the usefulness of developing these skills. Nevertheless, there is ample reason to consider these interventions so that adverse consequences of precursors of late-life depression, such as sadness and loneliness, can be prevented from becoming more serious outcomes.

BIPOLAR DISORDERS

In this chapter we have focused on late-life depression because this disorder occurs far more frequently than bipolar disorder in older adults. Nevertheless, a few words are in order about the latter. First, older adults with recurrent unipolar depression are less likely than younger adults to experience bipolar disorder. When bipolar disorder does emerge in late life, the symptoms are often atypical. Older adults in late life who do experience an episode of mania may be more irritable than happy. Anger, rather than excessive spending or expansive ideas, may dominate the clinical picture. At times, racing thoughts may be misinterpreted as a problem with memory or information processing. Once the diagnosis is made, however, the management is similar across the life cycle, and pharmacological management is the centerpiece of management. Lithium carbonate and valproic acid are the drugs of choice. Fortunately, they are often effective in doses much lower than those used when treating younger adults. For example, an older adult with bipolar disorder may be managed on 300 mg of lithium per day, with serum lithium levels between 0.2 and 0.5 mEq/L in comparison with a younger patient treated with 1,200 mg per day, with levels between 0.8 and 1.2 mEq/L. Other drugs that are used to treat bipolar disorders in older adults include lamotragine and clonazepam. Working with the family of the older patient with bipolar disorder can often assist in identifying an episode early and adjusting medications, so that hospitalization can be avoided.

CONCLUSIONS AND FUTURE DIRECTIONS

Basic scientists and clinical investigators have increased the extant empirical data on late-life depression at an almost dizzying pace over the past four decades. For example, the neurobiological substrate of late-life depression has emerged in increasing detail through both structural and functional scanning techniques. Studies of the phenomenology of late-life depression have enabled investigators to disaggregate the construct into potentially valuable subtypes, such as subthreshold depression, for future research. Therapies have been studied in much greater detail, especially the value of combined pharmacotherapy and psychotherapy over time. In summary, the diagnosis and treatment of late-life depression is now buttressed by an evidence base that was virtually absent three decades ago, except for the occasional clinical report.

Clinicians are therefore armed with a veritable textbook of important knowledge about the characteristics, origins, outcomes, and therapies for this most disabling and potentially fatal condition. Nevertheless, knowledge alone cannot render a clinician competent to care for an older adult with depression. That can only come through experience, and the experience needed is very clear. Clinicians must talk with their patients and with their patient's families. And they must talk with them through time. No journal article or review chapter can replace the living textbook of the client/patient who sits with the observant and caring clinician.

Despite the significant advances in our empirical understanding of the epidemiology, etiology, diagnosis, and treatment of late-life depression, many topics require further research. Three areas are illustrative. First, the subtypes of late-life depression must be better refined, so that therapies can be tailored better to phenotypes that more closely reflect neuro- and psychopathology. For example, the construct of vascular depression has emerged. Given the combined diagnostic requirements of clinical symptoms and signs on the MRI scan, this construct permits a more focused exploration of genetic predisposition, as well as potential environmental factors that may contribute to the cause of the disorder. Yet vascular depression is most certainly not a single, unitary construct; instead, it interacts with brain changes secondary to stress (e.g., hippocampal shrinkage), and perhaps other brain changes, such as those found with Alzheimer's disease.

Second, new pharmacotherapies and psychotherapies must be developed, and existing therapies must be studied so they can be applied optimally to increase both time to remission and achievement of as complete a remission as possible. Although the advent of the new generation of antidepressants has been a boon in treating late-life depression, the initial promise of a more potent therapy virtually without side effects has not stood the test of time. Many side effects that prevented treatment in the past have been alleviated through the use of the new medications, yet new side effects have emerged, some quite serious (e.g., the syndrome of inappropriate antidiuretic hormone secretion). We are far from having identified optimal agents for the pharmacological treatment of late-life depression. New psychotherapies currently being tested with older adults could lead to incremental yet important improvements or flexibility.

Third, the predictors of persistent depression must be studied further, for evidence has emerged that depression in late life can lead to many adverse outcomes, such as increased mortality secondary to cardiovascular disease and dementing disorders. There is no question that late-life depression has adverse effects on both short- and long-term physical and mental health. Yet the nuances of these adverse outcomes have yet to be discovered. These nuances could have major implications clinically in terms of managing the older adult with depression who is experiencing a chronic disease over time. In summary, we have learned much, but we still have much to learn.

REFERENCES

Alexopoulos, G., Meyers, B., Young, R., Kakuma, T., Feder, M., Einhorn, A., et al. (1996). Recovery in geriatric depression. *Archives of General Psychiatry, 53*, 305–312.

Alexopoulos, G., Meyers, B., Young, R., Mattis, S., & Kakuma, T. (1993). The course of geriatric depression with "reversible dementia": A controlled study. *American Journal of Psychiatry, 150*, 1693–1699.

American Psychiatric Association. (2000). *Diagnostic and statistical manual of mental disorders* (4th ed., text revision). Washington, DC: Author.

American Psychiatric Association. (2013). *Diagnostic and statistical manual of mental disorders* (5th ed.). Arlington, VA: Author.

Aquirre, I., Carretero, B., Ibarra, O., Kuhalainen, J., Martinez, J., Ferrer, A., et al. (2011). Age predicts low-frequency transcranial magnetic stimulation efficacy in major depression. *Journal of Affective Disorders, 130*, 466–469.

Arean, P., & Cook, B. (2002). Psychotherapy and combined psychotherapy/pharmacotherapy for late life depression. *Biological Psychiatry, 52*, 293–303.

Baltes, P., & Staudinger, U. (2000). Wisdom: A metaheuristic (pragmatic) to orchestrate mind and virtue toward excellence. *American Psychologist, 55*, 122–136.

Beck, A. (1987). Cognitive model of depression. *Journal of Cognitive Psychotherapy, 1*, 2–27.

Beekman, A., Deeg, D., & Geerlings, R. (2001). Emergence and persistence of late life depression:

A 3-year follow-up of the Longitudinal Aging Study Amsterdam. *Journal of Affective Disorders, 65*, 131–138.

Beekman, A., Geerlings, S., Deeg, D., Smit, J., Scoevers, R., de Beurs, E., et al. (2002). The natural history of late-life depression. *Archives of General Psychiatry, 59*, 605–611.

Berkman, L., Berkman, C., Kasl, S., Freeman, D., Leo, L., Ostfeld, A., et al. (1986). Depressive symptoms in relation to physical health and functioning in the elderly. *American Journal of Epidemiology, 124*, 372–388.

Black, S., Goodwin, J., & Markides, K. (1998). The association between chronic diseases and depressive symptomology in older Mexican Americans. *Journals of Gerontology: Medical Sciences, 53*, M118–M194.

Blazer, D. (1983). Impact of late-life depression on the social network. *American Journal of Psychiatry, 140*, 162–166.

Blazer, D. (1994). Dysthymia in community and clinical samples of older adults. *American Journal of Psychiatry, 151*, 1567–1569.

Blazer, D. (2002a). *Depression in late life* (3rd ed.). New York: Springer.

Blazer, D. (2002b). Self-efficacy and depression in late life: A primary prevention proposal. *Aging and Mental Health, 6*, 319–328.

Blazer, D., Bachar, J., & Hughes, D. (1987). Major depression with melancholia: A comparison of middle-aged and elderly adults. *Journal of the American Geriatrics Society, 35*, 927–932.

Blazer, D., Burchett, B., Service, C., & George, L. (1991). The association of age and depression among the elderly: An epidemiologic exploration. *Journals of Gerontology: Medical Sciences, 46*, M210–M215.

Blazer, D., Hughes, D., & George, L. (1987). The epidemiology of depression in an elderly community population. *Gerontologist, 27*, 281–287.

Blazer, D., & Hybels, C. (2005). Origins of depression in later life. *Psychological Medicine, 35*, 1241–1252.

Blazer, D., Moody-Ayers, S., Craft-Morgan, J., & Burchett, B. (2002). Depression in diabetes and obesity: Racial/ethnic/gender issues in older adults. *Journal of Psychosomatic Research, 52*, 1–4.

Brodaty, J., Luscombe, G., Peisah, C., Anstey, K., & Andrews, G. (2001). A 25-year longitudinal, comparison study of the outcome of depression. *Psychological Medicine, 31*, 1347–1359.

Bruce, M. (2001). Depression and disability in late life: Directions for future research. *American Journal of Geriatric Psychiatry, 9*, 102–112.

Carstensen, L., Mayr, U., Pasupathi, M., & Nesselroade, J. (2000). Emotional experience in everyday life across the adult life span. *Journal of Personality and Social Psychology, 79*, 644–655.

Conwell, Y., Duberstein, P., & Caine, E. (2002). Risk factors for suicide in later life. *Biological Psychiatry, 52*, 193–204.

Dakin, E. K., & Arean, P. (2013). Patient perspectives on the benefits of psychotherapy for late-life depression. *American Journal of Geriatric Psychiatry, 21*, 156–163.

de Beauvoir, S. (1973). *The coming of age* (P. O'Brian, Trans.). New York: Warner Paperback Library.

Devenand, D., Kim, M., Paykina, N., & Sackeim, H. (2002). Adverse life events in elderly patients with major depression or dysthymia and in healthy control subjects. *American Journal of Geriatric Psychiatry, 10*, 265–274.

Devenand, D., Noble, M., Singer, T., Kiersky, J., Turret, N., Roose, S., et al. (1994). Is dysthymia a different disorder in the elderly? *American Journal of Psychiatry, 151*, 1592–1599.

Eaton, W., Kramer, M., Anthony, J., Dryman, A., Shapiro, S., & Locke, B. (1989). The incidence of specific DIS/DSM-III mental disorders: Data from the NIMH Epidemiologic Catchment Area program. *Acta Psychiatrica Scandinavica, 79*, 109–125.

Erlangsen, A., Zarit, S., Tu, X., & Conwell, Y. (2006). Suicide among older psychiatric inpatients: An evidence-based study of a high-risk group. *American Journal of Geriatric Psychiatry, 14*, 734–741.

Flint, A., & Rifat, S. (1998). The treatment of psychotic depression in later life: A comparison of pharmacotherapy and ECT. *Journal of Geriatric Psychiatry, 13*, 23–28.

Folstein, M., Folstein, S., & McHugh, P. (1975). Mini-Mental State: A practical method for grading the cognitive state of patients for the clinician. *Journal of Psychiatric Research, 12*, 189–198.

Frank, E., Frank, N., & Cornes, C. (1993). Interpersonal psychotherapy in the treatment of late life depression. In G. Klerman & M. Weissman (Eds.), *New applications of interpersonal psychotherapy* (pp. 167–198). Washington, DC: American Psychiatric Press.

Fried, L. (1994). Frailty. In W. Hazzard, E. Bierman, J. Blass, W. Ettinger, Jr., & J. Halter (Eds.), *Principles of geriatric medicine and gerontology* (3rd ed., pp. 1149–1156). New York: McGraw-Hill.

Gallo, J., & Coyne, J. (2000). The challenge of depression in late life: Bridging science and service in primary care. *Journal of the American Medical Association, 284*, 1570–1572.

Gatz, M., Pedersen, N., Plomin, R., Nesselroade, J., & McClearn, G. (1992). Importance of shared genes and shared environments for symptoms of depression in older adults. *Journal of Abnormal Psychology, 101*, 701–708.

Gatz, M., & Zarit, S. (1999). A good old age: Paradox or possibility. In V. Bengtson, J. Ruth, & K. Schaie (Eds.), *Theories of gerontology* (pp. 396–416). New York: Springer.

Gaynes, B. N., Warden, D., Trivedi, M. H., Wisniewski, S. R., Fava, M., & Rush, A. J. (2009). What did STAR*D teach us?: Results from a large-scale, practical, clinical trial for patients with depression. *Psychiatric Services, 60*, 1439–1445.

Gonzalez, H. M., Tarraf, W., Whitfield, K. E., & Vega, W. A. (2010). The epidemiology of major depression and ethnicity in the United States. *Journal of Psychiatric Research, 44*, 1043–1051.

Gonzales-Salvador, T., Aragano, C., Lyketsos, C., & Barba, A. (1999). The stress and psychological morbidity of the Alzheimer patient caregiver. *International Journal of Geriatric Psychiatry, 14*, 701–710.

Gottfries, C. (1990). Neurochemical aspects on aging and diseases with cognitive impairment. *Journal of Neuroscience Research, 27*, 541–547.

Grant, B. F., Dawson, D. A., & Hasin, D. S. (2001). *The Alcohol Use Disorder and Associated Disabilities Interview Schedule—DSM-IV*. Bethesda, MD: National Institute on Alcohol Abuse and Alcoholism.

Gum, A. M., King-Kallimanis, B., & Kohn, R. (2009). Prevalence of mood, anxiety, and substance-abuse disorders for older Americans in the National Comorbidity Survey-Replication. *American Journal of Geriatric Psychiatry, 17*, 769–781.

Hasin, D., Goodwin, R., Stinson, F., & Grant, B. (2005). Epidemiology of major depressive disorder. *Archives of General Psychiatry, 62*, 1097–1106.

Henderson, A., Jorm, A., & MacKinnon, A. (1993). The prevalence of depressive disorders and the distribution of depressive symptoms in later life: A survey using draft ICD-10 and DSM-III-R. *Psychological Medicine, 23*, 719–729.

Hickie, I., Scott, E., Naismith, S., Ward, P., Turner, K., Parker, G., et al. (2001). Late-onset depression: Genetic, vascular and clinical contributions. *Psychological Medicine, 31*, 1403–1412.

Hinton, L., Zweifach, M., Oishi, S., Tang, L., & Unutzer, J. (2006). Gender disparities in the treatment of late-life depression: Qualitative and quantitative findings from the IMPACT trial. *American Journal of Geriatric Psychiatry, 14*, 884–892.

Hughes, D., Blazer, D., & George, L. (1988). Age differences in life events: A multivariate controlled analysis. *International Journal of Aging and Human Development, 127*, 207–220.

Hybels, C., Blazer, D., & Pieper, C. (2001). Toward a threshold for subthreshold depression: An analysis of correlates of depression by severity of symptoms using data from an elderly community survey. *Gerontologist, 41*, 357–365.

Hybels, C., Blazer, D., & Steffens, D. (2005). Predictors of partial remission in older patients treated for major depression: The role of comorbid dysthymia. *American Journal of Geriatric Psychiatry, 13*, 713–721.

Hybels, C. F., Landerman, L. R., & Blazer, D. G. (2012): Age differences in symptom expression in patients with major depression. *International Journal of Geriatric Psychiatry, 27,* 601–611.

Jacobson, S., Pies, R., & Katz, I. (2007). *Clinical manual of geriatric pharmacology.* Washington, DC: American Psychiatric.

Juurlink, D., Mamdani, M., Kopp, A., & Redelmeier, D. (2006). The risk of suicide with selective serotonin reuptake inhibitors in the elderly. *American Journal of Psychiatry, 163,* 813–821.

Kales, H. C., Hease, D. E., Sirey, J. A., Zivin, I. K., Kim, H. M., Kavanagh, J., et al. (2013). Racial differences in adherence to antidepressant treatment in later life. *American Journal of Geriatric Psychiatry, 21*(10), 999–1009.

Keller, M., Shapiro, R., Lavori, P., & Wolfe, N. (1982a). Recovery in major depressive disorder: Analyses with the life table. *Archives of General Psychiatry, 39,* 905–910.

Keller, M., Shapiro, R., Lavori, P., & Wolfe, N. (1982b). Relapse in major depressive disorder: Analysis with the life table. *Archives of General Psychiatry, 39,* 911–915.

Kennedy, G., Kelman, H., & Thomas, C. (1990). The emergence of depressive symptoms in late life: The importance of declining health and increasing disability. *Journal of Community Health, 15,* 93–104.

Kessler, R., Berglund, P., Demler, O., Jin, R., Merikangas, K., & Walters, E. (2005). Lifetime prevalence and age-of-onset distributions of DSM-IV disorders in the National Comorbidity Survey Replication. *Archives of General Psychiatry, 62,* 593–602.

Kessler, R. C., & Ustün, T. B. (2004). The World Mental Health (WMH) Survey Initiative version of the World Health Organization (WHO) Composite International Diagnostic Interview (CIDI). *International Journal of Methods in Psychiatric Research, 13,* 93–121.

Koenig, H., Meador, K., Cohen, H., & Blazer, D. (1988). Depression in elderly hospitalized patients with medical illness. *Archives of Internal Medicine, 148,* 1929–1936.

Kraaij, V., & de Wilde, E. (2001). Negative life events and depressive symptoms in the elderly: A life span perspective. *Aging and Mental Health, 5,* 84–91.

Krause, N. (1986). Stress and sex differences in depressive symptoms among older adults. *Journal of Gerontology, 41,* 727–731.

Krishnan, K. R., Hays, J., & Blazer, D. (1997). MRI-defined vascular depression. *American Journal of Psychiatry, 154,* 497–501.

Lee, S., Tsang, A., Zhang, M. Y., Huang, Y. O., He, Y. L., Liu, Z. R., et al. (2007). Lifetime prevalence and inter-cohort variation in DSM-IV disorders in metropolitan China. *Psychological Medicine, 37,* 61–73.

Li, Y., Meyer, J., & Thornby, J. (2001). Longitudinal follow-up of depressive symptoms among normal versus cognitively impaired elderly. *International Journal of Geriatric Psychiatry, 16,* 718–727.

Lyness, J., King, D., Conwell, Y., Cox, E., & Caine, E. (2000). Cerebrovascular risk factors and 1-year depression outcome in older primary care patients. *American Journal of Psychiatry, 157,* 1499–1501.

Lyness, J., King, D., Cox, C., Yoediono, Z., & Caine, E. (1999). The importance of subsyndromal depression in older primary care patients: Prevalence and associated functional disability. *Journal of the American Geriatrics Society, 47,* 647–652.

Mackin, R. S., Tosun, D., Mueller, S. G., Lee, J. Y., Insel, P., Schuff, N., et al. (2012). Patterns of reduced cortical thickness in late-life depression and relationship to psychotherapeutic response. *American Journal of Geriatric Psychiatry, 21*(8), 794–802.

Mazure, C., Maciejewski, P., Jacobs, S., & Bruce, M. (2002). Stressful life events interacting with cognitive/personality styles to predict late-onset major depression. *American Journal of Geriatric Psychiatry, 10,* 297–304.

Meyers, B. (1992). Geriatric delusional depression. *Clinics in Geriatric Medicine, 8,* 299–308.

Morley, J., & Kraenzle, D. (1994). Causes of weight loss in a community nursing home. *Journal of the American Geriatrics Society, 42,* 583–585.

Morse, J., & Lynch, T. (2004). A preliminary investigation of self-reported personality disorders in late life: Prevalence, predictors of depressive severity, and clinical correlates. *Aging and Mental Health, 8,* 307–315.

Murphy, E. (1982). Social origins of depression in old age. *British Journal of Psychiatry, 141,* 135–142.

National Center for Health Statistics. (2001). *Death rates for 72 selected causes by 5-year age groups, race, and sex: United States, 1979–1998.* Washington, DC: Author.

Nezu, A. (1987). A problem-solving formulation of depression: A literature review and proposal of a pluralistic model. *Clinical Psychological Reviews, 7,* 121–144.

Olin, J., Schneider, L., Katz, I., Meyers, B., Alexopoulos, G., Breitner, J., et al. (2002). Provisional diagnostic criteria for depression of Alzheimer disease. *American Journal of Geriatric Psychiatry, 10,* 125–128.

Palsson, S., Ostling, S., & Skoog, I. (2001). The incidence of first-onset depression in a population followed from the age of 70 to 85. *Psychological Medicine, 31,* 1159–1168.

Parmelee, P., Katz, I., & Lawton, M. (1989). Depression among institutionalized aged: Assessment and prevalence estimation. *Journals of Gerontology: Medical Sciences, 44,* M22–M29.

Patten, S., Wang, J., & Williams, J. (2006). Descriptive epidemiology of major depression in Canada. *Canadian Journal of Psychiatry, 51,* 84–90.

Penninx, B., Leveille, S., Ferrucci, L., van Eijk, J., & Guralnik, J. (1999). Exploring the effect of depression on physical disability: Longitudinal evidence from the established populations for epidemiologic studies of the elderly. *American Journal of Public Health, 89,* 1346–1352.

Radloff, L. (1977). The CES-D Scale: A self-report depression scale for research in the general population. *Applied Psychological Measures, 1,* 385–401.

Regier, D., Boyd, J., Burke, J., Rae, D., Myers, J., Kramer, M., et al. (1988). One-month prevalence of mental disorders in the United States: Based on five Epidemiologic Catchment Area sites. *Archives of General Psychiatry, 45,* 977–986.

Reynolds, C., Dew, M., Pollock, B., Mulsant, B., Frank, E., Miller, M., et al. (2006). Maintenance treatment of major depression in old age. *New England Journal of Medicine, 354,* 1130–1138.

Reynolds, C., Frank, E., Perel, J., Imber, S., Cornes, C., Miller, M., et al. (1999). Nortriptyline and interpersonal psychotherapy as maintenance therapies for recurrent major depression: A randomized controlled trial in patients older than 59 years. *Journal of the American Medical Association, 281,* 39–45.

Robins, L., Helzer, J., & Croughan, J. (1981). Diagnostic Interview Schedule: Its history, characteristics and validity. *Archives of General Psychiatry, 38,* 381–389.

Sapolsky, R. (2001). Depression, antidepressants, and the shrinking hippocampus. *Proceedings of the National Academy of Sciences of the USA, 98,* 12320–12323.

Schulz, R., Drayer, R., & Rollman, B. (2002). Depression as a risk factor for non-suicide mortality in the elderly. *Biological Psychiatry, 52,* 205–225.

Seripa, D., Panza, F., d'Onofrio, G., Paroni, G., Bizzarro, A., Fontana, A, et al. (2013). The serotonin transporter gene locus in late-life major depressive disorder. *American Journal of Geriatric Psychiatry, 21,* 67–77.

Sexton, C. E., Mackey, C. E., & Ebmeier, K. P. (2013): A systematic review and meta-analysis of magnetic resonance imaging studies in late-life depression. *American Journal of Geriatric Psychiatry, 21,* 184–195.

Sheline, Y., Mintun, M., Moerlein, S., & Snyder, A. (2002). Greater loss of 5-HT$_{2A}$ receptors in midlife than in late life. *American Journal of Psychiatry, 159,* 430–435.

Spitzer, R., Williams, J., Gibbon, M., & First, M. (1990). *Structured Clinical Interview for DSM-III-R.* New York: New York State Psychiatric Institute, Biometrics Research.

Taylor, W., Steffens, D., MacFall, J., McQuoid, D., Payne, M., Provenzale, J., et al. (2003). White matter hyperintensity progression and late-life depression outcomes. *Archives of General Psychiatry, 60,* 1090–1096.

Tedeschini, E., Levkovitz, Y., Iovieno, N., Ameral, V. E., Nelson, J. C., & Papakostas, G. I. (2011).

Efficacy of antidepressants for late-life depression: A meta-analysis and meta-regression of placebo-controlled randomized trials. *Journal of Clinical Psychiatry, 72*, 1660–1668.

Unutzer, J., Katon, W., Callahan, C. M., Williams, J., Hunkeler, E., Harpole, L., et al. (2002). Collaborative care management of late-life depression in the primary care setting. *Journal of the American Medical Association, 288*, 2836–2845.

Unutzer, J., Patrick, D., Simon, G., Grembowski, D., Walker, E., Rutter, C., et al. (1997). Depressive symptoms and the cost of health services in HMO patients 65+ years and older. *Journal of the American Medical Association, 277*, 1618–1623.

van den Kommer, T. N., Comijs, H. C., Aartsen, M. J., Huisman, M., Deeg, D. J. H., & Bekman, A. T. F. (2013): Depression and cognition: How do they interact in old age? *American Journal of Geriatric Psychiatry, 21*, 398–410.

Williams, S., Kasl, S., Heiat, A., Abramson, J., Krumholz, H., & Vaccarino, V. (2002). Depression and risk of heart failure among the elderly: A prospective community-based study. *Psychosomatic Medicine, 64*, 6–12.

Wright, B. M., Eiland, E. H., III, & Lorenz, R. (2013). Augmentation with atypical antipsychotics for depression: A review of evidence-based support from the medical literature. *Pharmacotherapy, 33*, 344–359.

Yaffe, K., Ettinger, B., & Pressman, A. (1998). Neuropsychiatric function and dehydroepiandrosterone sulfate in elderly women: A prospective study. *Biological Psychiatry, 43*, 694–700.

Yesavage, J., Brink, T., & Rose, T. (1983). Development and validation of a geriatric depression screening scale: A preliminary report. *Journal of Psychiatric Research, 17*, 37–49.

Zhang, X., Gainetdinov, R., Beaulieu, J., Sotnikova, T., Uhrch, L., Williams, R., et al. (2005). Loss-of-function mutation in tryptophan hydroxilae-2 identified in unipolar major depression. *Neuron, 45*, 11–16.

CHAPTER 24

Depression and Suicide

MATTHEW K. NOCK, ALEXANDER J. MILLNER,
CHARLENE A. DEMING, *and* CATHERINE R. GLENN

Suicide is the most concerning possible outcome associated with depression. It is one of the leading causes of death worldwide and is responsible for more fatalities each year than all wars, genocide, and interpersonal violence combined—meaning that we are each more likely to die by our own hand than by someone else's (Nock, Borges, & Ono, 2012). Given the scope and severity of this problem, suicide and suicidal behaviors (e.g., suicide attempts) are important outcomes to consider when studying, assessing, or treating depression. This chapter provides a review of the current state-of-the-science regarding suicide and suicidal behavior. We describe current approaches to classifying and defining these outcomes, their epidemiology, known risk and protective factors, and evidence-based approaches to assessment and intervention, and we outline some of the most promising directions for future research on this problem.

CLASSIFICATION AND DEFINITIONS OF SUICIDAL BEHAVIOR

When thinking about suicide, as with any area of scientific inquiry, it is important to be clear and consistent in the terms and definitions used to describe the constructs of interest. Unfortunately, researchers and clinicians sometimes use vague and inconsistently defined terms when describing suicidal behavior (e.g., *parasuicide, deliberate self-harm, suicidality*). Over the past several years, researchers and clinicians have proposed clearer and more specific terms for different forms of suicidal behavior (Silverman, Berman, Sanddal, O'Carroll, & Joiner, 2007a, 2007b) that are being used with increasing frequency in the literature. These include *suicide ideation*: thoughts of engaging in behavior intended to end one's life; *suicide plan*: formulation of a specific strategy to end one's life; *suicide attempt*: self-injurious behavior with some nonzero intention of dying; and *suicide*: intentional self-inflicted death. Given the relative infrequency of suicide and the difficulties inherent in studying people who have died by low base-rate events, a great deal of research focuses on studying the immediate precursors to suicide: nonfatal suicidal behaviors and thoughts (hereafter referred to collectively as *suicidal behavior*). Researchers and clinicians working in this area also distinguish between suicidal behavior and *nonsuicidal self-injury* (NSSI), which refers to direct and deliberate destruction of one's own body tissue in the absence of any intent to die. Research supports making a distinction between suicidal and nonsuicidal behaviors, as they have different prevalence rates, courses, correlates, and responsiveness to treatment (Nock, 2010). Although NSSI has been strongly linked with depression, this chapter focuses on a review of what is known about *suicidal behavior* specifically.

EPIDEMIOLOGY OF SUICIDAL BEHAVIOR

Prevalence

In the United States, suicide occurs in 12.4 per 100,000 persons, is the 10th leading cause of death, and accounts for 1.5% of all mortality (Centers for Disease Control and Prevention, 2013). Suicides occur much more frequently among men, who are approximately four times more likely to die by suicide (20.0 per 100,000) than are women (5.2 per 100,000). Suicide rates also are higher among males who are of white and Native American race (see Figure 24.1). Although there are occasional increases and decreases in the suicide rate among different subgroups (e.g., the suicide rate for men ages 45–64 years has increased over the past 10 years), the overall suicide rate in the United States has been quite stable over time. For instance, although there are ups and downs in the overall suicide rate, it was very similar in the year 2000 (10.4/100,000) to what it was in the year 1900 (10.2/100,000).

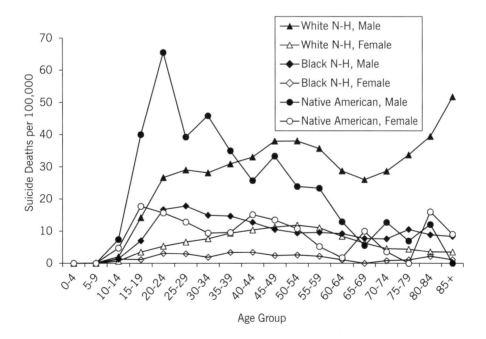

FIGURE 24.1. Rate of suicide death in the United States, 2010. Data from Centers for Disease Control and Prevention (2013). N-H, non-Hispanic.

Nonfatal suicidal behaviors are much more common than suicide deaths. In the United States, 15.6% of adults report a lifetime history of suicide ideation, 5.4% report a suicide plan, and 5.0% report that they have attempted to kill themselves (Nock, Borges, Bromet, Alonso, et al., 2008). Importantly, the sex differences flip in the case of nonfatal suicidal behaviors, with women being 40–70% more likely than men to report suicide ideation, plans, and attempts (Nock, Borges, Bromet, Alonso, et al., 2008). Research shows that males are more likely to make lethal attempts due to (1) a stronger intent to die; (2) the selection of quicker acting, lethal methods (e.g., males choose firearms, whereas females use poisoning); (3) differences in mental illness (e.g., males are more likely to have externalizing disorders with aggressive and impulsive characteristics, whereas females are more prone to internalizing disorders); (4) cultural bias and/or method choice in females leading to misclassification and/or underreporting of suicide; and (5) psychosocial differences, including one's likelihood of seeking help (Beautrais, 2002). Racial differences also are much less pronounced for nonfatal suicidal behaviors, with few significant differences across races.

Onset and Course

Suicidal behaviors (both fatal and nonfatal) are rare among children but show a rapid increase in onset during adolescence—a trend seen in the United States (Nock, Green, et al., 2013) and in countries around the world (Nock, Borges, Bromet, Alonso, et al., 2008). Approximately one-third of those who seriously consider suicide go on to make a suicide attempt, and the risk of this transition is highest in the first year after the initial onset of suicidal thinking (Nock, Borges, Bromet, Alonso, et al., 2008; Nock, Green, et al., 2013). Comprehensive epidemiological reviews of suicide are available elsewhere (Nock, Borges, Bromet, Cha, et al., 2008; Nock, Borges, & Ono, 2012).

RISK AND PROTECTIVE FACTORS FOR SUICIDAL BEHAVIOR

Given the alarming rates of suicide and suicidal behaviors, it is imperative to identify the risk and protective factors for these outcomes. A *risk factor* is a characteristic associated with increased odds of engaging in suicidal behavior, whereas a *protective factor* lessens the likelihood of suicidal behavior in the context of increased risk (Kraemer, Schmidt, & Ebert, 1997; Mrazek & Haggerty, 1994). In general, risk and protective factors are similar across gender and age groups, and therefore we describe risk and protective factors broadly, noting places in which research has shown important differences.

Risk Factors

Depression

Mood disorders are among the most commonly studied risk factors for suicidal behavior. Recent estimates suggest that approximately 23–95% (median: 50–60%) of people who die by suicide suffer from a mood disorder (broadly defined) at the time of their deaths (Appleby, Cooper, Amos, & Faragher, 1999; Brent et al., 1993; Cavanagh, Carson, Sharpe, & Lawrie, 2003; Chen & Dilsaver, 1996; Conwell et al., 1996; Foster, Gillespie, McClelland, & Patterson, 1999; Harwood, Hawton, Hope, & Jacoby, 2001; Houston, Hawton, & Shepperd, 2001; Lesage, et al., 1994; Marttunen, Aro, & Lönnqvist, 1993; Moskos, Olson, Halbern, Keller, & Gray, 2005; Vijayakumar & Rajkumar,

1999; Zonda, 2006) and approximately 2–8% of people with a mood disorder die by suicide (Blair-West, Cantor, Mellsop, & Eyeson-Annan, 1999; Bostwick & Pankratz, 2000; Inskip, Harris, & Barraclough, 1998). Studies examining major depressive disorder (MDD) specifically have found that 23–52% (median: ~30%) of those who die by suicide have a history of MDD (Appleby et al., 1999; Chen & Dilsaver, 1996; Conwell et al., 1996; Foster et al., 1999; Harwood et al., 2001; Houston et al., 2001; Lesage et al., 1994; Moskos et al., 2005; Vijayakumar & Rajkumar, 1999; Zonda, 2006) and that roughly 4–7% of those with MDD die by suicide (Nordentoft, Mortensen, & Pedersen, 2011).

MDD also is strongly linked to nonfatal suicidal behavior (Nock, Borges, Bromet, Alonso, et al., 2008; Nock, Hwang, Sampson, & Kessler, 2010). An estimated 12–19% of suicide ideators and 18–27% of suicide attempters have a prior history of MDD (Nock, Hwang, et al., 2009). Despite the importance of MDD in predicting suicidal behaviors, it should be noted that most people with MDD never experience suicidal thoughts. Less than half of those diagnosed with MDD report suicide ideation, and less than a fifth make a suicide attempt (Bottlender, Jäger, Strauss, & Möller, 2000; Chen & Dilsaver, 1996).

Recent research has sought to clarify the nature of the association between MDD and suicidal behavior. Several studies report that MDD is more severe among suicide attempters (Bulik, Carpenter, Kupfer, & Frank, 1990) and suicide decedents (Hawton, Casanas, Haw, & Saunders, 2013; Kessing, 2004), compared with control participants with depression; however, other studies find no such associations (Coryell & Young, 2005; Malone, Haas, Sweeney, & Mann, 1995; McGirr et al., 2007; Roy, 1993). In addition, some studies find that the first suicide attempt frequently occurs within the 2 years after depression onset (Malone et al., 1995; Roy, 1993; Vieta, Nieto, Gastó, & Cirera, 1992); however, the duration and number of depressive episodes are unrelated to suicide attempt or death (Ahrens, Berghöfer, Wolf, & Müller-Oerlinghausen, 1995; Bulik et al., 1990; Coryell & Young, 2005). Earlier age of onset of a depressive episode also has been associated with suicide attempts (Ahrens et al., 1995; Bulik et al., 1990; Roy, 1993), although here too research shows inconsistent results (Fowler, Tsuang, & Kronfol, 1979; Roy-Byrne, Post, Hambrick, Leverich, & Rosoff, 1988). In a meta-analysis, Hawton and colleagues reported that, among those with mood disorders, suicide death was preceded by increased hopelessness, the presence of alcohol or drug misuse, or a personality disorder (Hawton et al., 2013), all risk factors reported in general psychiatric populations (Mann, Waternaux, Haas, & Malone, 1999; Wenzel, et al., 2011). Notably, Hawton and colleagues (2013) also found that suicide risk was *not* increased in the presence of several specific depressive symptoms, including suicide ideation, guilt, reduced sleep, weight loss, psychomotor disturbance, and psychotic features (Hawton et al., 2013).

The precise mechanism by which MDD and suicide are related is currently unknown. It could be that, in a subset of people with depression, MDD alters adaptive psychological functioning (Nrugham, Holen, & Sund, 2012) or that MDD exacerbates underlying vulnerabilities (e.g., pessimism; Oquendo et al., 2004), which increases the likelihood of suicidal behavior. Alternatively, both MDD and suicidal behavior may be related to a third variable, such as hopelessness. Hopelessness has been found to prospectively predict future depressive episodes, suicide ideation, and suicide attempts (Smith, Alloy, & Abramson, 2006; Young et al., 1996). The intriguing proposition that suicide and depression are connected through a third variable would help to explain why only a subset of people with depression are also suicidal.

Interestingly, several recent papers reveal that MDD is the diagnosis most strongly associated with suicide ideation; however, among those with suicide ideation, MDD does not significantly predict who will make a suicide attempt. Instead, the transition from suicide ideation to attempt is predicted by disorders characterized by anxiety, agitation, and poor behavioral control (e.g., bipolar, anxiety, and substance use disorders; Bruf-faerts et al., 2010; Nock, Deming, et al., 2012; Nock, Hwang, et al., 2009), highlighting the importance of these other comorbid disorders in the occurrence of suicidal behavior.

Mental Disorders

Beyond depression, mental disorders more generally are shown to be significant risk fac-tors for suicidal behavior. Psychological autopsy studies estimate that greater than 90% of those dying by suicide have a prior history of a mental disorder (Cavanagh et al., 2003; Isometsä, 2001; Marttunen et al., 1993), most often a mood or substance use disorder (Isometsä, 2001). Comorbidity also is common among suicide decedents (Cavanagh et al., 2003). The majority of studies examining the association between mental disorders and suicide-related outcomes involve interviewing those with nonlethal suicidal behavior (Nock, Borges, Bromet, Cha, et al., 2008). For example, the World Health Organization World Mental Health Survey Initiative collected data on 16 mental disorders and suicidal behaviors from over 100,000 people across 21 countries (Nock, Borges, & Ono, 2012). This work indicates that approximately 40–50% of respondents who report thinking about suicide and 55–65% of those making a suicide attempt had a prior mental disorder. As with suicide death, comorbidity and multimorbidity (the presence of three or more disorders in one individual) significantly increase the risk of suicidal behavior (Nock, Hwang, et al., 2010).

Psychological Factors

Unfortunately, as with studies of MDD, research on mental disorders more broadly has failed to provide insight into *how* or *why* these factors lead to suicidal behavior. Exami-nation of psychological factors associated with suicidal behavior may provide insight into these questions. Theories of suicidal behavior suggest that when people experience extreme and seemingly unbearable psychological pain, they sometimes try to escape via suicide (Shneidman, 1996). It is possible that mental disorders are a proxy for psycho-logical factors, such as psychological pain (Mee et al., 2011) or feelings of intolerability that are especially likely to lead people to want to escape via suicide. Researchers also have proposed that psychological factors such as anhedonia and hopelessness increase the desire to kill oneself and that aggression and impulsiveness increase the likelihood of acting on suicidal thoughts (Fawcett, Busch, Jacobs, Kravitz, & Fogg, 1997; Mann et al., 1999). Therefore, the association between mental disorders and suicidal behavior may be explained by the combination of such factors.

Family History

There is consistent evidence for the familial transmission of risk for suicidal behavior. For instance, a recent meta-analytic review of suicide among individuals with depression revealed that a family history of mental illness was associated with a 40% increase in the odds of suicide among offspring and that a family history of suicidal behavior was associated with an 80% increase in the odds of offspring suicide (Hawton et al., 2013). Similar results have been found even after controlling for the presence of mental illness in offspring (Brent & Mann, 2005; Gureje et al., 2010), suggesting that the familial risk of suicidal behavior is not based solely on the transmission of mental illness (Brent & Mann, 2005). Potential mediators for the transmission of suicide risk include: impulsive aggression, neurocognitive deficits, and neuroticism (Brent & Melhem, 2008; Brent et al., 2003). Other plausible factors include cross-generational transmission of unhealthy family environments (e.g., abuse) and imitation.

Prior Self-Injurious Behavior

Prior history of either suicidal and nonsuicidal self-injurious behavior increase the likelihood that people will engage in future suicidal behavior. In fact, a history of prior suicidal behavior is one of the strongest predictors of future suicide attempts (Hawton et al., 2013). In addition, longitudinal studies indicate that NSSI is a strong independent risk factor for subsequent suicide attempts (Asarnow et al., 2011; Wilkinson, Kelvin, Roberts, Dubicka, & Goodyer, 2011).

Situational Factors

General situational factors also have been associated with increased risk for suicidal behavior. Some of these factors likely operate by increasing stress, such as being a sexual minority (Haas et al., 2011; Marshal et al., 2011) and being exposed to others' suicide (Haw, Hawton, Niedzwiedz, & Platt, 2013; Joiner, 2003; Swanson & Colman, 2013). Other factors include access to lethal means, such as use of hypnotic and sedative medications (Carlsten & Waern, 2009) and ease of access to and regular use of potentially lethal means (i.e., firearms among those in the military; Helmkamp, 1996; Mahon, Tobin, Cusack, Kelleher, & Malone, 2005). Finally, some situational risk factors are not clearly understood, such as the increased risk of suicide observed during the spring (Christodoulou et al., 2012; Dobbs, 2013; Petridou, Papadopoulos, Frangakis, Skalkidou, & Trichopoulos, 2002).

Stressors

Not surprisingly, research shows that the presence and frequency of stressful life events (both chronic and acute) are higher among suicidal individuals than among those who are not suicidal. Chronic stressors associated with suicide and suicidal behavior include physical pain (Braden & Sullivan, 2008) and illness (Druss & Pincus, 2000; Scott et al., 2010) and social disconnectedness (e.g., widowhood, loneliness, poor social support; Holt-Lunstad, Smith, & Layton, 2010). Many of these stressors are particularly relevant for older adults, including physical illness (e.g., those with five physical illnesses have a fivefold increase in suicide risk; Juurlink, Herrmann, Szalai, Kopp, & Redelmeier, 2004), pain (especially in males; Li & Conwell, 2010), functional capacity/impairment (Tsoh et al., 2005), and social disconnectedness (Fassberg et al., 2012; Van Orden & Conwell, 2011). Acute stressors related to suicide include: disciplinary/legal issues and interpersonal conflict (Phillips et al., 2002; Yen et al., 2005), childhood adversity (e.g., abuse, neglect; Bruffaerts et al., 2010; Dube et al., 2001), and trauma (particularly interpersonal and sexual violence; Stein, et al., 2010). Certain acute stressors are especially pertinent to adolescents, including bullying and peer victimization (Klomek et al., 2013), abuse, general family discord, and parental separation/divorce (Bursztein & Apter, 2008).

Notably, stressors may be particularly important in understanding suicide among military personnel, given the highly demanding and potentially disruptive nature of their jobs. Examples include relationship discord, military-related job stress (e.g., combat exposure), rank reduction, sleep issues, and traumatic brain injury (Hyman, Ireland,

Frost, & Cottrell, 2012; Logan, Skopp, Karch, Reger, & Gahm, 2012; Ribeiro, et al., 2012; Simpson & Tate, 2002; Teasdale & Engberg, 2001).

Protective Factors

Relative to risk factors, much less is known about factors that decrease the likelihood of suicidal behavior among those at risk. Religiosity has been found to protect against suicidal behavior, with religious/moral opposition to suicide, discouraged use of substances, and increased social support as possible explanations for this relation (Dervic et al., 2004; Gearing & Lizardi, 2009). Social support and connectedness appear to be protective against suicidal behavior among older adults (Fassberg et al., 2012; Van Orden & Conwell, 2011), and, relatedly, unit cohesion is believed to be protective among soldiers (Mitchell, Gallaway, Millikan, & Bell, 2012). Other research has examined well-being and positive response or "growth" in the face of stress and suggests the following may be protective: acceptance coping and positive reinterpretation (Park, Cohen, & Murch, 1996), emotional intelligence (Cha & Nock, 2009), and resilience traits (e.g., buffering via constructs such as positive attributional style and increased agency; Johnson, Wood, Gooding, Taylor, & Tarrier, 2011).

Theoretical/Conceptual Models of Suicidal Behavior

In summary, research on suicidal behavior continues to provide new information about an increasingly wide range of risk factors. What has been sorely lacking, however, is any firm understanding of how these risk factors work together to increase the likelihood of suicidal behavior. Vulnerability–stress models, such as the one shown in Figure 24.2, provide a general framework for synthesizing information about different risk factor

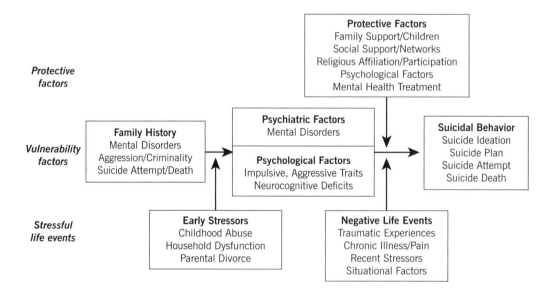

FIGURE 24.2. Vulnerability–stress model of suicidal behavior. From Nock, Deming, et al. (2013). Copyright 2013 by the Washington School of Psychiatry. Reprinted with permission from The Guilford Press.

domains. In this framework, *vulnerability factors* are distal influences that heighten the risk of suicidal behavior, and *stress factors* are proximal factors that trigger suicide outcomes among vulnerable individuals. However, these models are insufficiently specific, as risk factors increase the likelihood of a wide range of negative outcomes, and most people with these risk factors will never become suicidal. Several theoretical models of suicidal behavior have been proposed—many of which currently are being studied and tested (Baumeister, 1990; Joiner, 2005; Linehan, 1993a; Shneidman, 1993). These and other models provide promising ideas about how risk factors may work together to increase risk, but none has demonstrated an ability to accurately explain or predict suicidal behavior.

ASSESSMENT OF SUICIDAL BEHAVIOR

Understanding how risk and protective factors might influence suicidal behavior becomes especially important when attempting to assess the current presence, and future risk, of suicidal behavior. The assessment of suicidal behavior is a broad task that can be thought of as having three potential aims: assessing the presence of suicidal behavior, monitoring risk over time, and predicting imminent risk. It is important to note that suicide assessment relies on self-report instruments, which are limited because patients may fail to disclose their suicidal thoughts, plans, or intentions for fear of being stopped or hospitalized (Busch, Fawcett, & Jacobs, 2003).

Presence of Suicidal Behavior and Monitoring Risk over Time

A variety of methods have been developed for assessing the presence of suicidal behaviors, ranging from one-item measures built into larger scales (e.g., the suicide item from the Beck Depression Inventory; Beck, Steer, & Brown, 1996) to comprehensive interviews designed to thoroughly assess an individual's suicide history. Some widely used measures are highlighted here, and reviews of measures available for use with adults (Brown, 2001) and adolescents (Goldston, 2000) are discussed in greater detail elsewhere. The Scale for Suicide Ideation (SSI; Beck, Kovacs, & Weissman, 1979), a 21-item clinician-administered measure, and the Beck Scale for Suicide Ideation (Beck & Steer, 1991), a self-report version of the SSI, are commonly used to assess current suicidal thoughts, plans, and intentions to act. The Suicide Ideation Questionnaire (SIQ; Reynolds, 1987) is widely used to measure suicidal thoughts in youth. When more time is available, structured interviews, such as the Self-Injurious Thoughts and Behaviors Interview (Nock, Holmberg, Photos, & Michel, 2007) and the Suicide Attempt and Self-Injury Interview (Linehan, Comtois, Brown, Heard, & Wagner, 2006), can be useful for obtaining a thorough history of suicidal and nonsuicidal thoughts and behaviors. The Suicide Intent Scale (Beck, Schuyler, & Herman, 1974), a 15-item clinician-administered scale, assesses the intent and perceived lethality of the most recent attempt. Other scales, such as the Lethality Scales (Beck, Beck, & Kovacs, 1975) and Lethality of Suicide Attempt Rating Scale—Updated (Berman, Shepherd, & Silverman, 2003), measure the medical lethality of suicide attempts. In order to monitor risk and variations in suicidal thoughts, plans, and intentions over time, it is necessary to use measures that are sensitive to change. The Self-Monitoring Suicidal Ideation Scale (Clum & Curtin, 1993), and the ideation scales just discussed, have been used to assess changes in the duration and intensity of suicide ideation.

Assessing Imminent Risk

Ultimately, suicide risk assessment tools will be most useful if they can help determine whether an individual is at short-term or imminent risk of self-injury. That is, how likely is an individual to hurt him- or herself in the next minutes, hours, or days? Unfortunately, current assessment measures have demonstrated limited utility for predicting future suicidal behavior (Brown, 2001). In addition, there is currently no empirically supported method for combining information about known suicide risk and protective factors to determine an individual's level of suicide risk. Clinical judgment is currently used to synthesize this information and determine a patient's risk level.

TREATMENT OF SUICIDAL BEHAVIOR

Most people who experience suicidal behavior in the United States and other high-income countries receive some form of treatment for psychological or emotional problems; however, only a small minority of those with suicidal behavior (17%) in low-income countries receive any such care (Bruffaerts et al., 2011; Nock, Green, et al., 2013). Although it is good news that in many parts of the world the majority of people with suicidal behavior receive treatment, it is less clear whether such treatments have any positive impact. For instance, interventions that reduce depression have not proven particularly effective for decreasing suicide risk (Bruce et al., 2004), suggesting that treatments need to specifically target suicide-related outcomes. Although a variety of interventions have shown promise, there are currently no well-established treatments—psychological or pharmacological—for suicidal behavior. Some of the most promising treatments to date are reviewed next.

Psychological Treatment

Adults

In general, cognitive-behavioral therapies (CBT) appear to be most effective for reducing suicidal behavior among adults. Dialectical behavior therapy (DBT; Linehan, 1993b), which includes an intensive program of weekly individual sessions, group skills training, and phone coaching, has been found to significantly reduce suicidal thoughts (Pistorello, Fruzzetti, MacLane, Gallop, & Iverson, 2012; Turner, 2000) and attempts (Linehan, Comtois, Murray, et al., 2006). However, most studies of DBT have been conducted with female patients with borderline personality disorder (BPD), and it is unclear whether these treatments will generalize to depression or to male patients. Brief (10–12 session) CBT interventions also have shown some effects in reducing suicidal behavior (Brown et al., 2005; Raj, Kumaraiah, & Bhide, 2001; Slee, Garnefski, van der Leeden, Arensman, & Spinhoven, 2008). However, findings of problem-solving interventions for suicidal behavior have been mixed (Townsend et al., 2001). In addition to CBT, psychodynamic interventions (e.g., psychodynamic interpersonal therapy; Guthrie et al., 2001) and psychoanalytically oriented partial hospitalization (Bateman & Fonagy, 2001) have shown some promise for reducing suicidal behavior. Beyond standard treatments, brief interventions through which therapists maintain contact with patients via postcards, phone calls, or in-person visits have reduced suicide attempts (Hassanian-Moghaddam, Sarjami, Kolahi, & Carter, 2011; Vaiva et al., 2006) and suicide deaths (Fleischmann et al., 2008; Motto & Bostrom, 2001). Brief interventions may be particularly useful supplements to long-term care given the high-risk period for suicide shortly after hospital discharge (Qin & Nordentoft, 2005).

Adolescents

In randomized controlled trials (RCTs) with adolescents, two interventions have effectively reduced suicidal *thoughts*: a short, intensive version of interpersonal therapy for depressed adolescents (focused on alleviating interpersonal problems; Tang, Jou, Ko, Huang, & Yen, 2009) and attachment-based family therapy (focused on improving parent–adolescent relationships; Diamond et al., 2010). Only two interventions have been effective for reducing suicidal *behavior* in adolescents: integrated CBT (including individual skills training, family therapy, and parent training sessions; Esposito-Smythers, Spirito, Kahler, Hunt, & Monti, 2011) and multisystemic therapy (intensive home-based family treatment; Huey et al., 2004). However, each of these treatments has been examined only in a single RCT, and replications are needed before conclusions can be made about the effectiveness of these interventions. Finally, although initially promising (Wood, Trainor, Rothwell, Moore, & Harrington, 2001), group interventions with suicidal adolescents have been generally unsuccessful (Green et al., 2011; Hazell et al., 2009). Given the potential for social contagion of self-injury in adolescents (Prinstein et al., 2010), group treatments may be contraindicated in this population.

Older Adults

Although much research has focused on treatments for depression in older adults (Areán & Cook, 2002), few RCTs have examined interventions for reducing suicide risk. Preliminary research indicates that primary care interventions, such as the Prevention of Suicide in Primary Care Elderly: Collaborative Trial, may be effective for reducing suicide ideation in older adults (Bruce et al., 2004). In addition, CBT interventions, which have demonstrated positive results in younger adults, are currently being adapted for older populations (Bhar & Brown, 2012).

The Military

DBT was found to reduce suicide ideation in female veterans with BPD (Koons et al., 2001). In addition, the Collaborative Assessment and Management of Suicidality program, which uses an eclectic theoretical approach to understand the function of suicidal behavior for the individual, decreased the risk of suicidal behavior faster than treatment as usual in an Air Force sample (Jobes, Wong, Conrad, Drozd, & Neal-Walden, 2005). Finally, due to increased rates of suicide in the months following hospital discharge, short-term crisis management and treatment adherence programs have been created, such as the Suicide Assessment and Follow-up Engagement Veteran Emergency Treatment (SAFE VET) program—a two-part program that consists of crisis management, including safety planning (Stanley & Brown, 2012), in the emergency department and follow-up telephone contact as veterans transition to outpatient care (Knox et al., 2012). An initial feasibility study indicates that SAFE VET increases outpatient treatment compliance, but research examining its effectiveness for reducing suicidal behavior is still needed.

Pharmacological Treatment

There are currently no well-established pharmacological treatments for suicidal behavior. Antidepressant medications have received the most research, but also the most controversy. Based on evidence indicating a potential causal link between antidepressant medication and increased suicide risk in youth (Hammad, 2004), in 2004, the U.S. Food and Drug Administration issued a black-box warning about prescribing these medications to children and adolescents, which was extended to young adults in 2006. These black-box warnings decreased prescriptions of selective serotonin reuptake inhibitors (SSRIs) for youth and, notably, coincided with *increased* suicide rates in this population, suggesting that antidepressants may be more helpful than harmful for youth at risk for suicide (Gibbons et al., 2007). A recent meta-analysis suggests that antidepressants are effective for reducing suicidal behavior in adults and that this reduction may be mediated by decreased depressive symptoms (Gibbons, Brown, Hur, Davis, & Mann, 2012). Given the mixed evidence and continued debate, youth prescribed antidepressant medication should be closely monitored for increased suicide risk.

Meta-analytic reviews indicate that lithium also may be effective for reducing suicide risk in adults with unipolar mood disorders (Cipriani, Hawton, Stockton, & Geddes, 2013). There also is some evidence indicating that opioid antagonists, antipsychotics, anticonvulsants, and omega-3 fatty acids may be useful treatments for reducing self-injury (Plener, Libal, & Nixon, 2009). Electroconvulsive therapy may also help reduce short-term risk for suicide in adults (Sakinofsky, 2007). Finally, combined psychotherapy and medication interventions do not seem to provide unique treatment benefits over antidepressant medication alone in adolescents (Dubicka et al., 2010). Combined treatments in adults have demonstrated some efficacy for reducing depressive symptoms, compared with either intervention alone (Thase et al., 1997; von Wolff, Hölzel, Westphal, Härter, & Kriston, 2012); however, few studies have examined the effect of combined treatment on suicidal behavior.

FUTURE DIRECTIONS

How Should We Best Classify and Define Suicidal Behavior?

In the early days of the study of suicide, researchers and clinicians focused only on suicide death. Over the past 50 years, there has been a much larger focus on the immediate precursors to suicide: suicide ideation, plans, and attempts. Over the past 10 years, researchers have made even finer distinctions, placing more emphasis on the important differences between suicidal and nonsuicidal self-injury, as well as between different types of suicidal behavior (e.g., suicide attempt vs. interrupted attempt vs. aborted attempt). Future research must test whether these increasingly fine distinctions translate into more effective ways of understanding, predicting, and preventing suicide attempts and death.

Why Do People Try to Kill Themselves?

Considerable progress has been made in the mapping out of various risk and protective factors for suicidal behavior. However, although risk factors have been identified, we continue to have very little understanding of how they work together to produce suicidal behavior. Suicidal behavior undoubtedly results from the complex interaction of numerous risk factors operating at various levels of analysis (e.g., genetic, neurobiological, environmental). One of the most important next steps in suicide research is moving beyond simple tests of bivariate associations between putative risk factors and suicidal behavior and onto the examination of multivariate models that begin to help us understand how to combine information from different risk factor domains.

How Should We Measure Risk for Suicidal Behavior?

Perhaps the greatest limitation in the study of suicidal behavior is that virtually all methods of measuring suicidal behavior, both in scientific and in clinical settings, rely on the use of self-report. This is hugely problematic given that many, if not most, people who are considering suicide are motivated to deny or conceal their suicidal thoughts and intentions. Recent research has begun to search for objective biological and behavioral markers of suicide risk, with some early success. Biologically, recent studies suggest that blood and cerebrospinal fluid markers associated with stress, mood regulation, and impulsiveness are associated with suicide attempts and death (Le-Niculescu et al., 2013; Mann et al., 2006). Behaviorally, implicit associations with and attentional bias toward suicide-related stimuli have been shown to predict subsequent suicide attempts above and beyond clinician and patient prediction (Cha, Najmi, Park, Finn, & Nock, 2010; Nock, Park, et al., 2010). A related limitation is that virtually all data we have on suicidal behavior comes from long-term retrospective self-reports, and as such, we know very little about how suicidal thoughts and behaviors unfold in real time. New, real-time monitoring methods now allow researchers and clinicians to capture these events as they unfold (Nock, Prinstein, & Sterba, 2009), and the study of such data could lead to significant leaps forward in our understanding of suicidal behavior.

How Can We Predict and Ultimately Prevent Suicidal Behavior?

All that we have learned about suicidal behavior in the aforementioned areas must be brought to bear on efforts to improve our ability to predict and prevent suicidal behavior. There currently are no replicated, evidence-based methods available for predicting, treating, or preventing suicidal behavior, and so these continue to be among the most imperative directions for future research. As described in this chapter, recent research has provided some promising leads regarding effective treatments for suicidal behavior, but no firm solutions. Future research should continue to test promising treatments, but we also need novel interventions that build on recent advances in psychological science (e.g., MacLeod & Mathews, 2012; Neshat-Doost et al., 2013) and in any other areas that could provide a feasible means of better identifying and treating those at risk for this devastating and perplexing behavior.

REFERENCES

Ahrens, B., Berghöfer, A., Wolf, T., & Müller-Oerlinghausen, B. (1995). Suicide attempts, age and duration of illness in recurrent affective disorders. *Journal of Affective Disorders, 36*(1), 43–49.

Appleby, L., Cooper, J., Amos, T., & Faragher, B. (1999). Psychological autopsy study of suicides by people aged under 35. *British Journal of Psychiatry, 175*(2), 168–174.

Areán, P. A., & Cook, B. L. (2002). Psychotherapy and combined psychotherapy/pharmacotherapy for late life depression. *Biological Psychiatry, 52*(3), 293–303.

Asarnow, J. R., Porta, G., Spirito, A., Emslie, G., Clarke, G., Wagner, K. D., et al. (2011). Suicide attempts and nonsuicidal self-injury in the treatment of resistant depression in adolescents: Findings from the TORDIA study. *Journal of the American Academy of Child and Adolescent Psychiatry, 50*(8), 772–781.

Bateman, A., & Fonagy, P. (2001). Treatment of borderline personality disorder with psychoanalytically oriented partial hospitalization: An 18-month follow-up. *American Journal of Psychiatry, 158*(1), 36–42.

Baumeister, R. F. (1990). Suicide as escape from self. *Psychological Review, 97*(1), 90–113.

Beautrais, A. L. (2002). Gender issues in youth suicidal behaviour. *Emergency Medicine (Fremantle), 14*(1), 35–42.

Beck, A. T., Beck, R., & Kovacs, M. (1975). Classification of suicidal behaviors: I. Quantifying intent and medical lethality. *American Journal of Psychiatry, 132*(3), 285–287.

Beck, A. T., Kovacs, M., & Weissman, A. (1979). Assessment of suicidal intention: The Scale for Suicidal Ideation. *Journal of Consulting and Clinical Psychology, 47*(2), 343–352.

Beck, A. T., Schuyler, D., & Herman, I. (1974). Development of suicidal intent scales. In A. T. Beck, H. L. P. Resnik, & D. J. Lettieri (Eds.), *The prediction of suicide* (pp. 45–55). Bowie, MD: Charles Press.

Beck, A. T., & Steer, R. A. (1991). *Manual for the Beck Scale for Suicide Ideation.* San Antonio, TX: Psychological Corporation.

Beck, A. T., Steer, R. A., & Brown, G. K. (1996). *Manual for the Beck Depression Inventory—II.* San Antonio, TX: Psychological Corporation.

Berman, A. L., Shepherd, G., & Silverman, M. M. (2003). The LSARS II: Lethality of Suicide Attempt Rating Scale—Updated. *Suicide and Life-Threatening Behavior, 33*(3), 261–276.

Bhar, S. S., & Brown, G. K. (2012). Treatment of depression and suicide in older adults. *Cognitive and Behavioral Practice, 19*(1), 116–125.

Blair-West, G. W., Cantor, C. H., Mellsop, G. W., & Eyeson-Annan, M. L. (1999). Lifetime suicide risk in major depression: Sex and age determinants. *Journal of Affective Disorders, 55*(2–3), 171–178.

Bostwick, J. M., & Pankratz, V. S. (2000). Affective disorders and suicide risk: A reexamination. *American Journal of Psychiatry, 157*(12), 1925–1932.

Bottlender, R., Jäger, M., Strauss, A., & Möller, H. J. (2000). Suicidality in bipolar compared to unipolar depressed inpatients. *European Archives of Psychiatry and Clinical Neuroscience, 250*(5), 257–261.

Braden, J. B., & Sullivan, M. D. (2008). Suicidal thoughts and behavior among adults with self-reported pain conditions in the National Comorbidity Survey Replication. *Journal of Pain, 9*(12), 1106–1115.

Brent, D. A., & Mann, J. J. (2005). Family genetic studies, suicide, and suicidal behavior. *American Journal of Medical Genetics: Part C. Seminars in Medical Genetics, 133*C(1), 13–24.

Brent, D. A., & Melhem, N. (2008). Familial transmission of suicidal behavior. *Psychiatric Clinics of North America, 31*(2), 157–177.

Brent, D. A., Oquendo, M., Birmaher, B., Greenhill, L., Kolko, D., Stanley, B., et al. (2003). Peripubertal suicide attempts in offspring of suicide attempters with siblings concordant for suicidal behavior. *American Journal of Psychiatry, 160*(8), 1486–1493.

Brent, D. A., Perper, J. A., Moritz, G., Allman, C., Friend, A., Roth, C., et al. (1993). Psychiatric risk factors for adolescent suicide: A case-control study. *Journal of the American Academy of Child and Adolescent Psychiatry, 32*(3), 521–529.

Brown, G. K. (2001). A review of suicide assessment measures for intervention research with adults and older adults Available at *http://sbisrvntweb.uqac.ca/archivage/15290520.pdf.*

Brown, G. K., Ten Have, T., Henriques, G. R., Xie, S. X., Hollander, J. E., & Beck, A. T. (2005). Cognitive therapy for the prevention of suicide attempts: A randomized controlled trial. *Journal of the American Medical Association, 294*(5), 563–570.

Bruce, M. L., Ten Have, T. R., Reynolds, C. F., III, Katz, I. I., Schulberg, H. C., Mulsant, B. H., et al. (2004). Reducing suicidal ideation and depressive symptoms in depressed older primary care patients. *Journal of the American Medical Association, 291*(9), 1081–1091.

Bruffaerts, R., Demyttenaere, K., Borges, G., Haro, J. M., Chiu, W. T., Hwang, I., et al. (2010). Childhood adversities as risk factors for onset and persistence of suicidal behaviour. *British Journal of Psychiatry, 197*(1), 20–27.

Bruffaerts, R., Demyttenaere, K., Hwang, I., Chiu, W. T., Sampson, N., Kessler, R. C., et al. (2011). Treatment of suicidal people around the world. *British Journal of Psychiatry, 199,* 64–70.

Bulik, C. M., Carpenter, L. L., Kupfer, D. J., & Frank, E. (1990). Features associated with suicide attempts in recurrent major depression. *Journal of Affective Disorders, 18*(1), 29–37.

Bursztein, C., & Apter, A. (2008). Adolescent suicide. *Current Opinion in Psychiatry, 22,* 221–226.

Busch, K. A., Fawcett, J., & Jacobs, D. G. (2003). Clinical correlates of inpatient suicide. *Journal of Clinical Psychiatry, 64*(1), 14–19.

Carlsten, A., & Waern, M. (2009). Are sedatives and hypnotics associated with increased suicide risk of suicide in the elderly? *BMC Geriatrics, 9,* 20.

Cavanagh, J. T. O., Carson, A. J., Sharpe, M., & Lawrie, S. M. (2003). Psychological autopsy studies of suicide: A systematic review. *Psychological Medicine, 33*(3), 395–405.

Centers for Disease Control and Prevention. (2013). Injury prevention and control: Data and statistics (WISQARS). Retrieved March 5, 2013, from *www.cdc.gov/injury/wisqars/index.html*.

Cha, C. B., Najmi, S., Park, J. M., Finn, C. T., & Nock, M. K. (2010). Attentional bias toward suicide-related stimuli predicts suicidal behavior. *Journal of Abnormal Psychology, 119*(3), 616–622.

Cha, C. B., & Nock, M. K. (2009). Emotional intelligence is a protective factor for suicidal behavior. *Journal of the American Academy of Child and Adolescent Psychiatry, 48*(4), 422–430.

Chen, Y.-W., & Dilsaver, S. C. (1996). Lifetime rates of suicide attempts among subjects with bipolar and unipolar disorders relative to subjects with other axis I disorders. *Biological Psychiatry, 39*(10), 896–899.

Christodoulou, C., Douzenis, A., Papadopoulos, F. C., Papadopoulou, A., Bouras, G., Gournellis, R., et al. (2012). Suicide and seasonality. *Acta Psychiatrica Scandinavica, 125*(2), 127–146.

Cipriani, A., Hawton, K., Stockton, S., & Geddes, J. R. (2013). Lithium in the prevention of suicide in mood disorders: Updated systematic review and meta-analysis. *British Medical Journal, 346,* f3646.

Clum, G. A., & Curtin, L. (1993). Validity and reactivity of a system of self-monitoring suicide ideation. *Journal of Psychopathology and Behavioral Assessment, 15*(4), 375–385.

Conwell, Y., Duberstein, P. R., Cox, C., Herrmann, J. H., Forbes, N. T., & Caine, E. D. (1996). Relationships of age and axis I diagnoses in victims of completed suicide: A psychological autopsy study. *American Journal of Psychiatry, 153*(8), 1001–1008.

Coryell, W., & Young, E. A. (2005). Clinical predictors of suicide in primary major depressive disorder. *Journal of Clinical Psychiatry, 66*(4), 412–417.

Dervic, K., Oquendo, M. A., Grunebaum, M. F., Ellis, S., Burke, A. K., & Mann, J. J. (2004). Religious affiliation and suicide attempt. *American Journal of Psychiatry, 161*(12), 2303–2308.

Diamond, G. S., Wintersteen, M. B., Brown, G. K., Diamond, G. M., Gallop, R., Shelef, K., et al. (2010). Attachment-based family therapy for adolescents with suicidal ideation: A randomized controlled trial. *Journal of the American Academy of Child and Adolescent Psychiatry, 49*(2), 122–131.

Dobbs, D. (2013, June 24). Clues in the cycle of suicide. *New York Times.* Available at *http://well.blogs.nytimes.com/2013/06/24/clues-in-the-cycle-of-suicide/?smid=tw-nytimesscience&seid=auto*.

Druss, B., & Pincus, H. (2000). Suicidal ideation and suicide attempts in general medical illnesses. *Archives of Internal Medicine, 160*(10), 1522–1526.

Dube, S. R., Anda, R. F., Felitti, V. J., Chapman, D. P., Williamson, D. F., & Giles, W. H. (2001). Childhood abuse, household dysfunction, and the risk of attempted suicide throughout the life span: Findings from the Adverse Childhood Experiences Study. *Journal of the American Medical Association, 286,* 3089–3096.

Dubicka, B., Elvins, R., Roberts, C., Chick, G., Wilkinson, P., & Goodyer, I. M. (2010). Combined treatment with cognitive–behavioural therapy in adolescent depression: Meta-analysis. *British Journal of Psychiatry, 197*(6), 433–440.

Esposito-Smythers, C., Spirito, A., Kahler, C. W., Hunt, J., & Monti, P. (2011). Treatment of co-occurring substance abuse and suicidality among adolescents: A randomized trial. *Journal of Consulting and Clinical Psychology, 79*(6), 728–739.

Fassberg, M. M., van Orden, K. A., Duberstein, P., Erlangsen, A., Lapierre, S., Bodner, E., et al. (2012). A systematic review of social factors and suicidal behavior in older adulthood. *International Journal of Environmental Research and Public Health, 9*(3), 722–745.

Fawcett, J., Busch, K. A., Jacobs, D., Kravitz, H. M., & Fogg, L. (1997). Suicide: A four-pathway clinical–biochemical model. *Annals of the New York Academy of Sciences, 836*(1), 288–301.

Fleischmann, A., Bertolote, J. M., Wasserman, D., De Leo, D., Bolhari, J., Botega, N. J., et al. (2008). Effectiveness of brief intervention and contact for suicide attempters: A randomized control trial in five countries. *Bulletin of the World Health Organization, 86*(9), 703–709.

Foster, T., Gillespie, K., McClelland, R., & Patterson, C. (1999). Risk factors for suicide independent of DSM-III-R Axis I disorder: Case-control psychological autopsy study in Northern Ireland. *British Journal of Psychiatry, 175*(2), 175–179.

Fowler, R. C., Tsuang, M. T., & Kronfol, Z. (1979). Communication of suicidal intent and suicide in unipolar depression: A forty-year follow-up. *Journal of Affective Disorders, 1*(3), 219–225.

Gearing, R. E., & Lizardi, D. (2009). Religion and suicide. [Review]. *Journal of Religion and Health, 48*(3), 332–341.

Gibbons, R. D., Brown, C. H., Hur, K., Davis, J. M., & Mann, J. J. (2012). Suicidal thoughts and behavior with antidepressant treatment: Reanalysis of the randomized placebo-controlled studies of fluoxetine and venlafaxine. *Archives of General Psychiatry, 69*(6), 580–587.

Gibbons, R. D., Brown, C. H., Hur, K., Marcus, S. M., Bhaumik, D. K., Erkens, J. A., et al. (2007). Early evidence on the effects of regulators' suicidality warnings on SSRI prescriptions and suicide in children and adolescents. *American Journal of Psychiatry, 164*(9), 1356–1363.

Goldston, D. B. (2000). *Assessment of suicidal behaviors and risk among children and adolescents.* Bethesda, MD: National Institute of Mental Health.

Green, J. M., Wood, A. J., Kerfoot, M. J., Trainor, G., Roberts, C., Rothwell, J., et al. (2011). Group therapy for adolescents with repeated self-harm: Randomised controlled trial with economic evaluation. *British Medical Journal, 342*, 1–12.

Gureje, O., Oladeji, B., Hwang, I., Chiu, W. T., Kessler, R. C., Sampson, N. A., et al. (2010). Parental psychopathology and the risk of suicidal behavior in their offspring: Results from the World Mental Health surveys. *Molecular Psychiatry, 16*(12), 1221–1233.

Guthrie, E., Kapur, N., Mackway-Jones, K., Chew-Graham, C., Moorey, J., Mendel, E., et al. (2001). Randomised controlled trial of brief psychological intervention after deliberate self-poisoning. *British Medical Journal, 323*, 135–138.

Haas, A. P., Eliason, M., Mays, V. M., Mathy, R. M., Cochran, S. D., D'Augelli, A. R., et al. (2011). Suicide and suicide risk in lesbian, gay, bisexual, and transgender populations: Review and recommendations. *Journal of Homosexuality, 58*(1), 10–51.

Hammad, T. A. (2004). *Review and evaluation of clinical data.* Washington, DC: U.S. Food and Drug Administration.

Harwood, D., Hawton, K., Hope, T., & Jacoby, R. (2001). Psychiatric disorder and personality factors associated with suicide in older people: A descriptive and case-control study. *International Journal of Geriatric Psychiatry, 16*(2), 155–165.

Hassanian-Moghaddam, H., Sarjami, S., Kolahi, A. A., & Carter, G. L. (2011). Postcards in Persia: Randomised controlled trial to reduce suicidal behaviors 12 months after hospital-treated self-poisoning. *British Journal of Psychiatry, 198*(4), 309–316.

Haw, C., Hawton, K., Niedzwiedz, C., & Platt, S. (2013). Suicide clusters: A review of risk factors and mechanisms. *Suicide and Life-Threatening Behavior, 43*(1), 97–108.

Hawton, K., Casanas, I. C. C., Haw, C., & Saunders, K. (2013). Risk factors for suicide in individuals with depression: A systematic review. *Journal of Affective Disorders, 147*(1–3), 17–28.

Hazell, P. L., Martin, G., McGill, K., Kay, T., Wood, A., Trainor, G., et al. (2009). Group therapy for repeated deliberate self-harm in adolescents: Failure of replication of a randomized trial. *Journal of the American Academy of Child and Adolescent Psychiatry, 48*(6), 662–670.

Helmkamp, J. C. (1996). Occupation and suicide among males in the U.S. Armed Forces. *Annals of Epidemiology, 6*(1), 83–88.

Holt-Lunstad, J., Smith, T. B., & Layton, J. B. (2010). Social relationships and mortality risk: A meta-analytic review. *PLoS Medicine, 7*(7), e1000316.

Houston, K., Hawton, K., & Shepperd, R. (2001). Suicide in young people aged 15–24: A psychological autopsy study. *Journal of Affective Disorders, 63*(1–3), 159–170.

Huey, S. J., Jr., Henggeler, S. W., Rowland, M. D., Halliday-Boykins, C. A., Cunningham, P. B., Pickrel, S. G., et al. (2004). Multisystemic therapy effects on attempted suicide by youths presenting psychiatric emergencies. *Journal of the American Academy of Child and Adolescent Psychiatry, 43*(2), 183–190.

Hyman, J., Ireland, R., Frost, L., & Cottrell, L. (2012). Suicide incidence and risk factors in an active duty U.S. military population. *American Journal of Public Health, 102*(Suppl. 1), S138–146.

Inskip, H. M., Harris, E. C., & Barraclough, B. (1998). Lifetime risk of suicide for affective disorder, alcoholism and schizophrenia. *British Journal of Psychiatry, 172*(1), 35–37.

Isometsä, E. T. (2001). Psychological autopsy studies: A review. *European Psychiatry, 16*(7), 379–385.

Jobes, D. A., Wong, S. A., Conrad, A. K., Drozd, J. F., & Neal-Walden, T. (2005). The collaborative assessment and management of suicidality versus treatment as usual: A retrospective study with suicidal outpatients. *Suicide and Life-Threatening Behavior, 35*(5), 483–497.

Johnson, J., Wood, A. M., Gooding, P., Taylor, P. J., & Tarrier, N. (2011). Resilience to suicidality: The buffering hypothesis [Review]. *Clinical Psychology Review, 31*(4), 563–591.

Joiner, T. E. (2003). Contagion of suicidal symptoms as a function of assortative relating and shared relationship stress in college roommates. *Journal of Adolescence, 26*(4), 495–504.

Joiner, T. E. (2005). *Why people die by suicide.* Cambridge, MA: Harvard University Press.

Juurlink, D. N., Herrmann, N., Szalai, J. P., Kopp, A., & Redelmeier, D. A. (2004). Medical illness and the risk of suicide in the elderly. *Archives of Internal Medicine, 164*(11), 1179–1184.

Kessing, L. V. (2004). Severity of depressive episodes according to ICD-10: Prediction of risk of relapse and suicide. *British Journal of Psychiatry, 184*(2), 153–156.

Klomek, A. B., Kleinman, M., Altschuler, E., Marrocco, F., Amakawa, L., & Gould, M. S. (2013). Suicidal adolescents' experiences with bullying perpetration and victimization during high school as risk factors for later depression and suicidality. *Journal of Adolescent Health, 53*(1, Suppl.), S37–42.

Knox, K. L., Stanley, B., Currier, G. W., Brenner, L., Gharamanlou-Holloway, M., & Brown, G. (2012). An emergency department-based brief intervention for veterans at risk for suicide (SAFE VET). *American Journal of Public Health, 102*(Suppl. 1), S33–37.

Koons, C. R., Robins, C. J., Tweed, J. L., Lynch, T. R., Gonzalez, A. M., Morse, J. Q., et al. (2001). Efficacy of dialectical behavior therapy in women veterans with borderline personality disorder. *Behavior Therapy, 32*, 371–390.

Kraemer, G. W., Schmidt, D. E., & Ebert, M. H. (1997). The behavioral neurobiology of self-injurious behavior in rhesus monkeys: Current concepts and relations to impulsive behavior in humans. *Annals of the New York Academy of Science, 836*, 12–38.

Le-Niculescu, H., Levey, D. F., Ayalew, M., Palmer, L., Gavrin, L. M., Jain, N., et al. (2013). Discovery and validation of blood biomarkers for suicidality. *Molecular Psychiatry, 18*(12), 1249–1264.

Lesage, A. D., Boyer, R., Grunberg, F., Vanier, C., Morissette, R., Ménard-Buteau, C., et al. (1994). Suicide and mental disorders: A case-control study of young men. *American Journal of Psychiatry, 151*(7), 1063–1068.

Li, L. W., & Conwell, Y. (2010). Pain and self-injury ideation in elderly men and women receiving home care. *Journal of the American Geriatrics Society, 58*(11), 2160–2165.

Linehan, M. M. (1993a). *Cognitive-behavioral treatment of borderline personality disorder.* New York: Guilford Press.

Linehan, M. M. (1993b). *Skills training manual for treating borderline personality disorder.* New York, NY: Guilford Press.

Linehan, M. M., Comtois, K. A., Brown, M. Z., Heard, H. L., & Wagner, A. (2006). Suicide Attempt Self-Injury Interview (SASII): Development, reliability, and validity of a scale to assess suicide attempts and intentional self-injury. *Psychological Assessment, 18*(3), 303–312.

Linehan, M. M., Comtois, K. A., Murray, A. M., Brown, M. Z., Gallop, R. J., Heard, H. L., et al. (2006). Two-year randomized controlled trial and follow-up of dialectical behavior therapy vs. therapy by experts for suicidal behaviors and borderline personality disorder. *Archives of General Psychiatry, 63*(7), 757–766.

Logan, J., Skopp, N. A., Karch, D., Reger, M. A., & Gahm, G. A. (2012). Characteristics of suicides among U.S. army active duty personnel in 17 U.S. states from 2005 to 2007. *American Journal of Public Health, 102*(Suppl. 1), S40–44.

MacLeod, C., & Mathews, A. (2012). Cognitive bias modification approaches to anxiety. *Annual Review of Clinical Psychology, 8*, 189–217.

Mahon, M. J., Tobin, J. P., Cusack, D. A., Kelleher, C., & Malone, K. M. (2005). Suicide among regular-duty military personnel: A retrospective case-control study of occupation-specific risk factors for workplace suicide. *American Journal of Psychiatry, 162*(9), 1688–1696.

Malone, K. M., Haas, G. L., Sweeney, J. A., & Mann, J. J. (1995). Major depression and the risk of attempted suicide. *Journal of Affective Disorders, 34*(3), 173–185.

Mann, J. J., Currier, D., Stanley, B., Oquendo, M. A., Amsel, L. V., & Ellis, S. P. (2006). Can biological tests assist prediction of suicide in mood disorders? *International Journal of Neuropsychopharmacology, 9*(4), 465–474.

Mann, J. J., Waternaux, C., Haas, G. L., & Malone, K. M. (1999). Toward a clinical model of suicidal behavior in psychiatric patients. *American Journal of Psychiatry, 156*(2), 181–189.

Marshal, M. P., Dietz, L. J., Friedman, M. S., Stall, R., Smith, H. A., McGinley, J., et al. (2011). Suicidality and depression disparities between sexual minority and heterosexual youth: A meta-analytic review. *Journal of Adolescent Health, 49*(2), 115–123.

Marttunen, M. J., Aro, H. M., & Lönnqvist, J. K. (1993). Adolescence and suicide: A review of psychological autopsy studies. *European Child and Adolescent Psychiatry, 2*(1), 10–18.

McGirr, A., Renaud, J., Seguin, M., Alda, M., Benkelfat, C., Lesage, A., et al. (2007). An examination of DSM-IV depressive symptoms and risk for suicide completion in major depressive disorder: A psychological autopsy study. *Journal of Affective Disorders, 97*(1–3), 203–209.

Mee, S., Bunney, B. G., Bunney, W. E., Hetrick, W., Potkin, S. G., & Reist, C. (2011). Assessment of psychological pain in major depressive episodes. *Journal of Psychiatric Research, 45*(11), 1504–1510.

Mitchell, M. M., Gallaway, M. S., Millikan, A. M., & Bell, M. (2012). Interaction of combat exposure and unit cohesion in predicting suicide-related ideation among post-deployment soldiers. *Suicide and Life-Threatening Behavior, 42*(5), 486–494.

Moskos, M., Olson, L., Halbern, S., Keller, T., & Gray, D. (2005). Utah Youth Suicide Study: Psychological autopsy. *Suicide and Life-Threatening Behavior, 35*(5), 536–546.

Motto, J. A., & Bostrom, A. G. (2001). A randomized controlled trial of postcrisis suicide prevention. *Psychiatric Services, 52*(6), 828–833.

Mrazek, P. J., & Haggerty, R. J. (Eds.). (1994). *Reducing risks for mental disorders: Frontiers for prevention intervention research.* Washington, DC: National Academy Press.

Neshat-Doost, H. T., Dalgleish, T., Yule, W., Kalantari, M., Ahmadi, S. J., Dyregov, A., et al. (2013). Enhancing autobiographical memory specificity through cognitive training: An intervention for depression translated from basic science. *Clinical Psychological Science, 1*, 84–92.

Nock, M. K. (2010). Self-injury. *Annual Review of Clinical Psychology, 6*, 339–363.

Nock, M. K., Borges, G., Bromet, E. J., Alonso, J., Angermeyer, M., Beautrais, A., et al. (2008). Cross-national prevalence and risk factors for suicidal ideation, plans, and attempts in the WHO World Mental Health Surveys. *British Journal of Psychiatry, 192*, 98–105.

Nock, M. K., Borges, G., Bromet, E. J., Cha, C. B., Kessler, R. C., & Lee, S. (2008). Suicide and suicidal behavior. *Epidemiologic Reviews, 30*(1), 133–154.

Nock, M. K., Borges, G., & Ono, Y. (Eds.). (2012). *Suicide: Global perspectives from the WHO World Mental Health Surveys.* New York: Cambridge University Press.

Nock, M. K., Deming, C. A., Chiu, W. T., Hwang, I., Angermeyer, M., Borges, G., et al. (2012). Mental disorders, comorbidity, and suicidal behavior. In M. K. Nock, G. Borges, & Y. Ono (Eds.), *Suicide: Global perspectives from the WHO World Mental Health Surveys* (pp. 148–163). New York: Cambridge University Press.

Nock, M. K., Deming, C. A., Fullerton, C. S., Gilman, S. E., Goldenberg, M., Kessler, R. C., et al. (2013). Suicide among soldiers: A review of psychosocial risk and protective factors. *Psychiatry, 76*(2), 97–125.

Nock, M. K., Green, J. G., Hwang, I., McLaughlin, K. A., Sampson, N. A., Zaslavsky, A. M., et al. (2013). Prevalence, correlates, and treatment of lifetime suicidal behavior among adolescents: Results from the National Comorbidity Survey Replication Adolescent Supplement. *Journal of the American Medical Association Psychiatry, 70*(3), 300–310.

Nock, M. K., Holmberg, E. B., Photos, V. I., & Michel, B. D. (2007). Self-Injurious Thoughts and Behaviors Interview: Development, reliability, and validity in an adolescent sample. *Psychological Assessment, 19*(3), 309–317.

Nock, M. K., Hwang, I., Sampson, N., Kessler, R. C., Angermeyer, M., Beautrais, A., et al. (2009). Cross-national analysis of the associations among mental disorders and suicidal behavior: Findings from the WHO World Mental Health Surveys. *PLoS Medicine, 6*(8), e1000123.

Nock, M. K., Hwang, I., Sampson, N. A., & Kessler, R. C. (2010). Mental disorders, comorbidity, and suicidal behaviors: Results from the National Comorbidity Survey Replication. *Molecular Psychiatry, 15*(8), 868–876.

Nock, M. K., Park, J. M., Finn, C. T., Deliberto, T. L., Dour, H. J., & Banaji, M. R. (2010). Measuring the suicidal mind: Implicit cognition predicts suicidal behavior. *Psychological Science, 21*(4), 511–517.

Nock, M. K., Prinstein, M. J., & Sterba, S. K. (2009). Revealing the form and function of self-injurious thoughts and behaviors: A real-time ecological assessment study among adolescents and young adults. *Journal of Abnormal Psychology, 118*(4), 816–827.

Nordentoft, M., Mortensen, P. B., & Pedersen, C. B. (2011). Absolute risk of suicide after first hospital contact in mental disorder. *Archives of General Psychiatry, 68*(10), 1058–1064.

Nrugham, L., Holen, A., & Sund, A. M. (2012). Suicide attempters and repeaters. *Journal of Nervous and Mental Disease, 200*(3), 197–203.

Oquendo, M. A., Galfalvy, H., Russo, S., Ellis, S. P., Grunebaum, M. F., Burke, A., et al. (2004). Prospective study of clinical predictors of suicidal acts after a major depressive episode in patients with major depressive disorder or bipolar disorder. *American Journal of Psychiatry, 161*(8), 1433–1441.

Park, C. L., Cohen, L. H., & Murch, R. L. (1996). Assessment and prediction of stress-related growth. *Journal of Personality, 64*(1), 71–105.

Petridou, E., Papadopoulos, F. C., Frangakis, C. E., Skalkidou, A., & Trichopoulos, D. (2002). A role of sunshine in the triggering of suicide. *Epidemiology, 13*(1), 106–109.

Phillips, M. R., Yang, G., Zhang, Y., Wang, L., Ji, H., & Zhou, M. (2002). Risk factors for suicide in China: A national case-control psychological autopsy study. *Lancet, 360*, 1728–1736.

Pistorello, J., Fruzzetti, A. E., MacLane, C., Gallop, R., & Iverson, K. M. (2012). Dialectical behavior therapy (DBT) applied to college students: A randomized clinical trial. *Journal of Consulting and Clinical Psychology, 80*(6), 982–994.

Plener, P. L., Libal, G., & Nixon, M. K. (2009). Use of medication in the treatment of nonsuicidal self-injury in youth. In M. K. Nixon & N. L. Heath (Eds.), *Self-injury in youth: The essential guide to intervention and assessment* (pp. 275–308). New York: Routledge.

Prinstein, M. J., Heilbron, N., Guerry, J. D., Franklin, J. C., Rancourt, D., Simon, V., et al. (2010). Peer influence and nonsuicidal self-injury: Longitudinal results in community and clinically referred adolescent samples. *Journal of Abnormal Child Psychology, 38*(5), 669–682.

Qin, P., & Nordentoft, M. (2005). Suicide risk in relation to psychiatric hospitalization: Evidence based on longitudinal registers. *Archives of General Psychiatry, 62*(4), 427–432.

Raj, A. J., Kumaraiah, V., & Bhide, A. V. (2001). Cognitive-behavioral intervention in deliberate self-harm. *Acta Psychiatrica Scandinavica, 104*(5), 340–345.

Reynolds, W. M. (1987). *Suicidal Ideation Questionnaire: Professional Manual*. Lutz, FL: Psychological Assessment Resources.

Ribeiro, J. D., Pease, J. L., Gutierrez, P. M., Silva, C., Bernert, R. A., Rudd, M. D., et al. (2012). Sleep problems outperform depression and hopelessness as cross-sectional and longitudinal predictors of suicidal ideation and behavior in young adults in the military. *Journal of Affective Disorders, 136*(3), 743–750.

Roy, A. (1993). Features associated with suicide attempts in depression: A partial replication. *Journal of Affective Disorders, 27*(1), 35–38.

Roy-Byrne, P. P., Post, R. M., Hambrick, D. D., Leverich, G. S., & Rosoff, A. S. (1988). Suicide and course of illness in major affective disorder. *Journal of Affective Disorders, 15*(1), 1–8.

Sakinofsky, I. (2007). Treating suicidality in depressive illness: Part 2. Does treatment cure or cause suicidality? *Canadian Journal of Psychiatry, 52*(6, Suppl. 1), 85S–101S.

Scott, K. M., Hwang, I., Chiu, W. T., Kessler, R. C., Sampson, N. A., Angermeyer, M., et al. (2010). Chronic physical conditions and their association with first onset of suicidal behavior in the World Mental Health Surveys. *Psychosomatic Medicine, 72*(7), 712–719.

Shneidman, E. S. (1993). Suicide as psychache. *Journal of Nervous and Mental Disorders, 181*(3), 145–147.

Shneidman, E. S. (1996). *The suicidal mind*. New York: Oxford University Press.

Silverman, M. M., Berman, A. L., Sanddal, N. D., O'Carroll, P. W., & Joiner, T. E. (2007a). Rebuilding the tower of Babel: A revised nomenclature for the study of suicide and suicidal behaviors: Part 1. Background, rationale, and methodology. *Suicide and Life-Threatening Behavior, 37*(3), 248–263.

Silverman, M. M., Berman, A. L., Sanddal, N. D., O'Carroll, P. W., & Joiner, T. E. (2007b). Rebuilding the tower of Babel: A revised nomenclature for the study of suicide and suicidal behaviors: Part 2. Suicide-related ideations, communications, and behaviors. *Suicide and Life-Threatening Behavior, 37*(3), 264–277.

Simpson, G., & Tate, R. (2002). Suicidality after traumatic brain injury: Demographic, injury and clinical correlates. *Psychological Medicine, 32*(4), 687–697.

Slee, N., Garnefski, N., van der Leeden, R., Arensman, E., & Spinhoven, P. (2008). Cognitive-behavioural intervention for self-harm: Randomised controlled trial. *British Journal of Psychiatry, 192*(3), 202–211.

Smith, J. M., Alloy, L. B., & Abramson, L. Y. (2006). Cognitive vulnerability to depression, rumination, hopelessness, and suicidal ideation: Multiple pathways to self-injurious thinking. *Suicide and Life-Threatening Behavior, 36*(4), 443–454.

Stanley, B., & Brown, G. K. (2012). Safety planning intervention: A brief intervention to mitigate suicide risk. *Cognitive and Behavioral Practice, 19*(2), 256–264.

Stein, D. J., Chiu, W. T., Hwang, I., Kessler, R. C., Sampson, N., Alonso, J., et al. (2010). Cross-national analysis of the associations between traumatic events and suicidal behavior: Findings from the WHO World Mental Health Surveys. *PLoS One, 5*(5), e10574.

Swanson, S. A., & Colman, I. (2013). Association between exposure to suicide and suicidality outcomes in youth. *Canadian Medical Association Journal, 185*, 870–877.

Tang, T. C., Jou, S. H., Ko, C. H., Huang, S. Y., & Yen, C. F. (2009). Randomized study of school-based intensive interpersonal psychotherapy for depressed adolescents with suicidal risk and parasuicide behaviors. *Psychiatry and Clinical Neurosciences, 63*(4), 463–470.

Teasdale, T. W., & Engberg, A. W. (2001). Suicide after traumatic brain injury: A population study. *Journal of Neurology, Neurosurgery, and Psychiatry, 71*(4), 436–440.

Thase, M. E., Greenhouse, J. B., Frank, E., Reynolds, C. F., III, Pilkonis, P. A., Hurley, K., et al. (1997). Treatment of major depression with psychotherapy or psychotherapy–pharmacotherapy combinations. *Archives of General Psychiatry, 54*(11), 1009–1015.

Townsend, E., Hawton, K., Altman, D. G., Arensman, E., Gunnell, D., Hazell, P., et al. (2001). The efficacy of problem-solving treatments after deliberate self-harm: Meta-analysis of randomized controlled trials with respect to depression, hopelessness and improvement in problems. *Psychological Medicine, 31*(6), 979–988.

Tsoh, J., Chiu, H. F., Duberstein, P. R., Chan, S. S., Chi, I., Yip, P. S., et al. (2005). Attempted suicide in elderly Chinese persons: A multi-group, controlled study. *American Journal of Geriatric Psychiatry, 13*(7), 562–571.

Turner, R. M. (2000). Naturalistic evaluation of dialectical behavior therapy-oriented treatment for borderline personality disorder. *Cognitive and Behavioral Practice, 7*(4), 413–419.

Vaiva, G., Ducrocq, F., Meyer, P., Mathieu, D., Philippe, A., Libersa, C., et al. (2006). Effect of telephone contact on further suicide attempts in patients discharged from an emergency department: Randomised controlled study. *British Medical Journal, 332,* 1241–1245.

Van Orden, K., & Conwell, Y. (2011). Suicides in late life. *Current Psychiatry Reports, 13*(3), 234–241.

Vieta, E., Nieto, E., Gastó, C., & Cirera, E. (1992). Serious suicide attempts in affective patients. *Journal of Affective Disorders, 24*(3), 147–152.

Vijayakumar, L., & Rajkumar, S. (1999). Are risk factors for suicide universal?: A case-control study in India. *Acta Psychiatrica Scandinavica, 99*(6), 407–411.

von Wolff, A., Hölzel, L. P., Westphal, A., Härter, M., & Kriston, L. (2012). Combination of pharmacotherapy and psychotherapy in the treatment of chronic depression: A systematic review and meta-analysis. *BMC Psychiatry, 12*(1), 61.

Wenzel, A., Berchick, E. R., Tenhave, T., Halberstadt, S., Brown, G. K., & Beck, A. T. (2011). Predictors of suicide relative to other deaths in patients with suicide attempts and suicide ideation: A 30-year prospective study. *Journal of Affective Disorders, 132*(3), 375–382.

Wilkinson, P., Kelvin, R., Roberts, C., Dubicka, B., & Goodyer, I. (2011). Clinical and psychosocial predictors of suicide attempts and nonsuicidal self-injury in the Adolescent Depression Antidepressants and Psychotherapy Trial (ADAPT). *American Journal of Psychiatry, 168*(5), 495–501.

Wood, A., Trainor, G., Rothwell, J., Moore, A., & Harrington, R. (2001). Randomized trial of group therapy for repeated deliberate self-harm in adolescents. *Journal of the American Academy of Child and Adolescent Psychiatry, 40*(11), 1246–1253.

Yen, S., Pagano, M. E., Shea, M. T., Grilo, C. M., Gunderson, J. G., Skodol, A. E., et al. (2005). Recent life events preceding suicide attempts in a personality disorder sample: Findings from the collaborative longitudinal personality disorders study. *Journal of Consulting and Clinical Psychology, 73*(1), 99–105.

Young, M. A., Fogg, L. F., Scheftner, W., Fawcett, J., Akiskal, H., & Maser, J. (1996). Stable trait components of hopelessness: Baseline and sensitivity to depression. *Journal of Abnormal Psychology, 105*(2), 155–165.

Zonda, T. (2006). One hundred cases of suicide in Budapest. *Crisis: The Journal of Crisis Intervention and Suicide Prevention, 27*(3), 125–129.

PART IV

PREVENTION AND TREATMENT OF DEPRESSION

In recent years there have been significant developments in interventions for depression. This section includes six chapters that review the methods and evidence for the effectiveness of both prevention and treatment efforts. Importantly, these treatment chapters provide not only clinically useful guidelines for patient care but also state-of-the-art evaluations of the empirical status of interventions for major depressive disorder (MDD). Muñoz, Schueller, Barrera, Le, and Torres (Chapter 25) discuss prevention, its importance, and the diverse ways in which investigators have attempted to prevent development of depression or to reduce its impact in adults and children. Among typical treatments, pharmacotherapy is the most widely disseminated approach; in this context, both standard and innovative approaches to acute, continuation, and maintenance treatment are discussed by Gitlin (Chapter 26). Three of the most effective and well-validated psychotherapies for depression and bipolar disorder are discussed by authors who have contributed to its development and empirical evaluation. Cognitive-behavioral treatment is presented and reviewed by Hollon and Dimidjian (Chapter 27). Miklowitz (Chapter 28) reviews the literature on pharmacological and psychosocial interventions for bipolar disorder. Marital and family therapies, as well as interpersonal psychotherapy for depression, are discussed by Beach, Whisman, and Bodenmann (Chapter 29). Finally, Kaslow, Petersen-Coleman, and Alexander (Chapter 30) review the unique issues and methods applied to the treatment of depression in children and adolescents.

CHAPTER 25

Major Depression
Can Be Prevented
Implications for Research and Practice

RICARDO F. MUÑOZ, STEPHEN M. SCHUELLER,
ALINNE Z. BARRERA, HUYNH-NHU LE, *and* LEANDRO D. TORRES

In a recent article, "Major Depression Can Be Prevented," Muñoz, Beardslee, and Leykin (2012) argued that, as of the beginning of the 21st century, the preponderance of the research evidence indicates that major depressive episodes (MDE) can be prevented (Mrazek & Haggerty, 1994; Muñoz, Cuijpers, Smit, Barrera, & Leykin, 2010; O'Connell, Boat, & Warner, 2009). This is a major shift from the late 20th century, during which publications from the National Institute of Mental Health (NIMH) stated that "the onset of major depression cannot be prevented" (Lobel & Hirschfeld, 1984, p. 4). In this chapter, we discuss the meaning of the statement "major depression can be prevented"; argue that, with current knowledge, the goal of preventing 50% of new MDEs is feasible; and invite mental health professionals to consider the implications for research and practice.

Depression is a major public health problem. In the United States, 17% of adults experience at least one episode of major depression during their lives (Kessler et al., Chapter 1, this volume). The World Health Organization (WHO) reports that major depression is the number one cause of disability in the world, had the fourth highest impact of any disorder in 1990, and will come to have the second highest impact of any disorder by the year 2020 in terms of the burden of disease in the world, taking into account both disability and mortality (Murray & Lopez, 1996). For an epidemic of this scale, treatment is not enough (Le, Muñoz, Ippen, & Stoddard, 2003); it is necessary to dedicate a substantial portion of our resources to prevention (Albee, 1985).

Currently, most mental health resources are dedicated to treatment. In the case of major depression, however, treatment has serious limitations. It reaches very few and especially overlooks minorities: African American and Latino adults with depression are often less likely to use outpatient mental health services than are non-Hispanic whites (Hough et al., 1987; Ojeda & McGuire, 2006). Treatment is effective in only about two-thirds of those who adhere to treatment as directed (most do not; Depression Guideline Panel, 1993). Thus when we make the often-heard statement that "depression is a treatable disorder," we mean that most cases of major depression respond to psychological or pharmacological treatments.

Similarly, when we state that depression can be prevented, we mean that a substantial proportion of new episodes can be averted if we provide currently known interventions to those at risk. Many of the comparisons from published randomized controlled trials (RCTs) have yielded reductions in incidence greater than 50% (15 out of 42, or 36%); an additional 11 out of 42, or 26%, comparisons have yielded incidence reductions between 25 and 49%. Given that, even when treatment is effective, the chances of a recurrence of an MDE are 50% after one episode, 70% after two episodes, and 90% after three episodes (Judd, 1997), it is clear that preventing new episodes of major depression is essential. The ideal, of course, would be to prevent the first episode.

DELINEATING THE SCOPE OF PREVENTIVE INTERVENTIONS: THE INSTITUTE OF MEDICINE REPORT ON PREVENTING MENTAL DISORDERS

The Institute of Medicine (IOM) Report on Preventing Mental Disorders (Mrazek & Haggerty, 1994) was a spirited call for increased research on preventive interventions. The traditional, three-level public health definitions (primary, secondary, and tertiary prevention) were considered by the IOM Committee to confuse prevention and treatment. Therefore, the Committee proposed a more categorical definition (see Mrazek & Haggerty, 1994, Figure 2.1, p. 23): *Prevention* refers to interventions that occur *before the onset* of a disorder and that are designed to prevent its occurrence. *Treatment* refers to interventions that occur after onset and that are designed to bring a quick end to the clinical episode. *Maintenance* refers to interventions that occur after the acute episode has abated, in order to reduce likelihood of relapse, recurrence, or disability in patients who have received treatment. Within prevention, three sublevels were defined: *universal* (delivered widely regardless of risk), *selective* (targeted at individuals or groups who demonstrate a higher than average risk), and *indicated* (targeted at high-risk individuals with early signs or symptoms of a disorder; Mrazek & Haggerty, 1994).

In this chapter, we adhere to the IOM definitions. Specifically, we review RCTs designed to prevent MDEs—those trials that recruit participants who do not meet criteria for MDEs upon entry into the trial and that specifically compare rates of incidence in the experimental and comparison or control conditions. The outcome of interest is whether interventions result in significantly lower rates of new MDEs. We consider studies of both high-risk individuals identified in nonclinical settings (i.e., in an attempt to prevent the onset of major depression), and individuals with past major depression who have recovered for a long enough period (e.g., more than 8 weeks below criteria for full remission; Frank et al., 1991; Rush et al., 2006) that the MDE would be considered the onset of a new episode.

Many "prevention investigations" study the feasibility of reducing depressive symptoms in at-risk populations with the explicit or implicit expectation that doing so will eventually reduce incidence of MDEs. Although these are important studies, this chapter excludes those focused only on symptom reduction, as this may or may not lead to reduction in incidence (for a detailed discussion of studies focused on reducing depressive symptoms, see Barrera, Torres, & Muñoz, 2007; Muñoz, Le, Clarke, & Jaycox, 2002).

SPECIAL ISSUES INVOLVED IN PREVENTION RESEARCH

In treatment research trials, all participants meet diagnostic criteria for the disorder being treated. They either volunteer for treatment trials or seek psychological services and are thus fairly motivated for treatment. In contrast, participants in prevention trials, by definition, are not currently experiencing the disorder to be prevented. Thus, as part of outreach, it is crucial to provide a convincing rationale for attending the intervention, using the methods taught, and completing assessments over an extended period of time. This generally requires added attention to issues of recruitment and retention—particularly for minority groups, who heavily underutilize treatment services (Alegría et al., 2007). Therefore, providing preventive services that are accessible and acceptable to such groups is especially important. In addition, because individuals recovered from an MDE are at high risk for recurrence, they are a reasonable group to target for prevention of new episodes. For further discussions of issues in prevention research, see Muñoz and Ying (1993).

EMPIRICALLY TESTED
PREVENTIVE INTERVENTIONS THROUGH THE LIFE CYCLE

We now address three stages in the life cycle: adulthood, the school years, and the beginning of life. We begin with adulthood because the first depression prevention trials were conducted with adults and gradually moved to younger groups.

Preventing Depression in Adulthood

Strategies to prevent depression have often been developed from those used in the treatment of depression. We have much evidence that mood regulation skills are as effective as antidepressants in treating major depression and reducing the likelihood of relapse/recurrence (Segal et al., 2010; Teasdale et al., 2000). Why wait until someone is suffering from clinical depression to teach him or her these methods? The idea is logical, but is it practical? If we do not want to wait until people are sufficiently depressed to have to come to a mental health professional, how do we reach them ahead of time?

Randomized Trials Designed to Prevent MDEs

The San Francisco Depression Prevention Research Project, conducted from 1983 to 1986, was the first RCT intended to test whether new clinical episodes of major depression could be prevented (Muñoz & Ying, 1993; Muñoz, Ying, Armas, Chan, & Gurza, 1987). Participants were 150 English- and Spanish-speaking, predominantly minority primary care patients without any psychiatric disorder. Those in the intervention condition received 8 weekly group sessions of the Depression Prevention Course (Muñoz, 1984), a cognitive-behavioral approach grounded in social learning theory. Compared with control participants, participants in the intervention condition reported significantly lower depressive symptoms measured by the Beck Depression Inventory (BDI), but not by the Center for Epidemiologic Studies—Depression Scale (CES-D). At a 1-year follow-up, the reduction in incidence was in the expected direction (four cases in the control group and two in the experimental condition); however, given the low incidence, this difference was not statistically significant.

Other early trials focused on preventing depression in adults often recruited college students (e.g., Apex Project; Gillham et al., 1991), a group in transition and thus prone to depression. Recent trials, however, have expanded recruitment and dissemination, using Internet websites (Morgan, Jorm, & Mackinnon, 2012; O'Kearney, Kang, Christensen, & Griffiths, 2006) and recruiting from residential homes (Dozeman et al., 2012) and clinical settings (Godfrin & van Heeringen, 2010) to reach individuals in need. Results of preventive interventions with adults are mixed; some find little reduction in incidence (e.g., Seligman, Schulman, DeRubeis, & Hollon, 1999), whereas others produce significant reductions (e.g., Dozeman et al., 2012).

In summary, preventive interventions for adults are promising but do not consistently yield significant reductions in the incidence of MDEs. We discuss efforts to increase the potency of preventive interventions later in this chapter, but identifying groups with higher incidence is merited. It is also important to ask whether intervening earlier might be preferable. In the next section we focus on interventions for children in school.

Interventions during the School Years

Late childhood or early adolescence may be a particularly fruitful period for preventive efforts. Depression rates rise in early adolescence, especially for girls (Birmaher et al., 1996), with older adolescents reporting rates of depression close to those seen in adults (Lewinsohn, Hops, Roberts, Seeley, & Andrews, 1993). By age 18, as many as 20% of all adolescents will have experienced at least one MDE (Lewinsohn et al., 1993), which increases the risk of repeated episodes later in life (Lewinsohn, Rohde, Klein, & Seeley, 1999). Thus the school years are an important period for reducing depression risk (Horowitz & Garber, 2006; Merry, McDowell, Hetrick, Bir, & Muller, 2006). Despite this need, to date, studies focused on preventing MDEs during this period have been published only for adolescents, not grammar school children. Instead, programs for grammar school children have assessed only changes in depressive symptoms and not incidence of MDEs, and thus they are not included in our review.

Preventing Depression during Adolescence

PREVENTION IN YOUTH WITH ELEVATED SUBDIAGNOSTIC
DEPRESSIVE SYMPTOMS

Stice and colleagues examined the efficacy of a 6-session cognitive-behavioral (CB) intervention among high-risk (CES-D > 20) high school students. Students were randomized to one of four conditions: a CB group, a supportive–expressive group, bibliotherapy, or an assessment-only control. Compared with the control condition, a lower risk for MDE at the 6-month follow-up was found for the treatment conditions (Stice, Rohde, Seeley, & Gau, 2008), and at the 2-year follow-up for CB and bibliotherapy (Stice, Rohde, Gau, & Wade, 2010).

Clarke and colleagues (1995) identified youth with elevated symptoms (above the 75th percentile) using the CES-D. These youth ($n = 1,652$) were randomly assigned to either a 15-session cognitive group prevention intervention, focused on teaching adolescents to identify and challenge irrational and negative thoughts, or a usual-care control condition. Participants in the prevention condition reported significantly lower total incidence of MDEs over the follow-up period.

The Penn Resiliency Program (PRP) is a CB group intervention often delivered in school settings (Brunwasser, Gillham, & Kim, 2009), although it has also been used in primary care (Gillham, Hamilton, Freres, Patton, & Gallop, 2006). A meta-analysis of the impact of the PRP on preventing depression showed limited support, although it was effective in reducing depressive symptoms (Brunwasser et al., 2009). Similarly, two other large-scale school-based indicated prevention trials failed to reduce the incidence of MDE. The first trial examined a CB and problem-solving teacher-led intervention versus a monitoring control condition in high-risk youth (Spence, Sheffield, & Donovan, 2003). At 12 months the intervention group had a nonsignificantly lower incidence of MDE, but by the 4-year follow-up, 25% of all participants reported a depressive episode (Spence, Sheffield, & Donovan, 2005). The authors later examined a universal, indicated, and combined universal-indicated CB intervention approach in a sample of 13- to 15-year-old youth from 36 schools (Sheffield et al., 2006). Students with high symptoms ($n = 521$) were randomized to one of four conditions; the investigators found no significant group differences in MDE incidence over an 18-month period.

Young, Mufson, and Davies (2006) found a significant prevention effect throughout a 6-month follow-up when comparing a modified skills-training version of an interpersonal psychotherapy (IPT) group intervention for adolescents (IPT-A; Mufson, Gallagher, Dorta, & Young, 2004) to school counseling in a sample of inner-city adolescents with elevated depressive symptoms: 3.7% of the adolescents in the intervention ($n = 27$) reported a depression diagnosis compared with 28.6% of the comparison group ($n = 14$).

PREVENTION IN YOUTH WITH PARENTS WITH DEPRESSION

Promising results are available for prevention programs with adolescent children of parents with depression. ADAPT (Acceptance, Distraction, Activities, and Positive Thinking) is a 12-session family-group CB (FGCB) selective preventive intervention for children and parents (Compas et al., 2009) that focuses on teaching parenting skills, information about depressive disorders, and how to cope with the stressors associated with parental depression. The investigators randomized 111 families to either FGCB or a written information condition. Compas and colleagues (2011) found a lower incidence of MDE in offspring in FGCB from entry to 12- and 24-month follow-ups.

Clarke and colleagues (2001) recruited adults being treated for depression with offspring 13–18 years of age. Youth with subdiagnostic depressive symptoms or a past MDE were randomized to a 15-session group prevention program using cognitive therapy (CT) methods or usual health maintenance organization (HMO) care. Survival analyses indicated a significantly lower incidence of MDEs for the group CT condition than the usual-care control condition at 14-month follow-up. Garber and colleagues (2009) were interested in assessing the generalizability of these findings in a four-city, multicenter RCT with 13- to 17-year-old adolescent offspring of parent/caretakers with a current or past history of depression. Adolescents had reported high levels of depressive symptoms (CES-D > 20), had previously met criteria for an MDE, or both. Intent-to-treat analysis revealed a lower incidence of MDE at the 9-month follow-up for adolescents who received CT versus usual care.

Preventing Depression during the Prenatal and Perinatal Periods and Early Childhood

Many sequelae of maternal depression and other risk factors are already present before children begin school (O'Hara & Swain, 1996). Ideally, one would begin before birth, or even before conception. We now turn to work that focuses on the beginning of life.

INCIDENCE AND PREVALENCE OF MAJOR DEPRESSION
IN THE PRESCHOOL YEARS

The incidence of major depression for children younger than age 6 is not known (Luby, 2000). To understand the development of emotion dysregulation processes during early childhood, investigators have studied infants and children of parents with depression and the parents themselves (with a majority of these studies focusing on mothers; for reviews, see Le & Boyd, 2006; Gotlib & Colich, Chapter 13, this volume). Much of this research has documented that maternal (mostly postpartum) depression has detrimental consequences for the mother, her child (both during development and as he or she ages), and the quality of the mother–infant relationship (Weissman et al., 2006). Thus the focus of prevention of depression should begin with mothers-to-be with the goal of conferring benefits to the child.

PREVENTION OF MDEs
DURING THE PERINATAL PERIOD

A growing number of rigorous studies have focused on preventing perinatal depression. Brugha, Morrell, Slade, and Walters (2011) conducted a universal preventive intervention in the United Kingdom in which 101 primary care practices (clusters) were randomized to receive the intervention or care as usual. The intervention involved a health visitor trained to provide up to eight weekly individualized psychological (CB or person-centered therapy) sessions for low-risk postpartum women. At 6 and 12 months postpartum, women in the intervention group reported a lower significant incidence of depression than did those in the usual-care condition. These findings suggest that universal prevention can reduce the incidence of depression.

To date, 11 psychologically based RCTs have been conducted in women at high risk for depression. Despite varied approaches, all interventions generally included a psychoeducation component, teaching women about mood recognition and regulation and addressing the challenges of the transitional period. Austin (2003) reviewed five efficacy studies of prenatal interventions aimed at preventing postpartum depression (PPD) in high-risk women (Brugha et al., 2000; Buist, Westley, & Hill, 1999; Elliott et al., 2000; Stamp, Williams, & Crowther, 1995; Zlotnick, Johnson, Miller, Pearlstein, & Howard, 2001). Of the five studies, only two (Elliott et al., 2000; Zlotnick et al., 2001) reported significant results. Specifically, Elliott and colleagues (2000) reported that participating in an 11-session psychoeducational group significantly reduced PPD in first-time mothers from 39% in the control condition to 19% in the intervention. Zlotnick and colleagues (2001, 2006) found a similar effect using two brief interventions based on an IPT approach. An initial investigation of a small sample of at-risk pregnant women found that the intervention reduced PPD from 33% in the usual-care condition to 0% (Zlotnick et al., 2001), whereas a larger investigation found reductions from 20% in the control group to 4% in the intervention group (Zlotnick et al., 2006).

Muñoz and colleagues (2007) conducted a pilot RCT to evaluate the Mothers and Babies (MB) course, a 12-week CB group intervention conducted during pregnancy with 4 individual booster sessions in the first year postpartum in low-income, predominantly Mexican, women at high risk for PPD. Results at 1 year postpartum were not significant, although fewer women in the intervention (14%) developed MDEs compared with usual care (25%), with no differences in levels of depressive symptoms. Two additional RCTs have been conducted using modified versions of the MB course. First, Le, Perry, and

Stuart (2011) evaluated an 8-week group MB course[1] during pregnancy and three individual booster sessions in the first year postpartum in predominantly Central American at-risk pregnant women. Results indicate that intervention participants had significantly lower levels of depression and fewer cases of moderate depression postintervention, but these differences disappeared at 12 months postpartum. The cumulative incidence of MDEs did not differ between groups at 12 months postpartum. Second, Tandon, Perry, Mendelson, Kemp, and Leis (2011) adapted the MB course for low-income African American pregnant women and mothers at risk for depression who were receiving services in home visitation programs. Women were randomized to either a 6-week group MB course with home visit reinforcement of materials or to usual care. At 3 months postintervention, intervention participants' depressive symptoms declined at a significantly greater rate than did those of the usual-care participants. In addition, the intervention group had a significantly lower MDE incidence than did the usual-care group at both 3 months (Tandon et al., 2011) and 6 months postintervention (Tandon, Leis, Mendelson, Perry, & Edwards, 2014). A pilot Web-adapted version of the MB is currently in progress.

Lara, Navarro, and Navarrete (2010) conducted the first preventive RCT in Mexico, evaluating an 8-week group psychoeducational intervention in at-risk pregnant women. Among completers, the incidence of PPD was significantly lower in the intervention group than in the usual-care group. However, differential attrition of the two groups (57.6% of the intervention group vs. 7.8% of the control group never attended) limits the interpretability of this result.

Chabrol and colleagues (2002) designed and tested an innovative two-stage prevention and treatment program for at-risk pregnant women in France. A one-session CB preventive intervention was delivered over 2–5 days postpartum in the hospital. Participants were screened again, and those reporting elevated depressive symptoms during weeks 4–6 postpartum were invited to participate in the treatment intervention—composed of five to eight 1-hour weekly home visits. The prevention intervention was effective in significantly reducing the incidence of *probable* depression.

Taken together, the preceding investigations provide encouraging but limited evidence that brief preventive interventions are effective in reducing the incidence of depression during the perinatal period. Some evidence supports the effectiveness of these interventions for ethnically diverse women who are at risk for depression. Clearly, more research is warranted to elucidate the active ingredients of effective interventions and evaluate their long-term impact.

PREVENTING DEPRESSION RELAPSE AND RECURRENCE

Although the risk of recurrence increases with each additional episode (Solomon et al., 2000), recurrence is not inevitable. Mounting evidence suggests that medical (Frank et al., 1990; Geddes, et al., 2003) or psychological (Beshai, Dobson, Bockting, & Quigley, 2011; Piet & Hougaard, 2011) treatment can protect against recurrence. Per the IOM framework, such interventions are considered *maintenance*. It is critical, however, to differentiate relapse and recurrence, two distinct but related concepts (Beshai et al., 2011). As defined by Frank and colleagues (1991), an MDE occurring *before* full recovery is a *relapse*, whereas if full recovery is achieved, an MDE is considered a *recurrence* of the disorder. Full recovery requires a minimum period of time (i.e., 8 weeks) during which

---

[1] See Le, Zmuda, Perry, and Muñoz (2010) for a description of their cultural adaptation process.

criteria for MDE are not met and an individual remains below a symptom threshold (e.g., Hamilton Rating Scale for Depression < 8). Per this distinction, "relapse prevention" may resolve a partially abated episode rather than preventing a new one. "Recurrence prevention" is consistent with the IOM concept of prevention. Thus we review evidence for preventive effects on *new episodes* after an index episode has resolved.

Maintenance antidepressant medication (m-ADM) is the primary recurrence prevention strategy in psychiatric practice (American Psychiatric Association, 2000). Although m-ADM can prevent recurrence by as much as 70% (Frank et al., 1990; Geddes et al., 2003), sustained use is required. When m-ADM is withdrawn, the risk of recurrence can increase by 11 times, with approximately 40% of patients experiencing a recurrence within 6 months (Hollon et al., 2005; Kupfer et al., 1992).

In contrast, some psychological treatments might prevent subsequent recurrence without continued support. In two trials, patients with a history of three or more prior MDEs were treated to full remission with ADM. After 3–5 months of ADM treatment, Fava, Rafanelli, Cazzaro, Conti, and Grandi (1998) randomized 40 patients to 20 weeks of ADM plus clinical management or cognitive therapy (CT) plus ADM tapered to discontinuation. MDE rates were lower for patients in the CT group compared with the control-group patients over 2-year (25% vs. 80%) and 6-year (40% vs. 90%) follow-ups (Fava et al., 1998, 2004). Segal and colleagues (2010) randomized patients (n = 160) to either m-ADM, mindfulness-based cognitive therapy (m-MBCT), or placebo (m-PLA) after first achieving at least 7 months of remission. For patients who experienced increases in symptoms above the remission threshold during the period between initial remission and randomization, 18-month MDE rates for m-MBCT (28%) and m-ADM (27%) were less than for m-PLA (71%), but did not differ from each other. For patients who achieved a stable remission (no such increases in symptoms in the period between initial remission and randomization), there was no difference between the treatments in relapse rates.

Three trials that recruited individuals who had already achieved remission with a history of two (Bockting et al., 2005; Teasdale et al., 2000) or three (Kuyken et al., 2008) prior episodes also suggested that psychological treatments can prevent recurrence. For 187 participants in remission (≥ 10 weeks), 8 weeks of group CT reduced MDE rates compared with treatment as usual (TAU) at both 2 and 5.5 years follow-up. Difference in outcome was dependent on the number of previous MDEs. At the 2-year follow-up, patients with five or more previous episodes who received CT reported lower rates of MDEs than those receiving TAU (46 vs. 72%; Bockting et al., 2005). This difference was much smaller and not significant for patients with fewer than five previous episodes (63% for CT vs. 59% for TAU). At the 5.5-year follow-up, for patients with four or more previous episodes, receiving CT was associated with a 20% reduction in rates of MDE (75% for CT vs. 95% for TAU; Bockting et al., 2009). Again, this difference was smaller for patients with a history of fewer episodes (fewer than four episodes, 82% for CT, 79% for TAU). For 145 patients in remission (≥ 12 weeks), MBCT reduced MDE rates over 60 weeks compared with TAU (37 vs. 66%), but only for the 77% of the sample who had experienced at least three prior episodes (Teasdale et al., 2000). No differences in MDE rates were found between MBCT and m-ADM over 15 months (47 vs. 60%) in 123 participants in full or partial remission who had been treated earlier with ADM (Kuyken et al., 2008). A fourth trial with 89 college students with past (37% having at least two MDEs) but not current MDD found lower MDE rates over 18 months (33 vs. 51%) with a hybrid IPT/CT group compared with an assessment control (Sheets et al., 2013).

Investigations of the prevention of recurrence require careful scrutiny. Results may confound prevention with initial treatment response (Hollon et al., 2005). Additionally, many studies do not specify criteria for remission/recovery, do not require it prior to randomization, or recruit individuals with partial remission rather than full recovery (e.g., Dobson et al., 2008; Godfrin & van Heeringen, 2010; Hollon et al, 2005; Jarrett et al., 1998; Vittengl, Clark, & Jarrett, 2009). Such studies may reflect treatment of a partially abated MDE rather than prevention per se. Trials that recruit patients who have already achieved remission may thus reflect effects on relapse, not recurrence. Prevention of recurrence, however, has been demonstrated for as long as 5.5 years (Bockting et al., 2009) and might be useful regardless of duration of the index episode (Teasdale et al., 2000). Prevention of recurrence might be most useful for individuals who have experienced more MDEs in their lives (i.e., those with at least three prior MDEs), with the strongest evidence obtained from patients who still experience residual (Fava et al., 1998, 2004) or transient symptoms (Segal et al., 2010) during remission.

EVIDENCE THAT MAJOR DEPRESSION CAN BE PREVENTED

Until recently, clinicians believed that depression could not be prevented, but we now know that it can (Muñoz et al., 2012). Indeed, meta-analyses indicate that prevention programs for depression are quite effective, with an average reduction in incidence of 22% (Cuijpers, van Straten, Smit, Mihalopoulus, & Beekman, 2008). Reduction in incidence is even higher for some methods. For example, the Coping with Depression course, a widely used prevention program aimed at increasing pleasant activities, thoughts, and interpersonal interactions, has produced average reductions in incidence of 38%. Indeed, one of the highest reductions in incidence (50%) from a single study was obtained in a recent trial that implemented a stepped-care format in older primary care patients (van't Veer-Tazelaar et al., 2009). Thus, currently, incidence in depression can be reduced by 22% on average and by as much as 38–50% using the most potent methods.

These values set the stage for a reasonable goal for depression prevention. We suggest that the field aim for 50% reduction in incidence as a feasible target with current methods. This goal seems feasible, as several trials have yielded 50% reductions in incidence. As an illustration, Table 25.1 presents comparisons from RCTs of preventive programs in order of incidence reduction. Future advances could increase this proportion even further.

How might we reach this 50% goal? The first step is to identify and learn from the best practices in prevention programs. What are some of the characteristics of interventions that have yielded prevention rates above this 50% cutoff? First, many of the interventions target groups in specific stages of the lifespan or in role transition (e.g., pregnant women, adolescents, or older adults). This is not surprising, as these groups are typical targets for selective prevention. Second, none of programs yielding the highest effectiveness results involved universal prevention. Again, this is not surprising, as universal programs will generally not have sufficient statistical power to test reductions in incidence given the low base rate in the general population (Muñoz et al., 2010). At present, therefore, to have a reasonable chance to demonstrate statistically significant effects, preventive programs need to target those at risk; thus there is a need for improved screening. Lastly, these interventions include personalization, such as stepped-care programs, that match the level of intervention to an individual's needs (e.g., Dozeman et al., 2012; van't Veer-Tazelaar et al., 2009), emphasizing the importance of addressing the needs of those targeted. Such targeting and matching might also increase motivation to participate and devote effort to the strategies learned.

TABLE 25.1. Reduction in Incidence in Randomized Trials of Depression Prevention, Sorted by Reduction in Incidence

Study	Type of prevention	Target population	Inclusion criteria	Incidence (%) Tx	Incidence (%) Co	Reduction/ increase in incidence
			Studies showing a reduction of 50% or more in incidence			
Konnert et al. (2009)	Indicated	Nursing home residents (60+)	No MDE, GDS ≥ 9	0	8.7	–100.0%
Martinovic et al. (2006)	Selective	Adolescents (13–19) with epilepsy	sD; no current DD	0	20	–100.0%
Zlotnick et al. (2001)	Selective	Pregnant women	At least one of four risk indicators of PPD, no current MDD	0	33	–100.0%
Arnarson & Craighead (2009)	Indicated	Adolescents	CDI = 7th–90th percentile of CASQ ≥ 75th percentile	1.6	13.3	–87.9%
Young et al. (2006)	Indicated	Adolescents (15–16)	CES-D ≥16; two symptoms; no current MDD/ DYS	3.7	28.6	–87.1%
Stice et al. (2010) (CB bibliotherapy)	Indicated	High school students	CES-D ≥ 20, no MDE	3	23	–87.0%
Zlotnick et al. (2006)	Selective	Pregnant women	High score on risk survey, no current MDD	4	20	–80.0%
Clarke et al. (2001)	Indicated	Adolescents (13–18)	CES-D > 24; ≥ 1 DSM-IV criterion; parent with MDD	9.3	28.8	–67.8%
Lara et al. (2010)	Indicated	Pregnant women	CES-D ≥ 16 and/or self-report hx of MDD	10.7	25	–57.2%
Compas et al. (2011)	Selected	Children of parents with depression	Parents with current of past MDD during the lifetime of child	14.3	32.7	–56.3%
Godfrin & van Heeringen (2010)	Selective	Outpatients with a history of MDDs	Three or more past MDDs, no MDD in past 8 weeks, HAM–D < 14	30	68.1	–55.9%
Tandon et al. (2014)	Selective	Pregnant women	No current MDD, risk defined as CES-D ≥ 16 or life hx of MDE	14.6	32.4	–54.9%
Dozeman et al. (2012)	Indicated	Older adults in residential home	CES-D ≥ 8, no current MDD	6.5	14.1	–53.9%

480

Study	Type	Population	Criteria			
Brugha et al. (2000)	Selective	Pregnant women	Positive screen on a screening questionnaire	3	6	−50.0%
van't Veer–Tazelaar et al. (2009)	Indicated	Older adults in primary care	No current MDE; CES-D ≥ 16	12	24	−50.0%
Studies showing a reduction of 25–49% or more in incidence						
Muñoz et al. (2007)	Indicated	Pregnant Latina women	CES-D ≥ 16; hx of MDD	14	25	−44.0%
Clarke et al. (1995)	Indicated	Adolescents (15–16)	CES-D ≥ 24; no current MDD/DYS	14.5	25.7	−43.6%
Gillham et al. (2006)	Indicated	Early adolescents (11–12)	CDI ≥ 7/9; no current MDD/DYS	21	36	−41.7%
Muñoz et al. (1995)	Selective	General medical patients (minority; chronically ill)	No MDD in past 6 months	3	5	−40.0%
Stice et al. (2010) (group CB)	Indicated	High school students	CES-D ≥ 20, no MDE	14	23	−39.1%
Stice et al. (2010) (group supportive expressive)	Indicated	High school students	CES-D ≥ 20, no MDE	15	23	−34.8%
Garber et al. (2009)	Indicated	Adolescents (13–17) or parents with depression	Parent: hx of MDE; Adolescent: CES-D > 20 or 2 months remission from MDE or both	21.4	32.7	−34.6%
Willemse et al. (2004)	Indicated	Adults (16–85)	One MDD core symptom, no MDD in past 6 months	12	18	−33.3%
Dennis et al. (2009)	Indicated	New mothers (2 weeks postpartum)	High-risk mothers (EPDS > 9)	5	7	−28.6%
Robinson et al. (2008)	Selective	Poststroke patients	No current DD (major or minor), HAM-D < 11	25	35	−28.6%
Morgan et al. (2012)	Indicated	Internet-based recruitment using paid advertising and targeted advertising	Two to four symptoms on PHQ-9, no current MDD and not currently in depression treatment	12.7	16.8	−24.4%

(continued)

TABLE 25.1. (continued)

Study	Type of prevention	Target population	Inclusion criteria	Incidence (%) Tx	Incidence (%) Co	Reduction/increase in incidence
			Studies showing a reduction of less than 25% in incidence			
Le et al. (2011)	Indicated	Pregnant Latina women	CES-D ≥ 16; life or family hx of MDD	7.8	9.6	−18.8%
Compas et al. (2011)	Indicated	Parents with a history of depression	Current or past MDD during the lifetime of child	55.0	66.7	−17.5%
Seligman et al. (1999)	Selective	Undergraduate students	ASQ = bottom quartile, no current MDD	40	48	−16.7%
Robinson et al. (2008)	Selective	Poststroke patients	No current DD (major or minor), HAM–D < 11	31	35	−11.4%
Sheffield et al. (2006)	Universal	All students of 36 schools	High-symptom students (top 20% of CDI and CES-D), no current MDD/DYS	18	20	−10.0%
Sheffield et al. (2006)	Universal, indicated	All students of 36 schools	High-symptom students (top 20% of CDI and CES-D), no current MDD/DYS	18	20	−10.0%
Austin et al. (2008)	Selective	Antenatal women	Risk for depression (EPDS > 10 and/or ANRQ > 23 or hx of DD)	20	21	−4.8%
Seligman, Schulman, & Tyron (2007)	Selective	Undergraduates	Mild to moderate depressive sx (BDI = 9–24)	26	27	−3.7%
Priest et al. (2003)	Selective	All women, after delivery	No other inclusion criteria	18	18	0.0%

482

Studies showing an increase in incidence

Sheffield et al. (2006)	Indicated	All students of 36 schools	High-symptom students (top 20% of CDI and CES-D), no current MDD/DYS	21	20	5.0%
Schueller et al. (2013) (low-risk group)	Selective	Smokers visiting an Internet site	No current MDD, low-risk group	11.6	10.8	7.4%
Vázquez et al. (2012)	Indicated	Undergraduates	CES-D ≥ 16	8.6	7.9	8.8%
Allart–van Dam et al. (2007)	Indicated	Adults with sD	BDI ≥ 10; no current MDD	27.3	25	9.2%
Hagan et al. (2004)	Selective	Mothers of very preterm babies	No current DD	29	26	11.5%
Schueller et al. (2013) (high-risk group)	Selective	Smokers visiting an Internet site	No current MDD, high-risk group defined as CES-D ≥ 16 or life hx of MDE	32.8	26.6	23.3%
Spence et al. (2003)	Universal	All students of 18 high schools	No specific inclusion criteria	10	8	25.0%

Note. ANRQ, Antenatal Risk Questionnaire; ASQ, Attributional Style Questionnaire; BDI, Beck Depression Inventory; CASQ, Children's Attributional Style Questionnaire; CDI, Children's Depression Inventory; CES-D, Center for Epidemiologic Studies Depression Scale; Co, control; DD, depressive disorder; DSM-IV, *Diagnostic and Statistical Manual of Mental Disorders,* fourth edition; DYS, dysthymia; EPDS, Edinburgh Postnatal Depression Scale; GDS, Geriatric Depression Scale; HAM-D, Hamilton Depression Rating Scale, 17-item; hx, history; MDD, major depressive disorder; MDE, major depressive episode; PHQ-9, Patient Health Questionnaire, nine-item; PPD, postpartum depression; sD, subthreshold depression; sx, symptoms; Tx, treatment.

Other important considerations for creating more effective prevention programs need resolution. For example, a meta-analysis of the PRP found that the program produced larger effect sizes when conducted by research team leaders than by community leaders. In addition, longer follow-ups often correspond to lower reductions in incidence (Stice et al., 2008, 2010). These findings, in combination with the difficulties in showing statistically significant effects for universal prevention, bring up critical questions regarding program dissemination and implementation. Preventing 50% of depression cases is an ambitious goal that will require further research and creative applications. We next expand on recommendations for future work.

RECOMMENDATIONS FOR FUTURE RESEARCH AND PRACTICE

In summary, we have identified 35 published RCTs (with 42 comparisons) that test whether interventions reduced the incidence of MDEs. The state of the science as of 2013 is encouraging: 15 out of 42 trials (40%) have reported reductions of 50% or more in incidence of MDEs, and 10 out of 35 trials (29%) have reported reductions of 25–49%. Successful trials generally identify populations at risk for a high incidence of MDEs and provide interventions, such as IPT and CT approaches, that have been shown to be effective in the treatment of MDEs.

Following are three recommendations to further enhance research in the prevention of depression.

1. Future studies should utilize methods that (a) have successfully identified participants at high imminent risk of MDE; (b) provide a standardized measurement of new MDEs; and (c) use a sufficiently long follow-up period (at least 1 year) to provide reasonable tests of prevention. Studies should test specific, well-defined interventions, so that either positive or negative outcomes (e.g., Schueller, Pérez-Stable, & Muñoz, 2013) can inform the field about the impact of the intervention. Brown and Liao (1999) discuss design issues for prerandomization, intervention, and postintervention, focusing on different examples of prevention research as a primary strategy to prevent mental health problems. Prevention should ideally address healthy development, explicitly measuring effects on collateral public health problems (Muñoz, 2005) and on preventing psychopathology (Muñoz, 1998). Given the high comorbidity of depression with other mental disorders (see Mineka & Vrshek-Schallhorn, Chapter 5, this volume), prevention studies should also be designed to evaluate effects on additional disorders (e.g., see Seligman et al., 1999). Prevention studies should also explicitly target ethnically diverse populations and specific age groups. We must avoid a major weakness of the treatment outcome literature, in which there are few studies that test the efficacy of depression treatment with ethnic minority groups. In addition, we must address differences in participants' developmental stages: The literature is sorely lacking in the area of prevention of depression among very young children and older adults (Le & Boyd, 2006). Prevention studies are more likely to reach their intended audiences if they involve collaboration with community settings, such as the home, schools, health systems, religious networks, and so on.

2. Preventive interventions need to be delivered via innovative methods, not just by licensed professionals (Christensen, Miller, & Muñoz, 1978; Hollon et al., 2002). For example, interventions provided via television (Muñoz, Glish, Soo-Hoo, & Robertson, 1982) or the Internet (Muñoz et al., 2006) can reach many more people per year than

can face-to-face interventions (see O'Kearney et al., 2006). Given the need to reach larger groups with preventive interventions, we need to develop and test interventions that significantly reduce the usual ratio of professionals to consumers. Otherwise, we will have the same shortage of personnel to provide prevention as we do now to provide treatment.

3. Refinements in the definition of recovery tied to clinical outcomes are desirable (e.g., see Riso et al., 1997) in order to provide clearer targets for evaluating treatment and prevention (Keller, 2003). Given the high rates of subsequent MDEs after an initial episode, preventing recurrence may prove to be an efficient method of reducing the burden of depression. Research should establish the impact of episode history or the presence of symptoms during remission on recurrence prevention.

CONCLUDING REMARKS

Developing methods to prevent the onset of major depression is the next great challenge for the mental health field. The WHO has identified unipolar major depression as the number one cause of disability worldwide (Murray & Lopez, 1996). The IOM has determined that major depression is the best candidate for the first mental disorder that we will be able to prevent (Mrazek & Haggerty, 1994). The preponderance of the evidence shows that a 50% reduction in incidence of MDEs in high-risk individuals is feasible with current methods. It is time to start the journey toward a world without depression (Muñoz, 2001).

ACKNOWLEDGMENTS

We gratefully acknowledge support from the University of California Office of the President Committee on Latino Research for the University of California, San Francisco/San Francisco General Hospital Latino Mental Health Research Program; Drs. Cloyce Duncan and Gwendolyn Evans for their generous support of the Mothers and Babies Project; and the National Institute of Mental Health (NIMH; Grant Nos. MH 37992, MH 596056, and 5R34MH091231) for support of the Depression Prevention Research Project, the Mothers and Babies Intervention Development Project, and the Internet Intervention Project to Prevent Major Depressive Episodes (Ricardo F. Muñoz, Principal Investigator). Huynh-Nhu Le's work was supported by the Clinical Psychology Training Program and the NIMH-funded Psychology and Medicine Postdoctoral Fellowship (Nancy Adler, Principal Investigator), Department of Psychiatry, at the University of California, San Francisco, and by Grant No. R40 MC 02497 from the Maternal and Child Health Bureau (Title V, Social Security Act), Health Resources and Services Administration, U. S. Department of Health and Human Services.

REFERENCES

Albee, G. (1985). The argument for primary prevention. *Journal of Primary Prevention, 5,* 213–219.

Alegría, M., Mulvaney-Day, N., Woo, M., Torres, M., Gao, S., & Oddo, V. (2007). Correlates of past year mental health service use among Latinos: Results from the National Latino and Asian American Study. *American Journal of Public Health, 97,* 76–83.

Allart-van Dam, E., Hosman, C. M. H., Hoogduin, C. A. L., & Schaap, C. P. D. R. (2007). Prevention of depression in subclinically depressed adults: Follow-up effects on the "Coping with Depression" course. *Journal of Affective Disorders, 97,* 219–228.

American Psychiatric Association. (2000). Practice guideline for the treatment of patients with major depressive disorder (revision). *American Journal of Psychiatry, 157*(Suppl. 4), 1–45.

Arnarson, E., & Craighead, W. E. (2009). Prevention of depression among Icelandic adolescents. *Behaviour Research and Therapy, 47*, 577–585.

Austin, M. P. (2003). Targeted group antenatal prevention of postnatal depression: A review. *Acta Psychiatrica Scandinavica, 107*, 244–250.

Austin, M. P., Frilingos, M., Lumley, J., Hadzi-Pavlovic, D., Roncolato, W., Acland, S., et al. (2008). Brief antenatal cognitive behaviour therapy group intervention for the prevention of postnatal depression and anxiety: A randomised controlled trial. *Journal of Affective Disorders, 105*, 35–44.

Barrera, A. Z., Torres, L. D., & Muñoz, R. F. (2007). Prevention of depression: The state of the science at the beginning of the 21st century. *International Review of Psychiatry, 19*, 655–670.

Beshai, S., Dobson, K. S., Bockting, C. L. H., & Quigley, L. (2011). Relapse and recurrence prevention in depression: Current research and future prospects. *Clinical Psychology Review, 31*, 1349–1360.

Birmaher, B., Ryan, N. D., Williamson, D. E., Brent, D. A., Kaufman, J., Dahl, R. E., et al. (1996). Childhood and adolescent depression: A review of the past 10 years: Part I. *Journal of the American Academy of Child and Adolescent Psychiatry, 35*, 1427–1439.

Bockting, C. L. H., Schene, A. H., Spinoven, P., Koeter, M. W. J., Wouters, L., Huyser, J., et al. (2005). Preventing relapse/recurrence in recurrent depression with cognitive therapy: A randomized controlled trial. *Journal of Consulting and Clinical Psychology, 73*, 647–657.

Bockting, C. L. H., Spinhoven, P., Wouters, L. F., Koeter, M. W. J., Schene, A. H., & the DELTA Study Group. (2009). Long-term effect of preventive cognitive therapy in re current depression: 5.5-year follow-up. *Journal of Clinical Psychiatry, 70*, 1621–1628.

Brown, C. H., & Liao, J. (1999). Principles for designing randomized preventive trials in mental health: An emerging developmental epidemiology paradigm. *American Journal of Community Psychology, 27*, 673–710.

Brugha, T. S., Morrell, C. J., Slade, P., & Walters, S. J. (2011). Universal prevention of depression in women postnatally: Cluster randomized trial evidence in primary care. *Psychological Medicine, 41*, 739–748.

Brugha, T. S., Wheatley, S., Taub, N. A., Culverwell, A., Friedman, T., Kirwan, P., et al. (2000). Pragmatic randomized trial of antenatal intervention to prevent post-natal depression by reducing psychosocial risk factors. *Psychological Medicine, 30*, 1273–1281.

Brunwasser, S. M., Gillham, J. E., & Kim, E. S. (2009). A meta-analytic review of the Penn Resiliency Program's effect on depressive symptoms. *Journal of Consulting and Clinical Psychology, 77*, 1042–1054.

Buist, A. E., Westley, D., & Hill, C. (1999). Antenatal prevention of postnatal depression. *Archives of Women's Mental Health 1*(4), 167–173.

Chabrol, H., Teissedre, F., Saint-Jean, M., Teisseyre, N., Rogé, B., & Mullet, E. (2002). Prevention and treatment of post-partum depression: A controlled randomized study on women at risk. *Psychological Medicine, 32*, 1039–1047.

Christensen, A., Miller, W. R., & Muñoz, R. F. (1978). Paraprofessionals, partners, peers, paraphernalia, and print: Expanding mental health service delivery. *Professional Psychology, 9*, 249–270.

Clarke, G. N., Hawkins, W., Murphy, M., Sheeber, L. B., Lewinsohn, P. M., & Seeley, J. R. (1995). Targeted prevention of unipolar depressive disorder in an at-risk sample of high school adolescents: A randomized trial of a group cognitive intervention. *Journal of the American Academy of Child and Adolescent Psychiatry, 34*, 312–321.

Clarke, G. N., Hornbrook, M. C., Lynch, F. L., Polen, M., Gale, J., Beardslee, W. R., et al. (2001). A randomized trial of a group cognitive intervention for preventing depression in adolescent offspring of depressed parents. *Archives of General Psychiatry, 58*, 1127–1134.

Compas, B. E., Forehand, R., Keller, G., Champion, J. E., Rakwo, A., Reeslund, K. L., et al. (2009). Randomized controlled trial of a family cognitive-behavioral preventive intervention for children of depressed parents. *Journal of Consulting and Clinical Psychology, 77,* 1007–1020.

Compas, B. E., Forehand, R., Thigpen, J. C., Keller, G., Hardcastle, E., Cole, D. A., et al. (2011). Family group cognitive-behavioral preventive intervention for families of depressed parents: 18- and 24-month outcomes. *Journal of Consulting and Clinical Psychology, 79,* 488–499.

Cuijpers, P., van Straten, A., Smit, F., Mihalopoulus, C., & Beekman, A. (2008). Preventing the onset of depressive disorders: A meta-analytic review of psychological interventions. *American Journal of Psychiatry, 165,* 1272–1280.

Dennis, C. L., Hodnett, E., Kenton, L., Weston, J., Zupancic, J., Stewart, D. E., et al.(2009). Effect of peer support on prevention of postnatal depression among high-risk women: Multisite randomised controlled trial. *British Medical Journal, 338,* a3064.

Depression Guideline Panel. (1993). *Depression in primary care: Vol. 2. Treatment of major depression* (Clinical Practice Guideline No. 5, AHCPR Publication No. 93-0551). Rockville, MD: Department of Health and Human Services, Public Health Service, Agency for Health Care Policy and Research.

Dobson, K. S., Hollon, S. D., Dimidjian, S., Schmaling, K. B., Kohlenberg, R. J., Gallop, R. J., et al. (2008). Randomized trial of behavioral activation, cognitive therapy, and antidepressant medication in the prevention of relapse and recurrence in major depression. *Journal of Consulting and Clinical Psychology, 76,* 468–477.

Dozeman, E., van Marwijk, H. W. J., van Schaik, D. J. F., Smit, F., Stek, M. L., van der Horst, H. E., et al. (2012). Contradictory effects for prevention of depression and anxiety in residents in homes for the elderly: A pragmatic randomized controlled trial. *International Psychogeriatrics, 24,* 1242–1251.

Elliott, S. A., Leverton, T. J., Sanjack, M., Turner, H., Cowmeadow, P., Hopkins, J., et al. (2000). Promoting mental health after childbirth: A controlled trial of primary prevention of postnatal depression. *British Journal of Clinical Psychology, 39,* 223–241.

Fava, G. A., Rafanelli, C., Cazzaro, M., Conti, S., & Grandi, S. (1998). Well-being therapy: A novel psychotherapeutic approach for residual symptoms of affective disorders. *Psychological Medicine, 28,* 475–480.

Fava, G. A., Ruini, C., Rafanelli, C., Finos, L., Conti, S., & Grandi, S. (2004). Six-year outcome of cognitive behavior therapy for prevention of recurrent depression. *American Journal of Psychiatry, 161,* 1872–1876.

Frank, E., Kupfer, D. J., Perel, J. M., Cornes, C., Jarret, D. B., Mallinger, A. G., et al. (1990). Three-year outcomes for maintenance therapies in recurrent depression. *Archives of General Psychiatry, 47,* 1093–1099.

Frank, E., Prien, R. F., Jarrett, R. B., Keller, M. B., Kupfer, D. J., Lavori, P. W., et al. (1991). Conceptualization and rationale for consensus definitions of terms in major depressive disorder: Remission, recovery, relapse, and recurrence. *Archives of General Psychiatry, 48,* 851–855.

Garber, J., Clarke, G. N., Weersing, V. R., Beardslee, W. R., Brent, D. A., Gladstone, T. R. G., et al. (2009). Prevention of depression in at-risk adolescents: A randomized controlled trial. *Journal of the American Medical Association, 301,* 2215–2224.

Geddes, J. R., Carney, S. M., Davies, C., Furukawa, T. A., Kupfer, D. J., Frank, E., et al. (2003). Relapse prevention with antidepressant drug treatment in depressive disorders: A systematic review. *Lancet, 361,* 653–661.

Gillham, J. E., Hamilton, J., Freres, D. R., Patton, K., & Gallop, R. (2006). Preventing depression among early adolescents in the primary care setting: A randomized controlled study of the Penn Resiliency Program. *Journal of Abnormal Child Psychology, 34,* 203–219.

Gillham, J. E., Jaycox, L., Reivich, K., Hollon, S. D., Freeman, A., DeRubeis, R. J., et al. (1991). *The Apex Project manual for group leaders.* Unpublished manuscript.

Godfrin, K. A., & van Heeringen, C. (2010). The effects of mindfulness-based cognitive therapy of recurrence of depressive episodes, mental health, and quality of life: A randomized controlled study. *Behaviour Research and Therapy, 48,* 738–746.

Hagan, R., Evans, S. F., & Pope, S. (2004). Preventing postnatal depression in mothers of very preterm infants: A randomised controlled trial. *BJOG: An International Journal of Obstetrics and Gynaecology, 111*, 641–647.

Hollon, S. D., DeRubeis, R. J., Shelton, R. C., Amsterdam, J. D., Salomon, R. M., O'Reardon, J. P., et al. (2005). Prevention of relapse following cognitive therapy versus medication in moderate to severe depression. *Archives of General Psychiatry, 62*, 417–422.

Hollon, S. D., Muñoz, R. F., Barlow, D. H., Beardslee, W. R., Bell, C. C., Bernal, G., et al. (2002). Psychosocial intervention development for the prevention and treatment of depression: Promoting innovation and increasing access. *Biological Psychiatry, 52*, 610–630.

Horowitz, J. L., & Garber, J. (2006). The prevention of depressive symptoms in children and adolescents. *Journal of Consulting and Clinical Psychology, 74*, 401–415.

Hough, R. L., Landsverk, J. A., Karno, M., Burnam, A., Timbers, D. M., Escobar, J. I., et al. (1987). Utilization of health and mental health services by Los Angeles Mexican Americans and non-Hispanic whites. *Archives of General Psychiatry, 44*, 702–709.

Jarrett, R. B., Baco, M. R., Risser, R. C., Ramanan, J., Marwill, M., Kraft, D., et al. (1998). Is there a role for continuation phase cognitive therapy for depressed outpatients? *Journal of Consulting and Clinical Psychology, 66*, 1036–1040.

Judd, L. L. (1997). The clinical course of unipolar major depressive disorders. *Archives of General Psychiatry, 54*, 989–991.

Keller, M. B. (2003). Past, present and future directions for defining optimal treatment outcomes in depression: Remission and beyond. *Journal of the American Medical Association, 289*, 3152–3160.

Konnert, C., Dobson, K., & Stelmach, L. (2009). The prevention of depression in nursing home residents: A randomized clinical trial of cognitive-behavioral therapy. *Aging and Mental Health, 13*, 288–299.

Kupfer, D. J., Frank, E., Perel, J. M., Cornes, C., Mallinger, A. G., Thase, M. E., et al. (1992). Five-year outcome for maintenance therapies in recurrent depression. *Archives of General Psychiatry, 49*, 769–773.

Kuyken, W., Byford, S., Taylor, R. S., Watkins, E., Holden, E., White, K., et al. (2008). Mindfulness-based cognitive therapy to prevent relapse in recurrent depression. *Journal of Consulting and Clinical Psychology, 76*, 966–978.

Lara, M. A., Navarro, C. N., & Navarrete, L. (2010). Outcome results of a psycho-educational intervention in pregnancy to prevent PPD: A randomized control trial. *Journal of Affective Disorders, 122*, 109–117.

Le, H. N., & Boyd, R. C. (2006). Prevention of major depression: Early detection and early intervention in the general population. *Clinical Neuropsychiatry, 3*, 6–22.

Le, H. N., Muñoz, R. F., Ippen, C. G., & Stoddard, J. (2003). Treatment is not enough: We must prevent major depression in women. *Prevention and Treatment, 6*, Article 10.

Le, H. N., Perry, D. F., & Stuart, E. A. (2011). Evaluating a preventive intervention for perinatal depression in high-risk Latinas. *Journal of Consulting and Clinical Psychology, 79*, 135–141.

Le, H. N., Zmuda, J., Perry, D. F., & Muñoz, R. F. (2010). Transforming an evidence-based intervention to prevent perinatal depression for low-income Latina immigrants. *American Journal of Orthopsychiatry, 80*, 34–45.

Lewinsohn, P. M., Hops, H., Roberts, R. E., Seeley, J. R., & Andrews, J. A. (1993). Adolescent psychopathology: I. Prevalence and incidence of depression and other DSM-III-R disorders in high school students. *Journal of Abnormal Psychology, 102*, 133–144.

Lewinsohn, P. M., Rohde, P., Klein, D. N., & Seeley, J. R. (1999). Natural course of adolescent major depressive disorder: I. Continuity into young adulthood. *Journal of the American Academy of Child and Adolescent Psychiatry, 38*, 56–63.

Lobel, B., & Hirschfeld, R. M. A. (1984). *Depression: What we know* (DHHS Publication No. ADM 84-1318). Rockville, MD: National Institute of Mental Health.

Luby, J. L. (2000). Depression. In C. H. Zeanah (Ed.), *Handbook of infant mental health* (2nd ed., pp. 382–396). New York: Guilford Press.

Martinovic, Z., Simonovi, P., & Djoki, R. (2006). Preventing depression in adolescents with epilepsy. *Epilepsy Behavior, 9*, 619–624.

Merry, S., McDowell, H., Hetrick, S., Bir, J., & Muller, N. (2006). Psychological and/or educational interventions for the prevention of depression in children and adolescents. *Cochrane Database of Systematic Reviews, 3*, 1–107.

Morgan, A. J., Jorm, A. F., & Mackinnon, A. J. (2012). E-mail-based promotion of self-help for subthreshold depression: Mood memos randomised controlled trial. *British Journal of Psychiatry, 200*, 412–418.

Mrazek, P., & Haggerty, R. (1994). *Reducing risks for mental disorders: Frontiers for preventive intervention research.* Washington, DC: National Academy Press.

Mufson, L., Gallagher, T., Dorta, K. P., & Young, J. F. (2004). Interpersonal psychotherapy for adolescent depression: Adaptation for group therapy. *American Journal of Psychotherapy, 58*, 220–237.

Muñoz, R. F. (1984). *The depression prevention course.* Unpublished manuscript, University of California, San Francisco.

Muñoz, R. F. (1998, September). Preventing major depression by promoting emotion regulation: A conceptual framework and some practical tools. *International Journal of Mental Health Promotion*, pp. 23–40.

Muñoz, R. F. (2001). On the road to a world without depression. *Journal of Primary Prevention, 21*, 325–338.

Muñoz, R. F. (2005). *La depresión y la salud de nuestros pueblos* [Depression and the health of our communities]. *Salud Mental, 28*, 1–9. Retrieved February 24, 2007, from *www.inprf-cd.org.mx/pdf/sm2804/sm280401.pdf.*

Muñoz, R. F., Beardslee, W. R., & Leykin, Y. (2012). Major depression can be prevented. *American Psychologist, 67*, 285–295.

Muñoz, R. F., Cuijpers, P., Smit, F., Barrera, A. Z., & Leykin, Y. (2010). Prevention of major depression. *Annual Review of Clinical Psychology, 6*, 181–212.

Muñoz, R. F., Glish, M., SooHoo, T., & Robertson, J. L. (1982). The San Francisco Mood Survey Project: Preliminary work toward the prevention of depression. *American Journal of Community Psychology, 10*, 317–329.

Muñoz, R. F., Le, H. N., Clarke, G., & Jaycox, L. (2002). Preventing the onset of major depression. In I. H. Gotlib & C. L. Hammen (Eds.), *Handbook of depression* (p. 343–359). New York: Guilford Press.

Muñoz, R. F., Le, H. N., Ghosh Ippen, C., Diaz, M. A., Urizar, G. G., Soto, J., et al. (2007). Prevention of postpartum depression in low-income women: Development of the *Mamás y Bebés*/Mothers and Babies Course. *Cognitive and Behavioral Practice, 14*, 70–83.

Muñoz, R. F., Lenert, L. L., Delucchi, K., Stoddard, J., Pérez, J. E., Penilla, C., et al. (2006). Toward evidence-based Internet interventions: A Spanish/English Web site for international smoking cessation trials. *Nicotine and Tobacco Research, 8*, 77–87.

Muñoz, R. F., & Ying, Y. (1993). *The prevention of depression: Research and practice.* Baltimore, MD: Johns Hopkins University Press.

Muñoz, R. F., Ying, Y. W., Armas, R., Chan, F., & Gurza, R. (1987). The San Francisco Depression Prevention Research Project: A randomized trial with medical outpatients. In R. F. Muñoz (Ed.), *Depression prevention: Research directions* (pp. 199–215). Washington, DC: Hemisphere.

Muñoz, R. F., Ying, Y. W., Bernal, G., Pérez-Stable, E. J., Sorensen, J. L., Hargreaves, W. A., et al. (1995). Prevention of depression with primary care patients: A randomized controlled trial. *American Journal of Community Psychology, 23*, 199–222.

Murray, C. J. L., & Lopez, A. D. (1996). *The global burden of disease: Summary.* Boston, MA: Harvard University Press.

O'Connell, M. E., Boat, T., & Warner, K. E. (Eds.). (2009). *Preventing mental, emotional, and behavioral disorders among young people: Progress and possibilities.* Washington, DC: National Academies Press.

O'Hara, M. W., & Swain, A. M. (1996). Rates and risk of postpartum depression: A meta-analysis. *International Review of Psychiatry, 8*, 37–54.

Ojeda, V. D., & McGuire, T. G. (2006). Gender and racial/ethnic differences in use of outpatient mental health and substance use services by depressed adults. *Psychiatric Quarterly, 77*, 211–222.

O'Kearney, R., Kang, K., Christensen, H., & Griffiths, K. (2006). Effects of a cognitive-behavioral Internet program on depression, vulnerability to depression and stigma in adolescent males: A school-based controlled trial. *Cognitive Behavioral Therapy, 35*, 43–54.

Piet, J., & Hougaard, E. (2011). The effect of mindfulness-based cognitive therapy for prevention of relapse in recurrent major depressive disorder: A systematic review and meta-analysis. *Clinical Psychology Review, 31*, 1032–1040.

Priest, S. R., Henderson, J., Evans, S. F., & Hagan, R. (2003). Stress debriefing after childbirth: A randomised controlled trial. *Medical Journal of Australia, 178*, 542–545.

Riso, L. P., Thase, M. E., Howland, R. H., Friedman, E. S., Simons, A. D., & Tu, X. M. (1997). A prospective test of criteria for response, remission, relapse, recovery, and recurrence in depressed patients treated with cognitive behavior therapy. *Journal of Affective Disorders, 43*, 131–142.

Robinson, R. G., Jorge, R. E., Moser, D. J., Acion, L., Solodkin, A., Small, S. L., et al. (2008). Escitalopram and problem-solving therapy for prevention of poststroke depression. *Journal of the American Medical Association, 299*, 2391–2400.

Rush, A. J., Kraemer, H. C., Sackelm, H. A., Fava, M., Trivedi, M. H., Frank, E., et al. (2006). Report by the ACNP task force on response and remission in major depressive disorder. *Neuropsychopharmacology, 31*, 1841–1853.

Schueller, S. M., Pérez-Stable, E. J., & Muñoz, R. F. (2013). A mood management intervention in an Internet stop-smoking randomized controlled trial does not prevent depression: A cautionary tale. *Clinical Psychological Science, 1*, 401–412.

Segal, Z. V., Bieling, P., Young, T., MacQueen, G., Cooke, R., Martin, L., et al. (2010). Antidepressant monotherapy vs. sequential pharmacotherapy and mindfulness-based cognitive therapy, or placebo, for relapse prophylaxis in recurrent depression. *Archives of General Psychiatry, 67*, 1256–1264.

Seligman, M. E. P., Schulman, P., DeRubeis, R. J., & Hollon, S. D. (1999). The prevention of depression and anxiety. *Prevention and Treatment, 2*, Article 8. Available at *www.ppc.sas.upenn.edu/depprevseligman1999.pdf*.

Seligman, M. E. P., Schulman, P., & Tyron, A. M. (2007). Group prevention of depression and anxiety symptoms. *Behaviour Research and Therapy, 45*, 1111–1126.

Sheets, E. S, Craighead, L. W., Brosse, A. L., Hauser, M., Madsen, J. W., & Craighead, W. E. (2013). Prevention of recurrence of major depression among emerging adults by a group of cognitive-behavioral/interpersonal intervention. *Journal of Affective Disorders, 147*, 425–430.

Sheffield, J. K., Spence, S. H., Rapee, R. M., Kowalenko, N., Wignall, A., Davis, A., et al. (2006). Evaluation of universal, indicated, and combined cognitive-behavioral approaches to the prevention of depression among adolescents. *Journal of Consulting and Clinical Psychology, 74*, 66–79.

Solomon, D. A., Keller, M. B., Leon, A. C., Mueller, T. I., Lavori, P. W., Shea, M. T., et al. (2000). Multiple recurrences of major depressive disorder. *American Journal of Psychiatry, 157*, 229–233.

Spence, S. H., Sheffield, J. K., & Donovan, C. L. (2003). Preventing adolescent depression: An evaluation of the Problem Solving for Life Program. *Journal of Consulting and Clinical Psychology, 71*, 3–13.

Spence, S. H., Sheffield, J. K., & Donovan, C. L. (2005). Long-term outcome of a school-based, universal approach to prevention of depression in adolescents. *Journal of Consulting and Clinical Psychology, 73*, 160–167.

Stamp, G. E., Williams, A. S., & Crowther, C. A. (1995). Evaluation of antenatal and postnatal support to overcome postnatal depression: A randomized, controlled trial. *Birth, 22,* 138–143.

Stice, E., Rohde, P., Gau, J. M., & Wade, E. (2010). Efficacy trial of a brief cognitive-behavioral depression prevention program for high-risk adolescents: Effects at 1- and 2-year follow-up. *Journal of Clinical and Consulting Psychology, 78,* 856–867.

Stice, E., Rohde, P., Seeley, J. R., & Gau, J. M. (2008). Brief cognitive-behavioral depression prevention program for high-risk adolescents outperforms two alternative interventions: A randomized efficacy trial. *Journal of Clinical and Consulting Psychology, 76,* 595–606.

Tandon, S. D., Leis, J., Mendelson, T., Perry, D. F., & Edwards, K. (2014). Six-month outcomes from a randomized controlled trial to prevent perinatal depression in low-income home visiting clients. *Maternal and Child Health Journal, 18,* 873–881.

Tandon, S. D., Perry, D. F., Mendelson, T., Kemp, K., & Leis, J. A. (2011). Preventing perinatal depression in low-income home visiting clients: A randomized controlled trial. *Journal of Consulting and Clinical Psychology, 79,* 707–712.

Teasdale, J. D., Segal, Z. V., Williams, J. M. G., Ridgeway, V. A., Soulsby, J. M., & Lau, M. A. (2000). Prevention of relapse/recurrence in major depression by mindfulness-based cognitive therapy. *Journal of Consulting and Clinical Psychology, 68,* 615–623.

van't Veer-Tazelaar, P. J., van Marwijk, H. W. J., van Oppen, P., van Hout, H. P. J., van der Horst, H. E., Cuijpers, P., et al. (2009). Stepped-care prevention of anxiety and depression in late life: A randomized controlled trial. *Archives of General Psychiatry, 66,* 297–304.

Vázquez, F. L., Torres, A., Blaco, V., Díaz, O., Otero, P., & Hermida, E. (2012). Comparison of relaxation training with a cognitive-behavioural intervention for indicated prevention of depression in university students: A randomized controlled trial. *Journal of Psychiatric Research, 46,* 1456–1463.

Vittengl, J. R., Clark, L. A., & Jarrett, R. B. (2009). Continuation-phase cognitive therapy's effects on remission and recovery from depression. *Journal of Consulting and Clinical Psychology, 77,* 367–371.

Weissman, M. M., Wickramaratne, P., Nomura, Y., Warner, V., Pilowsky, D., & Verdeli, H. (2006). Offspring of depressed parents: 20 years later. *American Journal of Psychiatry, 163,* 1001–1008.

Willemse, G. R., Smit, F., Cuijpers, P., & Tiemens, B. G. (2004). Minimal-contact psychotherapy for sub-threshold depression in primary care: Randomised trial. *British Journal of Psychiatry, 185,* 416–421.

Young, J. F., Mufson, L., & Davies, M. (2006). Efficacy of Interpersonal Psychotherapy—Adolescent Skills Training: An indicated prevention intervention for depression. *Journal of Child Psychology and Psychiatry, 47,* 1254–1262.

Zlotnick, C., Johnson, S. L., Miller, I. W., Pearlstein, T., & Howard, M. (2001). Postpartum depression in women receiving public assistance: Pilot study of an interpersonal-therapy-oriented group intervention. *American Journal of Psychiatry, 158,* 638–640.

Zlotnick, C., Johnson, S. L., Miller, I. W., Pearlstein, T., & Howard, M. (2006). A preventive intervention for pregnant women on public assistance at risk for postpartum depression. *American Journal of Psychiatry, 163,* 1443–1445.

CHAPTER 26

Pharmacotherapy and Other Somatic Treatments for Depression

MICHAEL J. GITLIN

Antidepressants have been available for over half a century. After more than 30 years of very slow progress in the area, in 1987 the first agent of the second generation of antidepressants, fluoxetine (Prozac), was released. Since that time, 13 antidepressants (and a unique delivery system of an older agent) with a variety of biological effects, chemical structures, and differing side effects have been released, representing a minor explosion of treatment options. Yet there is no substantial evidence that any of our newer agents are more effective (as defined by response or remission rates; discussed in more detail later in the chapter) than imipramine, our original 1950s prototype. Additionally, none of these newer antidepressant medications has changed the field or created a sense of therapeutic excitement in the way that fluoxetine did. Over the last 5 years, the two most important advances in the somatic treatment of depression have been the increasing use of adjunctive treatments for depression—that is, medications added to an ineffective antidepressant to increase its efficacy—and the recent rapid development of non-pharmacological treatments, also described as neuromodulatory therapies. Aside from electroconvulsive therapy (ECT), which has been available for many decades, transcranial magnetic stimulation (TMS), vagal nerve stimulation (VNS), deep brain stimulation (DBS), and others have pointed in a very different direction in the somatic treatment of depression.

This chapter reviews the phases of treatment for depression with antidepressants; the choices of available agents; the advantages and disadvantages of the antidepressant classes and agents; the choices (especially adjunctive therapies) for treating nonresponsive patients; the use of the neuromodulatory treatments for depression; the use of antidepressants for special populations; and continuation and maintenance treatments. The chapter concludes with a summary of some of the current critical, clinical research questions in the area.

PHASES OF PHARMACOTHERAPY OF DEPRESSION

Antidepressants can be prescribed for any one of three goals or phases described as acute, continuation, and maintenance treatment. The goal of acute treatment is to alleviate the symptoms of an active depression. The goal of continuation treatment is to prevent a relapse into the same episode for which treatment was begun. By definition, continuation treatment begins at the time of remission from the acute depressive episode. Maintenance therapy is considered to begin when the goal is to prevent future recurrences of depressive episodes (or to prevent a recurrence of depressive symptoms following the successful treatment of a chronic depression). Given the recent data on the natural history of depression, consideration of maintenance treatment with antidepressants should commonly be discussed with patients. These phases of treatment flow naturally from one to another. This chapter focuses intensively on acute treatment, following which both the data and current clinical practice on continuation and maintenance treatment are presented.

ACUTE PHARMACOLOGICAL TREATMENT OF DEPRESSION

Table 26.1 shows the 26 antidepressants available in 2013, divided into pharmacological classes, with typical dose ranges. Table 26.2 lists the antidepressants by their side-effect profiles. No classification scheme is either consistent or comprehensive; each class is defined by different unifying characteristics, as described next.

Selective Serotonin Reuptake Inhibitors

The antidepressants in this class still dominate the treatment of depression in the United States. Selective serotonin reuptake inhibitors (SSRIs) share the common property of blocking the presynaptic reuptake of serotonin, which increases its availability to the postsynaptic neuron, thereby enhancing serotonergic function. Their popularity reflects their relatively benign side-effect profile, the fact that the initial dose is close to the therapeutic dose, and that generic preparations of all medications in this class are available, thereby making them easily affordable. The individual agents are not biologically identical, merely similar. As examples, citalopram (Celexa) is the most selective of the SSRIs, fluoxetine the least; sertraline (Zoloft) additionally blocks the reuptake of dopamine (albeit weakly). The clinical significance of these differences is unclear.

Side effects include (see Table 26.2) nausea, activation (insomnia, nervousness), sedation, and sexual side effects. In general, rates of nausea and sexual side effects are relatively similar across individual SSRI agents. Rates of sedation and activation, however, differ. Fluoxetine and sertraline are most commonly associated with activation effects, whereas paroxetine and fluvoxamine are more likely to cause sedation.

Bupropion

Bupropion (Wellbutrin) is a novel agent with effects on norepinephrine and dopamine and no serotonergic effects (Asher et al., 1995). Bupropion is a stimulating antidepressant, with the most common side effects of insomnia, anxiety, tremor, and headache. It is never sedating and is associated with virtually no sexual side effects and no weight gain. All bupropion preparations are available in generic form. The major safety concern is bupropion's propensity to cause seizures at a slightly higher rate than the other new

TABLE 26.1. Antidepressants

Class[a]	Typical starting dose (mg)	Usual dosage range (mg daily)
Selective serotonin reuptake inhibitors (SSRIs)		
Citalopram (Celexa)	10–20	20–60
S-citalopram (Lexapro)	5–10	10–30
Fluoxetine (Prozac)	10–20	10–80
Fluvoxamine (Luvox)	25–50	100–300
Paroxetine (Paxil)	10–20	20–60
Sertraline (Zoloft)	25–50	50–200
Novel antidepressants		
Bupropion (Wellbutrin)	100–150	300–450
Mirtazapine (Remeron)	15–30	15–60
Nefazodone (Serzone)[b]	50	400–600
Trazodone[c] (Desyrel)	50	150–400
Vilazodone (Viibryd)	10	40
Vortioxetine (Brintellix)	10	20
Dual-action agents		
Desvenlafaxine (Pristiq)	25	50–100
Duloxetine (Cymbalta)	20–30	60–120
Levomilnacipram (Fetzima)	20	40-120
Venlafaxine (Effexor)	37.5–75	150–300
Tricyclics + related compounds		
Amitriptyline (Elavil, Endep)	25–50	100–300
Amoxapine (Asendin)	50–100	150–400
Clomipramine (Anafranil)	25–50	100–250
Desipramine (Norpramin, Pertofrane)	25–50	100–300
Doxepin (Sinequan, Adapin)	25–50	100–300
Imipramine (Tofranil)	25–50	100–300
Maprotiline (Ludiomil)	25–50	100–225
Nortriptyline (Aventyl, Pamelor)	10–25	50–150
Protriptyline (Vivactil)	10	15–60
Trimipramine (Surmontil)	25–50	100–300
Monoamine oxidase inhibitors (MAOIs)		
Isocarboxazid (Marplan)	10–20	30–60
Phenelzine (Nardil)	15–30	30–90
Selegiline (Eldepryl)	10	20–60
Selegiline transdermal (Emsam patch)	6	6–12
Tranylcypromine (Parnate)	10–20	30–60

[a]Trade name is in parentheses.
[b]Branded product withdrawn from market; rarely prescribed.
[c]Rarely used as an antidepressant; prescribed more in low dose as a hypnotic.

TABLE 26.2. Common Side Effects of Antidepressants

Name[a]	Sedation	Stimulation	Postural effects	Anticholinergic	Other side effects
Selective serotonin reuptake inhibitors (SSRIs)					
Citalopram (Celexa)	+	+	0	0	Sexual
S-citalopram (Lexapro)	0±	+	0	0	Sexual
Fluoxetine (Prozac)	0±	+++	0	0	Sexual
Fluvoxamine (Luvox)	+	+	0	0	Sexual
Paroxetine (Paxil)	+	+	0	+	Sexual, weight gain
Sertraline (Zoloft)	0±	++	0	0	Sexual
Novel antidepressants					
Bupropion (Wellbutrin)	0	++	0	0	
Mirtazapine (Remeron)	+++	0	0	0	Weight gain
Nefazodone (Serzone)	+++	0	++	0	
Trazodone (Desyrel)	+++	0	+++	0	
Vilazodone (Viibryd)	0+	+	0	0	Nausea, diarrhea
Vortioxetine (Brintellix)	0	0	0	0	Nausea, constipation
Dual-action agents					
Desvenlafaxine (Pristiq)	+	+	0	0	
Duloxetine (Cymbalta)	0±	0±	0	0	Nausea, dry mouth, constipation
Levomilnacipran (Fetzima)	0	0	0	+	Sexual, nausea
Venlafaxine (Effexor)	+	+	0	0	Dose-related hypertension
Tricyclics and related compounds					
Amitriptyline (Elavil, Endep)	+++	0	+++	+++	
Amoxapine (Asendin)	+	0	++	+	
Clomipramine (Anafranil)	+++	0	+++	+++	
Desipramine (Norpramin, Pertofrane)	+	+	++	+	
Doxepin (Sinequan, Adapin)	+++	0	++	++	
Imipramine (Tofranil)	++	+	+++	++	
Maprotiline (Ludiomil)	++	+	+	+	
Nortriptyline (Aventyl, Pamelor)	++	0	+	+	
Protriptyline (Vivactil)	+	+	++	+++	
Trimipramine (Surmontil)	+++	0	++	+++	

(continued)

TABLE 26.2. (continued)

Name[a]	Sedation	Stimulation	Postural effects	Anticholinergic	Other side effects
Monoamine oxidase inhibitors (MAOIs)					
Isocarboxazid (Marplan)	++	+	+++	+	Weight gain, insomnia, sexual
Phenelzine (Nardil)	++	+	+++	+	Weight gain, insomnia, sexual
Selegiline (Eldepryl)	+	+	++	+	
Selegiline transdermal (Emsam)	0	+	+	0±	Skin reaction to patch
Tranylcypromine (Parnate)	+	+	+++	+	Insomnia, sexual

[a]Trade name is in parentheses.

antidepressants (Davidson, 1989). Bupropion is contraindicated in patients with seizure disorders or active eating disorders, such as bulimia nervosa or anorexia nervosa (which lower the seizure threshold, presumably via electrolyte abnormalities).

Dual-Action Agents: Venlafaxine, Duloxetine, Desmethylvenlafaxine

Dual-action agents should be considered equivalent in efficacy to SSRIs, but with a greater side-effect burden. In contrast to earlier studies, current evidence that dual-action agents are more effective than SSRIs as measured by either response or remission rates is weak (Schueler et al, 2011).

At low to moderate doses (up to 125 mg or so), venlafaxine (Effexor) is an SSRI with strong, selective effects on serotonin. As the dose is increased beyond that level, reuptake blockade of norepinephrine begins, giving venlafaxine a dual effect (Harvey, Rudolph, & Preskorn, 2000). The side-effect profile of venlafaxine is almost identical to that of the SSRIs. As venlafaxine doses increase, a dose-related hypertension may emerge, affecting up to 9% of treated patients at high dose (Thase, 1998). Duloxetine (Cymbalta) also blocks the reuptake of both norepinephrine and serotonin, but it does so in a more balanced manner, affecting both neurotransmitter systems at all prescribed doses. The clinical significance of this is unclear. Aside from its antidepressant efficacy (Kornstein, Wohlreich, Mallinckrodt, Watkin, & Stewart, 2006), duloxetine is both effective and commonly prescribed for neuropathic pain (e.g., diabetic neuropathy and postherpetic neuralgia; Goldstein, Lu, Detke, Lee, & Iyengar, 2005) and more nonspecific pain. Its side-effect profile differs somewhat from those of both the SSRIs and venlafaxine in that its most common side effects are nausea early in treatment, dry mouth, and constipation.

Mirtazapine

The presumed mechanism of antidepressant activity of mirtazapine (Remeron) is complex, with presynaptic noradrenergic blocking (thereby enhancing noradrenergic function) and secondary enhancement of serotonergic activity (Gorman, 1999). Because its most common side effects are sedation and weight gain, mirtazapine is most commonly prescribed to patients with depression, especially older adults with anorexia, agitation, and insomnia.

Vilazodone

Vilazodone's (Viibryd) mechanism of action includes both serotonin reuptake inhibition (similar to the SSRIs) and 5-HT_{1A} partial agonism (similar to the antianxiety agent buspirone [Buspar]; Frampton, 2011). It is associated with higher rates of nausea and diarrhea than other antidepressants but may be associated with fewer sexual side effects.

Levomilnacipran and Vortioxetine

The two most recently released antidepressants (early 2014) are levomilnacipran (Fetzima) and vortioxetine (Brintellix). Levomilnacipran is a norepinephrine-dominant dual-action agent with common side effects of nausea, constipation, and sweating. Vortioxetine is a serotonin modulator (with complex effects on different serotonin subreceptors). Its most common side effects are gastrointestinal.

Tricyclics

As the oldest class of antidepressants, the tricyclics, which increase norepinephrine, serotonin, or both, are still prescribed for depression but virtually never as first-line agents. These changes in prescribing practices reflect the relative side-effect profiles of the tricyclics versus the newer agents, not efficacy, because no newer antidepressant has shown greater efficacy than the tricyclics. The disadvantages of tricyclics include the need to increase the dose gradually to achieve full effect, a process that may take weeks; a substantial side-effect profile; and high lethality in overdose. Tricyclic antidepressants are especially difficult and potentially dangerous medications in the presence of cardiac disease because agents of this antidepressant class alter cardiac conduction and may either cause or exacerbate cardiac arrhthymias (Roose & Spatz, 1999).

Monoamine Oxidase Inhibitors

In general, monoamine oxidase inhibitors (MAOIs) have been relegated to third- or fourth-line antidepressants despite their unique utility for a subset of patients with depression. Their disfavor among clinicians and patients is due partly to their side-effect profile but more because the use of oral MAOIs requires strict dietary restrictions, without which severe, potentially life-threatening hypertensive reactions and a number of drug–drug interactions may occur. Because of these dangers, only responsible, compliant patients should take oral MAOIs. Although early studies seemed to indicate that MAOIs were not as effective as the tricyclics for severe, classic depression, this observation was due to the low, inadequate doses used in these studies. In later studies using higher doses, the MAOIs are equivalent in effectiveness to other antidepressant classes (Davis, Wang, & Janicak, 1993).

One of the MAOIs, selegiline, is available in a transdermal form (Emsam), administered as a daily patch. Because a transdermal preparation bypasses both gut and hepatic effects, the hypertensive effects of dietary tyramine are markedly diminished. Therefore, in low but still effective doses (6 mg patch), transdermal selegiline does not require any dietary restrictions and is the only MAOI preparation available in the United

States without these requirements. At 9- and 12-mg patch doses, dietary restrictions are required, although the risk of hypertensive reactions is still less than with oral MAOIs.

RATIONAL SELECTION OF AN ANTIDEPRESSANT

Table 26.3 shows the classic factors used by skillful clinicians to choose a specific antidepressant. Comparative efficacy is not a factor to be considered, as all antidepressants are relatively comparable in this regard (Gartlehner et al, 2011). Issues relating to side-effect profiles, which, it is assumed, relate partially to compliance, dominate the decision. Experienced clinicians use the differences among antidepressants of sedation–activation to benefit patients by typically prescribing activating agents to patients with depression, lethargy, and psychomotor retardation and sedating agents to individuals with more anxiety, agitation, and insomnia. However, in controlled trials, pretreatment anxiety is poorly predictive of antidepressant efficacy (Papakostas et al, 2008). Depressive subtypes are those that may predict response to one class of antidepressant more than another, such as atypical depression (see later discussion). Cost is only occasionally a factor in choosing an antidepressant because, at the time of this book's publication, all antidepressants except for vilazodone, desmethylvenlafaxine, and the patch version of selegiline will be available in generic form.

Among the secondary factors that determine choice of medications, no consistent data have shown that depressions can be subtyped by neurotransmitter effects (i.e., clinicians cannot categorize a patient as having a serotonergic vs. noradrenergic depression). Although family history of response is a commonsense approach to choosing a specific antidepressant, data supporting this approach are remarkably sparse (Malhotra, Murphy, & Kennedy, 2004). Safety/medical considerations were especially relevant in the gradual shift away from the tricyclics and MAOIs toward the newer antidepressants, which are medically safer. Given how infrequently older agents are prescribed for depression, safety/medical considerations are less primary concerns than in the past.

Although no single antidepressant is more or less effective than the others in double-blind studies of unselected patients with major depression, some clinical features or clinical subtypes (depression with psychotic features and atypical features) may predict differential responses and/or require different approaches.

Psychotic depression (DSM-IV/DSM-5 major depression with psychotic features) has been shown in a number of studies to respond less well to an antidepressant than to an antidepressant plus an antipsychotic or to electroconvulsive therapy (ECT; Farahani & Correll, 2012). Therefore, for most patients with psychotic depression, first-line recommendations are either an antidepressant/antipsychotic combination or ECT.

Atypical depression (DSM-IV/DSM-5 depression with atypical features) responds preferentially to MAOIs over tricyclics, with SSRIs likely to be as effective as MAOIs

---

TABLE 26.3. Considerations in Choosing a Specific Antidepressant

Primary	Secondary
• History of past response • Side-effect profile • Depressive subtype (e.g., atypical depression) • Cost	• Neurotransmitter specificity • Family history of response • Safety and medical issues

(Henkel et al, 2006). However, given the differential side-effect profiles, SSRIs are virtually always prescribed first for those with atypical depression.

GENERAL PRINCIPLES OF PHARMACOTHERAPY OF DEPRESSION

Response—usually defined as a 50% or more decrease in a depression rating scale—to a single antidepressant, derived from earlier studies, is more than 60%, compared with a placebo response rate of 30%, a difference of 30% (Klein, Gittelman-Klein, Quitkin, & Rifkin, 1980). Response rates from more recent studies hover around 50% (Papakostas & Fava, 2009). Drug–placebo differences have diminished even more over time, with studies since 2000 showing less than a 13% mean difference, due primarily to an increase in placebo response rates. Many studies, however, now utilize *remission* as the primary outcome variable. Typically, remission is defined as a Hamilton Depression Scale score < 7 or a parallel score on other rating scales. In the most representative of the recent studies, Sequenced Treatment Alternatives to Relieve Depression (STAR*D), using an open design of 2,876 patients in 41 sites, the remission rate to the first antidepressant prescribed was 28% after up to 14 weeks of treatment (Trivedi et al., 2006). Aside from the obvious goal of having the patient feel as well as possible, remission from an acute depressive episode predicts lower relapse rates (Rush et al., 2006).

Symptom changes based on self- or observer rating scales leading to response and remission rates are rather crude outcome measures and should be considered only one method of measuring outcome. Functional outcome—the individual's ability to participate in the core tasks of life such as primary role function (e.g., occupation, student, caregiver) and social roles (e.g., in a primary relationship, with family or social network)—is another less commonly measured outcome. Increasing evidence suggests that functional outcome lags behind symptomatic outcome for reasons that have not yet been elucidated (Mintz, Mintz, Arruda, & Hwang, 1992).

Classically, antidepressants were thought to work only after at least 2 weeks. However, more recent meta-analyses have demonstrated that antidepressant effects—regardless of the antidepressant class—are usually seen early, with continuing improvement over subsequent weeks (Posternak & Zimmerman, 2005). Over 60% of the improvement occurs within the first 2 weeks of treatment, and drug–placebo differences are the most pronounced during this time. Absence of a partial response within the first 2 weeks is a robust predictor of a poor response at 4–8 weeks (Szegedi et al., 2009)

The proper length of a full antidepressant trial has similarly undergone revisionist thinking. Classically, a full antidepressant trial was considered to be 6 weeks. However, in the STAR*D trial, mean time to remission was 6.7 weeks, with 40% of patients achieving remission between weeks 8 and 14 (Trivedi et al., 2006). Because STAR*D was not placebo controlled (it was meant to mimic real-world settings), it is difficult to interpret fully the time to remission data.

TREATMENT-RESISTANT DEPRESSION

With antidepressant response rates at 50%, and with many of those persons called responders still having residual symptoms, suggested approaches to nonresponders and nonremitters are multiple and varied. Unfortunately, the field still lacks a data-based approach to antidepressant treatment failures because the vast majority of studies in this area typically describe a pharmacotherapeutic approach compared with a placebo condition (Gitlin, 2005). Predictors of a poor response to antidepressant treatment include greater symptom severity, early onset of the depressive disorder, multiple prior episodes, comorbid anxiety disorders (especially panic disorder), and comorbid personality disorders (Gaynes et al., 2009). Clinically, however, it is important to note that *some* patients with any of these clinical and/or historical features will still respond to antidepressant therapy and should therefore be treated.

Pharmacological options for treatment resistance have been classically conceptually divided into optimization, switching, augmentation, or combination (Price, 1990). Optimization describes continuing to prescribe the original antidepressant but at higher dose or for a longer trial (e.g., the 14 weeks utilized in the STAR*D trial). Dose escalation beyond medium doses is more likely to be helpful for patients taking tricyclic antidepressants and venlafaxine and for some patients on MAOIs and is unlikely to be helpful with SSRIs (Adli, Baethge, Heinz, Langlitz, & Bauer, 2005). Switching to another antidepressant is a self-evident option. Augmentation is defined as adding a second agent that itself is not an antidepressant but that might augment the effect of the original medication. In combination treatment, a second agent that is itself an antidepressant is added.

The relative merits of switching within versus across an antidepressant class continue to be controversial. Practically, the usual clinical question is whether to switch to a second SSRI if a patient with depression has failed an adequate trial of the first SSRI or to switch to an agent from a different class, such as bupropion, venlafaxine, or others. Only a handful of well-designed, placebo-controlled studies have addressed this question, and, overall, no conclusive evidence suggests switching across versus within class (Souery et al., 2011). Once a full trial (i.e., an adequate dose for an adequate period of time) has been achieved, the clinical question is whether to switch to another antidepressant or to add another agent, whether an adjunctive agent or another antidepressant. Although the usual recommendations are to switch antidepressants in the case of nonresponse and to add a second agent when a patient partially responds, data on this question are inconclusive, and actual prescribing practices are dictated by local customs and individual practitioner experiences and treatment philosophies.

Options for adding a second agent are listed in Table 26.4. Lithium is the most well-studied agent, with 10 double-blind studies published. A meta-analysis of these studies demonstrates clear evidence of efficacy compared with placebo (Crossley & Bauer, 2007). Response typically occurs within 2 weeks and at doses that tend to be lower than those used in treating bipolar disorder. However, in the majority of the positive studies, tricyclics were the antidepressants used; in the smaller subset of SSRI/adjunctive lithium studies, the data are much weaker. Additionally, many clinicians feel negatively toward adjunctive lithium because of both a poorer observed response than is seen in published studies and the lack of patient acceptance due to side effects and the need for blood tests with lithium use.

TABLE 26.4. First-Line Adjunctive/Combination Strategies for Treatment-Resistant Depression

- Lithium
- Second-generation antipsychotic
- T_3
- Combination of two antidepressants[a]
- Stimulant

---

[a]Except for a strongly serotoninergic antidepressant plus MAO inhibitor.

Adding a second-generation antipsychotic, typically at low dose, has become a commonly used adjunctive treatment approach. Both aripiprazole (Abilify) and quetiapine (Seroquel) have Food and Drug Administration (FDA) indications for this purpose. A meta-analysis examining all controlled trials demonstrated clear efficacy of this approach (Nelson & Papakostas, 2009). Antipsychotic doses prescribed for adjunctive purposes are much lower than those used to treat either acute psychosis or mania.

T3 (triiodothyronine, marketed as Cytomel), a thyroid hormone, has been tested in five double-blind studies as an adjunctive antidepressant treatment, with positive response seen in some, but not all, studies (Aronson, Offman, Joffe, & Naylor, 1996). Prescribing T3 as an adjunctive agent is simple, with doses relatively low compared with situations in which it is prescribed for overt thyroid disease. Despite its simplicity, clinicians tend to use other adjunctive approaches before T3 because of a general clinical sense that it is often not effective enough.

Combining two antidepressants is a commonly employed strategy for refractory depression. Almost always, the second agent prescribed is from a different class than is the first antidepressant. Thus combining fluoxetine and paroxetine makes little sense; combining an SSRI with bupropion or mirtazapine is more common and is theoretically more reasonable. Despite the frequency of combination therapy, no substantial evidence has shown the efficacy of this approach compared with switching treatments (Thase, 2011).

Adjunctive stimulants such as methylphenidate (Ritalin), *d*-amphetamine (Dexedrine), and, more recently, modafinil (Provigil) and armodafinil (Nuvigil), are popular choices as adjunctive agents (Parker & Brotchie, 2010). Modest evidence for modafinil has been published. In neither of the two published studies examining the adjunctive efficacy of classic stimulants (extended-release methylphenidate in both studies) did drug separate from placebo. This result may reflect the relative low doses used in these studies. When stimulants work as adjunctive agents, they do so within a few days at most, which adds to their popularity.

Other adjunctive treatment approaches are either prescribed infrequently, have little data in support of their use, or both. These would include buspirone (Buspar; Landén, Björling, & Fahlén, 1998), the antianxiety agent, and lamotrigine (Barbee et al, 2011). Despite the lack of positive data, many clinicians prescribe lamotrigine for treatment-resistant depression.

A last option to consider for treatment-resistant depression is ketamine, an anesthetic agent with a primary mechanism of action as an antagonist of the NMDA (N-methyl-D-aspartate) glutamate receptor, resulting in increased excitatory neurotransmission (Kavalali & Monteggia, 2012). A number of small studies have demonstrated a rapid (typically after a single intravenous dose) and sustained (up to 2 weeks) antidepressant effect. However, its poor bioavailability when administered orally, its potential side effects of psychosis and dissociative symptoms, and its use as a street drug (called *K* or *special K*) makes it unlikely to be used with any frequency.

COMPLEMENTARY THERAPIES

Over the last decade, nonprescription (i.e., over the counter) agents have become areas of increasing clinical research and practice (Freeman et al, 2010). Omega-3 fatty acids–EPA (eicosapentanoic acid) and/or DHA (docosahexaenoic acid) have been evaluated as antidepressant treatments. A meta-analysis of studies on its efficacy in depression showed positive results (Sublette, Ellis, Geant, & Mann, 2011). Studies in which EPA provided at least 60% of the total dose were significantly more likely to show positive results. Usual doses are 1–2 grams daily, although far higher doses have also been used.

S-adenosyl methionine (SAM-E) is a methyl donor and may augment synthesis of a number of neurotransmitters. In the best recent trial, SAM-E showed efficacy in a double-blind, placebo-controlled study as an adjunctive therapy to ineffective antidepressant therapy (Papakostas, Mischoulon, Shyu, Alpert, & Fava, 2010). At the usual daily doses of 1200–1600 mg daily, side effects of SAM-E are minimal.

The most recent nutritional supplement used to treat depression is l-methylfolate (MHTF), the biologically active form of folate which regulates the formation of a critical cofactor in the synthesis of many neurotransmitters, including serotonin, dopamine, and norepinephrine. In one double-blind study, 15 mg of MHTF, but not 7.5 mg, was an effective adjunctive treatment when SSRIs were ineffective (Papakostas et al., 2010).

NEUROMODULATORY APPROACHES TO DEPRESSION

The newest area in the biological treatment of depression is the use of physical nonmedication treatments, sometimes referred to as neuromodulation therapies because they all modulate the activity of neural networks implicated in the pathophysiology of depression. By far, the oldest of these treatments is ECT, which is still commonly used today. Over the last decade, VNS, TMS, and DBS have been the subject of increasing numbers of clinical trials. VNS and TMS have FDA indications for depression, but DBS does not.

Electroconvulsive Therapy

ECT remains the most important approach for treatment-resistant depression. ECT is virtually never used as a first-line treatment for depression. Typically, it is recommended for patients who have failed multiple antidepressant therapies, especially if the depression is severe and associated with significant suicidal ideation and/or functional impairment. ECT may be the treatment of choice for depression with psychotic features. Classic remission rates with ECT, derived from clinical trial data, are usually given as 70–90% (Husain et al., 2004). However, naturalistic data from community settings suggest lower remission rates of 30–47% (Prudic, Olfson, Marcus, Fuller, & Sackeim, 2004) and a high relapse rate in 6 months for those who responded acutely. Predictors of a lower remission rate to ECT are comorbid personality disorders and inadequate length of treatment (i.e., treating to response instead of remission).

ECT is given as a series of treatments, two to three times weekly, with a total of 6–12 treatments (American Psychiatric Association Committee on Electroconvulsive Therapy, 2001). It may be given to inpatients or outpatients. Safety is ensured by the use of short-acting anesthesia, a muscle relaxant (to prevent broken bones, as in the past), and, in the better settings, electroencephalographic (EEG) monitoring. Bilateral lead placement and higher voltage are both associated with greater cognitive side effects but may be more effective for some patients. Results of the most systematic study suggested that high-voltage, unilateral ECT may be the best compromise to achieve efficacy with fewer cognitive side effects (Sackeim et al., 2000) with bilateral ECT reserved for those who fail to respond to at least six unilateral treatments.

After successful ECT, in order to avoid relapse, patients should be placed on either an aggressive preventive pharmacotherapy regimen (e.g., two agents from different classes) or be provided with maintenance ECT, in which the treatments are reduced in frequency to once monthly. In the only random assignment study, continuation ECT was as effective as a lithium–nortriptyline combination (Kellner et al., 2006). However, neither treatment was very effective or acceptable to patients because 54% in each group either relapsed or dropped out over 6 months.

Vagal Nerve Stimulation

VNS, an established treatment for treatment-resistant epilepsy, was approved by the FDA as a treatment for refractory depression in 2005. VNS is applied by a pulse-generating device implanted subcutaneously in the patient's chest (like a cardiac pacemaker), with a wire attached to the patient's left vagus nerve. The stimulator is then programmed externally. VNS's efficacy in depression is generally considered weak compared with other established treatments, and a meta-analysis confirmed its lack of significant efficacy differences in short-term studies compared with control conditions (Martin & Martin-Sanchez, 2012). Side effects with VNS are hoarseness (because the vagal nerve innervates the vocal chords), cough, and mild shortness of breath.

VNS has been infrequently utilized since its approval by the FDA. This reflects its relatively weak database, its need for surgical implantation, and its very high cost and rare approval by insurance companies.

Transcranial Magnetic Stimulation

Initially developed as a research tool for investigating cortical function and nerve conduction, TMS has evolved into a potential treatment alternative for depression. Although approved by the FDA for depression that was refractory to one full antidepressant treatment (a most narrow indication!), it is now used mostly off-label for patients with depression who are treatment resistant or treatment intolerant. TMS is administered by placing an electromagnetic coil over the scalp and creating a rapidly changing magnetic field that induces an electric current, stimulating the local underlying cortex. TMS is administered 5 days weekly for 4–6 weeks, with each treatment taking approximately 40 minutes. Because of the localized effect (it is typically placed over the left dorsolateral prefrontal cortex), many of the side effects seen with ECT, such as cognitive disturbance, are nonexistent with TMS. Additionally, TMS does not require anesthesia, providing another safety advantage. A meta-analysis of TMS studies for depression showed a statistically significant difference compared with sham TMS (Slotema, Blom, Hoek, & Sommer, 2010). In a large effectiveness trial sponsored by the National Institutes of Health (NIH), TMS was more effective than sham TMS in response and remission rates, but the percentages of remitters and responders were relatively low (George et al., 2010). Despite its frequent clinical use in treatment-resistant depression, TMS's efficacy for these patients is still unproven (Lisanby et al., 2009). Consistent with this finding, ECT is significantly more effective than TMS in the few head-to-head trials that exist (Berlim, Van den Eynde, & Daskalakis, 2013). Another concern with TMS is its cost (with a course of TMS costing $6,000–14,000) and its poor insurance coverage.

Deep Brain Stimulation

DBS has been used in neurology for treatment-refractory Parkinson's disease and dystonia. In DBS treatments, electrodes are implanted into specific anatomical structures, where continuous stimulation is applied via a device implanted subcutaneously under the clavicle. When used to treat depression, the most common location in which the electrodes are implanted is the subgenual cingulate gyrus. Open case series have shown consistently positive lasting results, with efficacy increasing up to 2 years in patients who were severely treatment resistant (Holtzheimer et al., 2012). No controlled studies have yet been published. Complications of DBS include intracranial infections and hemorrhages. As might be anticipated, DBS is very, very expensive, with costs in the hundreds of thousands of dollars. Nonetheless, the preliminary efficacy data are encouraging, and it may be a treatment for a very select group of individuals with severe treatment-resistant depression.

TREATING SPECIAL POPULATIONS

Two populations of patients with depression warrant separate discussions because of the unique considerations associated with their treatment: dysthymic disorder and depression during pregnancy and the postpartum period. Bipolar depression is covered by Miklowitz (Chapter 28, this volume).

Dysthymic Disorder

DSM-5 correctly combines dysthymic disorder with chronic major depression as persistent depressive disorder. Consistent with this notion, many, but not all, of the relatively few pharmacotherapy studies in this area have combined chronic major depression, dysthymic disorder, and double depression in their inclusion criteria. Response rates to antidepressants of major depression versus dysthymia are comparable, but dysthymic disorder responds less well to placebo, thereby yielding a greater drug–placebo difference (Levkovitz, Tedeschini, & Papakostas, 2011). As with major depression, no single agent is more consistently effective with dysthymia than any other. At this point, although chronicity itself is a negative predictor of antidepressant response, it should not preclude a thorough set of antidepressant trials.

Depression during Pregnancy or the Postpartum Period

Because the mean age of onset of depression and the age at which women are most likely to become pregnant commonly coincide, the problem of how to manage depression and antidepressants in preparation for, during, and following pregnancy is a critical issue in psychopharmacology. In the past, pregnancy was considered a time of unusually good mental health for women. Unfortunately, more recent studies contradict this older myth, and, at this point, there is little consistent evidence suggesting that women with mood disorders are particularly psychologically healthy during pregnancy (Cohen et al., 2006).

A key background consideration is the 2–4% base rate of major fetal malformations in women without depression on no medications (Stewart, 2011). Of note, depression itself may be associated with some negative pregnancy-related outcomes (such as lower birth weight or higher rates of preterm labor). Therefore, it is difficult at times to distinguish between the effects of the disorder (depression) and the medication(s) used to treat the disorder.

Four different types of potential negative effects of medications on fetuses/infants should be considered. The first reflects potential abnormalities in the overall course of the pregnancy, such as increased risk of miscarriage and higher rates of preterm birth and/or lower birthweight. The second is that of classic fetal malformations/abnormalities of structure, almost always due to first-trimester effects. This suggests the option, with some women, of discontinuing the medication before conception and restarting it in the beginning of the second trimester, thereby avoiding the chance of fetal malformations but not later pregnancy-related effects. The third group of potential negative effects of medication reflects toxic effects on the fetus or newborn, caused by third-trimester exposure. These would include abnormalities in the late stages of lung development, hypothyroidism caused by exposure to a thyrotoxic medication during pregnancy (such as lithium), and irritability in the neonate soon after birth as a side effect to a stimulating medication taken by the mother during pregnancy (and thereby exposing the fetus to the medication during pregnancy) or, conversely, caused by withdrawal from the psychotropic medication taken by the mother. The final potential negative effects are developmental in nature and would not be apparent for months or years. These include abnormalities in achieving developmental milestones, IQ, psychomotor coordination, attachment capabilities, and other possibilities. Of course, as with fetal malformations, in considering any of these potential outcomes, we must consider the inherent base rate of these abnormalities and the potential effect of untreated psychiatric disorders, as well as medication effects, as possible causes.

Overall, there is no evidence that antidepressants are consistently associated with increased fetal malformations or any specific malformation (Stewart et al., 2011). Some studies have shown a slightly higher risk of early miscarriage in women with depression who are taking antidepressants. Other studies have shown that women with depression who are taking antidepressants have higher rates of preterm birth (more prematurity) and lower birthweight in exposed infants compared with women with depression who were untreated (implying that the findings were due to the medications, not the depression; Ross et al., 2013). However, the long-term health implications of these slightly premature births are unclear. Finally, there is no consistent evidence (albeit with few studies) that in utero exposure to antidepressants causes any developmental delays (Nulman et al., 2012).

We have more safety data on SSRIs than on any other antidepressant class due to their greater use during a time of more careful monitoring. Overall, SSRIs are safe medications, and it is not considered a medication class associated with fetal malformations. The most cited concern is that of congenital heart defects, specifically that of the septal wall. Some, but not all, studies have specifically implicated paroxetine (Paxil) as being associated with higher rates of cardiac defects. Because of this, most experts recommend against the use of paroxetine as a new treatment for pregnancy-related depression.

The two later, third-trimester pregnancy-related concerns are: (1) increased risk of primary pulmonary hypertension (PPH) and (2) neonatal adaptation syndrome (Stewart, 2011). PPH is a syndrome at birth manifesting as difficulty breathing in the newborn. There is inconsistent evidence that PPH is more likely in SSRI-exposed neonates. Because a higher risk for PPH with SSRI-exposed neonates is still unclear, there are no recommendations to alter third-trimester antidepressant treatment due to this concern. Neonatal adaptation syndrome, characterized by irritability/jitteriness, weak crying, temperature instability, and alterations in muscle tone, is seen in a minority of neonates exposed to SSRIs during the third trimester. The cause of this syndrome is unclear and may reflect antidepressant withdrawal effects, antidepressant toxicity, or other unknown causes. These symptoms typically spontaneously resolve within 2 weeks.

Much less information is available about the potential effects of other modern antidepressants on pregnancy. With the limited information we have, there are no known concerns regarding any of these medications, such as dual-action agents venlafaxine (Effexor), duloxetine (Cymbalta), mirtazapine (Remeron), or bupropion (Wellbutrin). Given the smaller amount of safety data with these medications during pregnancy, it is generally recommended that they be continued if an antidepressant is needed but that they should not be the first antidepressant selected for pregnancy-related depression.

Tricyclic antidepressants are not known to be associated with negative effects on pregnant women and fetuses, but they are not typically used because of their overall side-effect profile. If a tricyclic is prescribed, desipramine (Norpramin) and nortriptyline (Pamelor) are generally preferred due to lower rates of weight gain, sedation, and blood pressure changes.

MAOIs should generally be avoided during pregnancy due to animal studies suggesting fetal growth abnormalities and concerns about the risk of hypertensive episodes associated with their use. Given the infrequency of their use in the community in general, this issue rarely arises.

Given the current conflicting data regarding SSRI safety, there is no clear consensus on treatment recommendations for pregnant women with depression. The ultimate decision on how best to manage depression for any individual woman should, of course, be discussed between the prescribing physician, the pregnant woman (preferably in anticipation of pregnancy), the father (if present), and the therapist. Possible strategies include withdrawing the antidepressant before conception, discontinuing the antidepressant when pregnancy is confirmed, avoiding medication during the first trimester, discontinuing the antidepressant midway through pregnancy (given the concerns about late pregnancy effects), or continuing the medication throughout the pregnancy. The severity of the depression, its recurrent nature, whether the woman has previously been able to withdraw from antidepressants without depressive relapse for some time, and the availability and efficacy of psychotherapeutic intervention are all important factors to weigh in the decision.

Whether to breast-feed is another issue for women on antidepressants. The context of this decision is the high risk of postpartum depression in women with a prior history of depression (Viguera et al., 2011). Overall, antidepressants have a relatively benign side-effect profile in breast-feeding. All antidepressants are excreted into breast milk in measurable levels. Yet the blood levels of these antidepressants in breast-fed infants are very low to undetectable. Consistent with this, the great majority of breast-fed infants show no negative effects from maternal antidepressants. Occasional individual case reports describe an infant with both high blood levels of antidepressants and/or symptoms consistent with antidepressant side effects such as either sedation or colic and crying. These, however, are exceptions to the general finding of low blood levels and no side effects (Davanzo, Copertino, De Cunto, Minen, & Amaddeo, 2011).

CONTINUATION TREATMENT AND MAINTENANCE TREATMENT

The goal of continuation treatment is, as noted earlier, to prevent a relapse soon after improvement from the acute depressive episode. Clinically, continuation treatment begins when patient and clinician agree that the patient is conclusively better and that further changes in medications to control symptoms are not needed. Continuation treatment with antidepressants, using the acute treatment dose, is associated with reduced relapse rates compared with switching to placebo. Only two studies—one evaluating a tricyclic and the other an SSRI—have specifically examined the optimal length of continuation period (Prien & Kupfer, 1986; Reimherr et al., 1998). In both studies, continuation therapy was more effective than placebo in preventing relapse. The usual recommendation for 4–9 months of continuation treatment fits the available data.

If long-term maintenance treatment is clinically unnecessary (see the next section) and the antidepressant is to be discontinued, common sense dictates that it be tapered rather than stopped suddenly. Should depressive symptoms return during tapering, they are typically milder, and treatment can be more easily reinstated compared with a full, sudden recurrence, which is more likely to occur if the antidepressant is stopped precipitously. Additionally, discontinuation/withdrawal symptoms may be seen with a variety of antidepressants and are also avoided with medication tapering. The optimal time period for medication tapering after continuation therapy is unstudied, but a reasonable time period is 4–8 weeks.

Because, in the majority of patients, depression is either a recurrent or a chronic disorder (see Klein & Allmann, Chapter 4, this volume), long-term preventative treatment should be considered. Factors in deciding which individuals with depression are appropriate candidates for maintenance therapy are based more on common sense than on data. They include the number of depressive episodes over a lifetime, the frequency of depressive episodes, the severity of the depressions (including both symptom severity and functional consequences), the responsiveness of episodes to prior treatments, the speed with which episodes have emerged, and insight into emerging depressive symptoms (Gitlin, 1996).

Many patients are concerned about potential long-term side effects of antidepressants on body organs, such as the liver, the kidneys, and especially the brain. Although definitive studies do not exist, there is no evidence whatsoever that antidepressants as a class (available for over 50 years) or SSRIs specifically (available for 20 years) are associated with any long-term negative effects on organ function or physiology. Virtually all maintenance studies with tricyclic or SSRI antidepressants have demonstrated greater efficacy of active agents compared with placebo in preventing depressive recurrences. There is no evidence that any single antidepressant prevents future episodes better than any other. Few studies have addressed the question of optimal antidepressant doses in maintenance treatment. Based on extrapolation from two studies that were not designed specifically to answer this question (Frank et al., 1993; Prien et al., 1984), the current consensus is that patients in maintenance treatment should remain on their acute treatment doses.

CONCLUSIONS AND FUTURE DIRECTIONS FOR RESEARCH

In the narrow sense, antidepressant treatments could be seen as a well-established area with few to no great improvements over the last decade. Since the last edition of this book, only two new antidepressants have been released, and neither can be considered a breakthrough drug in any meaningful sense. Furthermore, most of the antidepressants in the research pipeline that are being considered for release in the next few years seem not too dissimilar in either biological profile or efficacy compared with the currently available agents. A number of these new agents are triple-uptake inhibitors, blocking the norepinephrine, serotonin, and dopamine transporters—interesting, but not dramatically different from currently available agents. Another medication considered for release in the next few years is agomelatine, which has a different mechanism of action as a melatonin agonist. It is available in Europe, but its release in the United States has been slowed by less than optimal efficacy trials.

Yet there is interest and excitement in three important areas in the biological treatment of depression with both the availability of new treatments and the promise of further research leading to the development of other new treatments. These areas are the ketamine data, the potential use of genetic markers for improving diagnosis and treatment, and the proliferation of neuromodulatory approaches. The studies that have demonstrated the efficacy of ketamine in treatment-resistant depression—both unipolar and bipolar—are exciting in themselves. What makes these results even more interesting are:

1. The rapidity of response, in which a single intravenous ketamine dose results in marked improvement in depressive symptoms within hours. Because all currently available antidepressants work far more slowly, this suggests a different mechanism of action for antidepressant effects. This also suggests the possible use of ketamine (or other similar agents) to treat suicidal ideation in an emergency setting, with the hope/goal of diminishing depressive symptoms and suicidality rapidly (Murrough & Charney, 2012).

2. The sustained nature of the antidepressant effects, as a single dose of ketamine continued to separate from placebo for up to a few weeks. Aside from replications of these early data, ongoing studies are evaluating ketamine's effects in treating acute suicidality and in developing a paradigm for maintaining the clinical effect by either repeated ketamine administrations or the use of other glutamatergic agents (aan het Rot, Zarate, Charney, & Mathew, 2012).

Realistically, ketamine will never become a first-line treatment. The requirement for intravenous or intranasal use, its capacity for abuse, and its side-effect profile of dissociative and psychotic symptoms will preclude its general use. But the positive preliminary data point to a (hopefully) fruitful research direction—that of glutamatergic antidepressants and clarification of a new mechanism of action that may provide more rapid efficacy than is seen with currently available agents.

The elucidation of the human genome has created hope that knowledge of genetic markers could help in a variety of areas relevant to psychiatric disorders and treatment. These areas include: more accurate diagnosis; prediction of treatment response; and prediction of side effects and correlates of innate capacity to metabolize medications, which may then predict blood levels, thereby suggesting optimal doses for individual patients (Miller & O'Callaghan, 2013).The greatest progress has been made in the area of predicting optimal doses, as it is now possible to genotype patients as rapid, intermediate, or slow metabolizers of medications. Unfortunately, this test is expensive and, so far, has been less clinically useful than hoped. Nonetheless, the use of genetic markers in psychiatry will be the subject of much more work in the foreseeable future.

The third exciting area of clinical research surrounds the dramatic expansion of neuromodulatory techniques in treating depression. Aside from the well-established ECT, VNS and TMS are now FDA-approved treatments. Although the current database for TMS suggests reasonable efficacy, it is difficult to justify a very expensive and time-consuming treatment that is no more effective than generically available, inexpensive antidepressants. However, TMS may have a very specific role in treating pregnant women with depression (because it is theoretically safer for the fetus than any antidepressant) or patients with treatment intolerance (because TMS's side-effect profile is so benign).

Beyond the currently available neuromodulatory techniques are a host of others currently under investigation. These include: transcranial direct current stimulation, transcranial low voltage pulsed electromagnetic fields, magnetic seizure therapy, and trigeminal nerve therapy (Cook et al, 2013; Holtzheimer & Mayberg, 2012). All these techniques share the capacity to alter local neuronal conduction with downstream effects throughout the neural network that is presumed to underlie depressive symptoms and syndromes. The holy grail for all these techniques is antidepressant efficacy, hopefully parallel with ECT but without the side effects, cumbersomeness, and cost. Over the next number of years, we will see some of these techniques achieve clinical utility if they satisfy these goals, whereas others will fade away. The work goes on.

REFERENCES

aan het Rot, M., Zarate, C. A., Jr., Charney, D. S., & Mathew, S. J. (2012). Ketamine for depression: Where do we go from here? *Biological Psychiatry, 72*, 537–547.

Adli, M., Baethge, C., Heinz, A., Langlitz, N., & Bauer, M. (2005). Is dose escalation of antidepressants a rational strategy after a medium-dose treatment has failed?: A systematic review. *European Archives of Psychiatry and Clinical Neuroscience, 255*(6), 387–400.

American Psychiatric Association Committee on Electroconvulsive Therapy. (2001). *The practice of electroconvulsive therapy: Recommendations for treatment, training, and privileging* (2nd ed.). Washington, DC: American Psychiatric Association.

Aronson, R., Offman, H. J., Joffe, R. T., & Naylor, C. D. (1996). Triiodothyronine augmentation in the treatment of refractory depression. *Archives of General Psychiatry, 53*, 842–848.

Asher, J. A., Cole, G. O., Colin, J. N., Feighner, J. P., Ferris, R. M., Fibiger, H. C., et al. (1995). Bupropion: A review of its mechanisms of antidepressant activity. *Journal of Clinical Psychiatry, 56*, 395–401.

Barbee, J. G., Thompson, T. R., Jamhour, N. J., Stewart, J. W., Conrad, E. J., Reimherr, F. W., et al. (2011). A double-blind placebo-controlled trial of lamotrigine as an antidepressant augmentation agent in treatment-refractory unipolar depression. *Journal of Clinical Psychiatry, 72*(10), 1405–1412.

Berlim, M. T., Van den Eynde, F., & Daskalakis, Z. J. (2013). Efficacy and acceptability of high frequency repetitive transcranial magnetic stimulation (rTMS) versus electroconvulsive therapy (ECT) for major depression: A systematic review and meta-analysis of randomized trials. *Depression and Anxiety, 30*, 614–623.

Cohen, L. S., Altshuler, L. L., Harlow, B. L., Nonacs, R., Newport, D. J., Viguera, A. C., et al. (2006). Relapse of major depression during pregnancy in women who maintain or discontinue antidepressant treatment. *Journal of the American Medical Association, 295*(5), 499–507.

Cook, I. A., Schrader, L. M., DeGiorgio, C. M., Miller, P. R., Maremont, E. R., & Leuchter, A. F (2013). Trigeminal nerve stimulation in major depressive disorder: Acute outcomes in an open pilot study. *Epilepsy and Behavior, 28*, 221–226.

Crossley, N. A., & Bauer, N. (2007). Acceleration and augmentation of antidepressants with lithium for depressive disorders: Two meta-analyses of randomized, placebo-controlled trials. *Journal of Clinical Psychiatry, 68*, 935–940.

Davanzo, R., Copertino, M., De Cunto, A., Minen, F., & Amaddeo, A. (2011). Antidepressant drugs and breastfeeding: A review of the literature. *Breastfeeding Medicine, 6*(2), 89–98.

Davidson, J. R. T. (1989). Seizures and bupropion: A review. *Journal of Clinical Psychiatry, 50*, 256–261.

Davis, J. M., Wang, Z., & Janicak, P. G. (1993). A quantitative analysis of clinical drug trials for the treatment of affective disorders. *Psychopharmacological Bulletin, 29*, 175–181.

Farahani, A., & Correll, C. U. (2012). Are antipsychotics or antidepressants needed for psychotic depression?: A systematic review and meta-analysis of trials comparing antidepressant or antipsychotic monotherapy with combination treatment. *Journal of Clinical Psychiatry, 73*(4), 486–496.

Frampton, J. E. (2011). Vilazodone in major depressive disorder. *CNS Drugs, 25*(7), 615–627.

Frank, E., Kupfer, D. J., Perel, J. M., Cornes, C., Mallinger, A. G., Thase, M. E., et al. (1993). Comparison of full-dose versus half-dose pharmacotherapy in the maintenance treatment of recurrent depression. *Journal of Affective Disorders, 27*, 139–145.

Freeman, M. P., Fava, M., Lake, J., Trivedi, M. H., Wisner, K. L., & Mischoulon, D. (2010). Complementary and alternative medicine in major depressive disorder: The American Psychiatric Association task force report. *Journal of Clinical Psychiatry, 71*(6), 669–681.

Gartlehner, G., Hansen, R. A., Morgan, L. C., Thaler, K., Lux, L., Van Noord, M., et al. (2011). Comparative benefits and harms of second-generation antidepressants for treating major depressive disorder: An updated meta-analysis. *Annals of Internal Medicine, 155*, 772–785.

Gaynes, B. N. (2009). Identifying difficult-to-treat depression: Differential diagnosis, subtypes, and comorbidities. *Journal of Clinical Psychiatry, 70*(Suppl. 6), 10–15.

George, M. S., Lisanby, S. H., Avery, D., McDonald, W. M., Durkalski, V., Pavlicova, M., et al. (2010). Daily left prefrontal transcranial magnetic stimulation therapy for major depressive disorder: A sham-controlled randomized trial. *Archives of General Psychiatry, 67*(5), 507–516.

Gitlin, M. (1996). *The psychotherapist's guide to psychopharmacology* (2nd ed.). New York: Free Press.

Gitlin, M. (2005). Treatment of refractory depression. In J. Licinio & M. Wong (Eds.), *Biology of depression* (pp. 387–412). Weinheim, Germany: Wiley-VCH.

Goldstein, D. J., Lu, Y., Detke, M. J., Lee, T. C., & Iyengar, S. (2005). Duloxetine vs. placebo in patients with painful diabetic neuropathy. *Pain, 116*(1–2), 109–118.

Gorman, J. M. (1999). Mirtazapine: Clinical overview. *Journal of Clinical Psychiatry, 60*(Suppl. 17), 9–13.

Harvey, A. T., Rudolph, R. L., & Preskorn, S. H. (2000). Evidence of the dual mechanisms of action of venlafaxine. *Archives of General Psychiatry, 57*, 503–509.

Henkel, V., Mergl, R., Allgaier, A., Kohnen, R., Moller, H., & Hegerl, U. (2006). Treatment of depression with atypical features: A meta-analytic approach. *Psychiatry Research, 141*, 89–101.

Holtzheimer, P. E., Kelley, M. E., Gross, R. E., Filkowski, M. M., Garlow, S. J., Barrocas, A., et al. (2012). Subcallosal cingulate deep brain stimulation for treatment-resistant unipolar and bipolar depression. *Archives of General Psychiatry, 69*(2), 150–158.

Holtzheimer, P. E., & Mayberg, H. S. (2012). Neuromodulation for treatment-resistant depression. *F1000 Medicine Reports, 4*(22), 1–10.

Husain, M. M., Rush, A. J., Fink, M., Knapp, R., Petrides, G., Rummans, T., et al. (2004). Speed of response and remission in major depressive disorder with acute electroconvulsive therapy (ECT): A Consortium for Research in ECT (CORE) report. *Journal of Clinical Psychiatry, 65*(4), 485–491.

Kavalali, E. T., & Monteggia, L. M. (2012). Synaptic mechanisms underlying rapid antidepressant action of Ketamine. *American Journal of Psychiatry, 69*, 1150–1156.

Kellner, C. H., Knapp, R. G., Petrides, G., Rummans, T. A., Husain, M. M., Rasmussen, K., et al. (2006). Continuation electroconvulsive therapy vs. pharmacotherapy for relapse prevention in major depression: A multisite study from the Consortium for Research in Electroconvulsive Therapy (CORE). *Archives of General Psychiatry, 63*(12), 1337–1344.

Klein, D. F., Gittelman-Klein, R., Quitkin, F. M., & Rifkin, A. (1980). *Diagnosis and drug treatment of psychiatric disorders*. Baltimore: Williams & Wilkins.

Kornstein, S. G., Wohlreich, M. M., Mallinckrodt, C. H., Watkin, J. G., & Stewart, D. E. (2006). Duloxetine efficacy for major depressive disorder in male vs. female patients: Data from seven randomized, double-blind, placebo-controlled trials. *Journal of Clinical Psychiatry, 67*(5), 761–770.

Landén, M., Björling, G., & Fahlén, T. (1998). A randomized, double-blind placebo-controlled trial of buspirone in combination with an SSRI in patients with treatment-refractory depression. *Journal of Clinical Psychiatry, 59*, 664–668.

Levkovitz, Y., Tedeschini, E., & Papakostas, G. I. (2011). Efficacy of antidepressants for dysthymia: A meta-analysis of placebo-controlled randomized trials. *Journal of Clinical Psychiatry, 72*(4), 509–514.

Lisanby, S. H., Husain, M. M., Rosenquist, P. B., Maixner, D., Gutierrez, R., Krystal, A., et al. (2009). Daily left prefrontal repetitive transcranial magnetic stimulation in the acute treatment of major depression: Clinical predictors of outcome in a multisite, randomized controlled clinical trial. *Neuropsychopharmacology, 34*(2), 522–534.

Malhotra, A. K., Murphy, G. M., Jr., & Kennedy, J. L. (2004). Pharmacogenetics of psychotropic drug response. *American Journal of Psychiatry, 161*(5), 780–796.

Martin, J. L. R., & Martin-Sanchez, E. (2012). Systematic review and meta-analysis of vagus nerve stimulation in the treatment of depression: Variable results based on study designs. *European Psychiatry, 27,* 147–155.

Miller, D. B., & O'Callaghan, J. P. (2013). Personalized medicine in depression: Opportunities and pitfalls. *Metabolism, 52*(Suppl. 1), S34–S39.

Mintz, J., Mintz, L. I., Arruda, M. J., & Hwang, S. S. (1992): Treatments of depression and the functional capacity to work. *Archives of General Psychiatry 49*(10), 761–768.

Murrough, J. W., & Charney, D. S. (2012). Is there anything really novel on the antidepressant horizon? *Current Psychiatry Reports, 14,* 643–649.

Nelson, J. C., & Papakostas, G. I. (2009). Atypical antipsychotic augmentation in major depressive disorder: A meta-analysis of placebo-controlled randomized trials. *American Journal of Psychiatry, 166,* 980–991.

Nulman, I., Koren, G., Rovet, J., Barrera, M., Pulver, A., Streiner, D., et al. (2012). Neurodevelopment of children following prenatal exposure to venlafaxine, selective serotonin reuptake inhibitors, or untreated maternal depression. *American Journal of Psychiatry, 169,* 1165–1174.

Papakostas, G. I., & Fava, M. (2009). Does the probability of receiving placebo influence clinical trial outcome?: A meta-regression of double-blind, randomized clinical trials in MDD. *European Neuropsychopharmacology, 19,* 34–40.

Papakostas, G. I., Mischoulon, D., Shyu, I., Alpert, J. E., & Fava, M. (2010). S-adenosyl methionine (SAMe) augmentation of serotonin reuptake inhibitors for antidepressant nonresponders with major depressive disorder: A double-blind, randomized clinical trial. *American Journal of Psychiatry, 167*(8), 942–948.

Papakostas, G. I., Shelton, R. C., Zajecka, J. M., Etemad, B., Rickels, K., Clain, A., et al. (2012). L-methylfolate as adjunctive therapy for SSRI-resistant major depression: Results of two randomized, double-blind, parallel-sequential trials. *American Journal of Psychiatry, 169*(12), 1267–1274.

Papakostas, G. I., Stahl, S. M., Krishen, A., Seifert, B. A., Tucker, V. L., Goodale, E. P., et al. (2008). Efficacy of bupropion and the selective serotonin reuptake inhibitors in the treatment of major depressive disorder with high levels of anxiety (anxious depression): A pooled analysis of 10 studies. *Journal of Clinical Psychiatry, 69*(8), 1287–1292.

Parker, G., & Brotchie, H. (2010). Do the old psychostimulant drugs have a role in managing treatment resistant depression? *Acta Psychiatrica Scandinavica, 121,* 308–314.

Posternak, M. A., & Zimmerman, M. (2005). Is there a delay in the antidepressant effect?: A meta-analysis. *Journal of Clinical Psychiatry, 66*(2), 148–158.

Price, L. H. (1990). Pharmacological strategies in refractory depression. In A. Tasman, S. Goldfinger, & C. Kaufmann (Eds.), *Review of psychiatry* (Vol. 9, pp. 116–131). Washington, DC: American Psychiatric Press.

Prien, R. F., & Kupfer, D. J. (1986). Continuation drug therapy for major depressive episodes: How long should it be maintained? *American Journal of Psychiatry, 143*(1), 18–23.

Prien, R. F., Kupfer, D. J., Mansky, P. A., Small, J. G., Tuason, U. B., Voss, C. B., et al. (1984). Drug therapy in the prevention of recurrences in unipolar and bipolar affective disorders: A report of the NIMH Collaborative Study Group comparing lithium carbonate, imipramine and a lithium carbonate–imipramine combination. *Archives of General Psychiatry, 41,* 1096–1104.

Prudic, J., Olfson, M., Marcus, S. C., Fuller, R. B., & Sackeim, H. A. (2004). Effectiveness of electroconvulsive therapy in community settings. *Biological Psychiatry, 55*(3), 301–312.

Reimherr, F. W., Amsterdam, J. D., Quitkin, F. M., Rosenbaum, J. F., Fava, M. F., Zajecka, J., et al. (1998). Optimal length of continuation therapy in depression: A prospective assessment during long-term fluoxetine treatment. *American Journal of Psychiatry, 155*(9), 1247–1253.

Roose, S. P., & Spatz, E. (1999). Treating depression in patients with ischemic heart disease. *Drug Safety, 20,* 459–465.

Ross, L. E., Grigoriadis, S., Mamisashvili, L., VonderPorten, E. H., Roerecke, M., Rehn, J., et al. (2013). Selected pregnancy and delivery outcomes after exposure to antidepressant medication. *Journal of the American Medical Association Psychiatry, 70*(4), 436–443.

Rush, A. J., Trivedi, M. H., Wisniewski, S. R., Nierenberg, A. A., Stewart, J. W., Warden, D., et al. (2006). Acute and longer-term outcomes in depressed outpatients requiring one or several treatment steps: A STAR*D report. *American Journal of Psychiatry, 163*(11), 1905–1917.

Sackeim, H. A., Prudic, J., Devanand, D. P., Nobler, M. S., Lisanby, S. H., Peyser, S., et al. (2000). A prospective, randomized, double-blind comparison of bilateral and right unilateral electroconvulsive therapy at different stimulus intensities. *Archives of General Psychiatry, 57,* 425–434.

Schueler, Y.-B., Koesters, M., Wieseler, B., Grouven, U., Kromp, M., Kerekes, M. F., et al. (2011). A systematic review of duloxetine and venlafaxine in major depression, including unpublished data. *Acta Psychiatrica Scandinavica, 123,* 247–265.

Slotema, C. W., Blom, J. D., Hoek, H. W., & Sommer, I. E. C. (2010). Should we expand the toolbox of psychiatric treatment methods to include repetitive transcranial magnetic stimulation (rTMS)?: A meta-analysis of the efficacy of rTMS in psychiatric disorders. *Journal of Clinical Psychiatry, 71*(7), 873–884.

Souery, D., Serretti, A., Calati, R., Oswald, P., Massat, I., Konstantinidis, A., et al. (2011). Switching antidepressant class does not improve response or remission in treatment-resistant depression. *Journal of Clinical Psychopharmacology, 31*(4), 512–516.

Stewart, D. E. (2011). Depression during pregnancy. *New England Journal of Medicine, 365,* 1605–1611.

Sublette, M. E., Ellis, S. P., Geant, A. L., & Mann, J. J. (2011). Meta-analysis of the effects of eicosapentaenoic acid (EPA) in clinical trials in depression. *Journal of Clinical Psychiatry, 72*(12), 1577–1584.

Szegedi, A., Jansen, W. T., van Willigenburg, A. P. P., van der Meulen, E., Stassen, H. H., & Thase, M. E. (2009). Early improvement in the first 2 weeks as a predictor of treatment outcome in patients with major depressive disorder: A meta-analysis including 6562 patients. *Journal of Clinical Psychiatry, 70*(3), 344–353.

Thase, M. E. (1998). Effects of venlafaxine on blood pressure: A meta-analysis of original data from 3,744 depressed patients. *Journal of Clinical Psychiatry, 59*(10), 502–508.

Thase, M. E. (2011). Antidepressant combinations: Widely used, but far from empirically validated. *Canadian Journal of Psychiatry, 56*(6), 317–323.

Trivedi, M. H., Rush, A. J., Wisniewski, S. R., Nierenberg, A. A., Warden, D., Ritz, L., et al. (2006). Evaluation of outcomes with citalopram for depression using measurement-based care in STAR*D: Implications for clinical practice. *American Journal of Psychiatry, 163*(1), 28–40.

Viguera, A. C., Tondo, L., Koukopoulos, A. E., Reginaldi, D., Lepri, B., & Baldessarini, R. J. (2011). Episodes of mood disorders in 2,252 pregnancies and postpartum periods. *American Journal of Psychiatry, 168*(11), 1179–1185.

CHAPTER 27

Cognitive and Behavioral Treatment of Depression

STEVEN D. HOLLON *and* SONA DIMIDJIAN

The cognitive and behavioral therapies are among the most widely used treatments for depression. These approaches have been shown to be as efficacious as medications and quite possibly longer lasting (Hollon, Thase, & Markowitz, 2002). There are even indications that they can prevent the onset of depressive episodes in at-risk adolescents, including those who have never yet had depression (Garber et al., 2009).

This chapter focuses on the nature and efficacy of the various cognitive and behavioral interventions. These include cognitive therapy and the related cognitive-behavioral interventions, along with the more purely behavioral interventions such as behavioral activation. These approaches often overlap in the procedures that they use but differ in other respects with regard to both theory and practice. Whether these differences matter with respect to the outcomes they produce remains to be seen, but they have implications for the nature of the patients treated and the ease with which the respective treatments can be disseminated.

COGNITIVE THERAPY AND RELATED INTERVENTIONS

Cognitive therapy (CT) is the earliest and best established of the cognitive-behavioral interventions (Hollon & Beck, 2013). CT is based on the notion that the way people interpret life experiences influences how they feel about those events and what they do to attempt to cope with them behaviorally (Beck, 2005). According to cognitive theory, people who are prone to depression are unduly negative in their perceptions of themselves, their worlds, and their futures (the negative cognitive triad) and are susceptible to a host of information-processing distortions that make it difficult for them to benefit from positive experience. Their thinking is seen as being dominated by negative *cognitive schemas*, organized knowledge structures that contain both core beliefs and underlying assumptions and that dictate the operation of biases in information processing. These schemas often function as "silent" *diatheses* (risk factors) that are activated by negative life events; for patients with more chronic distress, the schemas may be in a state of continuous activation.

Cognitive Model and Theory of Change

CT is predicated on the notion that teaching patients to recognize and correct negative beliefs and maladaptive information-processing proclivities helps them reduce their distress and enables more effective coping with life's challenges (Beck, Rush, Shaw, & Emery, 1979). The primary role of the therapist is to teach patients a set of skills used to examine the accuracy of their beliefs and to modify their behaviors. The ultimate goal of therapy is to help clients learn to use these tools independently. Such skills are not only important for symptom relief but also for relapse or recurrence prevention.

A successful course of CT accomplishes these goals through a structured, collaborative process that includes three distinct but interrelated components. The first component comprises a thorough *exploration* of the patient's dysfunctional beliefs or, more generally, his or her personal meaning system. A careful *examination* of that well-articulated belief system constitutes the second component of the therapy process. In this process, evidence speaking for and against the belief is reviewed, alternative explanations or interpretations are considered, and the consequences that might ensue if the belief were true are considered and put in a realistic perspective. Finally, active *experimentation*, designed specifically to "test" the validity of the maladaptive belief systems, is the third component of the therapeutic endeavor. Patients are first encouraged to engage in behavioral experiments to test specific predictions and then trained to examine the accuracy of their beliefs and finally to explore the larger meaning systems in which they are embedded.

The Structure of CT within and across Sessions

Individual sessions typically begin with the therapist and patient working together to set an agenda to prioritize matters of importance and ensure that their time together is spent efficiently. Once areas of difficulty are delineated, the therapist uses a series of gentle, thoughtful questions to bring to light the dysfunctional thoughts and beliefs that may be driving the patient's distress and maladaptive behaviors. This process of exploring negative automatic thoughts and their underlying core beliefs has been referred to as *Socratic questioning* and is assumed to be critical to successful CT. By its very nature, it avoids confrontation because the goal is to discover whether those negative thoughts and beliefs are serving the patient well rather than to expose him or her as a "faulty thinker." A failure to fully understand the patient's personal meaning system can hinder progress. In particular, it is important to "follow the affect." To the extent that the theory is correct, any strong affect should be associated with thoughts and beliefs that would make the reaction understandable (and universal) if they were true. The question then is whether those beliefs are as true as they first seemed to the patient. If the therapist cannot imagine feeling what the patient feels if he or she believed what the patient believes, then still more of the meaning system needs to be explored.

From the first session on, therapist and patient collaboratively generate assignments for the patient to complete between sessions. These assignments, which can be written or behavioral, often incorporate the experimental component of the therapeutic process. They allow the patient and therapist to test the patient's negative beliefs and predictions and to gather evidence necessary for cognitive change.

As therapy continues, the therapist and the patient work collaboratively to examine whether the patient's interpretations of events and beliefs about self, world, and future are accurate or adaptive. Progress is regularly and systematically assessed in terms of concrete behavioral outcomes. As patient and therapist gain a better understanding of the patient's worldview and as problematic core beliefs and underlying assumptions begin to change, they may revisit goals. New techniques are introduced throughout therapy, but all serve to address the same concept: the testing of negative beliefs and expectations.

CT emphasizes the links among thoughts, feelings, and behavior. As a result, many effective techniques incorporate behavioral interventions in the service of testing specific automatic negative thoughts and underlying beliefs or assumptions (Bennett-Levy et al., 2004). For example, patients with depression often feel overwhelmed and believe that they are unable to cope with life's demands. In fact, patients may indeed be facing serious demands in a number of different areas, including problems in relationships, financial difficulties, and difficulties at work. Such patients might be encouraged to "brainstorm" possible generic solutions (things that someone else might do), then to break large tasks into smaller constituent steps.

Patients then are encouraged to run an experiment to see whether they can get things done by focusing on accomplishing just one step at a time. After doing this *graded task assignment*, patients often find that they can more easily complete the larger tasks they set for themselves because they are less likely to be overwhelmed by their own negative thinking. This experience of success is used to disconfirm patients' negative expectations and to question underlying beliefs in their own incompetence.

Use of the various techniques depends on patients' goals and symptoms. Some techniques, such as the graded task assignment just described or scheduling in advance activities to complete across a given period of time (*activity scheduling*), are particularly useful early in therapy. Such concrete behavioral assignments allow patients to learn the observational and problem-solving skills they will be using throughout therapy and motivate them to take an active approach to problem solving and the pursuit of goals.

As therapy progresses, the focus turns to more explicitly cognitive techniques. For example, patients are taught to ask themselves a series of questions to examine the accuracy of their negative beliefs:

1. What is the *evidence* for and against that belief?
2. Are there *alternative explanations* for that event other than the one that first occurred to me?
3. What are the real *implications* if that belief is true?

The Dysfunctional Thoughts Record (DTR) is a formalized way to help patients learn to identify and respond to their negative automatic thoughts in a written format. The DTR comprises separate columns for recording the specific event that triggered a negative belief and the consequent feelings. The patient is encouraged to record each aspect of the problematic situation, to explore the larger meaning system in which that negative belief is embedded, and then to examine the accuracy of the belief using the three questions just described and perhaps collecting more information or running a behavioral experiment to test those beliefs. Additional techniques include teaching problem-solving and decision-making skills, developing flash cards with important phrases as patient self-reminders, and in-session role play to practice real-life interactions.

The Course of CT and Schema-Focused Modifications

CT is designed to be an efficient, structured, short-term form of treatment. For patients with uncomplicated depressions—that is, for people with recurrent depressions who have an essentially adaptive view of the self when not depressed—this might mean a treatment length of 10–20 sessions over 12–16 weeks (Beck, 2011). In contrast, patients with long-standing histories of rigid dysfunctional beliefs (usually patients with chronic histories or depressions secondary to personality disorders) may need a considerably longer course of treatment. For such patients, the inaccurate beliefs and related maladaptive behaviors often are deeply entrenched and may represent the only way they have ever thought about themselves or their world. As a result, more exploration and examination of the faulty belief system and more experimentation designed to modify those beliefs often are required. Thus, regardless of the persistence of depressive symptoms, it is the patient's particular set of maladaptive or dysfunctional beliefs that is the primary target of CT.

In recent years, CT has evolved with respect to its approach to the treatment of long-standing symptoms and personality disorders (Beck, Freeman, Davis, & Associates, 2003). The process of providing a cognitive conceptualization was always a central organizing principle of the approach, but early efforts with episodic patients focused more exclusively on applying cognitive and behavioral techniques to the resolution of negative thoughts and maladaptive behaviors in response to life difficulties "in the here and now." Attention to earlier life events and childhood antecedents that contributed to the development of these underlying schemas was reserved for later sessions, after the patient was largely free of symptoms. In a similar fashion, attention was paid to the therapeutic relationship only when problems arose in the working alliance.

Over recent decades, it has become clear that patients with histories of chronic depression or with depressions superimposed on long-standing character disorders have no other way of thinking about themselves and often need help to construct completely new schemas to guide thinking and behavior. For these patients, Beck uses the metaphor of a "three-legged stool" to describe his approach to the implementation of CT. According to this metaphor, the three "legs" include exploring (1) the thoughts and feelings that surround some particular current life concern, (2) the historical antecedents that gave rise to those beliefs, and (3) the way in which those beliefs manifest themselves in the ongoing therapeutic relationship.

This process seems to help the patient recognize that much of his or her distress stems from these long-standing maladaptive beliefs and not just from events. Moreover, it further helps to recognize that these beliefs often were acquired early in life, before the patient developed the capacity to make the kinds of reasoned judgments that come with greater maturity. Most important, it helps to make sense out of the habitual and self-defeating patterns of behavior (*compensatory strategies*) that such patients adopt to deal with perceived imperfections and dangers specified by those beliefs. Dealing with the manifestations of these attitudes and beliefs and the maladaptive behaviors they engender in the context of the therapeutic relationship provides an opportunity to try out new behaviors in a somewhat safer interpersonal context. Although many of these strategies are reminiscent of more dynamic therapies, the discussion is always brought back around to just how these beliefs can be tested in current life situations, and no presumption is made that unconscious sexual or aggressive drives are at the core of the patient's difficulties.

Evidence for Efficacy and Comparisons to Medication

CT has been one of the most extensively studied of the psychosocial interventions, and it has typically fared well in comparisons with minimal treatment controls and other psychosocial interventions (DeRubeis & Crits-Christoph, 1998). Early studies suggested that CT was superior to medications, but they were flawed with respect to the way that pharmacotherapy was implemented (Blackburn, Bishop, Glen, Whalley, & Christie, 1981; Rush, Beck, Kovacs, & Hollon, 1977). Subsequent studies that did a better job of implementing both interventions adequately found CT to be about as efficacious as medications (Hollon, DeRubeis, Evans, et al., 1992; Murphy, Simons, Wetzel, & Lustman, 1984). In the National Institute of Mental Health (NIMH) Treatment of Depression Collaborative Research Program (TDCRP), however, CT was less efficacious than medications and no more efficacious than pill placebo among patients with more severe depressions (Elkin et al., 1995). Given the size of this study and the fact that it was the first placebo-controlled comparison with medication, the TDCRP had a major impact on the field and led to the recommendation that CT not be used alone in the treatment of patients with severe depression (American Psychiatric Association, 2000).

It is important to note, however, that differences among the sites in their prior experience with CT mirrored differences in efficacy of the approach (Jacobson & Hollon, 1996a). At the two sites with less prior experience with the modality, CT did no better than pill placebo, whereas at a third site, with greater prior experience in the approach, CT did as well as medications (Jacobson & Hollon, 1996b). This suggests that the TDCRP may have failed to implement CT in an adequate fashion at each of its sites, just as some of the earlier comparative trials may have failed to implement drug treatment adequately.

It now appears that the TDCRP was something of an anomaly. Subsequent studies have found that CT is as efficacious as medications and both superior to pill placebo when each is adequately implemented (DeRubeis et al., 2005; Jarrett et al., 1999). Therapist competence appears to be a key, especially with more severe or complicated patients, something that represents a limitation to the approach, as we discuss later.

Does CT Have an Enduring Effect?

There are consistent indications that CT has an enduring effect that lasts beyond the end of treatment (Hollon, Stewart, & Strunk, 2006). Several studies have shown that patients treated to remission with CT are considerably less likely to relapse following treatment termination than patients treated to remission with medications (Blackburn, Eunson, & Bishop, 1986; Kovacs, Rush, Beck, & Hollon, 1981; Simons, Murphy, Levine, & Wetzel, 1986) and that the magnitude of this enduring effect is at least as great as that when patients are kept on continuation medications (David, Szentagotai, Lupu, & Cosman, 2008; Dobson et al., 2008; Evans et al., 1992; Hollon et al., 2005). The only two studies that have not found such an enduring effect for prior CT involved a small pilot sample of atypical patients (Jarrett et al., 2000) and the follow-up to the NIMH TDCRP, in which such nonsignificant differences as were apparent favored prior CT (Shea et al., 1992). A recent meta-analysis found that prior CT prevented one relapse for every 5 patients treated relative to medication withdrawal and one relapse prevented for every 10 patients treated with continuation medications (Cuijpers et al., 2013). Given that most patients with recurrent or chronic depressions are now kept on medications indefinitely, this enduring effect represents a major advantage that CT has over medication treatment (Hollon, 2011).

Klein (1996) has argued that such findings could be an artifact of differential attrition because high-risk patients may need medications to improve and low-risk patients may be unable to tolerate medications' side effects, therefore dropping out of treatment at a differential rate. Such proclivities could lead acute treatment to serve as a "differential sieve" that systematically biases subsequent comparisons against medication treatment if a greater proportion of high-risk patients completed and responded to medication than to CT. It is noteworthy, however, that several studies that first treated patients to remission or recovery with medications and subsequently randomized patients to CT or related interventions also have shown an enduring effect that could not be attributed to differential attrition (Bockting et al., 2005; Fava, Rafanelli, Grandi, Conti, & Belluardo, 1998; Paykel et al., 1999; Teasdale et al., 2002). Moreover, there are indications that cognitive-behavioral interventions can be used to prevent the onset of symptoms in people at risk who do not currently have depression (Garber et al., 2009; Seligman, Schulman, DeRubeis, & Hollon, 1999).

Who Responds to CT?

There is an important distinction to be made between prognostic and prescriptive indices. *Prognostic indices* tell you which patients do better than others in a given treatment (or in treatment in general), whereas *prescriptive indices* tell you what treatment is best for a given patient. Prescriptive indices also are known as moderators and typically are detected on the basis of patient-by-treatment interactions (Kraemer, Wilson, Fairburn, & Agras, 2002). Patients with chronic depression, those who are older, and those who are less intelligent did worse than other patients in either CT or medication treatment in a recent placebo-controlled trial (Fournier et al., 2009). Although such prognostic indices might indicate who needs more intensive or longer treatment, they do not provide a basis for choosing one treatment over another. However, Fournier and colleagues (2009) found that patients who were married or unemployed or who had more prior precipitating life events did better in CT than they did in medication treatment. If replicated, such prescriptive indices could be used as a basis for treatment selection. All the prescriptive indices were ordinal in nature; that means that patients with those characteristics did better in one treatment than they did in another (in each instance CT was superior to medications), whereas patients without those characteristics responded comparably to each. The only prescriptive characteristic that showed a disordinal interaction was presence of an Axis II personality disorder; patients with personality disorders did better on medications than they did in CT, whereas patients without personality disorders showed the opposite pattern (Fournier et al., 2008). Although patients with Axis II disorders were more likely to respond to medications than to CT, they were particularly likely to relapse when those medications were taken away, whereas those patients who responded to CT tended not to relapse following treatment termination regardless of whether they had an Axis II disorder.

One of the purely prognostic indices warrants particular mention because of its possible implications for the underlying nature of medication treatment. The more prior medication exposures a patient had, the worse the patient did in medication treatment; no such relation was evident for cognitive therapy (Leykin et al., 2007). This is not the first time that this prognostic pattern has been observed with respect to medication treatment, and it has at least two possible explanations. First, it may simply be that those patients who are less likely to respond to medications are going to be switched from one to another in hopes of finding one to which they respond. This is the *individual differences* explanation. The second possibility is somewhat more pernicious. There are concerns that being exposed to active medications may generate a kind of *progressive resistance* such that patients become increasingly less likely to respond with each subsequent exposure. *Tachyphylaxis* is the term used in the medical literature to refer to the progressive loss of response with subsequent or extended exposure. Furthermore, there is a growing concern that active medications may suppress symptoms at the expense of worsening the course of the underlying disorder (Whitaker, 2010); in essence, patients may stay "in episode" for as long as they stay on medications (Fava, 1994) and be at elevated risk for relapse at whatever point they are taken off (El-Mallakh, Waltrip, & Peters, 1999). Along that line, it has been shown that the extent to which a given antidepressant medication perturbs the biogenic amine neurotransmitter systems (serotonin and norepinephrine especially) determines the likelihood of relapse when they are discontinued (Andrews et al., 2011). For all these reasons, some in the field are starting to reconsider the wisdom of routinely combining CT with medications, preferring instead to use the psychosocial intervention alone (Forand, DeRubeis, & Amsterdam, 2013).

There also are indications that patients with less severe depressions respond largely for nonspecific reasons; drug–placebo differences are evident only among patients with more severe depressions (Fournier et al., 2010), and the same appears to be true for psychotherapy (Driessen, Cuijpers, Hollon, & Dekker, 2010). What this means is that patients with less severe depressions are likely to get better regardless of the type of treatment they receive and that treatments that mobilize specific causal mechanisms are required only for patients with more severe depressions (Driessen et al., 2010). However, that relation appears to hold only with respect to acute response; there is no indication that severity moderates the enduring effect of treatment. Given that medication treatment does not separate from pill placebo among patients with less severe depressions (the majority of patients who meet criteria for major depressive disorder) and that medications produce noxious side effects not found for the psychosocial interventions, a case can be made that CT with its enduring effect should be preferred over medications as the first line of treatment for all nonpsychotic unipolar depressions, especially if concerns that medications worsen the course of the underlying disorder are founded (Hollon, 2011).

MECHANISMS OF CHANGE AND PREVENTION

It is useful to distinguish between the active ingredients of a given intervention and the mechanisms in the patient through which they work. Both can be considered mediators, and logically they have to occur in a sequential order (active ingredients engage causal mechanisms to produce clinical change). With respect to the active ingredients in CT, DeRubeis and colleagues have shown that the extent to which therapists utilize behavioral and cognitive change strategies in early sessions predicts subsequent change in depression, whereas the quality of the working alliance (a nonspecific aspect of the therapeutic relationship) was more a consequence than a cause of symptom change (DeRubeis & Feeley, 1990; Feeley, DeRubeis, & Gelfand, 1999). This suggests that it may not be necessary to build the relationship before trying to produce change; rather, working to produce change may build a sense of trust and collaboration. Both behavioral and cognitive strategies predicted change, a point we return to when we talk about behavioral interventions.

Cognitive theory suggests that disconfirming negative expectations may be the most efficient way to reduce existing distress, whereas changing underlying explanatory style or self-concept may be more central to the prevention of future episodes (Abramson, Metalsky, & Alloy, 1989). Patients treated with medications alone often show as much change in specific expectations and beliefs as patients treated with CT. However, the patterns of change over time between the two modalities tend to be quite different; change in expectations drives change in depression in CT, whereas change in depression drives change in expectations in medication treatment (DeRubeis et al., 1990). This suggests that cognitive change plays a causal role in CT, whereas it is a consequence of change in symptoms brought about by biological means in medication.

At the same time, changes in core beliefs and information-processing proclivities may be central to the prevention of subsequent relapse and recurrence. In an earlier trial, change in explanatory style was specific to CT and predictive of subsequent freedom from relapse following treatment termination (Hollon, Evans, & DeRubeis, 1990). Whereas change in expectations was nonspecific and occurred in conjunction with change in depression (whether cause or consequence), change in explanatory style occurred only in CT and then only later in the course of therapy, well after the bulk of the change in depression. This suggests that change in these underlying proclivities is not necessary for initial symptom reduction but may be central to the prevention of subsequent symptom return. The acquisition of skills in recognizing and disputing negative beliefs predicted freedom from relapse in one study (Strunk, DeRubeis, Chiu, & Alvarez, 2007) and "insight" into the role of cognition in driving affect preceded sudden gains in treatment that in turn predicted freedom from subsequent relapse and recurrence in another (Tang, DeRubeis, Hollon, Amsterdam, & Shelton, 2007). The fact that medications do little to reduce these cognitive diatheses is consistent with the finding that they do little to reduce subsequent risk for relapse or recurrence once their use is terminated. Although it is unclear whether patients treated with CT change in some way that redresses underlying vulnerabilities or whether they develop compensatory skills that they must continue to apply, it is apparent that risk is reduced (Barber & DeRubeis, 1989).

All cognition and behavior rests on an underlying neural substrate (Beck, 2008). It is likely that CT works from the "top down" through cortical mechanisms to produce its enduring change in depression, whereas medications work from the "bottom up" through their effects on the brain stem and limbic system (DeRubeis, Siegle, & Hollon, 2008). Patients with depression typically show hyperactivity in the limbic regions that are important to perceiving emotional aspects of information (especially the amygdala) and hypoactivity in areas of the prefrontal cortex that exert inhibitory control over those limbic regions (Drevets, 2000; Gotlib & Hamilton, 2008). Imaging studies are consistent with this formulation with differential change in exactly those regions as a function of differential treatment with CT versus medications (Kennedy et al., 2007). These differential changes have not yet been related to subsequent relapse and recurrence, but Maier, Amat, Baratta, Paul, and Watkins (2006) have shown not only that cortically mediated "learned resilience" in the rat has a direct inhibitory effect on stress reactivity mediated in the limbic system and brain stem but also that this mechanism has an enduring effect that lasts over time and reduces reactivity to future stress.

PROBLEMS IN DISSEMINATION AND ROBUSTNESS ACROSS TRIALS

Despite its apparent efficacy and evidence of enduring effects, CT has not been easy to disseminate and has suffered from a lack of robustness across trials. The TDCRP stands as one clear example of a study in which experienced therapists had trouble learning to apply CT (Elkin et al., 1995), and a subsequent comparison with a more purely behavioral activation (BA) represents another (Dimidjian et al., 2006). In each of these studies, CT was outperformed by medications and one other psychosocial intervention (interpersonal psychotherapy [IPT] in the first instance and BA in the second) in the treatment of patients with more severe depression. A third study found a significant site × treatment interaction in which CT did better than medications at the site with more experienced therapists and less well than medications at the site with the less experienced CT therapists (DeRubeis et al., 2005). These studies raise questions as to just how easy it is for therapists to learn to use the approach, especially when working with patients with more complicated disorders (Coffman, Martell, Dimidjian, Gallop, & Hollon, 2007). Findings with respect to CT's enduring effect are more robust (Dobson et al., 2008; Hollon et al., 2005; but see Shea et al., 1992). We return to these issues when we discuss the more purely behavioral interventions.

MINDFULNESS-BASED COGNITIVE THERAPY

Mindfulness-based cognitive therapy (MBCT) represents an integration of meditation with more conventional CT. Patients are trained to observe thinking patterns that characterize depressive states and to develop a new mode of responding to such patterns, thus preventing negative emotions from escalating into more enduring affective states (Segal, Williams, & Teasdale, 2002). MBCT prevents subsequent relapse or recurrence significantly more than treatment as usual (Bondolfi et al., 2010; Godfrin & van Heeringen, 2010; Ma & Teasdale, 2004; Teasdale et al., 2000) and comparably to maintenance medication (Kuyken et al., 2008; Segal et al., 2010). The magnitude of the effect produced by MBCT appears to be greatest for more vulnerable patients, including those with more recurrent depressions or unstable patterns of remission. Recently, MBCT also has been examined in controlled trials as an intervention for patients with acute or residual depression (e.g., Chiesa, Mandelli, & Serretti, 2012; Geschwind, Peeters, Huibers, van Os, & Wichers, 2012).

NOVEL DELIVERY FORMATS

Finally, recent years have witnessed an expansion of interest in novel delivery formats for CT interventions such as online and telephone-administered approaches. Although such interventions do not differ from CT in underlying theory or specific strategies used, the emphasis on self-guided treatment or minimal therapist coaching differs from standard CT or cognitive-behavioral therapy (CBT) approaches. Both online programs (e.g., Christensen, Griffiths, & Jorm, 2004; Clarke et al., 2005; Proudfoot et al., 2004; Richards & Richardson, 2012) and telephone-administered treatments (e.g., Mohr, Vella, Hart, Heckman, & Simon, 2008; Mohr et al., 2012; Simon, Ludman, Tutty, Operskalski, & VonKorff, 2004) have fared well in clinical trials.

MORE PURELY BEHAVIORAL INTERVENTIONS

There also exist a number of more purely behavioral approaches to depression. Problem-solving therapy (PST) is predicated on the notion that deficits in coping skills contribute to the onset and maintenance of depression (D'Zurilla & Nezu, 1982). It seeks to teach patients how to define life problems in ways that facilitate finding a solution and helps them to generate and to choose among several possible alternatives. PST has been found to be superior to no treatment and nonspecific controls in a pair of studies with symptomatic community volunteers (Nezu, 1986; Nezu & Perri, 1989). More recently, investigators in England found a brief PST to be comparable to drugs and superior to placebo in the treatment of depression in a general practice sample (Mynors-Wallace, Gath, Day, & Baker, 2000; Mynors-Wallace, Gath, Lloyd-Thomas, & Tomlinson, 1995). These studies suggest that PST has considerable merit.

More purely behavioral interventions based on operant theory typically also have fared well in controlled trials. Hersen, Bellack, Himmelhoch, and Thase (1984) found no differences between social skills training (combined with either drugs or pill placebo) and drugs alone or a brief dynamic psychotherapy in a sample of female outpatients with depression. McLean and Hakstian (1979) found a modest advantage for a behavioral intervention based on contingency management relative to either medications alone or to a brief dynamic psychotherapy in the treatment of outpatients with depression. O'Leary and Beach (1990) found that behavioral marital therapy was as efficacious as CT and superior to a wait-list control in the treatment of depression in couples with marital distress. Similarly, Jacobson, Dobson, Fruzzetti, Schmaling, and Salusky (1991) found that behavioral marital therapy was as efficacious as CT in reducing depression in women with marital distress but less efficacious than CT for women without such marital problems.

Behavioral Activation and Other Activation-Oriented Treatments

Work on purely behavioral treatments for depression stagnated somewhat before publication of a component analysis study by Jacobson, Dobson, and colleagues (1996) in which the BA component of CT produced as much change as did the full treatment package. Moreover, there were no differences in subsequent rates of relapse following treatment termination (Gortner, Gollan, Dobson, & Jacobson, 1998). These findings were so unexpected that Jacobson, Martell, and Dimidjian (2001) developed a more comprehensive version of the approach rooted in the work of Lewinsohn (1974) and Ferster (1973, 1981), both of whom highlighted the centrality of context and activity in understanding depression.

The BA approach emphasizes the role of life contexts that are characterized by low levels of positive reinforcement and high levels of aversive control in precipitating or maintaining depression. In addition, an individual's tendency to respond to such contexts with avoidance and withdrawal is highlighted. The BA approach emphasizes that such responses are natural and understandable; however, they also prevent contact with experiences that could improve mood and hinder active problem solving. Guided activation is proposed as a general approach to help to disrupt the context–activity–mood relations that maintain depression.

The implementation of BA is highly idiographic; a careful assessment of the factors that maintain a particular patient's depression helps a therapist to individualize the general model and guides the selection of treatment strategies. Therapists work with clients to define and to describe key problems specifically and to examine the behavioral patterns that prompt or maintain such problems. Self-monitoring is a key tool, and treatment focuses heavily on helping patients identify contingent relations among situations, activities, and moods.

Like CT, BA is highly structured. Therapists work collaboratively with patients to set and to follow an agenda each session, to clearly review progress since previous sessions, and to use patient ratings on self-report symptom severity questionnaires to assess change. Assigning and reviewing homework is a major focus of BA, and therapists spend considerable time anticipating and troubleshooting potential barriers and working with clients to maximize their commitment to action.

Over the course of treatment, therapists utilize a small set of strategies and maintain an overriding focus on activation. Primary strategies include developing activation assignments that increase pleasure and mastery and approach behavior (as opposed to avoidance). Therapists work with clients to schedule activities and frequently break larger activities down into their constituent parts and sequence them to increase likelihood of success. BA therapists frequently work with patients to generate and to evaluate solutions to problems and may teach skills as appropriate (e.g., assertive communication). Therapists in BA do not target the direct modification of thoughts or beliefs, as do cognitive therapists. Although BA therapists may assess negative or ruminative thoughts, treatment strategies emphasize highlighting the consequences of ruminative thinking, practice in engaging with direct and immediate experience, and refocusing on immediate goals. In general, a primary treatment goal of BA is to encourage patients to act proactively instead of engaging in avoidance behaviors.

Research on BA has expanded substantially in recent years (Dimidjian, Barrera, Martell, Muñoz, & Lewinsohn, 2011). BA has been compared with CT and with pharmacotherapy (paroxetine) in a randomized, placebo-controlled clinical trial (Dimidjian et al. 2006). Among patients with more severe depression, BA was comparable in outcomes to pharmacotherapy and significantly outperformed CT; among patients with less severe depression, no differences among the treatments were observed. Patients treated with BA also did as well with respect to the prevention of relapse as those treated with CT or continued on their medication over the follow-up period, although only those previously treated with CT demonstrated significant advantage compared with those whose medications were discontinued (Dobson et al., 2008). These findings suggest that BA also has promise with respect to enduring effects.

The encouraging findings associated with BA are consistent with other trials investigating related activation approaches to depression. An early dismantling study among older adults, for instance, also found no differences between a purely behavioral and a cognitive bibliotherapy intervention, with both significantly outperforming a control intervention (Scogin, Jamison, & Gochneaur, 1989). A related behavioral activation model has shown promise in the treatment of depression among cancer patients (Hopko, Bell, Armento, Hunt, & Lejuez, 2005) and among psychiatric inpatients (Hopko, Lejuez, LePage, Hopko, & McNeil, 2003). Exercise-based interventions have also accumulated increasing support in the treatment of depression (Stathopoulou, Powers, Berry, Smits, & Otto, 2006).

Early findings on BA appear to be robust across recent studies and meta-analyses (e.g., Cuijpers, van Straten, & Warmerdam, 2007; Ekers, Richards, & Gilbody, 2008; Mazzucchelli, Kane, & Rees, 2009). Such results may well revive interest in more purely behavioral interventions (Hollon, 2001). These interventions may be considerably easier to apply and may lend themselves more readily to dissemination than either CT or more traditional psychotherapeutic approaches. Initial studies with nonspecialist providers or non-Western populations support such hypotheses (Ekers, Richards, McMillan, Bland, & Gilbody, 2011; Moradveisi, Huibers, Renner, Arasteh, & Arntz, 2013). If such findings are replicated across settings and other care providers, the public health benefit of BA may be significant.

CONCLUSIONS AND FUTURE DIRECTIONS

Cognitive and behavioral interventions are clearly efficacious in the treatment of depression. Moreover, they appear to have enduring effects that reduce subsequent risk. CT may work by teaching patients to identify and to test their negative beliefs and information-processing strategies, although the success of more purely behavioral interventions raises the question as to whether it is necessary to focus on cognition to produce symptom change. At the least, imparting a set of strategies that patients can use to relieve their own distress produces lasting change. It does appear that these strategies can be extended to patients with more severe and complicated depressions, although questions remain about how robust CT is in that regard. It is possible that more purely behavioral approaches will prove to be easier to disseminate than CT.

Recent studies further suggest that simpler and more concrete behavioral interventions are efficacious for many patients with affective distress, including those with severe or chronic depression. To the extent that this is true, it may facilitate the dissemination of these approaches to the clinical practice community, which is increasingly coming to rely on less extensively trained practitioners and shorter treatment intervals. If they prove to have enduring effects (as early studies suggest), they will generate real enthusiasm in the field.

Even more critically, it remains to be seen whether the enduring effect produced by the cognitive and possibly the behavioral interventions extends to the prevention of recurrence. Any such enduring effect would be more interesting theoretically and more important pragmatically if it worked to prevent the onset of wholly new episodes. As effective as medications are (and they are largely safe and effective), there is no evidence that they do anything to reduce subsequent risk once their use is discontinued (Hollon, 1996). Because depression tends to be a chronic episodic disorder, any treatment that can reduce subsequent risk would be a real boon to the field, both in terms of the reduction of human misery and the savings in costs to society.

Closely related is the notion of primary prevention. Not only do the cognitive and (possibly) the behavioral interventions appear to have an enduring effect, but there also reason to believe that they may have a preventive effect in at-risk adolescents, including those who have not yet had their first episode (Garber et al., 2009). Throughout the history of medical science, major public health advances have occurred more as a consequence of prevention than of treatment (Hollon, DeRubeis, & Seligman, 1992). Much of this work will need to take place outside of traditional service delivery settings, most likely in schools and in general practice settings (Rotheram-Boras, Swendeman, & Chorpita, (2012). Nonetheless, it is clear that the technology already exists both to detect persons at risk and to provide them with tools they can use to reduce subsequent risk (Gillham, Shatte, & Freres, 2000).

Much of this progress has occurred in conjunction with a growing understanding of the basic processes that underlie the nature and expression of depression. Depression is a disorder that is clearly affected by biological, psychological, and sociological factors, and important advances in treatment both draw upon and feedback to advances in basic research (Hollon, Muñoz, et al., 2002). The cognitive-behavioral interventions in particular have benefited from advances in understanding of basic cognitive processes and our growing understanding of information processing (Hollon & Garber, 1990; see Joormann & Arditte, Chapter 14, this volume). The direct links between basic and applied research are not always clear, but they are important.

In this regard, several questions seem particularly important. For example, depression often involves disruptions in social bonds, yet medications and the cognitive and behavior therapies are among its most efficacious interventions (along with IPT). Similarly, biological processes often trigger affective distress, and both genes and environmental events appear to confer risk for subsequent distress (Caspi et al., 2003). Maladaptive beliefs and behaviors can be acquired through either route and further amplify risk for those who are so predisposed. Nonetheless, we have little clear understanding of how these processes relate to one another nor of exactly how our treatments work when they work. The brain is an organ designed to mediate interaction with the environment, and there is reason to believe that it is capable of responding to external contingencies within the constraints set by biology (Davidson, Pizzagalli, Nitschke, & Putnam, 2002). Clearly, more needs to be done to explore the ways in which cognitive and interpersonal processes interface with basic biology in determining the nature and expression of depression.

REFERENCES

Abramson, L. Y., Metalsky, G. I., & Alloy, L. B. (1989). Hopelessness depression: A theory-based subtype of depression: A metatheoretical analysis with implications for psychopathology research. *Psychological Review, 96,* 358–372.

American Psychiatric Association. (2000). Practice guideline for the treatment of patients with major depressive disorder (revision). *American Journal of Psychiatry, 157*(Suppl. 4), 1–45.

Andrews, P. W., Kornstein, S. G., Halberstadt, L. J., Gardner, C. O., & Neale, M. C. (2011). Blue again: Perturbational effects of antidepressants suggest monoaminergic homeostasis in major depression. *Frontiers in Psychology, 2,* 159. Available at *www.ncbi.nlm.nih.gov/pmc/articles/PMC3133866/.*

Barber, J. P., & DeRubeis, R. J. (1989). On second thought: Where the action is in cognitive therapy for depression. *Cognitive Therapy and Research, 13,* 441–457.

Beck, A. T. (2005). The current state of cognitive therapy: A 40-year retrospective. *Archives of General Psychiatry, 62,* 953–959.

Beck, A. T. (2008). The evolution of the cognitive model of depression and its neural correlates. *American Journal of Psychiatry, 165,* 969–977.

Beck, A. T., Freeman, A., Davis, D. D., & Associates. (2003). *Cognitive therapy of personality disorders* (2nd ed.). New York: Guilford Press.

Beck, A. T., Rush, A. J., Shaw, B. F., & Emery, G. (1979). *The cognitive therapy of depression.* New York: Guilford Press.

Beck, J. S. (2011). *Cognitive therapy: Basics and beyond* (2nd ed.). New York: Guilford Press.

Bennett-Levy, J., Butler, G., Fennell, M., Hackmann, A., Mueller, M., & Westbrook, D. (2004). *Oxford guide to behavioural experiments in cognitive therapy.* Oxford, UK: Oxford University Press.

Blackburn, I. M., Bishop, S., Glen, A. I. M., Whalley, L. J., & Christie, J. E. (1981). The efficacy of cognitive therapy in depression: A treatment trial using cognitive therapy and pharmacotherapy, each alone and in combination. *British Journal of Psychiatry, 139,* 181–189.

Blackburn, I. M., Eunson, K. M., & Bishop, S. (1986). A two-year naturalistic follow-up of depressed patients treated with cognitive therapy, pharmacotherapy and a combination of both. *Journal of Affective Disorders, 10,* 67–75.

Bockting, C. L., Schene, A. H., Spinhoven, P., Koeter, M. W. J., Wouters, L. F., Huyser, J., et al. (2005). Preventing relapse/recurrence in recurrent depression with cognitive therapy: A randomized controlled trial. *Journal of Consulting and Clinical Psychology, 73,* 647–657.

Bondolfi, G., Jermann, F., der Linden, M. V., Gex-Fabry, M., Bizzini, L., Rouget, B. W., et al.

(2010). Depression relapse prophylaxis with mindfulness-based cognitive therapy: Replication and extension in the Swiss health care system. *Journal of Affective Disorders, 122*(3), 224–31.

Caspi, A., Sugden, K., Moffitt, T. E., Taylor, A., Craig, I. W., Harrington, H., et al. (2003). Influence of life stress on depression: Moderation by a polymorphism in the *5-HTT* gene. *Science, 301*, 386–389.

Chiesa, A., Mandelli, L., & Serretti, A. (2012). Mindfulness-based cognitive therapy versus psycho-education for patients with major depression who did not achieve remission following antidepressant treatment: A preliminary analysis. *Journal of Alternative and Complementary Medicine, 18*(8), 756–760.

Christensen, H., Griffiths, K. M., & Jorm, A. F. (2004). Delivering interventions for depression by using the Internet: Randomised controlled trial. *British Medical Journal, 328*, 265.

Clarke, G., Eubanks, D., Reid, E., Kelleher, C., O'Connor, E., DeBar, L. L., et al. (2005). Overcoming depression on the Internet (ODIN): 2. A randomized trial of a self-help depression skills program with reminders. *Journal of Medical Internet Research, 7*, e16.

Coffman, S., Martell, C. R., Dimidjian, S., Gallop, R., & Hollon, S. D. (2007). Extreme nonresponse in cognitive therapy: Can behavioral activation succeed where cognitive therapy fails? *Journal of Consulting and Clinical Psychology, 75*, 531–541.

Cuijpers, P., Hollon, S. D., van Straten, A., Bockting, C., Berking, M., & Andersson, G. (2013). Does cognitive behavior therapy have an enduring effect that is superior to keeping patients on continuation pharmacotherapy? *BMJ Open, 3*(4), e002542. Available at *www.ncbi.nlm.nih.gov/pmc/articles/PMC3641456/*.

Cuijpers, P., van Straten, A., & Warmerdam, L. (2007). Behavioral activation treatments of depression: A meta-analysis. *Clinical Psychology Review, 27*, 318–326.

David, D., Szentagotai, A., Lupu, V., & Cosman, D. (2008). Rational emotive behavior therapy, cognitive therapy, and medication in the treatment of major depressive disorder: A randomized clinical trial, posttreatment outcomes, and six-month follow-up. *Journal of Clinical Psychology, 64*, 728–746.

Davidson, R. J., Pizzagalli, D., Nitschke, J. B., & Putnam, K. (2002). Depression: Perspectives from affective neuroscience. *Annual Review of Psychology, 35*, 545–574.

DeRubeis, R. J., & Crits-Christoph, P. (1998). Empirically supported individual and group psychological treatments for adult mental disorders. *Journal of Consulting and Clinical Psychology, 66*, 37–52.

DeRubeis, R. J., Evans, M. D., Hollon, S. D., Garvey, M. J., Grove, W. M., & Tuason, V. B. (1990). How does cognitive therapy work?: Cognitive change and symptom change in cognitive therapy and pharmacotherapy for depression. *Journal of Consulting and Clinical Psychology, 58*, 862–869.

DeRubeis, R. J., & Feeley, M. (1990). Determinants of change in cognitive therapy for depression. *Cognitive Therapy and Research, 14*, 469–482.

DeRubeis, R. J., Hollon, S. D., Amsterdam, J. D., Shelton, R. C., Young, P. R., Salomon, R. M., et al. (2005). Cognitive therapy vs. medications in the treatment of moderate to severe depression. *Archives of General Psychiatry, 62*, 409–416.

DeRubeis, R. J., Siegle, G. J., & Hollon, S. D. (2008). Cognitive therapy versus medication for depression: Treatment outcomes and neural mechanisms. *Nature Reviews Neuroscience, 9*, 788–796.

Dimidjian, S., Barrera, M., Jr., Martell, C., Muñoz, R. F., & Lewinsohn, P. M. (2011). The origins and current status of behavioral activation treatments for depression. *Annual Review of Clinical Psychology, 7*, 1–38.

Dimidjian, S., Hollon, S. D., Dobson, K. S., Schmaling, K. B., Kohlenberg, R. J., Addis, M. E., et al. (2006). Behavioral activation, cognitive therapy, and antidepressant medication in the acute treatment of major depression. *Journal of Consulting and Clinical Psychology, 74*, 658–670.

Dobson, K. S., Hollon, S. D., Dimidjian, S., Schmaling, K. B., Kohlenberg, R. J., Gallop, R., et al. (2008). Behavioral activation, cognitive therapy, and anti-depressant medication in the treatment of major depression: Prevention of relapse effects. *Journal of Consulting and Clinical Psychology, 76,* 468–477.

Driessen, E., Cuijpers, P., Hollon, S. D., & Dekker, J. J. M. (2010). Does pretreatment severity moderate the efficacy of psychological treatment of adult outpatient depression?: A meta-analysis. *Journal of Consulting and Clinical Psychology, 78,* 668–680.

Driessen, E., & Hollon, S. D. (2010). Cognitive behavioral therapy for mood disorders: Efficacy, moderators and mediators. *Psychiatric Clinics of North America, 33,* 537–555.

Drevets, W. C. (2000). Neuroimaging studies of mood disorders. *Biological Psychiatry, 48,* 813–829.

D'Zurilla, T. J., & Nezu, A. (1982). Social problem solving in adults. In P. C. Kendall (Ed.), *Advances in cognitive-behavioral research and therapy* (Vol. 1, pp. 202–274). New York: Academic Press.

Ekers, D., Richards, D., & Gilbody, S. (2008). A meta-analysis of randomized trials of behavioural treatment of depression. *Psychological Medicine, 38,* 611–623.

Ekers, D., Richards, D., McMillan, D., Bland, J. M., & Gilbody, S. (2011). Behavioural activation delivered by the non-specialist: Phase II randomized controlled trial. *British Journal of Psychiatry, 198,* 66–72.

Elkin, I., Gibbons, R. D., Shea, T., Sotsky, S. M., Watkins, J. T., Pilkonis, P. A., et al. (1995). Initial severity and differential treatment outcome in the National Institute of Mental Health Treatment of Depression Collaborative Research Program. *Journal of Consulting and Clinical Psychology, 63,* 841–847.

El-Mallakh, R. S., Waltrip, C., & Peters, C. (1999). Can long-term antidepressant use be depressogenic? *Journal of Clinical Psychiatry, 60,* 263–264.

Evans, M. D., Hollon, S. D., DeRubeis, R. J., Piasecki, J., Grove, W. M., Garvey, M. J., et al. (1992). Differential relapse following cognitive therapy and pharmacotherapy for depression. *Archives of General Psychiatry, 49,* 802–808.

Fava, G. (1994). Do antidepressant and antianxiety drugs increase chronicity in affective disorders? *Psychotherapy and Psychosomatics, 61,* 125–131.

Fava, G. A., Rafanelli, C., Grandi, S., Conti, S., & Belluardo, P. (1998). Prevention of recurrent depression with cognitive behavioral therapy: Preliminary findings. *Archives of General Psychiatry, 55,* 816–820.

Feeley, M., DeRubeis, R. J., & Gelfand, L. A. (1999). The temporal relation of adherence and alliance to symptom change in cognitive therapy for depression. *Journal of Consulting and Clinical Psychology, 67,* 578–582.

Ferster, C. B. (1973). A functional analysis of depression. *American Psychologist, 28,* 857–870.

Ferster, C. B. (1981). A functional analysis of behavior therapy. In L. P. Rehm (Ed.), *Behavior therapy for depression: Present status and future directions* (pp. 181–196). New York: Academic Press.

Forand, N. R., DeRubeis, R. J., & Amsterdam, J. A. (2013). Combining medication and psychotherapy in the treatment of major mental disorders. In M. J. Lambert (Ed.), *Garfield and Bergin's Handbook of psychotherapy and behavior change* (6th ed., 735–774). New York: Wiley.

Fournier, J. C., DeRubeis, R. J., Hollon, S. D., Dimidjian, S., Amsterdam, J. D., Shelton, R. C., et al. (2010). Antidepressant drug effects and depression severity: A patient-level meta-analysis. *Journal of the American Medical Association, 303,* 47–53.

Fournier, J. C., DeRubeis, R. J., Shelton, R. C., Gallop, R., Amsterdam, J. D., & Hollon, S. D. (2008). Cognitive therapy vs. antidepressant medications in the treatment of depressed patients with and without personality disorder. *British Journal of Psychiatry, 192,* 124–129.

Fournier, J. C., DeRubeis, R. J., Shelton, R. C., Hollon, S. D., Amsterdam, J. D., & Gallop, R. (2009). Prediction of response to medication and cognitive therapy in the treatment of moderate to severe depression. *Journal of Consulting and Clinical Psychology, 77,* 775–787.

Garber, J., Clarke, G. N., Weersing, V. R., Beardslee, W. R., Brent, D. A., Gladstone, T. R. G., et al. (2009). Prevention of depression in at-risk adolescents: A randomized controlled trial. *Journal of the American Medical Association, 301*, 2215–2224.

Geschwind, N., Peeters, F., Huibers, M., van Os, J., & Wichers, M. (2012). Efficacy of mindfulness-based cognitive therapy in relation to prior history of depression: Randomised controlled trial. *British Journal of Psychiatry, 201*, 320–325.

Gillham, J. E., Shatte, A. J., & Freres, D. R. (2000). Preventing depression: A review of cognitive-behavioral and family interventions. *Applied and Preventive Psychology, 9*, 63–88.

Godfrin, K. A., & van Heeringen, C. (2010). The effects of mindfulness-based cognitive therapy on recurrence of depressive episodes, mental health, and quality of life: A randomized controlled study. *Behavior Research and Therapy, 48*(8), 738–746.

Gortner, E. T., Gollan, J. K., Dobson, K. S., & Jacobson, N. S. (1998). Cognitive-behavioral treatment for depression: Relapse prevention. *Journal of Consulting and Clinical Psychology, 66*, 377–384.

Gotlib, I. H., & Hamilton, J. P. (2008). Neuroimaging and depression: Current status and unresolved issues. *Current Directions in Psychological Science, 17*, 159–163.

Hersen, M., Bellack, A. S., Himmelhoch, J. M., & Thase, M. E. (1984). Effects of social skill training, amitriptyline, and psychotherapy in unipolar depressed women. *Behavior Therapy, 15*, 21–40.

Hollon, S. D. (1996). The efficacy and effectiveness of psychotherapy relative to medications. *American Psychologist, 51*, 1025–1030.

Hollon, S. D. (2001). Behavioral activation treatment for depression: A commentary. *Clinical Psychology: Science and Practice, 8*, 271–273.

Hollon, S. D. (2011). Cognitive and behavior therapy in the treatment and prevention of depression. *Depression and Anxiety, 28*, 263–266.

Hollon, S. D., & Beck, A. T. (2013). Cognitive and cognitive-behavioral therapies. In M. J. Lambert (Ed.), *Garfield and Bergin's Handbook of psychotherapy and behavior change* (6th ed., 393–442). New York: Wiley.

Hollon, S. D., DeRubeis, R. J., Evans, M. D., Wiemer, M. J., Garvey, M. J., Grove, W. M., et al. (1992). Cognitive therapy and pharmacotherapy for depression: Singly and in combination. *Archives of General Psychiatry, 49*, 774–781.

Hollon, S. D., DeRubeis, R. J., & Seligman, M. E. P. (1992). Cognitive therapy and the prevention of depression. *Applied and Preventive Psychology, 1*, 89–95.

Hollon, S. D., DeRubeis, R. J., Shelton, R. C., Amsterdam, J. D., Salomon, R. M., O'Reardon, J. P., et al. (2005). Prevention of relapse following cognitive therapy versus medications in moderate to severe depression. *Archives of General Psychiatry, 62*, 417–422.

Hollon, S. D., Evans, M. D., & DeRubeis, R. J. (1990). Cognitive mediation of relapse prevention following treatment for depression: Implications of differential risk. In R. E. Ingram (Ed.), *Psychological aspects of depression* (pp. 114–136). New York: Plenum Press.

Hollon, S. D., & Garber, J. (1990). Cognitive therapy of depression: A social-cognitive perspective. *Personality and Social Psychology Bulletin, 16*, 58–73.

Hollon, S. D., Muñoz, R. F., Barlow, D. H., Beardslee, W. R., Bell, C. C., Bernal, G., et al. (2002). Psychosocial intervention development for the prevention and treatment of depression: Promoting innovation and increasing access. *Biological Psychiatry, 52*, 610–630.

Hollon, S. D., Stewart, M. O., & Strunk, D. (2006). Cognitive behavior therapy has enduring effects in the treatment of depression and anxiety. *Annual Review of Psychology, 57*, 285–315.

Hollon, S. D., Thase, M. E., & Markowitz, J. C. (2002). Treatment and prevention of depression. *Psychological Science in the Public Interest, 3*, 39–77.

Hopko, D. R., Bell, J. L., Armento, M. E. A., Hunt, M. K., & Lejuez, C. W. (2005). Behavior therapy for depressed cancer patients in primary care. *Psychotherapy: Theory, Research, Practice and Training, 42*, 236–243.

Hopko, D. R., Lejuez, C. W., LePage, J. P., Hopko, S. D., & McNeil, D. W. (2003). A brief behavioral activation treatment for depression: A randomized pilot trial within an inpatient psychiatric hospital. *Behavior Modification, 27,* 458–469.

Jacobson, N. S., Dobson, K., Fruzzetti, A. E., Schmaling, K. B., & Salusky, S. (1991). Marital therapy as a treatment for depression. *Journal of Consulting and Clinical Psychology, 59,* 547–557.

Jacobson, N. S., Dobson, K. S., Truax, P. A., Addis, M. E., Koerner, K., Gollan, J. K., et al. (1996). A component analysis of cognitive-behavior treatment for depression. *Journal of Consulting and Clinical Psychology, 64,* 295–304.

Jacobson, N. S., & Hollon, S. D. (1996a). Cognitive-behavior therapy versus pharmacotherapy: Now that the jury's returned its verdict, it's time to present the rest of the evidence. *Journal of Consulting and Clinical Psychology, 64,* 74–80.

Jacobson, N. S., & Hollon, S. D. (1996b). Prospects for future comparisons between drugs and psychotherapy: Lessons from the CBT-versus-pharmacotherapy exchange. *Journal of Consulting and Clinical Psychology, 64,* 104–108.

Jacobson, N. S., Martell, C., & Dimidjian, S. (2001). Behavioral activation treatment for depression: Returning to contextual roots. *Clinical Psychology: Science and Practice, 8,* 255–270.

Jarrett, R. B., Kraft, D., Schaffer, M., Witt-Browder, A., Risser, R., Atkins, D. H., et al. (2000). Reducing relapse in depressed outpatients with atypical features: A pilot study. *Psychotherapy and Psychosomatics, 69,* 232–239.

Jarrett, R. B., Schaffer, M., McIntire, D., Witt-Browder, A., Kraft, D., & Risser, R. C. (1999). Treatment of atypical depression with cognitive therapy or phenelzine: A double-blind, placebo-controlled trial. *Archives of General Psychiatry, 56,* 431–437.

Kennedy, S. H., Konarski, J. Z., Segal, Z. V., Lau, M. A., Bieling, P. J., McIntyre, R. S., et al. (2007). Differences in brain glucose metabolism between responders to CBT and venlafaxine in a 16-week randomized controlled trial. *American Journal of Psychiatry, 164,* 778–788.

Klein, D. F. (1996). Preventing hung juries about therapy studies. *Journal of Consulting and Clinical Psychology, 64,* 81–87.

Kovacs, M., Rush, A. J., Beck, A. T., & Hollon, S. D. (1981). Depressed outpatients treated with cognitive therapy or pharmacotherapy. *Archives of General Psychiatry, 38,* 33–39.

Kraemer, H. C., Wilson, G. T., Fairburn, C. G., & Agras, W. S. (2002). Mediators and moderators of treatment effects in randomized clinical trials. *Archives of General Psychiatry, 59,* 877–883.

Kuyken, W., Byford, S., Taylor, R. S., Watkins, E., Holden, E., White, K., et al. (2008). Mindfulness-based cognitive therapy to prevent relapse in recurrent depression. *Journal of Consulting and Clinical Psychology, 76,* 966–978.

Lewinsohn, P. M. (1974). A behavioral approach to depression. In R. M. Friedman & M. M. Katz (Eds.), *The psychology of depression: Contemporary theory and research* (pp. 157–185). New York: Wiley.

Leykin, Y., Amsterdam, J. D., DeRubeis, R. J., Gallop, R., Shelton, R. C., & Hollon, S. D. (2007). Progressive resistance to selective serotonin reuptake inhibitor but not to cognitive therapy in the treatment of major depression. *Journal of Consulting and Clinical Psychology, 75,* 267–276.

Ma, S. H., & Teasdale, J. D. (2004). Mindfulness-based cognitive therapy for depression: Replication and exploration of differential relapse prevention effects. *Journal of Consulting and Clinical Psychology, 72*(1), 31–40.

Maier, S. F., Amat, J., Baratta, M. V., Paul, E., & Watkins, L. R. (2006). Behavioral control, the medial prefrontal cortex, and resilience. *Dialogues in Clinical Neuroscience, 8,* 353–373.

Mazzucchelli, T., Kane, R., & Rees, C. (2009). Behavioral activation treatments for depression in adults: A meta-analysis and review. *Clinical Psychology: Science and Practice, 16*(4), 383–411.

McLean, P. D., & Hakstian, A. R. (1979). Clinical depression: Comparative efficacy of outpatient treatments. *Journal of Consulting and Clinical Psychology, 47,* 818–836.

Mohr, D. C., Ho, J., Duffecy, J., Reifler, D., Sokol, L., Burns, M. N., et al. (2012). Effect of telephone-administered vs. face-to-face cognitive behavioral therapy on adherence to therapy and depression outcomes among primary care patients: A randomized trial. *Journal of the American Medical Association, 307,* 2278–2285.

Mohr, D. C., Vella, L., Hart, S., Heckman, T., & Simon, G. (2008). The effect of telephone-administered psychotherapy on symptoms of depression and attrition: A meta-analysis. *Clinical Psychology: Science and Practice, 15*(3), 243–253.

Moradveisi, L., Huibers, M. J. H., Renner, F., Arasteh, M., & Arntz, A. (2013). Behavioural activation vs. antidepressant medication for treatment depression in Iran: Randomised trial. *British Journal of Psychiatry, 202*(3), 204–211.

Murphy, G. E., Simons, A. D., Wetzel, R. D., & Lustman, P. J. (1984). Cognitive therapy and pharmacotherapy, singly and together, in the treatment of depression. *Archives of General Psychiatry, 41,* 33–41.

Mynors-Wallis, L. M., Gath, D., Day, A., & Baker, F. (2000). Randomised controlled trial of problem-solving treatment, antidepressant medication and combined treatment for major depression in primary care. *British Medical Journal, 320,* 26–30.

Mynors-Wallis, L. M., Gath, D. H., Lloyd-Thomas, A. R., & Tomlinson, D. (1995). Randomised controlled trial comparing problem solving treatment with amitriptyline and placebo for major depression in primary care. *British Medical Journal, 310,* 441–445.

Nezu, A. M. (1986). Efficacy of a social problem-solving therapy approach for unipolar depression. *Journal of Consulting and Clinical Psychology, 54,* 196–202.

Nezu, A. M., & Perri, M. G. (1989). Social problem-solving therapy for unipolar depression: An initial dismantling investigation. *Journal of Consulting and Clinical Psychology, 57,* 408–413.

O'Leary, K. D., & Beach, S. R. H. (1990). Marital therapy: A viable treatment for depression and marital discord. *American Journal of Psychiatry, 147,* 183–186.

Paykel, E. S., Scott, J., Teasdale, J. D., Johnson, A. L., Garland, A., Moore, R., et al. (1999). Prevention of relapse in residual depression by cognitive therapy. *Archives of General Psychiatry, 56,* 829–835.

Proudfoot, J., Ryden, C., Everitt, B., Shapiro, D. A., Goldberg, D., Mann, A., et al. (2004). Clinical efficacy of computerised cognitive-behavioural therapy for anxiety and depression in primary care: Randomised controlled trial. *British Journal of Psychiatry, 185,* 46–54.

Richards, D., & Richardson, T. (2012). Computer-based psychological treatments for depression: A systematic review and meta-analysis. *Clinical Psychology Review, 32*(4), 329–342.

Rotheram-Boras, M. J., Swendeman, D., & Chorpita, B. F. (2012). Disruptive innovations for designing and diffusing evidence-based interventions. *American Psychologist, 67,* 463–476.

Rush, A. J., Beck, A. T., Kovacs, M., & Hollon, S. D. (1977). Comparative efficacy of cognitive therapy and pharmacotherapy in the treatment of depressed outpatients. *Cognitive Therapy and Research, 1,* 17–38.

Scogin, F., Jamison, C., & Gochneaur, K. (1989). Comparative efficacy of cognitive and behavioral bibliotherapy for mildly and moderately depressed older adults. *Journal of Consulting and Clinical Psychology, 57,* 403–407.

Segal, Z. V., Bieling, P., Young, T., MacQueen, G., Cooke, R., Martin, L., et al. (2010). Antidepressant monotherapy vs. sequential pharmacotherapy and mindfulness-based cognitive therapy, or placebo, for relapse prophylaxis in recurrent depression. *Archives of General Psychiatry, 67,* 1256–1264.

Segal, Z. V., Williams, J. M. G., & Teasdale, J. D. (2002). *Mindfulness-based cognitive therapy for depression.* New York: Guilford Press.

Seligman, M. E. P., Schulman, P., DeRubeis, R. J., & Hollon, S. D. (1999). The prevention of depression and anxiety. *Prevention and Treatment, 2,* Article 8.

Shea, M. T., Elkin, I., Imber, S. D., Sotsky, S. M., Watkins, J. T., Collins, J. F., et al. (1992). Course of depressive symptoms over follow-up: Findings from the National Institute of Mental Health Treatment of Depression Collaborative Research Program. *Archives of General Psychiatry, 49,* 782–787.

Simon, G. E., Ludman, E. J., Tutty, S., Operskalski, B., & VonKorff, M. (2004). Telephone psychotherapy and telephone care management for primary care patients starting antidepressant treatment: A randomized trial. *Journal of the American Medical Association, 292,* 935–942.

Simons, A. D., Murphy, G. E., Levine, J. E., & Wetzel, R. D. (1986). Cognitive therapy and pharmacotherapy for depression: Sustained improvement over one year. *Archives of General Psychiatry, 43,* 43–49.

Stathopoulou, G., Powers, M. B., Berry, A. C., Smits, J. A. J., & Otto, M. W. (2006). Exercise interventions for mental health: A quantitative and qualitative review. *Clinical Psychology: Science and Practice, 13,* 179–193.

Strunk, D. R., DeRubeis, R. J., Chiu, A. W., & Alvarez, J. (2007). Patients' competence in and performance of cognitive therapy skills: Relation to the reduction of relapse risk following treatment for depression. *Journal of Consulting and Clinical Psychology, 75,* 523–529.

Tang, T. Z., DeRubeis, R. J., Hollon, S. D., Amsterdam, J. D., & Shelton, R. C. (2007). Sudden gains in cognitive therapy of depression and relapse/recurrence. *Journal of Consulting and Clinical Psychology, 75,* 404–408.

Teasdale, J. D., Moore, R. G., Hayhurst, H., Pope, M., Williams, S., & Segal, Z. V. (2002). Metacognitive awareness and prevention of relapse in depression: Empirical evidence. *Journal of Consulting and Clinical Psychology, 70,* 275–287.

Teasdale, J. D., Segal, Z., Williams, J. M. G., Ridgeway, V. A., Soulsby, J. M., & Lau, M. A. (2000). Prevention of relapse/recurrence in major depression by mindfulness-based cognitive therapy. *Journal of Consulting and Clinical Psychology, 68*(4), 615–623.

Whitaker, R. (2010). *Anatomy of an epidemic: Magic bullets, psychiatric drugs, and the astonishing rise of mental illness in America.* New York: Crown.

CHAPTER 28

Pharmacotherapy and Psychosocial Treatments for Bipolar Disorder

DAVID J. MIKLOWITZ

Bipolar disorder is a reasonably common and highly debilitating illness. Bipolar I and II disorder affect as many as 1 in 50 persons; when its spectrum variants are included, the rate goes up to 4.5% in epidemiological samples (Merikangas et al., 2007). In a sample of 61,392 adults in 11 countries, lifetime prevalence rates were 0.6% for bipolar I disorder, 0.4% for bipolar II, and 1.4% for subthreshold bipolar disorder (Merikangas, et al., 2011). Between 50 and 67% of patients have the first onset of illness before age 18, and between 13 and 28% before age 13 (Perlis et al., 2004). The disorder is highly recurrent and disabling, leading to unemployment or lost days of work, high rates of divorce, legal problems, and low quality of life. The direct and indirect costs of bipolar disorder were estimated to be $151 billion in the United States alone (Dilsaver, 2011).

The evidence that lithium and, more recently, the anticonvulsants and second-generation antipsychotics (SGAs) are effective in controlling manic or depressive episodes is substantial (e.g., Correll, Sheridan, & DelBello, 2010; Geddes, Burgess, Hawton, Jamison, & Goodwin, 2004). However, full and rapid recovery from episodes, notably bipolar depressive episodes, is often unattainable with pharmacotherapy alone. In a 26-week randomized trial involving 22 sites (the Systematic Treatment Enhancement Program for Bipolar Disorder [STEP-BD]), recovery from a bipolar depressive episode occurred in only 21–27% of patients receiving mood stabilizers (Sachs et al., 2007). In a 4-year follow-up of children with bipolar I disorder (mean age, 10.8 years) with manic episodes, most of whom were undergoing pharmacotherapy, duration of episodes (without recovery) averaged 79 weeks (Geller, Tillman, Craney, and Bolhofner, 2004).

The effectiveness of pharmacotherapy alone is even more questionable when one examines the long-term course of the disorder. In Geller and colleagues' (2004) 4-year follow-up, children with bipolar disorder spent an average of 57% of their total weeks with diagnosable mania or hypomania and 47% of the total weeks with major or minor depression or dysthymia. In a study of 1,469 adults with bipolar I and II disorders followed over 1 year, 49% had recurrences of their disorders; twice as many of these recurrences were for depressive episodes as for manic episodes (Perlis et al., 2006). Patients with bipolar disorder experience significant impairment in work, social, and family functioning, especially if they have treatment-resistant depressive symptoms (Altshuler et al., 2006; Gitlin, Mintz, Sokolski, Hammen, & Altshuler, 2011). Functional impairment is associated with earlier illness recurrence independently of symptom states (e.g., Weinstock & Miller, 2008).

Two integrated treatment avenues are essential to providing optimal outcomes for bipolar patients—flexible pharmacotherapy (allowing for changes in drug or dosage patterns as patients relapse or remit) and psychosocial interventions. This biopsychosocial approach to treatment is gaining traction and is now favored in the majority of international treatment guidelines (e.g., Goodwin & Consensus Group of the British Association for Psychopharmacology, 2009; Yatham et al., 2012).

This chapter reviews the literature on drug and psychosocial treatments. Because there are comprehensive reviews of the pharmacotherapy literature (e.g., Correll et al., 2010; Malhi, Adams, & Berk, 2009), this chapter places greater emphasis on psychosocial interventions. A final section offers recommendations for future research.

PHARMACOTHERAPY FOR BIPOLAR DISORDER

Pharmacological studies have generally been focused on the acute stabilization of manic or depressive episodes, whereas psychosocial studies have focused on maintenance treatment (prevention of recurrence and mitigation of residual symptoms). These different emphases reflect in part the more rapid response of patients to pharmacotherapy than to psychotherapy. In the following sections, findings from large-scale clinical trials are reviewed, and gaps in the literature are highlighted.

Proper Diagnosis

The effectiveness of drug or psychosocial treatment can be undermined when patients are misdiagnosed with other conditions or have unrecognized comorbid disorders. The most straightforward example is the misdiagnosis of bipolar depression as unipolar depression. Patients with depression who have unrecognized bipolar syndromes are often given antidepressants alone, which can precipitate affective switches or cycle acceleration (Thase, 2006a, 2006b). Conversely, misdiagnosing persons with major depression as having bipolar disorder may lead to unnecessary treatment with medications that have significant metabolic side effects (Correll et al., 2009). Until biomarkers specific to the pathophysiology of bipolar disorder are identified, accurate diagnoses through structured clinical interviews and personal histories are essential to successful treatment.

What Is a Mood Stabilizer?

Mood stabilizers are drugs that are effective in treating or preventing manic, mixed, and/or depressive episodes without triggering new episodes of the opposite polarity (Keck et al., 2004). Psychiatrists increasingly are substituting divalproex sodium, lamotrigine, or SGAs for lithium or combining these agents to control or prevent manic, mixed, or depressive episodes. This change in practice is generally attributed to the more tolerable side-effect profiles among anticonvulsant or SGA agents in contrast to lithium. There is, however, little evidence that these alternative agents are more effective than lithium.

The following medications have been approved by the Food and Drug Administration (FDA) for the treatment of bipolar disorder: lithium; the anticonvulsants divalproex sodium (valproic acid; marketed in the United States as Depakote), lamotrigine (Lamictal), and carbamazepine (Tegretol); the atypical antipsychotics (olanzapine [Zyprexa], aripiprazole [Abilify], quetiapine [Seroquel], risperidone [Risperdal], ziprasidone [Geodon]), and asenapine [Saphris]); the combination of olanzapine and fluoxetine (Prozac), also called OFC or Symbyax; and the traditional antipsychotic chlorpromazine (Thorazine). These medications are often combined with antidepressants or anxiolytic agents. Lithium, risperidone, olanzapine, aripiprazole, and quetiapine are approved for treating mania in children and adolescents.

These drugs have multiple mechanisms of action. Lithium and valproate both inhibit the protein kinase C signal transduction pathway. Lithium also has inhibitory effects on calcium, glutamate, and guanine nucleotide-binding proteins (G-proteins), all components of the intracellular signaling cascade (Manji et al., 2003). Lithium has neuroprotective effects in preventing apoptosis (cell death) through inhibiting glycogen synthase kinase-3 (GSK3) and other mechanisms (Li, Frye, & Shelton, 2012). The SGAs selectively block dopamine and serotonin receptors, thus having broad effects on mood, anxiety, and psychosis. The various antidepressants alleviate depression primarily through serotonergic, dopaminergic, and noradrenergic mechanisms. They may also reduce the output of glucocorticoids, which, if overproduced, can lead to the destruction of hippocampal cells (Sapolsky, 2000).

Anticonvulsants such as divalproex may have "antikindling" effects through diminishing excitation and enhancing inhibition in the mesolimbic system and other neural circuits responsible for emotion regulation (Post, 2007). Lamotrigine and carbamazepine reduce the outflow, the presynaptic release, or the postsynaptic uptake of excitatory amino acids such as glutamate.

Evidence for Drug Efficacy in Randomized Clinical Trials

Treatment of Mania

Lithium remains the mainstay of treatment for adults, although its use in children is overshadowed by prescriptions for divalproex sodium. Approximately 60–70% of persons with bipolar disorder show a remission of manic symptoms on lithium (Keck et al., 2004). The benefits of lithium do not come without costs: Common side effects include somnolence, nausea, diarrhea, cognitive dulling, weight gain, stomach irritation, thirst, motor tremors, acne, and a long-term risk of kidney clearance problems and hypothyroidism.

Lithium is impressive as a prophylactic agent in maintenance treatment. A meta-analysis that included 770 participants in five placebo-controlled randomized controlled trials (RCTs) concluded that lithium was effective in reducing manic relapses (average of 14 vs. 24% placebo relapse rate), but its effects in preventing depressive relapses failed to reach statistical significance (25 vs. 32%; Geddes et al., 2004). Thus lithium significantly reduces overall rates of relapse, but patients continue to have "breakthrough" episodes.

Divalproex sodium appears to be as effective as lithium in controlling manic episodes but may have a milder side-effect profile. Side effects of divalproex include nausea, stomach pain, fatigue, weight gain, elevated liver enzymes, and depression of platelet counts. It is not clear which patient characteristics moderate the efficacy of lithium versus divalproex. A large trial in the United Kingdom found that lithium was more effective than divalproex in prevention of mood episodes and that combining lithium with divalproex was more effective than valproate alone (Geddes et al., 2010). In an 18-month maintenance trial involving 60 children with bipolar disorder, no differences emerged between lithium and divalproex in time to recurrence (Findling et al., 2005).

In a meta-analysis of 24 trials (*N* = 6,187), SGAs were significantly superior to placebo in treating acute episodes of mania and were just as effective as mood stabilizers. The most efficacious treatment for mania was the combination of SGAs and mood stabilizers (e.g., quetiapine plus divalproex; Scherk, Pajonk, & Leucht, 2007). In a meta-analysis of 68 RCTS (*N* = 16,073), antipsychotics appeared to be superior to anticonvulsants and lithium in treating acute manic episodes (Cipriani et al., 2011). SGAs are often given as short-term treatment for mania but are usually tapered or discontinued during maintenance because of side effects such as weight gain, metabolic disturbances, and sedation.

Treatment of Depression

Lithium and divalproex are the recommended first-line options for mild to moderate episodes of bipolar depression. Lithium did as well as the combination of lithium and antidepressants in one study, especially when patients were maintained on blood levels of 0.8 mEq/L or higher (Nemeroff et al., 2001). Also, lithium appears to have strong antisuicide benefits. A study of over 21,000 patients with bipolar disorder found that patients treated with lithium were less likely to attempt or to complete suicide than patients who received divalproex or carbamazepine (Goodwin et al., 2003).

Depression generally has a slower recovery trajectory than mania, and mood stabilizers more effectively treat and prevent manic than depressive episodes (Moller, Grunze, & Broich, 2006). As a result, many psychiatrists augment mood stabilizers with other agents to enhance recovery. There is considerable debate about whether mood stabilizers should be augmented with antidepressants given their propensity to cause affective switches or rapid cycling. When used alone, antidepressants can induce mania and accelerate mood cycling in 20–40% of patients (Goodwin et al., 2009). However, there is less evidence that antidepressants cause cycle acceleration when used in combination with adequate dosages of mood stabilizers.

A naturalistic study found that bipolar patients who were successfully treated for depression with mood stabilizers and SSRIs were less likely to develop depression if they continued antidepressants for 6 months after remission (Altshuler et al., 2003). In contrast, the STEP-BD study found no differences in time to recovery among 366 patients with bipolar depression randomly assigned to mood stabilizers plus antidepressants (buproprion or paroxetine) or mood stabilizers plus placebo (Sachs et al., 2007). Neither study found an association between antidepressant usage and the likelihood of treatment-emergent mania or hypomania.

Current treatment guidelines recommend adjunctive antidepressants only when other agents have failed in the treatment of bipolar depression, and then only in combination with a mood stabilizing or atypical antipsychotic agent (e.g., Yatham et al., 2012).

Lamotrigine, the only agent other than lithium approved by the FDA as a maintenance agent in bipolar I disorder, appears to be efficacious in the acute and maintenance treatment of bipolar depression (Bowden et al., 2003). A meta-analysis of five trials of lamotrigine in bipolar depression reported modest effects for episode stabilization, with stronger effects among patients with higher initial depression severity (Geddes, Calabrese, & Goodwin, 2009). A randomized trial involving patients with bipolar depression who had failed on at least two antidepressants found that patients treated with lamotrigine had lower depression severity ratings over 16 weeks than patients treated with inositol or risperidone (Nierenberg et al., 2006). Adverse reactions to lamotrigine can include a serious skin rash in about 5–10% of patients that, in about 0.1% of cases, can progress into Stevens–Johnson syndrome, a potentially fatal dermatological reaction (Thase, 2006b).

Patients with bipolar depression can be stabilized more effectively with a fixed-dose preparation combining olanzapine and fluoxetine (OFC, or Symbyax) than with olanzapine alone (Tohen et al., 2003). OFC was associated with faster depression response rates and a greater reduction in mania symptoms than lamotrigine in one 7-week trial (Brown et al., 2006). However, patients had fewer side effects on lamotrigine than on OFC.

Evidence is building for the efficacy of the SGA quetiapine; it is more effective in the acute treatment of bipolar depression than placebo, paroxetine, and lithium (De Fruyt et al., 2012). A 2-year maintenance trial of 1,226 patients with bipolar depression who had responded to quetiapine during acute treatment reported longer time to recurrence for quetiapine than placebo, although switching to lithium during the continuation phase was equally effective (Weisler et al., 2011). A newer antipsychotic agent, lurasidone, is also showing promise as an acute treatment for bipolar I depression (Loebel et al., 2014).

Issues in the Pharmacotherapy of Bipolar Disorder in Childhood and Adolescence

Child and adolescent bipolar disorder is particularly difficult to assess, diagnose, and treat, in part because of the lack of consensus on its boundaries. Preadolescent and adolescent mania appear to be characterized by lengthy episodes, psychosis, frequent polarity shifts, and a highly recurrent course (Birmaher et al., 2006; Geller et al., 2004). Episodic mania has been recognized as early as the preschool years (Luby, Tandon, & Belden, 2009). A central controversy in the diagnosis of pediatric-onset mania is how to characterize children with persistent irritability. Children with mania based on episodic periods of irritability and activation usually develop elated mood or grandiosity at some point in their illness (Hunt et al., 2013). Children with nonepisodic irritability, however, are at risk for later depression but not bipolar disorder. These youths are better characterized as having *severe mood dysregulation* (Leibenluft, Cohen, Gorrindo, Brook, & Pine, 2006), a unique category that has features of oppositional defiant disorder and attention-deficit/hyperactivity disorder (ADHD).

A meta-analysis of placebo-controlled trials indicated that SGAs may have greater benefit for stabilization of pediatric mania than mood stabilizers (Correll et al., 2010). Among 279 children and adolescents in a manic episode, responses to the SGA risperidone were higher than to lithium or divalproex, although risperidone also produced more serious side effects (Geller et al., 2012). Quetiapine is effective alone or in conjunction with divalproex in stabilizing pediatric mania (DelBello, Schwiers, Rosenberg, & Strakowski, 2002; DelBello et al., 2006). In contrast, in a 28-day trial, divalproex did not differ from placebo in controlling mania symptoms in children (Wagner et al., 2009). Few data exist on the treatment of bipolar depression in children, with at least one negative trial for quetiapine (DelBello et al., 2009).

Weight gain and other metabolic side effects from atypical antipsychotics pose unacceptable health risks to younger patients. The difficulty in balancing effective treatment and side effects has prompted the development of treatment guidelines for pediatric bipolar disorder (Pfeifer, Kowatch, & DelBello, 2010). These guidelines favor beginning with a mood-stabilizing agent and/or adding an SGA and augmenting with another mood stabilizer or SGA if response is only partial. Newer agents for adults with bipolar depression—such as ketamine (Zarate et al., 2012)—have not been studied in pediatric samples.

Methodological Limitations of Bipolar Treatment Studies

Two issues stand out as methodological shortcomings in pharmacological and psychotherapy trials for bipolar disorder. First is the near-exclusive focus on symptomatic improvement to the neglect of functional (i.e., vocational, relationship) improvement or quality of life. Patients with bipolar disorder have ongoing problems in social and occupational functioning, even once they are symptomatically remitted (Gitlin et al., 2011).

Second, inconsistency in patients' medication usage patterns is one of the major reasons for the ineffectiveness of drug treatments for bipolar disorder. Laboratory-based drug efficacy and effectiveness trials often differ in results due to the high rate of medication discontinuation in everyday practice (Colom et al., 2000). Patients who rapidly discontinue mood stabilizers are at an increased risk for recurrence and suicide (Tondo & Baldessarini, 2000). However, few drug or psychosocial studies examine medication adherence as a moderator or mediator of treatment outcomes.

Nonadherence is a serious problem for all long-lasting medical conditions with intermittent symptoms. Beyond this, medication issues associated with bipolar disorder include side effects (e.g., weight gain, fatigue, cognitive dulling), dislike of having one's moods controlled by a medication, lack of family or social supports, poor doctor–patient relationships, and lack of information about the disorder. The patients at highest risk for nonadherence are younger, have more severe illnesses, and are more likely to have comorbid personality or substance use disorders (Colom et al., 2000).

Thus future drug or psychosocial studies would benefit from including functional improvement as a key outcome criterion. Examining the mediating effects of medication adherence is critical to determining the effectiveness of both classes of treatments.

PSYCHOSOCIAL TREATMENTS FOR BIPOLAR DISORDER

Psychosocial treatments are considered as adjuncts to medications during stabilization and maintenance. The majority of RCTs for psychosocial treatment are maintenance trials oriented toward relapse prevention and management of residual symptoms, but more recent studies have considered the value of adjunctive psychotherapy in stabilizing acute episodes of depression.

Modern psychosocial approaches are based in research showing that psychosocial stressors have a role in eliciting episodes of bipolar disorder (see Johnson, Cuellar, & Peckham, Chapter 17, this volume). There is prognostic evidence for three types of psychosocial stress: (1) life-events stress, notably events that engage the patient in goal pursuit (Johnson et al., 2008) or that disrupt sleep–wake cycles and other circadian rhythms (Malkoff-Schwartz et al., 1998); (2) high family expressed emotion (EE) or family discord (e.g., Miklowitz, Biuckians, & Richards, 2006; Miklowitz, Goldstein, Nuechterlein, Snyder, & Mintz, 1988); and (3) early childhood adversity in the form of sexual or physical abuse or parental neglect (Dienes, Hammen, Henry, Cohen, & Daley, 2006; Post & Leverich, 2006). Among preadolescent and adolescent patients with bipolar disorder, life stressors (Kim, Miklowitz, Biuckians, & Mullen, 2007), family EE (Miklowitz et al., 2006), and low parental warmth (Geller et al., 2004) are prospectively associated with symptom severity and recurrence.

Moderators of the effects of life stress, which would be quite informative for the development of psychosocial interventions, have not been identified. Events that involve goal attainment may be particularly potent in eliciting manic symptoms among vulnerable persons with high behavioral activation (e.g., novelty seeking) or reward sensitivity (Alloy et al., 2012; Johnson et al., 2008).

Despite theories of kindling (Post & Leverich, 2006), life events do not appear to be more potent in provoking initial episodes than later episodes in either adult (Hammen & Gitlin, 1997; Hlastala et al., 2000) or adolescent (Hillegers et al., 2004) samples. There is better evidence for a stress reactivity hypothesis, in which certain subgroups of patients become more vulnerable to stress with repeated episodes or due to antecedent vulnerabilities (Hammen & Gitlin, 1997). For example, one study found that early childhood adversity moderated the relationship between life stress and recurrence among adults with bipolar disorder such that patients with more severe early adversity (particularly parental neglect) reported lower levels of stress prior to recurrences than did patients with less severe early adversity (Dienes et al., 2006).

Many of the existing psychotherapy studies cite these stress–outcome studies as justifications for their approach. However, few studies have examined whether the effects of different forms of psychotherapy are moderated by stressful events or circumstances or are mediated by changes in patients' ability to cope with stressors. The examination of moderators and mediators is a major gap in this literature, as elaborated later in the chapter.

Cognitive-Behavioral Therapy

Cognitive-behavioral therapy (CBT) approaches to bipolar disorder are similar to the models used in major depression and comprise behavioral activation followed by cognitive restructuring and modifying core dysfunctional beliefs. CBT for bipolar disorder also includes restructuring hyperpositive thinking and monitoring daily activities to reduce overstimulation. There have been several RCTs of CBT (the STEP-BD trial, which focused on depression recovery, is covered later). Lam, Hayward, Watkins, Wright, and Sham (2005) randomly assigned 103 euthymic patients with bipolar disorder to CBT (12–18 sessions) plus pharmacotherapy versus usual care and pharmacotherapy. The 1-year results were positive: 44% of the patients in CBT relapsed versus 75% of those in usual care; patients in CBT also spent fewer days in mood episodes. The results were weakened over 30 months: Patients in CBT no longer differed from patients in usual care in time to recurrence, but they had fewer days in mood episodes and an increased ability to recognize early warning signs of recurrence.

Two large-scale community trials have raised questions about the effectiveness of adjunctive CBT in relapse prevention. Scott and associates (2006) examined CBT (22 sessions) versus treatment as usual (TAU) in 253 bipolar patients in a variety of symptom states. Over 18 months, no differential effects were found for CBT on time to recurrence. A post hoc analysis revealed that patients with < 12 episodes were less likely to have recurrences if treated with CBT than with TAU, but patients with 12 or more episodes were more likely to have recurrences in CBT than in TAU. These results suggest two possibilities: CBT is best suited to the earlier phases of the disorder, or CBT may be unsettling and agitating to patients who have had numerous episodes. In a multisite Canadian trial of 204 patients in full or partial remission, participants were randomly assigned to 20 sessions of individual CBT or 6 sessions of group psychoeducation with pharmacotherapy (Parikh et al., 2012). No differences emerged over 1.5 years in symptom severity or recurrence rates.

Thus the evidence for adjunctive CBT in relapse prevention is inconclusive. Future studies should consider the addition of mindfulness meditation strategies for highly chronic patients. Open trials of mindfulness-based CBT have observed positive effects on depression and anxiety symptoms in patients with bipolar disorder (Deckersbach et al., 2012; Miklowitz, Alatiq, et al., 2009; Weber et al., 2010).

Interpersonal and Social Rhythm Therapy

Interpersonal and social rhythm therapy (IPSRT), an adaptation of the interpersonal psychotherapy of depression, consists of problem solving, clarification, and interpretation to help patients resolve issues related to grief, role transitions, role disputes, or interpersonal deficits. IPSRT emphasizes the role of social and circadian rhythm dysregulation in the onset of manic episodes. The IPSRT is based on the Ehlers, Kupfer, Frank, and Monk (1993) notions of social zeitgebers (timekeepers) and zeitstorers (time disturbers). Life events that disrupt social zeitgebers are believed to precipitate episodes of depression or mania, whereas treatments or lifestyle changes that help strengthen zeitgebers are expected to help stabilize moods. Direct tests of this model have established a role for social rhythm disruption in the onset of manic episodes, but not in the onset of depressive episodes (Malkoff-Schwartz et al., 1998).

Unlike CBT, IPSRT has been tested primarily with patients with bipolar disorder who began treatment shortly after an acute episode of mania or depression. In the Pittsburgh Maintenance Therapies for Bipolar Disorder (MTBD) trial (Frank et al., 2005), 175 patients were randomly assigned during acute treatment to weekly IPSRT plus protocol pharmacotherapy or clinical management plus protocol pharmacotherapy. Once patients had recovered, they were rerandomized to IPSRT or active clinical management on a monthly basis for up to 2 years. IPSRT in the acute phase was associated with longer survival time prior to recurrences in the maintenance phase than was clinical management. The effects of IPSRT during maintenance were mediated by whether patients were able to stabilize their social routines and sleep–wake cycles during the acute phase. However, continued treatment with IPSRT during maintenance did not affect recurrence rates during the maintenance phase.

Family-Focused Therapy

Family-focused therapy (FFT) is a 9-month, 21-session outpatient treatment for patients and their immediate family members (spouse, parents, siblings). It consists of psychoeducation about bipolar disorder, communication enhancement training, and problem-solving skills training (Miklowitz, 2010). Given in conjunction with pharmacotherapy during the postepisode period, FFT aims to hasten stabilization and reduce the likelihood of early recurrences. It seeks to (1) increase the family's understanding of mood disorder episodes, (2) identify early signs of recurrence, (3) enhance the patient's adherence to medications, (4) help the patient and family members distinguish personality variables from signs of the disorder, (5) assist the patient and family members in coping with stressors that may precipitate episodes, and (6) increase the protective effects of family relationships.

In adult patients with bipolar disorder, FFT has been tested in two open trials with historical comparison groups (Miklowitz, George, Richards, Simoneau, & Suddath, 2003; Miklowitz & Goldstein, 1990), two 2-year maintenance RCTs (Miklowitz et al., 2003; Rea et al., 2003), and the 1-year STEP-BD trial focused on stabilization of depressive episodes (Miklowitz, Otto, Frank, Reilly-Harrington, Kogan, et al., 2007; Miklowitz, Otto, Frank, Reilly-Harrington, Wisniewski, et al., 2007). There are also two RCTs in adolescents with bipolar disorder (Miklowitz, Axelson, et al., 2008; Miklowitz et al., in press) and one in children and adolescents at risk for bipolar disorder (Miklowitz et al., 2013). The results are depicted in Table 28.1. Overall, FFT is associated with a 35–40% reduction in recurrence rates over 2 years and a 48% increase in recovery rates over 1

TABLE 28.1. Recovery, Relapse, and Rehospitalization Rates in Family-Focused Treatment versus Comparison Groups

Study	Sample	Type of trial	Clinical state	Comparison group	Key findings
Miklowitz & Goldstein (1990)	32 adults	Open (9 months)	Manic episode in prior 3 months	TAU (historical controls)	FFT, 11% relapse rate; comparison, 61%
Miklowitz, George, Richards, Simoneau, & Suddath (2003)	101 adults	RCT (2 years)	Depressed or manic episode in prior 3 months	Crisis management (2 family psychoeducation sessions)	54% survival rate in FFT versus 17% in crisis management
Rea et al. (2003)	53 adults	RCT (2–3 years)	Manic episode in prior 3 months	Individual therapy (21 sessions)	36% rehospitalization rate in FFT; 60% in individual therapy
Miklowitz, George, et al. (2003)	100 adults	Open (1 year)	Depressed or manic episode in prior 3 months	Crisis management (historical controls)	FFT plus interpersonal therapy associated with longer delays to relapse and less severe depression than crisis management
Miklowitz, Otto, Frank, Reilly-Harrington, Kogan, et al. (2007); Miklowitz, Otto, Frank, Reilly-Harrington, Wisniewski, et al. (2007)	293 adults	RCT (1 year)	Current episode of depression	Collaborative care (3 psychoeducation sessions)	77% recovered in FFT in 1 year; 65% in IPT; 60% in CBT; 52% in collaborative care; better social functioning in FFT and IPT
Miklowitz, Biuckians, & Richards (2006)	20 adolescents	Open	Various states	None	Adolescents showed significant improvement over 2 years in depression, mania, and problem behaviors

540

Study	Sample	Design	Inclusion criteria	Comparison condition	Findings
Miklowitz, Axelson, et al. (2008)	58 adolescents	RCT (2 years)	Mood episode in prior 3 months; acutely or subsyndromally ill	3 education sessions	Adolescents in FFT recovered from depression 7 weeks faster than adolescents in brief psychoeducation
Miklowitz et al. (2011)	13 children (ages 9–17) with bipolar parents	Open (1 year)	Depression or subthreshold manic or hypomanic symptoms	None	Youth in FFT showed significant improvements in depression, mania, and global functioning scores
Perlick et al. (2010)	Caregivers of 46 adults with bipolar I disorder, 1 year	RCT (4.7 months)	Various states	8- to 12-session health program	Caregivers and patients in FFT had decreases in depressive symptoms
Miklowitz et al. (2013)	40 children (ages 9–17) wit bipolar relatives	RCT (1 year)	Depression or subthreshold manic or hypomanic symptoms	TAU (1–2 sessions of family education)	Children in FFT recovered from depression 8 weeks faster, and spent more time in remission over 1 year than children in TAU
Miklowitz et al. (2014)	145 adolescents (ages 12–17)	RCT (2 years)	Mood episode in last 3 months; currently symptomatic	Enhanced care (three sessions of family education)	No differences in time to recovery or recurrence; patients in FFT had less severe manic symptoms in second study year

Note. TAU, treatment as usual; RCT, randomized controlled trial; FFT, family-focused therapy; IPT, interpersonal psychotherapy.

year. The effects of FFT have been less consistent in bipolar adolescents than among adults (Miklowitz et al., in press). In several trials, effect sizes for FFT (in comparison with brief treatment) have been stronger in patients from high-EE than low-EE families (Kim & Miklowitz, 2004; Miklowitz, Axelson, et al., 2009; Miklowitz et al., 2013), suggesting that patients in high-intensity–high-conflict families may show the greatest benefits from FFT.

In one study, FFT was associated with an increase in the use of positive verbal and nonverbal communication in family interactions measured at a pretreatment baseline and again at 9 months. These improvements were correlated with mood improvements of patients over the same interval (Simoneau, Miklowitz, Richards, Saleem, & George, 1999). Patients in FFT were also more likely than patients in brief treatment to be consistent with their lithium and/or anticonvulsant regimens, which in turn predicted the stabilization of mania symptoms over 2 years. Because of the design of the study, it was not possible to establish the direction of these associations (e.g., whether patients improved symptomatically first and then communicated better with their relatives, or the reverse).

FFT as Early Intervention for High-Risk Youth

A follow-up of children with subthreshold bipolar disorder (i.e., those with brief and recurrent hypomanic or manic episodes that did not meet DSM-IV episode criteria) and a positive family history of mania found that up to half developed full DSM-IV bipolar I or II disorder over 5 years (Axelson et al., 2011). FFT has been adapted for children and adolescents (ages 9–17) who are at risk for developing bipolar disorder, including those with depression or hypomania and at least one first- or second-degree relative with bipolar I or II disorder. In a 1-year RCT, 40 high-risk children (ages 9–17) with either major depressive disorder (MDD), cyclothymic disorder, or bipolar disorder–not otherwise specified were randomly assigned to FFT, high-risk version (FFT-HR), or a one- to two-session control treatment (Miklowitz et al., 2013). Participants in FFT-HR recovered more rapidly from their depressive symptoms, had more weeks in remission over 1 year, and showed greater improvement in hypomania symptoms over 1 year than participants in the control treatment.

There are other family treatment models that have shown promise in pediatric bipolar disorder. In a large (N = 165) wait-list trial, Fristad, Verducci, Walters, and Young (2009) found that children with mood disorders who were assigned to multifamily groups improved to a greater extent than children on a waiting list over 6 months. A 12-session family-focused cognitive-behavioral program has been developed for school-age children with bipolar disorder, with positive effects on mood symptoms and psychosocial functioning (West & Weinstein, 2012). Thus family interventions—administered in single-family or group formats—may enhance symptom stabilization in adult and childhood bipolar samples.

Group Treatment

Group psychoeducation appears to be a highly effective adjunct to pharmacotherapy in relapse prevention in bipolar samples. Colom and associates (2003) randomly assigned 120 patients with remitted bipolar disorder to a 21-session structured psychoeducation group or 21 sessions of an unstructured support group, both with pharmacotherapy. Results at the end of a 5-year follow-up indicated a lower relapse rate and better psychosocial functioning in the psychoeducation group than in the unstructured group. The reduction in number of hospital days translated into a cost savings of approximately $6,500 for each patient in psychoeducation (Scott et al., 2009).

Two large-scale randomized trials have examined the effectiveness of group psycho-education within the context of multicomponent care management plans. Bauer and colleagues (2006) examined a "collaborative care" program for patients with bipolar disorder at 11 Veterans Administration (VA) sites. The intervention included mood monitoring by a nurse care coordinator and group treatment to improve patients' self-management and relapse prevention skills. Over a 3-year period, patients in the care treatment program spent fewer weeks in manic episodes than patients who received usual VA care (*N* = 306). Improvements in the collaborative care group were also observed in social functioning, quality of life, and treatment satisfaction. There were no significant effects of collaborative care on manic and depressive symptoms over the 3-year period.

In the largest randomized trial of a psychosocial treatment for bipolar disorder (*N* = 441) to date, Simon, Ludman, Bauer, Unutzer, and Operskalski (2006) compared a similar 2-year multicomponent care intervention to TAU among patients in a health care network. Over 2 years, patients in the multicomponent program had significantly lower mania scores and spent less time in manic or hypomanic episodes than those in the comparison group. There were no effects on depressive symptoms. In both studies, group psychoeducation was one component of a larger collaborative care program. Thus dismantling studies will be necessary to determine the unique contribution of group psychoeducation to outcomes.

An adaptation of group psychoeducation—functional remediation treatment—emphasizes improving patients' cognitive functioning through memory, attention, problem solving, and organizational skills. In a 10-site RCT in Spain, 268 euthymic patients with bipolar disorder were assigned to 21 weekly group sessions of functional remediation, 21 sessions of standard group psychoeducation, or TAU (Torrent et al., 2013). Patients in functional remediation showed greater changes in occupational and social functioning than those in TAU, but differed only modestly from patients in the standard psychoeducation groups.

Overall, group psychoeducation appears to be a viable and cost-effective alternative to individual or family approaches in the stabilization of manic symptoms, although their role in controlling depressive symptoms is unclear. Research on the processes that mediate the effectiveness of group psychoeducation—decreased social isolation, medication adherence, the ability to recognize oncoming episodes, or support against the stigma of the disorder—may contribute to the development of group models with greater longevity of effects.

Comparison of Psychosocial Approaches: The STEP-BD Study

Many of the studies cited earlier were single-center studies at the universities in which the treatments were developed. The STEP-BD study examined pharmacological and psychosocial interventions in a "practical" clinical trial across 22 U.S. centers (Sachs et al., 2007). In one part of the program, 293 patients with bipolar I and II depression from 15 sites were randomly assigned to pharmacotherapy and (1) one of three intensive psychosocial treatments (defined as 30 sessions of FFT, IPSRT, or CBT over 9 months) or (2) a control treatment. The control involved three educational sessions over 6 weeks and focused on developing a relapse prevention plan. Over 1 year, being in any of the intensive psychotherapies was associated with more frequent (and more rapid) recovery from depression (64.4%; 25% median: 169 days) than being in the control treatment (51.5%;

25% median: 279 days; Miklowitz, Otto, Frank, Reilly-Harrington, Wisniewski, et al., 2007). Patients in intensive treatment were also 1.6 times more likely than patients in collaborative care to be clinically well in any given study month. Rates of recovery over 1 year were as follows: FFT, 77% (20/26); IPSRT, 65% (40/62); CBT, 60% (45/75); and collaborative care, 52%. The positive effects of intensive psychosocial intervention extended to functional outcomes (relationship functioning and life satisfaction) as well (Miklowitz, Otto, Frank, Reilly-Harrington, Kogan, et al., 2007). The STEP-BD study suggests that psychotherapy is a vital part of the effort to stabilize episodes of depression in bipolar illness and that patients with acute depression may require more intensive psychotherapy than is typically offered in community mental health centers.

Psychosocial Treatment for Bipolar Disorder: Common Ingredients

The commonalities among the existing psychosocial approaches to bipolar disorder are more striking than their differences. Miklowitz, Goodwin, Bauer, and Geddes (2008) designed a Therapist Strategies Questionnaire to tabulate common and specific elements of psychotherapies for bipolar disorder. In analyses of data obtained from 31 clinicians who participated in one of 14 RCTs, several common factors were identified: psychoeducation about symptoms, etiology, course and treatment; resolving key interpersonal and family problems; enhancing coping with the stigma of mental illness; and community advocacy (assisting patients in obtaining services). Beyond these common elements were specific ingredients that were featured in some modalities and not others: self-rated mood monitoring, relapse prevention planning, enhancing adherence with medications, pleasant events scheduling, cognitive restructuring, regulating sleep–wake routines, and involvement of family members in skills training. Research has not established whether these common or specific elements are more or less important in bringing about therapeutic change. Possibly, future RCTs might use dismantling strategies to identify the most effective components of these treatments and develop "hybrid" models of psychotherapy that emphasize these most effective elements.

CONCLUSIONS AND FUTURE DIRECTIONS

Practical Trials

Many questions remain to be resolved in future studies of drug and psychosocial treatments for bipolar disorder. First, pharmacotherapy trials and psychosocial treatment trials have largely developed independently. What is needed are large-scale "practical trials" that evaluate pharmacotherapy with psychotherapy decisions at different phases of the illness cycle. For example, when attempting to stabilize bipolar depression, psychotherapy should be evaluated as an alternative to adding an antidepressant, a second mood stabilizer, or an SGA. Studies may examine whether patients who respond to psychotherapy in acute treatment are able to taper one or more of their medications during the maintenance phase.

Contrary to previous thinking, patients with bipolar II depression may respond to antidepressants alone, without a heightened risk of manic switching (Amsterdam, Wang, & Shults, 2010). Moreover, a small-scale RCT showed that bipolar II depression could be stabilized just as rapidly with interpersonal therapy alone as with quetiapine monotherapy (Swartz, Frank, & Cheng, 2012). Thus some patients with bipolar disorder may benefit from simplified algorithms for depression, although we do not currently know who these patients are or what level of improvement can be expected from each treatment component. Future practical trials may be able to address these questions.

Moderators and Mediators

Considerable work is needed to identify moderators and mediators of treatment effects (Kraemer, Wilson, Fairburn, & Agras, 2002). Few moderators of effects have been identified for pharmacological or psychosocial modalities. Frank and colleagues (2005) found that patients without medical comorbidities did better with IPSRT than with active clinical management, whereas the reverse was true of patients who had medical comorbidities. Scott and colleagues (2006) found that CBT was more effective in preventing recurrences among patients with < 12 episodes. It appears that EE is a moderator of the effects of FFT in bipolar disorder in both adult and childhood samples (Kim & Miklowitz, 2004; Miklowitz, Axelson, et al., 2009; Miklowitz et al., 2013).

The end goal of moderator analyses is to provide pragmatic clinical data on who will be most likely to benefit from which treatments. Nonetheless, studies of moderators must be powered with adequate sample sizes to identify treatment by moderator interactions reliably. Typically, clinical trials—notably, pharmacotherapy trials—have not been designed with moderators in mind, and exploratory examinations of moderators have sometimes capitalized on chance. For example, lamotrigine has been found to be more effective in patients with more severe bipolar depression than in those with less severe depression, despite its preferential use for patients with milder depression in clinical practice (Geddes et al., 2009). Replication of treatment by moderator interactions in subsequent trials, or meta-regression models that examine interactions across studies, will be necessary to translate subgroup findings into clinical recommendations.

Mediators are typically "change variables" that are measured before, during, and after treatment and that help explain how treatments work (Kraemer et al., 2002). In studies of FFT, treatment-associated changes in mania scores were mediated by improvements in medication adherence, whereas changes in depressive symptoms were related to improvements in patient–relative interactions (Miklowitz, George, et al., 2003; Simoneau et al., 1999). In the Pittsburgh IPSRT trial, stabilization of sleep–wake rhythms during an acute treatment phase mediated the success of IPSRT in delaying recurrences during a maintenance phase (Frank et al., 2005). To date, no consistent mediators have been identified in studies of CBT or group psychoeducation.

Early-Onset Bipolar Disorder and Prodromal Phenotypes

As noted earlier, patients with early-onset bipolar disorder are at risk for a host of adverse outcomes. Given the disadvantages of polypharmacy for the younger age groups (e.g., significant weight gain), effective psychosocial interventions are critical. Possibly, effective psychosocial therapy could reduce the number of medications needed to stabilize patients with early onset. The development of structured psychosocial approaches for childhood bipolar disorder is just beginning to receive attention.

Extending this rationale further, psychosocial interventions may have a role in staving off the initial onset of bipolar disorder. A study of FFT as an early intervention for subthreshold youth with first-degree relatives with bipolar disorder indicated that depressive and hypomanic symptoms could be stabilized over 1 year (Miklowitz et al., 2013). It is unclear whether early stabilization of mood symptoms has downstream effects that contribute to the delay or prevention of first onsets of mania, or in turn whether preventing first episodes arrests the neurotoxic effects of repeated mood episodes during development. A multisite trial of FFT for youth at risk for bipolar disorder is currently under way at the University of California Los Angeles (D. Miklowitz, Principal Investigator), University of Colorado (C. Schneck, Principal Investigator), and Stanford University (K. Chang, Principal Investigator) and should help clarify these questions.

Finally, there is a significant gap in the treatment dissemination literature. How does one teach pharmacological strategies or psychosocial interventions to practicing clinicians and make their use sustainable in community mental health settings? The appearance of practice parameters and multisite effectiveness trials, such as STEP-BD, are a move in the right direction. However, more needs to be done to ensure that training materials are widely available, training seminars are convenient and low cost, and incentives are given to clinicians who use these empirically supported strategies. Technology-based interventions, including mood monitoring via text messaging or webform e-mail, may assist clinicians in monitoring patients who do not consistently attend treatment (Miklowitz, et al., 2012). "Bench-to-bedside" approaches will be essential in maintaining the recent gains of treatment research in this highly debilitating disorder.

REFERENCES

Alloy, L. B., Bender, R. E., Whitehouse, W. G., Wagner, C. A., Liu, R. T., Grant, D. A., et al. (2012). High Behavioral Approach System (BAS) sensitivity, reward responsiveness, and goal-striving predict first onset of bipolar spectrum disorders: A prospective behavioral high-risk design. *Journal of Abnormal Psychology, 121*(2), 339–351.

Altshuler, L., Suppes, T., Black, D., Nolen, W. A., Keck, P. E. J., Frye, M. A., et al. (2003). Impact of antidepressant discontinuation after acute bipolar depression remission on rates of depressive relapse at 1-year follow-up. *American Journal of Psychiatry, 160*, 1252–1262.

Altshuler, L. L., Post, R. M., Black, D. O., Keck, P. E. J., Nolen, W. A., Frye, M. A., et al. (2006). Subsyndromal depressive symptoms are associated with functional impairment in patients with bipolar disorder: Results of a large, multisite study. *Journal of Clinical Psychiatry, 67*(10), 1551–1560.

Amsterdam, J. D., Wang, G., & Shults, J. (2010). Venlafaxine monotherapy in bipolar type II depressed patients unresponsive to prior lithium monotherapy. *Acta Psychiatrica Scandinavaca, 121*(3), 201–208.

Axelson, D. A., Birmaher, B., Strober, M. A., Goldstein, B. I., Ha, W., Gill, M. K., et al. (2011). Course of subthreshold bipolar disorder in youth: Diagnostic progression from bipolar disorder not otherwise specified. *Journal of the American Academy of Child and Adolescent Psychiatry, 50*(10), 1001–1016.

Bauer, M. S., McBride, L., Williford, W. O., Glick, H., Kinosian, B., Altshuler, L., et al. (2006). Cooperative Studies Program 430 Study Team: Collaborative care for bipolar disorder: Part II. Impact on clinical outcome, function, and costs. *Psychiatric Services, 57*, 937–945.

Birmaher, B., Axelson, D., Strober, M., Gill, M. K., Valeri, S., Chiappetta, L., et al. (2006). Clinical course of children and adolescents with bipolar spectrum disorders. *Archives of General Psychiatry, 63*(2), 175–183.

Bowden, C. L., Calabrese, J. R., Sachs, G., Yatham, L. N., Asghar, S. A., Hompland, M., et al. (2003). A placebo-controlled 18-month trial of lamotrigine and lithium maintenance treatment in recently manic or hypomanic patients with bipolar I disorder. *Archives of General Psychiatry, 60*, 392–400.

Brown, E. B., McElroy, S. L., Keck, P. E. J., Deldar, A., Adams, D. H., Tohen, M., et al. (2006). A 7-week, randomized, double-blind trial of olanzapine/fluoxetine combination versus lamotrigine in the treatment of bipolar I depression. *Journal of Clinical Psychiatry, 67*(7), 1025–1033.

Cipriani, A., Barbui, C., Salanti, G., Rendell, J., Brown, R., Stockton, S., et al. (2011). Comparative efficacy and acceptability of antimanic drugs in acute mania: A multiple-treatments meta-analysis. *Lancet, 378*, 1306–1315.

Colom, F., Vieta, E., Martinez-Aran, A., Reinares, M., Benabarre, A., & Gasto, C. (2000). Clinical factors associated with treatment noncompliance in euthymic bipolar patients. *Journal of Clinical Psychiatry, 61*, 549–555.

Colom, F., Vieta, E., Martinez-Aran, A., Reinares, M., Goikolea, J. M., Benabarre, A., et al. (2003). A randomized trial on the efficacy of group psychoeducation in the prophylaxis of recurrences in bipolar patients whose disease is in remission. *Archives of General Psychiatry, 60*, 402–407.

Correll, C. U., Manu, P., Olshanskiy, V., Napolitano, B., Kane, J. M., & Malhotra, A. K. (2009). Cardiometabolic risk of second-generation antipsychotic medications during first-time use in children and adolescents. *Journal of the American Medical Association, 302*, 1765–1773.

Correll, C. U., Sheridan, E. M., & DelBello, M. P. (2010). Antipsychotic and mood stabilizer efficacy and tolerability in pediatric and adult patients with bipolar I mania: A comparative analysis of acute, randomized, placebo-controlled trials. *Bipolar Disorders, 12*(2), 116–141.

De Fruyt, J., Deschepper, E., Audenaert, K., Constant, E., Floris, M., Pitchot, W., et al. (2012). Second-generation antipsychotics in the treatment of bipolar depression: A systematic review and meta-analysis. *Journal of Psychopharmacology, 26*(5), 603–617.

Deckersbach, T., Hölzel, B. K., Eisner, L. R., Stange, J. P., Peckham, A. D., Dougherty, D. D., et al. (2012). Mindfulness-based cognitive therapy for nonremitted patients with bipolar disorder. *CNS Neuroscience and Therapeutics, 18*(2), 133–141.

DelBello, M. P., Chang, K., Welge, J. A., Adler, C. M., Rana, M., Howe, M., et al. (2009). A double-blind, placebo-controlled pilot study of quetiapine for depressed adolescents with bipolar disorder. *Bipolar Disorders, 11*(5), 483–493.

DelBello, M. P., Kowatch, R. A., Adler, C. M., Stanford, K. E., Welge, J. A., Barzman, D. H., et al. (2006). A double-blind randomized pilot study comparing quetiapine and divalproex for adolescent mania. *Journal of the American Academy of Child and Adolescent Psychiatry, 45*(3), 305–313.

DelBello, M. P., Schwiers, M. L., Rosenberg, H. L., & Strakowski, S. M. (2002). A double-blind, randomized, placebo-controlled study of quetiapine as adjunctive treatment for adolescent mania. *Journal of the American Academy of Child and Adolescent Psychiatry, 41*, 1216–1223.

Dienes, K. A., Hammen, C., Henry, R. M., Cohen, A. N., & Daley, S. E. (2006). The stress sensitization hypothesis: Understanding the course of bipolar disorder. *Journal of Affective Disorders, 95*(1–3), 43–49.

Dilsaver, S. C. (2011). An estimate of the minimum economic burden of bipolar I and II disorders in the United States: 2009. *Journal of Affective Disorders, 129*(1–3), 79–83.

Ehlers, C. L., Kupfer, D. J., Frank, E., & Monk, T. H. (1993). Biological rhythms and depression: The role of zeitgebers and zeitstorers. *Depression, 1*, 285–293.

Findling, R. L., McNamara, N. K., Youngstrom, E. A., Stansbrey, R. J., Gracious, B. L., Reed, M. D., et al. (2005). Double-blind 18-month trial of lithium versus divalproex maintenance treatment in pediatric bipolar disorder. *Journal of the American Academy of Child and Adolescent Psychiatry, 44*(5), 409–417.

Frank, E., Kupfer, D. J., Thase, M. E., Mallinger, A. G., Swartz, H. A., Fagiolini, A. M., et al. (2005). Two-year outcomes for interpersonal and social rhythm therapy in individuals with bipolar I disorder. *Archives of General Psychiatry, 62*(9), 996–1004.

Fristad, M. A., Verducci, J. S., Walters, K., & Young, M. E. (2009). Impact of multifamily psychoeducational psychotherapy in treating children aged 8 to 12 years with mood disorders. *Archives of General Psychiatry, 66*(9), 1013–1021.

Geddes, J. R., Burgess, S., Hawton, K., Jamison, K., & Goodwin, G. M. (2004). Long-term lithium therapy for bipolar disorder: Systematic review and meta-analysis of randomized controlled trials. *American Journal of Psychiatry, 161*(2), 217–222.

Geddes, J. R., Calabrese, J. R., & Goodwin, G. M. (2009). Lamotrigine for treatment of bipolar depression: Independent meta-analysis and meta-regression of individual patient data from five randomised trials. *British Journal of Psychiatry, 194*(1), 4–9.

Geddes, J. R., Goodwin, G. M., Rendell, J., Azorin, J. M., Cipriani, A., Ostacher, M. J., et al. (2010). Lithum plus valproate combination therapy versus monotherapy for relapse prevention in bipolar I disorder (BALANCE): A randomised open-label trial. *Lancet, 375,* 385–395.

Geller, B., Luby, J. L., Joshi, P., Wagner, K. D., Emslie, G., Walkup, J. T., et al. (2012). A randomized controlled trial of risperidone, lithium, or divalproex sodium for initial treatment of bipolar I disorder, manic or mixed phase, in children and adolescents. *Archives of General Psychiatry, 69*(5), 515–528.

Geller, B., Tillman, R., Craney, J. L., & Bolhofner, K. (2004). Four-year prospective outcome and natural history of mania in children with a prepubertal and early adolescent bipolar disorder phenotype. *Archives of General Psychiatry, 61,* 459–467.

Gitlin, M. J., Mintz, J., Sokolski, K., Hammen, C., & Altshuler, L. L. (2011). Subsyndromal depressive symptoms after symptomatic recovery from mania are associated with delayed functional recovery. *Journal of Clinical Psychiatry, 72*(5), 692–697.

Goodwin, F. K., Fireman, B., Simon, G. E., Hunkeler, E. M., Lee, J., & Revicki, D. (2003). Suicide risk in bipolar disorder during treatment with lithium and divalproex. *Journal of the American Medical Association, 290*(11), 1467–1473.

Goodwin, G. M., & Consensus Group of the British Association for Psychopharmacology. (2009). Evidence-based guidelines for treating bipolar disorder: Revised second edition—recommendations from the British Association for Psychopharmacology. *Journal of Psychopharmacology, 23*(4), 346–388.

Hammen, C., & Gitlin, M. J. (1997). Stress reactivity in bipolar patients and its relation to prior history of the disorder. *American Journal of Psychiatry, 154,* 856–857.

Hillegers, M. H., Burger, H., Wals, M., Reichart, C. G., Verhulst, F. C., Nolen, W. A., et al. (2004). Impact of stressful life events, familial loading and their interaction on the onset of mood disorders. *British Journal of Psychiatry, 185,* 97–101.

Hlastala, S. A., Frank, E., Kowalski, J., Sherrill, J. T., Tu, X. M., Anderson, B., et al. (2000). Stressful life events, bipolar disorder, and the "kindling model." *Journal of Abnormal Psychology, 109,* 777–786.

Hunt, J. I., Case, B. G., Birmaher, B., Stout, R. L., Dickstein, D. P., Yen, S., et al. (2013). Irritability and elation in a large bipolar youth sample: Relative symptom severity and clinical outcomes over 4 years. *Journal of Clinical Psychiatry, 74*(1), 110–117.

Johnson, S. L., Cuellar, A., Ruggero, C., Perlman, C., Goodnick, P., White, R., et al. (2008). Life events as predictors of mania and depression in bipolar I disorder. *Journal of Abnormal Psychology, 117,* 268–277.

Keck, P. E., Jr., Perlis, R. H., Otto, M. W., Carpenter, D., Docherty, J. P., & Ross, R. (2004). Expert Consensus Guideline Series: Treatment of bipolar disorder. *Postgraduate Medicine Special Report,* 1–108.

Kim, E. Y., & Miklowitz, D. J. (2004). Expressed emotion as a predictor of outcome among bipolar patients undergoing family therapy. *Journal of Affective Disorders, 82,* 343–352.

Kim, E. Y., Miklowitz, D. J., Biuckians, A., & Mullen, K. (2007). Life stress and the course of early-onset bipolar disorder. *Journal of Affective Disorders, 99*(1), 37–44.

Kraemer, H. C., Wilson, T., Fairburn, C. G., & Agras, W. S. (2002). Mediators and moderators of treatment effects in randomized clinical trials. *Archives of General Psychiatry, 59,* 877–883.

Lam, D. H., Hayward, P., Watkins, E. R., Wright, K., & Sham, P. (2005). Relapse prevention in patients with bipolar disorder: Cognitive therapy outcome after 2 years. *American Journal of Psychiatry, 162,* 324–329.

Leibenluft, E., Cohen, P., Gorrindo, T., Brook, J. S., & Pine, D. S. (2006). Chronic vs. episodic irritability in youth: A community-based, longitudinal study of clinical and diagnostic associations. *Journal of Child and Adolescent Psychopharmacology, 16*(4), 456–466.

Li, X., Frye, M. A., & Shelton, R. C. (2012). Review of pharmacological treatment in mood disorders and future directions for drug development. *Neuropsychopharmacology, 37*, 77–101.

Loebel, A., Cucchiaro, J., Silva, R., Kroger, H., Hsu, J., Sarma, K., et al. (2014). Lurasidone monotherapy in the treatment of bipolar I depression: a randomized, double-blind, placebo-controlled study. *American Journal of Psychiatry, 171*, 160–168.

Luby, J. L., Tandon, M., & Belden, A. (2009). Preschool bipolar disorder. *Child and Adolescent Psychiatric Clinics of North America, 18*(2), 391–403.

Malhi, G. S., Adams, D., & Berk, M. (2009). Medicating mood with maintenance in mind: Bipolar depression pharmacotherapy. *Bipolar Disorders, 11*(Suppl. 2), 55–76.

Malkoff-Schwartz, S., Frank, E., Anderson, B., Sherrill, J. T., Siegel, L., Patterson, D., et al. (1998). Stressful life events and social rhythm disruption in the onset of manic and depressive bipolar episodes: A preliminary investigation. *Archives of General Psychiatry, 55*, 702–707.

Manji, H. K., Quiroz, J. A., Payne, J. L., Singh, J., Lopes, B. P., Viegas, J. S., et al. (2003). The underlying neurobiology of bipolar disorder. *World Psychiatry, 2*(3), 136–146.

Merikangas, K. R., Akiskal, H. S., Angst, J., Greenberg, P. E., Hirschfeld, R. M. A., Petukhova, M., et al. (2007). Lifetime and 12-month prevalence of bipolar spectrum disorder in the National Comorbidity Survey Replication. *Archives of General Psychiatry, 64*, 543–552.

Merikangas, K. R., Jin, R., He, J. P., Kessler, R. C., Lee, S., Sampson, N. A., et al. (2011). Prevalence and correlates of bipolar spectrum disorder in the World Mental Health Survey initiative. *Archives of General Psychiatry, 68*(3), 241–251.

Miklowitz, D. J. (2010). *Bipolar disorder: A family-focused treatment approach* (2nd ed.). New York: Guilford Press.

Miklowitz, D. J., Alatiq, Y., Goodwin, G. M., Geddes, J. R., Fennell, M. V. F., Dimidjian, S., et al. (2009). A pilot study of mindfulness-based cognitive therapy for bipolar disorder. *International Journal of Cognitive Therapy, 2*(4), 373–382.

Miklowitz, D. J., Axelson, D. A., Birmaher, B., George, E. L., Taylor, D. O., Schneck, C. D., et al. (2008). Family-focused treatment for adolescents with bipolar disorder: Results of a 2-year randomized trial. *Archives of General Psychiatry, 65*(9), 1053–1061.

Miklowitz, D. J., Axelson, D. A., George, E. L., Taylor, D. O., Schneck, C. D., Sullivan, A. E., et al. (2009). Expressed emotion moderates the effects of family-focused treatment for bipolar adolescents. *Journal of the American Academy of Child and Adolescent Psychiatry, 48*, 643–651.

Miklowitz, D. J., Biuckians, A., & Richards, J. A. (2006). Early-onset bipolar disorder: A family treatment perspective. *Development and Psychopathology, 18*(4), 1247–1265.

Miklowitz, D. J., Chang, K. D., Taylor, D. O., George, E. L., Singh, M. K., Schneck, C. D., et al. (2011). Early psychosocial intervention for youth at risk for bipolar disorder: A 1-year treatment development trial. *Bipolar Disorders, 13*(1), 67–75.

Miklowitz, D. J., George, E. L., Richards, J. A., Simoneau, T. L., & Suddath, R. L. (2003). A randomized study of family-focused psychoeducation and pharmacotherapy in the outpatient management of bipolar disorder. *Archives of General Psychiatry, 60*, 904–912.

Miklowitz, D. J., & Goldstein, M. J. (1990). Behavioral family treatment for patients with bipolar affective disorder. *Behavior Modification, 14*, 457–489.

Miklowitz, D. J., Goldstein, M. J., Nuechterlein, K. H., Snyder, K. S., & Mintz, J. (1988). Family factors and the course of bipolar affective disorder. *Archives of General Psychiatry, 45*, 225–231.

Miklowitz, D. J., Goodwin, G. M., Bauer, M. S., & Geddes, J. (2008). Common and specific elements of psychosocial treatments for bipolar disorder: A survey of clinicians participating in randomized trials. *Journal of Psychiatric Practice, 14*, 1–9.

Miklowitz, D. J., Otto, M. W., Frank, E., Reilly-Harrington, N. A., Kogan, J. N., Sachs, G. S., et al. (2007). Intensive psychosocial intervention enhances functioning in patients with bipolar depression: Results from a 9-month randomized controlled trial. *American Journal of Psychiatry, 164*, 1340–1347.

Miklowitz, D. J., Otto, M. W., Frank, E., Reilly-Harrington, N. A., Wisniewski, S. R., Kogan, J. N., et al. (2007). Psychosocial treatments for bipolar depression: A 1-year randomized trial from the Systematic Treatment Enhancement Program. *Archives of General Psychiatry, 64,* 419–427.

Miklowitz, D. J., Price, J., Holmes, E. A., Rendell, J., Bell, S., Budge, K., et al. (2012). Facilitated integrated mood management (FIMM) for adults with bipolar disorder. *Bipolar Disorders, 14*(2), 185–197.

Miklowitz, D. J., Schneck, C. D., George, E. L., Taylor, D. O., Sugar, C. A., Birmaher, B., et al. (in press). Pharmacotherapy and family-focused treatment for adolescents with bipolar I and II disorders: A 2-year randomized trial. *American Journal of Psychiatry.*

Miklowitz, D. J., Schneck, C. D., Singh, M. K., Taylor, D. O., George, E. L., Cosgrove, V. E., et al. (2013). Early intervention for symptomatic youth at risk for bipolar disorder: A randomized trial of family-focused therapy. *Journal of the American Academy of Child and Adolescent Psychiatry, 52*(2), 121–131.

Moller, H. J., Grunze, H., & Broich, K. (2006). Do recent efficacy data on the drug treatment of acute bipolar depression support the position that drugs other than antidepressants are the treatment of choice?: A conceptual review. *European Archives of Psychiatry and Clinical Neuroscience, 256*(1), 1–16.

Nemeroff, C. B., Evans, D. L., Gyulai, L., Sachs, G. S., Bowden, C. L., Gergel, I. P., et al. (2001). Double-blind, placebo-controlled comparison of imipramine and paroxetine in the treatment of bipolar depression. *American Journal of Psychiatry, 158*(6), 906–912.

Nierenberg, A. A., Ostacher, M. J., Calabrese, J. R., Ketter, T. A., Marangell, L., Miklowitz, D. J., et al. (2006). Treatment-resistant bipolar depression: A STEP-BD equipoise randomized effectiveness trial of antidepressant augmentation with lamotrigine, inositol or risperidone. *American Journal of Psychiatry, 163*(2), 210–216.

Parikh, S. V., Zaretsky, A., Beaulieu, S., Yatham, L. N., Young, L. T., Patelis-Siotis, I., et al. (2012). A randomized controlled trial of psychoeducation or cognitive-behavioral therapy in bipolar disorder: A Canadian Network for Mood and Anxiety Treatments (CANMAT) study. *Journal of Clinical Psychiatry, 73*(6), 803–810.

Perlick, D., Miklowitz, D. J., Lopez, N., Chou, J., Kalvin, C., Adzhiashvili, V., et al. (2010). Family-focused treatment for caregivers of patients with bipolar disorder. *Bipolar Disorders, 12*(6), 627–637.

Perlis, R. H., Miyahara, S., Marangell, L. B., Wisniewski, S. R., Ostacher, M., DelBello, M. P., et al. (2004). Long-term implications of early onset in bipolar disorder: Data from the first 1,000 participants in the Systematic Treatment Enhancement Program for Bipolar Disorder (STEP-BD). *Biological Psychiatry, 55,* 875–881.

Perlis, R. H., Ostacher, M. J., Patel, J., Marangell, L. B., Zhang, H., Wisniewski, S. R., et al. (2006). Predictors of recurrence in bipolar disorder: Primary outcomes from the Systematic Treatment Enhancement Program for Bipolar Disorder (STEP-BD). *American Journal of Psychiatry, 163*(2), 217–224.

Pfeifer, J. C., Kowatch, R. A., & DelBello, M. P. (2010). Pharmacotherapy of bipolar disorder in children and adolescents: Recent progress. *CNS Drugs, 24*(7), 575–593.

Post, R. M. (2007). Kindling and sensitization as models for affective episode recurrence, cyclicity, and tolerance phenomena. *Neuroscience and Biobehavioral Review, 31*(6), 858–873.

Post, R. M., & Leverich, G. S. (2006). The role of psychosocial stress in the onset and progression of bipolar disorder and its comorbidities: The need for earlier and alternative modes of therapeutic intervention. *Development and Psychopathology, 18*(4), 1181–1211.

Rea, M. M., Tompson, M., Miklowitz, D. J., Goldstein, M. J., Hwang, S., & Mintz, J. (2003). Family focused treatment vs. individual treatment for bipolar disorder: Results of a randomized clinical trial. *Journal of Consulting and Clinical Psychology, 71,* 482–492.

Sachs, G. S., Nierenberg, A. A., Calabrese, J. R., Marangell, L. B., Wisniewski, S. R., Gyulai, L., et al. (2007). Effectiveness of adjunctive antidepressant treatment for bipolar depression. *New England Journal of Medicine, 356,* 1–12.

Sapolsky, R. M. (2000). The possibility of neurotoxicity in the hippocampus in major depression: A primer on neuron death. *Biological Psychiatry, 48,* 755–765.

Scherk, H., Pajonk, F. G., & Leucht, S. (2007). Second-generation antipsychotic agents in the treatment of acute mania: A systematic review and meta-analysis of randomized controlled trials. *Archives of General Psychiatry, 64*(4), 442–455.

Scott, J., Colom, F., Popova, E., Benabarre, A., Cruz, N., Valenti, M., et al. (2009). Long-term mental health resource utilization and cost of care following group psychoeducation or unstructured group support for bipolar disorders: A cost–benefit analysis. *Journal of Clinical Psychiatry, 70*(3), 378–386.

Scott, J., Paykel, E., Morriss, R., Bentall, R., Kinderman, P., Johnson, T., et al. (2006). Cognitive behaviour therapy for severe and recurrent bipolar disorders: A randomised controlled trial. *British Journal of Psychiatry, 188*, 313–320.

Simon, G. E., Ludman, E. J., Bauer, M. S., Unutzer, J., & Operskalski, B. (2006). Long-term effectiveness and cost of a systematic care program for bipolar disorder. *Archives of General Psychiatry, 63*(5), 500–508.

Simoneau, T. L., Miklowitz, D. J., Richards, J. A., Saleem, R., & George, E. L. (1999). Bipolar disorder and family communication: Effects of a psychoeducational treatment program. *Journal of Abnormal Psychology, 108*, 588–597.

Swartz, H. A., Frank, E., & Cheng, Y. (2012). A randomized pilot study of psychotherapy and quetiapine for the acute treatment of bipolar II depression. *Bipolar Disorders, 14*(2), 211–216.

Thase, M. E. (2006a). Bipolar depression: Diagnostic and treatment challenges. *Development and Psychopathology, 18*(4), 1213–1230.

Thase, M. E. (2006b). Pharmacotherapy of bipolar depression: An update. *Current Psychiatry Reports, 8*(6), 478–488.

Tohen, M., Vieta, E., Calabrese, J., Ketter, T. A., Sachs, G., Bowden, C., et al. (2003). Efficacy of olanzapine and olanzapine–fluoxetine combination in the treatment of bipolar I depression. *Archives of General Psychiatry, 60*, 1079–1088.

Tondo, L., & Baldessarini, R. J. (2000). Reducing suicide risk during lithium maintenance treatment. *Journal of Clinical Psychiatry, 61*(Suppl. 9), 97–104.

Torrent, C., del Mar Bonnin, C., Martinez-Aran, A., Valle, J., Amann, B. L., González-Pinto, A., et al. (2013). Efficacy of functional remediation in bipolar disorder: A multicenter randomized controlled study. *American Journal of Psychiatry, 170*(8), 852–859.

Wagner, K. D., Redden, L., Kowatch, R. A., Wilens, T. E., Segal, S., Chang, K., et al. (2009). A double-blind, randomized, placebo-controlled trial of divalproex extended-release in the treatment of bipolar disorder in children and adolescents. *Journal of the American Academy of Child and Adolescent Psychiatry, 48*(5), 519–532.

Weber, B., Jermann, F., Gex-Fabry, M., Nallet, A., Bondolfi, G., & Aubry, J. M. (2010). Mindfulness-based cognitive therapy for bipolar disorder: A feasibility trial. *European Psychiatry, 25*(6), 334–337.

Weinstock, L. M., & Miller, I. W. (2008). Functional impairment as a predictor of short-term symptom course in bipolar I disorder. *Bipolar Disorders, 10*(3), 437–442.

Weisler, R. H., Nolen, W. A., Neijber, A., Hellqvist, A., Paulsson, B., & Trial 144 Study Investigators. (2011). Continuation of quetiapine versus switching to placebo or lithium for maintenance treatment of bipolar I disorder (Trial 144: A randomized controlled study). *Journal of Clinical Psychiatry, 72*(11), 1452–1464.

West, A. E., & Weinstein, S. M. (2012). A family-based psychosocial treatment model. *Israeli Journal of Psychiatry and Related Sciences, 49*(2), 86–93.

Yatham, L. N., Kennedy, S. H., Parikh, S. V., Schaffer, A., Beaulieu, S., Alda, M., et al. (2012). Canadian Network for Mood and Anxiety Treatments (CANMAT) and International Society for Bipolar Disorders (ISBD) collaborative update of CANMAT guidelines for the management of patients with bipolar disorder: Update 2013. *Bipolar Disorders, 15*(1), 1–44.

Zarate, C. A. J., Brutsche, N. E., Ibrahim, L., Franco-Chaves, J., Diazgranados, N., Cravchik, A., et al. (2012). Replication of ketamine's antidepressant efficacy in bipolar depression: A randomized controlled add-on trial. *Biological Psychiatry, 71*(11), 939–946.

CHAPTER 29

Couple, Parenting, and Interpersonal Therapies for Depression in Adults

Toward Common Clinical Guidelines within a Stress-Generation Framework

Steven R. H. Beach, Mark A. Whisman, *and* Guy Bodenmann

Problems in family relationships are common and prominent for many depressed persons (Beach & Whisman, 2012), as are concerns about other interpersonal problems (Joiner & Coyne, 1999), concerns about lack of connection and support (Bodenmann, Widmer, Charvoz, & Bradbury, 2004), concerns about bereavement (Paykel, 2003), and other interpersonal role problems. As a consequence, clinicians working with patients with depression, regardless of their initial approach, are often confronted with complex decisions about which patients to recommend for adjunctive treatment with an interpersonal focus, as well as questions about whether to begin therapy with an interpersonal focus, initiate a focus on interpersonal problems concurrently with other interventions they are using, or wait until after an initial round of treatment has been completed in the hope that interpersonal and family problems will remit as the episode of depression remits. In this chapter we suggest that a stress-generation framework can provide a useful clinical framework within which to organize the broad and complicated literature on casual connections between interpersonal processes and depression and so provide an empirically grounded foundation for clinical decision making.

We begin by briefly documenting the interpersonal impact of depression, as well as the impact of interpersonal stressors on depression. We then briefly review the association of couple, family, and interpersonal problems with clinical outcomes in depression. In doing so, we lay the groundwork for thinking about bidirectional causation between interpersonal problems and depression in the context of clinical intervention for depression. Ultimately, we place this broad literature within the organizing framework of stress generation and so highlight key interpersonal relationships that may be stress generating and that are therefore potentially important as targets for intervention in the treatment of depression. We next provide a brief overview of the outcome literature for currently available efficacious couple, family, and interpersonal intervention modalities for adult depression, providing a menu of readily available efficacious intervention and referral options, and we propose preliminary referral guidelines. Using the example of couple relationship distress, for which issues related to clinical utility have been more fully explored, we examine briefly the potential for development of an empirically grounded set of binary decision-making rules that could guide clinical decision making as well as referral by clinicians who may not be expert in intervention on particular interpersonal domains. Finally, we examine several issues that need to be addressed in future research.

INTERPERSONAL PROBLEMS AND DEPRESSION

Social Impairment and Depression

Depression has the potential to disrupt the lives of both sufferers and their family members, producing substantial social and economic costs (Greenberg et al., 2003; Simon, 2003; see also Kessler et al., Chapter 1, this volume). Role impairment is often quite noticeable among patients with depression and is particularly likely to be present in longer lasting episodes of depression (Kessler et al., 2003). Depression-related impairment has become a leading cause of disability worldwide, leading to calls to make prevention of depression a global priority (Cuijpers, Beekman, & Reynolds, 2012). At the same time, disability is also well predicted by concurrent relationship problems, and the effect of relationship distress on disability goes beyond its association with primary diagnosis (Whisman & Uebelacker, 2006). Accordingly, addressing relationship problems effectively, particularly those identified as stress generating, will be required as one aspect of prevention and treatment efforts to reduce the long-term disability associated with depression.

Relationship Distress and Depression

There is a highly replicable association between relationship distress and depressive symptoms that hovers around $r = .40$ (Whisman, 2001b) and parallels a similar observed correlation between relationship distress and the broader construct of well-being (Proulx, Helms, & Buehler, 2007), suggesting that the magnitude of the association is robust across different measures of mental health and well-being. Furthermore, people with depressive disorders report lower relationship quality than do people without such disorders (e.g., Whisman, 1999, 2007). The moderate association reflects the fact that the intimate relationships of men and women with depression are often (but not always) distressed and that the correlation is consistent with unidirectional or bidirectional patterns of causation. Suggesting that causality may go from relationship discord to depression, as well as the reverse, severe interpersonal stressors, such as partner infidelity and threats of relationship dissolution, confer increased risk of later onset of depression (e.g., Cano & O'Leary, 2000). Similarly, relationship conflict with physical abuse predicts increased later depressive symptoms even after earlier depressive symptoms and relationship distress are controlled (Beach et al., 2004). Likewise, longitudinal investigations have demonstrated that relationship distress predicts onset of depressive episodes (e.g., Whisman & Bruce, 1999) and increases in depressive symptoms (e.g., Beach, Katz, Kim, & Brody, 2003). Finally, Whisman and Uebelacker (2009) found that the impact of baseline relationship distress on subsequent depressive symptoms was not significantly different from the impact of baseline depressive symptoms on subsequent relationship distress, providing strong evidence of bidirectional longitudinal effects

A bidirectional relation between depression and couple, family, and interpersonal problems creates the potential for such problems that are present at the outset of treatment to influence treatment response. In addition, it raises the potential for couple, family, or interpersonal problems present at the end of treatment to predict poorer long-term functioning and prognosis. Unfortunately, current evidence does not support the hypothesis that interpersonal problems, such as relationship distress, routinely remit in response to pharmacological or psychosocial interventions (for a review, see Whisman, 2001b). As a result, clinicians are often confronted with cases in which an individual with depression expresses concerns about important interpersonal relationships at the beginning of treatment and continues to do so at the end of treatment, raising the practical issue of whether such interpersonal problems should have been addressed earlier in treatment or whether it is reasonable to wait until after the conclusion of an initial course of treatment for depression before making interpersonal problems a focus of treatment. For example, for outpatients with depression treated by psychotherapy (cognitive therapy, interpersonal psychotherapy) or medication, poorer relationship adjustment at posttreatment predicted higher relapse rates following treatment (Kung & Elkin, 2000; Whisman, 2001a), and relationship distress at baseline was associated with a lower remission rate for outpatients with chronic depression treated with the cognitive-behavioral analysis system of psychotherapy (CBASP) or medication, singly or in combination (Denton et al., 2010). Likewise, when conflict in key relationships is not resolved by the end of treatment, allowing high levels of expressed emotion (EE; critical comments, hostility, or emotional involvement) in primary relationships during the posttreatment phase, this may increase the risk for subsequent relapse (cf. Hooley, 2007). Similarly, a study by Meuwly, Bodenmann, and Coyne (2012) indicated that dysfunctional thinking in the patient with depression can be triggered by negative attitudes of the partner, thus increasing the individual's depressive symptoms and so providing a potential mechanism linking interpersonal problems to relapse.

Complicating the work of clinicians, however, not all patients with depression assessed for family and interpersonal problems prior to intervention require a focus on relationship problems. Research by O'Leary, Riso, and Beach (1990), for example, found that among women who perceived their relationship problems as coming *after the onset of their depression*, there was little evidence of need to routinely address relationship issues. These women showed good improvement in their relationship problems as their depression remitted in response to individual therapy. Conversely, women who reported that their relationship difficulties preceded the onset of their depressive episode did require direct attention to relationship problems. For these women, the absence of direct attention to relationship problems resulted in substantial additional deterioration in relationship functioning by the end of treatment despite improvement in depressive symptoms. Accordingly, appropriate therapeutic decision making requires attention to the presence of distress in the relationship at pretreatment assessment, as well as some basis for determining whether the distress can reasonably be expected to remit upon successful treatment of the depressive episode. Thus neither routine referral nor routine neglect is an acceptable approach to clinical management of interpersonal problems occurring in the context of depression. These considerations suggest that routine assessment to identify those in need of direct attention to couple, family, and interpersonal problems is critical, at least at the initiation and at the end of treatment for depression.

Partner Support and Depression

In addition to relationship distress, there is also often strong erosion of positive aspects of relationships and an accumulation of sources of felt burden among patients with depression and their partners (Benazon & Coyne, 2000; Coyne, Thompson, & Palmer, 2002). Persons with depression are less effective at providing or eliciting support (Rook, Pietromonaco, & Lewis, 1994). In addition, when partners experience stress from outside the relationship, it can prompt an experience of stress inside the relationship as well, sometimes manifested as conflict and sometimes as withdrawal (Pasch & Bradbury, 1998; Randall & Bodenmann, 2009). The stress that arises within the relationship in this manner may also be characterized as a stress-generating process. Illustrating this dynamic in action, Davila, Bradbury, Cohan, and Tochluk (1997) examined negative support behaviors (e.g., criticism, rejection, blaming, exaggerating problems, inattentiveness) and found that wives with greater levels of depressive symptoms showed more negative support behaviors and expectations and that negative support behaviors mediated the effect of prior depressive symptoms on later relationship stress. In turn, relationship stress predicted more depressive symptoms.

Accordingly, there is good reason to examine support behavior in marriage as a potential target of intervention. Relationship support was negatively associated with depressive symptoms, even after statistically adjusting for genetic and shared environmental selection effects (Beam et al., 2011), suggesting it is a viable additional potential avenue for intervention to reduce stress generation in couples in which one member has or has had depression in the past (Bodenmann et al., 2008). A focus on increasing partner support requires considering the partner without depression in the therapy process and strengthening both partners' resources by encouraging mutual support (dyadic coping). More recent studies indicate that providing support, and not just receiving it, is often more beneficial and covaries with better well-being and lower mortality (e.g., Brown, Nesse, Vinokur, & Smith, 2003), underscoring the value of encouraging mutual support.

Parenting and Depression

Given the interconnected nature of family subsystems and the strong connection of depression to family and interpersonal dysfunction, it is not surprising that there is also a link between parenting behavior and depression. Observational studies of the parenting behavior of women with depression (Lovejoy, Graczyk, O'Hare, & Neuman, 2000) suggest that mothers with depression are more withdrawn, as well as more negative, than are other parents. These depression-associated changes in parental behavior can lead to increased problems and disruptive behaviors in children (e.g., Conger, Patterson, & Ge, 1995; Hoffman, Crnic, & Baker, 2006) and decreases children's emotional self-regulation (Hoffman et al., 2006), further exacerbating difficulties in the parent–child relationship (e.g., Webster-Stratton & Spitzer, 1996) and contributing to the elevated rates of psychiatric disorder documented to be present among children of parents with depression relative to other children (Beardslee & Podorefsky, 1988; see Gotlib & Colich, Chapter 13, this volume). Indeed, poorer maternal parenting quality appears to confer much of the risk for future problems among offspring of parents with depression (Goodman, 2007). These considerations suggest strong potential for reciprocal influences between child problems and parental depression. Accordingly, although there is less documentation of a link between parenting problems at the beginning of treatment and outcomes, available data are consistent with the literature on intimate relationships in depression in suggesting that many, but not all, persons with depression with child-rearing responsibilities experience difficulties in parenting and in the parent–child relationship and that these difficulties could present an obstacle to effective intervention in some cases and pose risks for relapse and continuing functional impairment among some adults with depression when not successfully addressed.

Grief

Loss events, most of which are social in nature and which also are particularly common in depression, also deserve attention as potentially potent stressful experiences. Loss events sometimes may be processed more flexibly in an individual format than in dyadic or relationship-specific formats, suggesting good potential for depressive episodes triggered by loss and bereavement to be addressed by individual approaches such as interpersonal psychotherapy (IPT) or its derivatives (e.g., Shear, 2005). Death of a partner, in particular, is associated with a ninefold increase in major depression and a fourfold increase in depressive symptoms among recently bereaved older adults (Turvey, Carney, & Arndt, 1999), suggesting additional potential directions for interpersonal intervention. Likewise, complicating predictive models, the effect of bereavement is especially pronounced for those lacking social support (Wortman, Wolff, & Bonanno, 2004). At the same time, when the loss event involves someone other than the spouse, dyadic coping may provide another approach for intervention.

STRESS GENERATION: AN ORGANIZING FRAMEWORK FOR UNDERSTANDING INTERPERSONAL PROBLEMS

The stress-generation model has been developed over a number of years to help characterize the way in which certain types of stress may be self-generated and yet function to exacerbate or maintain a depressive episode (Hammen, 1991). The available evidence suggests that individuals with depression (and perhaps those with mental health problems other than depression) experience worse symptoms when they experience stress but that they are also more likely to behave in ways that increase the probability of additional events in their lives (e.g. Kercher, Rapee, & Schniering, 2009; Moos, Schutte, Brennan, & Moos, 2005; Trombello, Schoebi, & Bradbury, 2011). The self-generating nature of some stressors leads to a key distinction in stress generation between *dependent* and *independent* stressful events. Of great clinical interest is the observation that dependent events—those to which the person may have contributed—contribute more to the prediction of depression than do independent events—those to which the individual could not plausibly have contributed (Kendler, Karkowski, & Prescott, 1999). Dependent events are particularly likely to be relational in nature and include most stressors in the couple and parenting domains.

Individuals with current or former depression appear to be vulnerable to stress generation, and the model has received considerable support across ages and symptom levels (e.g., Hammen, 2006; Liu & Alloy, 2010). It is possible that stress generation operates in a stronger fashion for women (see Lui & Alloy, 2010). In addition, because stress generation may occur outside of the depressive episode, it can confer increased risk even during periods of subsyndromal symptoms (e.g., Joiner, Wingate, Gencoz, & Gencoz, 2005). Similarly, *chronic stressors*—those that have continued for a year or more—are as predictive as or more predictive of depression than are brief, acute stressors (McGonagle & Kessler, 1990). Because relationship problems often fall into the chronic category, events in the interpersonal domain often may be part of a larger vicious cycle serving to maintain depressive symptoms.

WHICH INTERVENTIONS INTERRUPT STRESS-GENERATING INTERPERSONAL PROBLEMS?

Stress generation serves not only to maintain a current episode of depression but also to increase risk for future symptoms and episodes of depression even among people with subsyndromal symptoms. Accordingly, stress-generating processes may be an essential target of intervention among some patients who have current depression as well as among patients with remitted depression if they continue to report serious difficulties in key family and interpersonal domains. Couple, family, and other interpersonal relationships may provide excellent points of therapeutic intervention for persons with depression if (1) the stress-generating behaviors in the domain are amenable to change; (2) the person with current or former depression can make the necessary changes in response to treatment; (3) there is evidence that successful intervention produces a reduction in depressive symptoms, indicating that processes linked to depression maintenance have been influenced; and (4) changes in stress-generating behaviors can be maintained over time (e.g., Halford, 2011).

Well-Established Interventions for Relational Problems

Are there potentially effective interventions for relationship distress, parenting difficulties, and other interpersonal stress generators? For relationship distress, well-specified approaches already have been shown to be efficacious and easily accessible to clinicians. For example, several approaches to couple therapy have been found to be efficacious, including behavioral couple therapy, cognitive-behavioral couple therapy, emotion-focused therapy for couples, and insight-oriented couple therapy (for a review, see Snyder, Castellani, & Whisman, 2006). Parent management training (Patterson, Reid, & Dishion, 1992), which targets the coercive and maladaptive patterns of parent–child interaction characteristic of children presenting with oppositional behavior, has been identified as a well-established treatment for disruptive behavior disorders (e.g., oppositional defiant disorder, conduct disorder) in children (Kazdin, 2005). In addition to modifying parent and child behavior, we review evidence suggesting that a welcome side effect of parent management training is the alleviation of parental depression. Likewise, IPT provides an additional well-studied, interpersonal approach that focuses on conflicts and interpersonal transitions, but unlike couple and parenting interventions, it typically involves only the patient with depression in therapy, as do several other approaches introduced over the past decade, including an individually focused intervention for couples (Halford, 2011) and IPT modified for resolution of complicated grief reactions (Shear, Frank, Houk, & Reynolds, 2005). Because each of these interpersonal problem areas appears to have substantial potential to become stress generating, we briefly review efficacy data for these approaches next.

Well-Established Couple Therapy Approaches

In this section we review the outcome data for several couple therapy approaches that have been shown to be effective in treating relationship distress and depression. There are several other approaches to couple therapy that have been developed specifically for individuals with depression; for a more extensive review of the outcome research associated with these approaches, see Beach and Whisman (2012) and Whisman, Johnson, BE, and Li (2012).

Three studies have compared behavioral couple therapy (BCT) with individual therapy with similar results (Beach & O'Leary, 1992; Emanuels-Zuurveen & Emmelkamp, 1996; Jacobson, Dobson, Fruzzetti, Schmaling, & Salusky, 1991). In all three studies, BCT and individual therapy yielded equivalent outcomes when the dependent variable was depressive symptoms; and BCT therapy was superior to individual cognitive therapy (CT) in improving couple functioning. In addition, BCT was found to be significantly better than the wait-list control (Beach & O'Leary, 1992). Dessaulles, Johnson, and Denton (2003) compared the efficacy of emotionally focused therapy (EFT) for couples with pharmacotherapy in a small clinical trial. Results from the study indicated that both EFT and pharmacotherapy led to clinically significant reductions in depression. The benefit of a support-focused couples approach was demonstrated by Bodenmann and colleagues (2008). Coping-oriented couple therapy (COCT) was found to have similar effects on depression recovery to individual-oriented interventions but also to show a significant impact on negative attitudes (EE) and a lower relapse rate within 1.5 years. Partners in the COCT condition showed substantial declines in criticism, and these changes were not observed in either IPT or CT.

Cast within a stress-generation framework, the results of these studies suggest several important conclusions. First, it is clear that efficacious forms of therapy focused on the enhancement of the intimate relationship can be safely and usefully applied to a depressed population. Second, BCT has been shown in three independent studies to produce significant change in relationship distress in a discordant and depressed population, and in each case it has outperformed a control group and/or an alternative intervention, allowing it to be considered a specific and efficacious treatment for relationship distress. Third, because the intimate relationship appears to be an important context for stress generation, successful intervention of this sort can be viewed as particularly promising and provides a strong rationale for recommending relationship intervention, where appropriate, with patients with depression. Fourth, work focused on training partners to provide effective social support in the context of marriage (Bodenmann et al., 2008) suggests the potential to supplement the focus on conflict reduction by including an additional focus on support provision. Bodenmann and colleagues' (2008) study expands on other couple-based treatments by adding a focus on coping with external stressors and documenting an impact of treatment on EE. It also departs from the bulk of the prior literature in not focusing on distressed couples. For cases in which low support and high EE are primary issues, it may prove particularly useful. In future research, it will be important to determine whether the addition of a focus on support is additive in its impact on depression. Given the promising effects on reduction of depressive symptoms to date, it is important that work continue to specify the conditions under which couple therapy may serve as a treatment for depression in its own right, as well as a means of complementing other interventions by reducing stress-generation processes that might otherwise limit their impact on depression.

Well-Established Approaches to Parent Training

Because compromised parenting is common among parents with depression and because parent-focused intervention reduces a number of stress-generating processes (Sandler, Wolchik, Winslow, & Schenck, 2006), approaches that target parenting behavior and the quality of parent–child relationships are also of interest as a potential means of reducing stress generation for parents with depression. Illustrating work in this area, Hutchings,

Lane, and Kelly (2004) examined the efficacy of behavioral parent training compared with standard mental health service treatment for parents of 2- to 10-year-old children who presented for conduct problems. The parent training intervention included observation and coding of parent–child interactions, instruction and practice on more adaptive parenting strategies, and homework and found that mothers in the parenting intervention reported significantly lower levels of depression at 6-month and 4-year follow-ups than did mothers in the standard treatment group (Hutchings et al., 2004). Likewise, the effect on depression of Triple P (Positive Parenting Program), a universal prevention program developed by researchers in Australia to enhance child behavior and parenting efficacy, was also found to be associated with significant declines in parental depressive symptoms pre- to posttreatment (Gallart & Matthey, 2005). Building on these findings, Beach and colleagues (2008) examined the effects of a prevention-oriented parenting intervention on 163 mothers with elevated depression scores. Compared with participation in the control group, participation in the parenting program was associated with reduced depressive symptoms, enhanced parenting, and improvements in youth behavior. Changes in parenting (consistent discipline, child monitoring, open communication), but not in youth intrapersonal competencies, were found to mediate intervention effects on mothers' depression. Results suggest the importance of enhanced parenting efficacy in alleviating their depressive symptoms.

Examining parenting at an earlier stage of development, Gelfand, Teti, Seiner, and Jameson (1996) evaluated a multicomponent intervention program in which registered nurses visited depressed mothers of infants at their homes to assess mothers' parenting skills, to enhance mothers' self-confidence, and to reinforce their existing parenting techniques. Mothers diagnosed with major depression were assigned to the parenting intervention group (i.e., needs assessment, modeling of warm mother–infant interactions, reinforcement of positive parenting skills) or the usual mental health care group (i.e., ongoing treatment with referral source). Results suggested that mothers in the intervention group demonstrated significantly greater improvement in depressive symptoms than did those in usual care.

Sanders and McFarland (2000) also examined behavioral parenting training for parental depression. Families in which the mother met diagnostic criteria for major depression and in which at least one child met diagnostic criteria for either conduct disorder or oppositional defiant disorder were randomly assigned either to traditional behavioral family intervention (BFI), focused on instruction, role playing, feedback, and coaching in the use of social learning principles, or to a cognitively enhanced BFI condition (CBFI) that focused on traditional behavioral skills, as well as cognitive skills such as identification and interruption of dysfunctional child-related cognitions and automatic thoughts, along with increasing relaxation. Although both interventions were associated with significant change in child behavior problems, significantly more mothers in the CBFI condition (72%) than in the BFI condition (35%) were not depressed at follow-up. The studies reviewed here suggest that parenting approaches are promising for alleviating parental depressive symptoms, as well as enhancing child outcomes, and that incorporating components designed to alter common, problematic interpretations and reactions to child behavior may increase their impact.

Well-Established Approaches to Interpersonal Therapy, Intervention for Grief, and Individual Approaches to Couple Problems

Because it is focused on individuals, IPT may have important practical advantages as a vehicle for interpersonal intervention in many cases. In addition, when maintained, IPT has the potential to prevent recurrence and relapse (Frank et al., 1990). Recent expansion of IPT has refined its capacity to alleviate complicated grief reactions (Shear et al., 2005), providing an enhanced positive response to intervention. Likewise, the development of individual approaches to deal with relationship problems (Halford, Osgarby, & Kelly, 1996) suggests an expanding range of potentially useful approaches to interrupt stress-generating processes.

There are likely to be individuals with depression who would benefit from attention to interpersonal problems or interpersonal stress-generation processes but who, nonetheless, are not good candidates for dyadic therapies or who do not see themselves as having relationship or parenting problems. Such individuals may be particularly good candidates for IPT or for other individual formats that allow a focus on interpersonal and relationship concerns but do not require additional family members to attend sessions. For example, some persons with depression may need to attend therapy as individuals for practical reasons, due to the unavailability of a partner or other family member. IPT may also help to resolve a wider range of difficult interpersonal transitions and/or interpersonal losses than would typically be handled in parenting or couple-focused approaches. IPT has been reviewed in detail by Westen and Morrison (2001), who indicate that IPT may be an efficacious treatment for depression, and is probably best viewed as having effects that are not significantly different from the effects of alternative psychosocial interventions for depression (e.g., CT). It is not currently known, however, whether IPT reliably changes interpersonal functioning and whether it can be viewed as an intervention that directly interrupts interpersonal stress-generation processes.

Decision Rules for Selecting Among Well-Established Relational Interventions

Suggesting the promise of decision rules that prompt referral for various stress-generating problem areas when they are present, Segel, Vincent, and Levitt (2002) found that adding additional interventions following pharmacotherapy has the potential to convert partial responders to full response. Likewise, the preceding selective review of the effectiveness of several types of couple, family, supportive, interpersonal, and partner psychoeducational approaches suggests great promise for utilization of these approaches when appropriate. Looking across literatures and findings, one can conclude that well-established relational approaches, when indicated, can help relieve depressive symptoms or even relieve residual symptoms following the conclusion of other forms of treatment. In addition, it appears possible to intervene in an efficacious manner on potentially stress-generating processes even in the context of significant concurrent depressive symptoms. These findings suggest the potential utility of either concurrent or crossover interventions combining couple, family, or other interpersonal intervention approaches with pharmacotherapy. Consistent with this perspective, Denton, Wittenborn, and Golden (2012) evaluated the impact of augmenting pharmacotherapy with EFT for couples in a sample of women with depression. Compared with women who received medication management only, those who additionally received couple therapy experienced significantly more improvement in relationship quality, although there were no differences between groups in severity of depressive symptoms.

One approach to the development of decision rules to guide referral is to focus on areas of salience to the patient with depression. Couple interventions, and perhaps other family and interpersonal approaches, appear to work best when the problem area is salient to the individual (Beach & O'Leary, 1992; Weissman, Markowitz, & Klerman,

2000) or when the person with depression believes that the difficulties preceded or caused his or her current episode of depression (O'Leary et al., 1990). Because loss of positive interactions is common in depression, approaches focused on the enhancement of support may also provide a useful approach for individuals with depression who do not see their relationships as distressed.

Although the research on predictors of differential response is less well developed in the case of parent training as an intervention for individuals with depression, one might hypothesize that similar patterns will emerge as additional work accumulates. If so, one would expect to find better response to parent training when the child's behavior problems are salient and are seen as serious (e.g., Sanders & McFarland, 2000) or, alternatively, when the child's problem behavior, or conflict with the child, is viewed as a major source of concern or leaves the parent with very low parenting efficacy. This suggests the value of parent training when the child carries a diagnosis of a disruptive behavior disorder, including oppositional defiant disorder or conduct disorder, or when the adult with depression is at a key transition that might render the parenting relationship more salient and foster doubts about parenting ability, such as the birth of a child or the child's transition to adolescence.

Brief Decision Rules for Referral from a Stress-Generation Perspective

The foregoing considerations suggest that therapists should explore current areas of interpersonal dysfunction, with particular attention to couple functioning, parenting, erosion of support, broader interpersonal functioning, and grief. If any of these areas are salient and stressful for the patient with depression, they should be carefully monitored. In cases in which the interpersonal distress precedes the onset of the depression or is seen as contributing to the maintenance of the depression, a referral for concurrent intervention should be considered when feasible. In all cases, if interpersonal dysfunction is still present at the end of treatment, referral for intervention within an efficacious format targeted to the particular form of distress that is present is recommended.

Are Dichotomous Decisions Possible?

Treatment and referral decisions are inherently dichotomous, raising questions about possible cut points and criteria to aid in clinical decision making. Such decisions are further complicated by the fact that often multiple concurrent areas of interpersonal difficulty are reported by persons with depression. If most problems are distributed in a continuous manner, it may be difficult to specify an empirically supported, nonarbitrary cut point that identifies a group in need of intervention on one and only one interpersonal dimension and a different group that is not in need of intervention. Two solutions to this conundrum are possible. First, in keeping with long-standing practice in IPT, patients with depression can be asked to provide guidance to clinicians regarding the areas that are most salient and pressing for them. When these areas can be addressed with efficacious interventions, the framework described previously could be applied without specification of cut points for referral to deal with particular problem areas. Thus, if someone presents with both relationship problems and interpersonal conflict in other settings, the focus of intervention might be guided primarily by an assessment of which area is seen by the patient as most troubling and stressful. If an efficacious intervention is available for the identified problem area, it would be offered.

An alternative approach, or a supplemental source of decision-making guidance, would be to attempt to identify nonarbitrary cut points in each problem domain in order to characterize for a given individual that particular areas were "above" threshold for referral. Intervention would then be preferentially directed toward those areas that were "elevated." Taxometrics (Waller & Meehl, 1998) has been used to examine the distribution of scores related to relationship distress and determine whether there is a nonarbitrary breaking point that separates two qualitatively different groups: "distressed" versus "nondistressed" couples. Beach, Fincham, Amir, and Leonard (2005) found taxonicity in a sample of recently married individuals who were assessed with the Marital Adjustment Test. Replicating and extending this finding, Whisman, Beach, and Snyder (2008) examined a nationally representative sample of 1,020 couples who were assessed with the Marital Satisfaction Inventory—Revised (MSI-R; Snyder, 1997), and also found a taxonic result. Based on these findings, the authors developed and made available self-report and interview-based screening tools (Whisman, Snyder, & Beach, 2009), designed to distinguish distressed and nondistressed couples. Similar simple interview-based measures have been developed for a number of other areas of family functioning (Foran, Beach, Heyman, Slep, & Wamboldt, 2012), suggesting the potential for development of cut points to guide referral for problems in other interpersonal areas as well.

CONCLUSIONS AND DIRECTIONS FOR FUTURE RESEARCH

Some work has suggested that the families most in need of treatment for depression do not have ready access to, or fail to seek, mental health services. In addition, barriers to effective treatment may result from individuals being dissimilar in important ways to the populations on which the therapeutic approaches have been tested, rendering some aspects of the presentation or clinical approach less relevant to them or, in the worst case, off-putting. Thus insuring the relevance and effectiveness of couple, parenting, and interpersonal therapies for depression for the diverse populations who may be in need of such services requires further consideration of the diversity of individuals and families. In addition, association between relationship quality and physical health outcomes suggest potential opportunities for broadening the scope of couple and family approaches to health outcomes.

Socioeconomic Status, Ethnicity, Single-Parent Status

Those with lower socioeconomic status (SES) are at elevated risk of having depression (Lorant, Deliege, & Eaton, 2003; see Kessler et al., Chapter 1, this volume). As might be expected, much of the risk attributable to low SES is conferred by financial disadvantage, unemployment, low education, and low material standard of living (Fryers, Melzer, & Jenkins, 2003), all of which are sources of chronic stress. This suggests the potential value of interventions that enhance coping. Likewise, some of the effect of low SES is also conferred by decreased social support (Turner & Marino, 1994), and the impact of the lack of high-quality social relationships may be stronger for those disadvantaged by low SES (Turner, Lloyd, & Roszell, 1999), considerations that further support use of interpersonal interventions to address depression occurring in the context of low SES.

Couple, parenting, and interpersonal interventions for depression in the context of low SES are likely to involve special considerations, modifications, and accommodations. In particular, widespread dissemination of efficacious interventions for couple and parenting difficulties to low-SES families requires that they be offered in a manner that lowers cost to consumers and makes programs more easily accessible. Thus an important challenge for future research is that of packaging efficacious interventions and developing delivery systems that can meet the needs of individuals with depression in economically stressed circumstances. Fortunately, the need to address low SES and ethnically diverse groups more effectively has been the focus of recent discussion both in the couple area (Hawkins et al., 2013; Johnson, 2012) and in the parenting domain (Cowan & Cowan, 2002), suggesting that this is an area that will be receiving increasing empirical attention. At a minimum, establishing trust and offering couple therapy approaches, parenting programs, or other interpersonal interventions that take into consideration the racial, socioeconomic, and regional characteristics of the populations served are critical to meet the needs of many currently underserved groups (Beach et al., 2008; Hurt et al., 2006).

It is noteworthy that risk of onset of a depressive episode is greater among single mothers than among married mothers (Brown & Moran, 1997), perhaps reflecting the combined effect of several sources of stress with lack of support. These findings underscore the potential importance of working to strengthen coparenting and other close relationships among single mothers with depression and particularly to focus on strengthening supportive transactions between those helping with caregiving. Thus, in many cases, a focus on coparenting may be more relevant for single mothers than a focus on a romantic relationship.

Aging and Later Life

Compared with younger individuals, depression in older adults appears to differ in prevalence, presentation, etiology, risk and protective factors, and potential outcomes (see Blazer & Hybels, Chapter 23, this volume). Interpersonal functioning may be particularly important for the well-being of older individuals. According to the tenets of socioemotional selectivity theory (Carstensen, Isaacowitz, & Charles, 1999), emotionally close relationships are increasingly valued as people age and realize they are gradually approaching the end of life. Consequently, problems in close relationships may be more strongly associated with the mental health of older persons relative to younger individuals. Consistent with this perspective, age moderated the association between relationship distress and major depressive disorder in a population-based sample of adults 18 years and older, such that the strength of the association increased with increasing age (Whisman, 2007).

To date, couple, family, and other interpersonally oriented treatments such as IPT have not yet been studied as stand-alone treatments for depression in older adults. The use of these treatments for older adults, including the adaptation of treatments to the specific needs of older persons (e.g., problems associated with physical illness and disability, bereavement, caregiving), is an important topic for future research. Furthermore, because a large proportion of older adults with depression do not receive treatment of any kind, clinicians may want to consider ways of maximizing access to psychological services for older adults with depression, including delivering treatment in primary care settings (see Fiske, Wetherell, & Gatz, 2009).

Health

The association of relationship quality with a range of specific health problems suggests that stress-generation models may be useful for organizing a broader literature on health effects and may be useful in guiding application of couple and family interventions. Marital relationships appear to have a substantial influence on health outcomes, particularly for women (Kiecolt-Glaser & Newton, 2001). Likewise, effects of relationship quality have been documented on the physical health of older couples (Bookwala, 2005), with greater negative spousal behavior predicting more physical symptoms, more chronic health problems, greater physical disability, and poorer perceived health. Supporting a focus on the impact of negative interactions with the partner, Umberson, Williams, Powers, Liu, and Needham (2006) found that negative marital encounters sped up declines in self-rated health over time. Likewise, Holt-Lunstad, Birmingham, and Jones (2008) showed that lower marital quality was associated with higher blood pressure and higher stress. In addition, the impact of relationship quality on health has also been documented for unmarried couples (Simon & Barrett, 2010).

Accordingly, satisfying, supportive, romantic relationships are positively associated with physical well-being, but discordant, unsupportive relationships are associated with less physical well-being, and this may account for some of the overlap between depression and physical health outcomes. These considerations suggest the potential value of research that examines the longer term associations of romantic relationship functioning with physical health outcomes and the way that depression may mediate or moderate these effects. In addition, these data suggest the utility of further exploration of couple, family, and interpersonal treatments as a means for influencing physical health outcomes. Again, because focus on romantic relationship quality is not currently a well-established component of preventive care, clinicians may need to find new ways to work with primary care physicians to develop successful intervention delivery models for couples with depression, distress, and physical illness.

The Future of Couple, Family, and Interpersonal Interventions for Depression

Although current progress should not be overstated, it is clear that a substantial conceptual and empirical foundation grounded in a stress-generation framework is available to guide referral decisions for couple, family, and interpersonal interventions with patients with depression. A large and robust literature indicates that couple, parenting, and other interpersonal relationships are often problematic for persons with depression and may create a stress-generating context unless successfully addressed. From the perspective of the stress-generation framework, difficulties in the area of couple and parenting relationships and the likelihood that these processes will continue even after successful individual treatment are troubling. At the same time, there is good evidence that these problematic relationships can be successfully addressed using empirically supported interventions, and it seems appropriate to recommend an efficacious, targeted intervention when problems are identified.

The stress-generation framework suggests that targeted, efficacious interventions have the potential to break the vicious cycles that may serve to maintain depression or limit gains to partial rather than full remission. If so, interventions that include attention to problematic couple and family relationships may decrease future distress and the risk for, or severity of, future episodes. This promise, however, awaits a conclusive demonstration. Continuing efforts to document the conditions under which couple and parenting interventions are efficacious in relieving an episode of depression are warranted, as are efforts to directly assess the added value of interpersonal interventions in various contexts and at various points in the treatment process. In the meantime, both couple and parenting interventions can claim to be efficacious interventions for important sources of stress generation in depression, and it seems likely that the same is true for areas addressed by IPT, treatment of complicated grief, and COCT.

The stress-generation framework also highlights the potential for particular areas of individual vulnerability, such as experiences of childhood adversity, to lead to increased difficulty with stress generation (Hammen, Henry, & Daley, 2000), as well as the potential for individual differences in genetic factors to contribute to depression (Hammen, Brennan, Keenan-Miller, Hazel, & Najman, 2010). As the connection between particular areas of individual vulnerability and interpersonal stress generation is more clearly mapped, it may be possible to develop new interpersonal approaches that combine attention to both individual history and genetic vulnerability to better tailor interventions to the circumstances of particular couples and families. In particular, stress-generation theory lends itself to increasingly refined models and corresponding refinements of intervention, allowing for the type of bench-to-bedside dialogue that is most likely to lead to sustained progress in intervention. The stress-generation framework also provides an excellent "neutral" framework within which researchers of various backgrounds and orientations can share information and innovative suggestions for intervention and an excellent framework for generalization across contexts and perhaps across additional health outcomes. To the extent that we value an empirical foundation broad enough to encompass couple, parenting, and interpersonal interventions for depression, it may be increasingly useful to adopt stress-generation theory as a way to summarize empirical findings and guide the development of new interventions.

REFERENCES

Beach, S. R. H., Fincham, F. D., Amir, N., & Leonard, K. E. (2005). The taxometrics of marriage: Is marital discord categorical? *Journal of Family Psychology, 19*, 276–285.

Beach, S. R. H., Katz, J., Kim, S., & Brody, G. H. (2003). Prospective effects of marital satisfaction on depressive symptoms in established marriages: A dyadic model. *Journal of Social and Personal Relationships, 20*, 355–371.

Beach, S. R. H., Kim, S., Cercone-Keeney, J., Gupta, M., Arias, I., & Brody, G. (2004). Physical aggression and depressive symptoms: Gender asymmetry in effects? *Journal of Social and Personal Relationships, 21*, 341–360.

Beach, S. R. H., Kogan, S. M., Brody, G. H., Chen, Y., Lei, M., & Murry, V. M. (2008). Change in caregiver depression as a function of the Strong African American Families Program. *Journal of Family Psychology, 22*, 241–252.

Beach, S. R. H., & O'Leary, K. D. (1992). Treating depression in the context of marital discord: Outcome and predictors of response for marital therapy versus cognitive therapy. *Behavior Therapy, 23*, 507–258.

Beach, S. R. H., & Whisman, M. A. (2012). Affective disorders. *Journal of Marital and Family Therapy, 38*, 201–219.

Beam, C. R., Horn, E. E., Hunt, S. K., Emery, R. E., Turkheimer, E., & Martin, N. (2011). Revisiting the effect of marital support on depressive symptoms in mothers and fathers: A genetically informed study. *Journal of Family Psychology, 25*, 336–344.

Beardslee, W. R., & Podorefsky, D. (1988). Resilient adolescents whose parents have serious affective and other psychiatric disorders: The importance of self-understanding and relationships. *American Journal of Psychiatry, 145*, 63–69.

Benazon, N. R., & Coyne, J. C. (2000). Living with a depressed spouse. *Journal of Family Psychology, 14*, 71–79.

Bodenmann, G., Plancherel, B., Beach, S. R. H., Widmer, K., Gabriel, B., Meuwly, N., et al.

(2008). Effects of coping-oriented couple therapy on depression: A randomized clinical trial. *Journal of Consulting and Clinical Psychology, 76,* 944–954.

Bodenmann, G., Widmer, K., Charvoz, L., & Bradbury, T. N. (2004). Differences in individual and dyadic coping in depressed, non-depressed and remitted persons. *Journal of Psychopathology and Behavioral Assessment, 26,* 75–85.

Bookwala, J. (2005). The role of marital quality in physical health during the mature years. *Journal of Aging and Health, 17,* 85–104.

Brown, G. W., & Moran, P. M. (1997). Single mothers, poverty, and depression. *Psychological Medicine, 27,* 21–33.

Brown, S. L., Nesse, R. M., Vinokur, A. M., & Smith, D. M. (2003). Providing social support may be more beneficial than receiving it: Results from a prospective study of mortality. *Psychological Science, 14,* 320–327.

Cano, A., & O'Leary, K. D. (2000). Infidelity and separations precipitate major depressive episodes and symptoms of non-specific depression and anxiety. *Journal of Consulting and Clinical Psychology, 68,* 774–781.

Carstensen, L. L., Isaacowitz, D. M., & Charles, S. T. (1999). Taking time seriously: A theory of socioemotional selectivity. *American Psychologist, 54,* 165–181.

Conger, R., Patterson, G., & Ge, X. (1995). It takes two to replicate: A mediational model of the impact of parents' stress on adolescent adjustment. *Child Development, 66,* 80–97.

Cowan, P. A., & Cowan, C. P. (2002). Strengthening couples to improve children's well-being. *Poverty Research News, 3,* 18–20.

Coyne, J. C., Thompson, R., & Palmer, S. C. (2002). Marital quality, coping with conflict, marital complaints, and affection in couples with a depressed wife. *Journal of Family Psychology, 16*(1), 26–37.

Cuijpers, P., Beekman, A. T. F., & Reynolds, C. F. (2012). Preventing depression: :A global priority. *Journal of the American Medical Association, 307*(10), 1033–1034.

Davila, J., Bradbury, T. N., Cohan, C. L., &Tochluk, S. (1997). Marital functioning and depressive symptoms: Evidence for a stress generation model. *Journal of Personality and Social Psychology, 73,* 849–861.

Denton, W. H., Carmody, T. J., Rush, A. J., Thase, M. E., Trivedi, M. H., Arnow, B. A., et al. (2010). Dyadic discord at baseline is associated with lack of remission in the acute treatment of chronic depression. *Psychological Medicine, 40,* 415–424.

Denton, W. H., Wittenborn, A. K., & Golden, R. N. (2012). Augmenting antidepressant medication treatment of depressed women with emotionally focused therapy for couples: A randomized pilot study. *Journal of Marital and Family Therapy, 38,* 23–38.

Dessaulles, A., Johnson, S. M., & Denton, W. H. (2003). Emotion-focused therapy for couples in the treatment of depression: A pilot study. *American Journal of Family Therapy, 31,* 345–353.

Emanuels-Zuurveen, L., & Emmelkamp, P. M. (1996). Individual behavioral-cognitive therapy vs. marital therapy for depression in maritally distressed couples. *British Journal of Psychiatry, 169,* 181–188.

Fiske, A., Wetherell, J. L., & Gatz, M. (2009). Depression in older adults. *Annual Review of Clinical Psychology, 5,* 363–389.

Foran, H. M., Beach, S. R. H., Heyman, R. E., Slep, A. S., & Wamboldt, M. (2012). *Family problems and family violence: Reliable assessment and the ICD-11.* New York: Springer.

Frank, E., Kupfer, D. J., Perel, J. M., Cornes, C., Jarrett, D. B., Mallinger, A. G., et al. (1990). Three-year outcomes for maintenance therapies in recurrent depression. *Archives of General Psychiatry, 47,* 1093–1099.

Fryers, T., Melzer, D., & Jenkins, R. (2003). Social inequalities and the common mental disorders: A systematic review of the evidence. *Social Psychiatry and Psychiatric Epidemiology, 38,* 229–237.

Gallart, S. C., & Matthey, S. (2005). The effectiveness of group Triple P and the impact of four telephone contacts. *Behavior Change, 22,* 71–80.

Gelfand, D. M., Teti, D. M., Seiner, S. A., & Jameson, P. B. (1996). Helping mothers fight depression: Evaluation of a home-based intervention for depressed mothers and their infants. *Journal of Clinical Child Psychology, 24,* 406–422.

Goodman, S. H. (2007). Depression in mothers. *Annual Review of Clinical Psychology, 3,* 107–135.

Greenberg, P. E., Kessler, R. C., Birnbaum, H. G., Leong, S. A., Lowe, S. W., Berglund, P., et al. (2003). The economic burden of depression in the United States: How did it change between 1990 and 2000? *Journal of Clinical Psychiatry, 64,* 1465–1475.

Halford, W. K. (2011). *Marriage and relationship education: What works and how to provide it.* New York: Guilford Press.

Halford, W. K., Osgarby, S., & Kelly, A., (1996). Brief behavioral couples therapy: A preliminary evaluation. *Behavioral and Cognitive Psychotherapy, 24,* 263–273.

Hammen, C. (1991). Generation of stress in the course of unipolar depression. *Journal of Abnormal Psychology, 100,* 555–561.

Hammen, C. (2006). Stress generation in depression: Reflections on origins, research, and future directions. *Journal of Clinical Psychology, 62*(9), 1065–1082.

Hammen, C., Brennan, P. A., Keenan-Miller, D., Hazel, N. A., & Najman, J. M. (2010). Chronic and acute stress, gender, and serotonin transporter gene-environment interactions predicting depression symptoms in youth. *Journal of Child Psychology and Psychiatry, 51*(2), 180–187.

Hammen, C., Henry, R., & Daley, S. E. (2000). Depression and sensitization to stressors among young women as a function of childhood adversity. *Journal of Consulting and Clinical Psychology, 68,* 782–787.

Hawkins, A. J., Stanley, S. M., Cowan, P. A., Fincham, F. D., Beach, S. R. H., Cowan, C. P., et al. (2013). A more optimistic perspective on government-supported marriage and relationship education programs for lower income couples. *American Psychologist, 67,* 110–111.

Hoffman, C., Crnic, K. A., & Baker, J. K. (2006). Maternal depression and parenting: Implications for children's emergent emotion regulation and behavioral functioning. *Parenting: Science and Practice, 6,* 271–295.

Holt-Lunstad, J., Birmingham, W., & Jones, B. Q. (2008). Is there something unique about marriage?: The relative impact of marital status, relationship quality, and network social support on ambulatory blood pressure and mental health. *Annals of Behavioral Medicine, 35,* 239–244.

Hooley, J. M. (2007). Expressed emotion and relapse of psychopathology. *Annual Review of Clinical Psychology, 3,* 329–352.

Hurt, T. R., Franklin, K. J., Beach, S. R. H., Murry, V. B., Brody, G. H., McNair, L. D., et al. (2006). Dissemination of couples interventions among African American populations: Experiences from ProSAAM. *Couples Research and Therapy Newsletter, 12,* 13–16.

Hutchings, J., Lane, E., & Kelly, J. (2004). Comparison of two treatments for children with severely disruptive behaviors: A four-year follow-up. *Behavioral and Cognitive Psychotherapy, 32,* 15–30.

Jacobson, N. S., Dobson, K., Fruzzetti, A. E., Schmaling, K. B., & Salusky, S. (1991). Marital therapy as a treatment for depression. *Journal of Consulting and Clinical Psychology, 59,* 547–557.

Johnson, M. D. (2012). Healthy marriage initiatives: On the need for empiricism in policy implementation. *American Psychologist, 67,* 296–308.

Joiner, T. E., & Coyne, J. C. (1999). *The interactional nature of depression.* Washington, DC: American Psychological Association.

Joiner, T. E., Jr., Wingate, L. R., Gencoz, T., & Gencoz, F. (2005). Stress generation in depression: Three studies on its resilience, possible mechanism, and symptom specificity. *Journal of Social and Clinical Psychology, 24*(2), 236–253.

Kazdin, A. E. (2005). *Parent management training: Treatment for oppositional, aggressive, and antisocial behavior in children and adolescents.* New York: Oxford University Press.

Kiecolt-Glaser, J. K., & Newton, T. L. (2001). Marriage and health: His and hers. *Psychological Bulletin, 127,* 472–503.

Kendler, K. S., Karkowski, L. M., & Prescott, C. A. (1999). The assessment of dependence in the study of stressful life events: Validation using a twin design. *Psychological Medicine, 29,* 1455–1460.

Kercher, A., Rapee, R. M., & Schniering, C. A. (2009). Neuroticism, life events, and negative thoughts in the development of depression in adolescent girls. *Journal of Abnormal Child Psychology, 37,* 903–915.

Kessler, R. C., Berglund, P., Demler, O., Jin, R., Koretz, D., Merikangas, K. R., et al.(2003). The epidemiology of major depressive disorder: : Results from the National Comorbidity Survey Replication (NCS-R). *Journal of the American Medical Association, 289,* 3095–3105.

Kung, W. W., & Elkin, I. (2000). Marital adjustment as a predictor of outcome in individual treatment of depression. *Psychotherapy Research, 10,* 267–278.

Lorant, V., Deliege, D., & Eaton, W. (2003). Socioeconomic inequalities in depression: A meta-analysis. *American Journal of Epidemiology, 157,* 98–112.

Lovejoy, M. C., Graczyk, P. A., O'Hare, E., & Neuman, G. (2000). Maternal depression and parenting behavior: A meta-analytic review. *Clinical Psychology Review, 20,* 561–592.

Liu, R. T., & Alloy, L. B. (2010). Stress generation in depression: A systematic review of the empirical literature and recommendations for future study. *Clinical Psychology Review, 30,* 582–593.

McGonagle, K. A., & Kessler, R. C. (1990). Chronic stress, acute stress, and depressive symptoms. *American Journal of Community Psychology, 18*(5), 681–706.

Meuwly, N., Bodenmann, G., & Coyne, J. C. (2012). The association between partners' expressed emotion and depression: Mediated by patients' dysfunctional attitudes? *Journal of Social and Clinical Psychology, 31,* 690–706.

Moos, R. H., Schutte, K. K., Brennan, P., & Moos, B. S. (2005). The interplay between life stress and depressive symptoms among older adults. *Journal of Gerontology: Series B. Psychological Sciences and Social Sciences, 60B,* 199–206.

O'Leary, K. D., Riso, L. P., & Beach, S. R. H. (1990). Attributions about the marital discord/depression link and therapy outcome. *Behavior Therapy, 21,* 413–422.

Pasch, L. A., & Bradbury, T. N. (1998). Social support, conflict, and the development of marital dysfunction. *Journal of Consulting and Clinical Psychology, 66,* 219–230.

Patterson, G. R., Reid, J. B., & Dishion, T. J. (1992). *Antisocial boys.* Eugene, OR: Castilia.

Paykel, E. S. (2003). Life events and affective disorders. *Acta Psychiatrica Scandinavica, 108,* 61–66.

Proulx, C. M., Helms, H. M., & Buehler, C. (2007). Marital quality and personal well-being: A meta-analysis. *Journal of Marriage and Family, 69,* 576–593.

Randall, A. K., & Bodenmann, G. (2009). The role of stress in close relationships and marital satisfaction. *Clinical Psychology Review, 29,* 105–115.

Rook, K. S., Pietromonaco, P. R., & Lewis, M. (1994). When are depressives distressing to others and vice-versa?: Effects of friendship, similarity, and interaction task. *Journal of Personality and Social Psychology, 67,* 548–559.

Sanders, M. R., & McFarland, M. (2000). Treatment of depressed mothers with disruptive children: A controlled evaluation of cognitive-behavioral family intervention. *Behavior Therapy, 31,* 89–112.

Sandler, I. N., Wolchik, S. A., Winslow, E. B., & Schenck, C. (2006). Prevention as the promotion of healthy parenting following parental divorce. In S. R. H. Beach, M. Z. Wamboldt, N. J. Kaslow, R. E. Heyman, M. B. First, L. G. Underwood, & Reiss, D. (Eds.), *Relational processes and DSM-V: Neuroscience, assessment, prevention, and treatment* (pp. 195–209). Washington: DC: American Psychiatric Publishing.

Segel, Z., Vincent, P., & Levitt, A. (2002). Efficacy of combined sequential and cross-over psychotherapy and pharmacotherapy in improving outcomes in depression. *Journal of Psychiatry Neuroscience, 27*(4), 281–290.

Shear, K. (2005). Symposium monograph supplement: Bereavement-related depression in the elderly. *CNS Spectrums, 10*(8), 3–5.

Shear, K., Frank, E., Houk, P. R., & Reynolds, C. F. (2005). Treatment of complicated grief: A randomized controlled trial. *Journal of the American Medical Association, 293,* 2601–2608.

Simon, G. E. (2003). Social and economic burden of mood disorders. *Biological Psychiatry, 54*(3), 208–215.

Simon, R. W., & Barrett, A. E. (2010). Nonmarital romantic relationships and mental health in early adulthood: Does the association differ for men and women? *Journal of Health and Social Behavior. 51,* 168–182.

Snyder, D. K. (1997). *Marital Satisfaction Inventory—Revised (MSI-R).* Torrance, CA: Western Psychological Services.

Snyder, D. K., Castellani, A. M., & Whisman, M. A. (2006). Current status and future directions in couple therapy. *Annual Review of Psychology, 57,* 317–344.

Trombello, J. M., Schoebi, D., & Bradbury, T. N. (2011). Relationship functioning moderates the association between depressive symptoms and life stressors. *Journal of Family Psychology, 25*(1), 58–67.

Turner, J., Lloyd, D. A., & Roszell, P. (1999). Personal resources and the social distribution of depression. *American Journal of Community Psychology, 27,* 643–672.

Turner, R. J., & Marino, F. (1994). Social support and social structure: A descriptive epidemiology. *Journal of Health and Social Behavior, 35,* 193–212.

Turvey, C., Carney, C., & Arndt, S. (1999). Conjugal loss and syndromal depression in a sample of elders aged 70 years or older. *American Journal of Psychiatry, 156,* 1596–1601.

Umberson, D., Williams, K., Powers, D., Liu, H., & Needham, B. (2006). You make me sick: Marital quality and health over the life course. *Journal of Health and Social Behavior, 47,* 1–16.

Waller, N. G., & Meehl, P. E. (1998). *Multivariate taxometric procedures: Distinguishing types from continua.* Thousand Oaks, CA: Sage

Webster-Stratton, C., & Spitzer, A.(1996). Parenting a young child with conduct problems: New insights using qualitative methods. In T. H. Ollendick & R. H. Prinz (Eds.), *Advances in clinical child psychology* (Vol. 18, pp. 1–62). New York: Plenum Press.

Weissman, M. M., Markowitz, J. C., & Klerman, G. L. (2000).*Comprehensive guide to interpersonal psychotherapy.* New York: Basic Books.

Westen, D., & Morrison, K. (2001). A multidimensional meta-analysis of treatments for depression, panic, and generalized anxiety disorder: An empirical examination of the status of empirically supported therapies. *Journal of Consulting and Clinical Psychology, 69,* 875–899.

Whisman, M. A. (1999). Marital dissatisfaction and psychiatric disorders in a community sample: Results from the National Comorbidity Survey. *Journal of Abnormal Psychology, 108,* 701–706.

Whisman, M. A. (2001a). Marital adjustment and outcome following treatments for depression. *Journal of Consulting and Clinical Psychology, 69,* 125-129.

Whisman, M. A. (2001b). The association between depression and marital dissatisfaction. In S. R. H. Beach (Ed.), *Marital and family processes in depression* (pp. 3–24). Washington, DC: American Psychological Association.

Whisman, M. A. (2007). Marital distress and DSM-IV psychiatric disorders in a population-based national survey. *Journal of Abnormal Psychology, 116,* 638–643.

Whisman, M. A., Beach, S. R. H., & Snyder, D. K. (2008). Is marital discord taxonic and can taxonic status be assessed reliably?: Results from a national, representative sample of married couples. *Journal of Consulting and Clinical Psychology, 76,* 745–755.

Whisman, M. A., & Bruce, M. L. (1999). Marital distress and incidence of major depressive episode in a community sample. *Journal of Abnormal Psychology, 108,* 674–678.

Whisman, M. A., Johnson, D. P., BE, D., & Li, A. (2012). Couple-based interventions for depression. *Couple and Family Psychology: Research and Practice, 1,* 185–198.

Whisman, M. A., Snyder, D. K., & Beach, S. R. H. (2009). Screening for marital and relationship discord. *Journal of Family Psychology, 23,* 247–254.

Whisman, M. A., & Uebelacker, L. A. (2006). Impairment and distress associated with relationship discord in a national sample of married or cohabiting adults. *Journal of Family Psychology, 20,* 369–377.

Whisman, M. A., & Uebelacker, L. A. (2009). Prospective associations between marital discord and depressive symptoms in middle-aged and older adults. *Psychology and Aging, 24,* 184–189.

Wortman, C. B., Wolff, K., & Bonanno, G. A. (2004). Loss of an intimate partner through death. In D. J. Mashek & A. P. Aron (Eds.), *Handbook of closeness and intimacy* (pp. 305–320). Mahwah, NJ: Erlbaum.

CHAPTER 30

Biological and Psychosocial Interventions for Depression in Children and Adolescents

Nadine J. Kaslow, Marissa N. Petersen-Coleman,
and Ashley Maehr Alexander

Depression in youth is a serious, disabling public health problem associated with academic and social difficulties and negative health and behavioral consequences, including an increased risk of suicidal behavior (Meredith et al., 2009; Spirito, Esposito-Smythers, Wolff, & Uhl, 2011). Youth with depression utilize health care, school, and other social services more than youth without depression (Lyon & Clarke, 2006). The past two decades have witnessed increased attention to evidence-based programs to treat and prevent depression in youth. There is modest support for pharmacological, psychosocial, and combined interventions (Brent et al., 2008; Coyle et al., 2003; David-Ferdon & Kaslow, 2008; Dubicka et al., 2010; Melvin et al., 2006; Spirito et al., 2011; Varley, 2006; Vitiello, 2011). A meta-analysis found that, overall, there were no benefits of combined treatment over antidepressants alone after brief treatment or at follow-up (Dubicka et al., 2010). However, there was an advantage of combined treatment in the acute stages. Another meta-analysis found a small effect size for psychotherapeutic interventions (Weisz, McCarty, & Valeri, 2006). There is some evidence that combined interventions are the most cost-effective (Domino et al., 2009; Lynch et al., 2011). Yet depression in youth is underdiagnosed and undertreated (Ma, Lee, & Stafford, 2005; Merikangas, He, Rapoport, Vitiello, & Olfson, 2013). This chapter reviews the evidence-based intervention and prevention programs for children and adolescents (David-Ferdon & Kaslow, 2008; Vitiello, 2011; Weisz et al., 2006). Mediators, moderators, and predictors of treatment outcome are addressed (Nilsen, Eisemann, & Kvernmo, 2013). Existing treatment guidelines are presented, and guiding principles for treating youth with depression are proffered.

BIOLOGICAL TREATMENTS

Pharmacological Interventions

Antidepressant medications often are prescribed, alone or in combination with psychosocial treatments (Delate, Gelenberg, Simmons, & Motheral, 2004). Findings on rates of antidepressant use vary. A retrospective cohort study using claims data from United States managed care plans revealed widespread use of antidepressants (Czaja & Valuck, 2012). In contrast, another cross-sectional survey found that only a minority of adolescents with depression were prescribed antidepressants (Merikangas et al., 2013).

Though knowledge about antidepressant treatments in youth is limited, large National Institute of Mental Health (NIMH) studies have informed our understanding of the impact of medication in treating major depressive disorder (MDD). Overall, efficacy and safety data about tricyclic antidepressants (TCAs) are not favorable (Mann et al., 2006; Michael & Crowley, 2002). Selective serotonin reuptake inhibitors (SSRIs) have become the first-line pharmacological intervention (Emslie, 2012). SSRI safety data are mixed but more positive than for TCAs (Cheung, Emslie, & Mayes, 2005; Whittington et al., 2004). Despite the high use of SSRIs, the U.S. Food and Drug Administration (FDA) has approved only two SSRIs for pediatric MDD: fluoxetine (Prozac) and escitalopram (Lexapro; Tao, Emslie, & Mayes, 2010).

Efficacy Trials

No randomized controlled trials (RCTs) have focused solely on children and SSRI use. RCTs have examined SSRIs with combined samples of children and adolescents or adolescents alone. One RCT found a 50–60% reduction rate of depressive symptoms to a first antidepressant with MDD, and 40–50% who failed one antidepressant responded to a second (Brent et al., 2008). The most incontrovertible evidence is for fluoxetine (Emslie et al., 2002; March et al., 2004). Analyses indicate that fluoxetine has a role in treating pediatric depression (Kratochvil et al., 2006; Ryan, 2005) and most (Emslie, Kratochvil, et al., 2006) have argued for its safety.

After findings from only one RCT (Wagner, Jonas, Findling, Ventura, & Saikali, 2006), escitalopram also received FDA approval. Suicide-related events were observed in one patient treated with escitalopram and in two patients treated with placebo. Despite positive findings from this RCT, some research suggests that escitalopram should be a "second-line" option (Carandang, Jabbal, MacBride, & Elbe, 2011). There is mixed evidence for the following SSRIs: citalopram (Celexa; von Knorring, Olsson, Thomsen, Lemming, & Hulten, 2006; Wagner et al., 2004), sertraline (Zoloft; Melvin et al., 2006; Wagner et al., 2003), and paroxetine (Paxil; Berard, Fong, Carpenter, Thomason, & Wilkinson, 2006; Emslie, Wagner, et al., 2006).

No non-SSRI medications have proven effective (Emslie, 2012). There are mixed findings regarding serotonin–norepinepherine reuptake inhibitors (SNRIs): nefazadone (Serzone), venlafaxine (Effexor), and mirtrazapine (Remeron; Cheung et al., 2005; Cheung, Emslie, & Mayes, 2006; Emslie et al., 2002; Emslie, Findling, Yeung, Kunz, & Li, 2007; Mann et al., 2006). Evidence for SNRIs is insufficient to support their use.

Some medications help prevent relapse (Emslie et al., 2004). Other medications (fluoxetine, bupropion sustained release [Wellbutrin]) effectively treat depression that co-occurs with other disorders (Cornelius et al., 2001; Daviss et al., 2001).

Combined Pharmacotherapy and Psychosocial Interventions

Treatment for Adolescents with Depression Study

The Treatments for Adolescents with Depression Study (TADS), a multisite trial sponsored by NIMH, offers evidence for combined pharmacotherapy and psychotherapy for adolescents with MDD and for medications alone (Curry et al., 2006, 2011; Emslie, Kratochvil, et al., 2006; Kennard et al., 2006; Kennard, Silva, Mayes, et al., 2009; Kennard, Silva, Tonev, et al., 2009; Kratochvil et al., 2006; March et al., 2004; March, Silva, Vitiello, & the TADS Team, 2006; March & Vitiello, 2009; the Treatment for Adolescents with Depression Study Team, 2003, 2005; Vitiello et al., 2006, 2009). This RCT evaluated the effectiveness of cognitive-behavioral therapy (CBT), fluoxetine, a combination of CBT and fluoxetine (combined), and placebo pill.

The 12-week, 15-session CBT-skills-based psychoeducational program focused on depression and its causes, goal setting, mood monitoring, increasing pleasant activities, social problem solving, cognitive restructuring, and enhancing social skills. Two parent sessions offered information. Conjoint sessions addressed parent and adolescent concerns. The SSRI condition used a flexible dosing schedule; youth were able to receive up to 40 milligrams per day of fluoxetine by week 8. Adolescents met for six visits over 12 weeks with a pharmacotherapist, who provided monitoring and encouragement. Youth in the combined treatment received all components of CBT and medication alone. Youth in the placebo group received a sugar pill following the same dosage and monitoring patterns as the fluoxetine group.

Following acute treatment, 71% no longer met diagnostic criteria (responders), 50% had residual symptoms, and 23% reached remission. The combined treatment was most effective in reducing depressive symptoms and suicidal ideation. The superiority of the combined intervention was further supported by effect sizes; endpoint data related to 16 outcomes; global functioning, health outcomes, and quality of life; remission rates; response rate times; and probability of sustained early response. Fluoxetine was superior to CBT alone, but CBT was not more effective than placebo. This pattern held true for youth with mild to moderate depression; however, for severely depressed youth, there was no evidence that adding CBT was helpful.

A few additional findings are noteworthy. The youth's level of cognitive distortions and family income status influenced treatment outcome. Suicidal events were twice as common in adolescents treated with fluoxetine alone than in youth in the combined or CBT groups. Youth who received fluoxetine, alone or in combination, endorsed physical symptoms at a rate twice that of the placebo group. CBT was associated with the fewest adverse events and fluoxetine alone was related to the most.

Follow-up and longitudinal data suggested the benefit of longer initial treatment in the remission and maintenance of gains (Curry et al., 2011; Kennard, Silva, Tonev, et al., 2009; March & Vitiello, 2009). Youth treated with combined fluoxetine plus CBT or CBT alone achieved greater response maintenance than those treated with fluoxetine alone. At week 36, the rate of recovery was 65% and 71%, respectively, for acute and continuation phase remitters; this was true across conditions. Longer term treatment resulted in more sustained improvement, even following the discontinuation of active treatment. Residual symptoms at termination of the acute phase were associated with failure to achieve remission.

Follow-up data revealed that 96% recovered from their index MDD episode (Curry et al., 2011). Recovery at 2-year follow-up occurred more often for short-term treatment than for partial or nonresponders. Among the adolescents who met criteria for recovery, 47% had a recurrence, predicted by initial nonresponse and gender (female).

A cost-effectiveness examination revealed that CBT was most costly (Domino et al., 2009). However, those in the fluoxetine-only condition had higher direct and indirect costs. The combined condition was the most cost-effective.

Treatment of SSRI-Resistant Depression in Adolescents

The Treatment of SSRI-Resistant Depression in Adolescents (TORDIA) study was a multisite RCT with 334 12- to 18-year-olds with a primary diagnosis of MDD who had not responded to a 2-month initial SSRI treatment (Brent et al., 2008). Youth were randomly assigned to switch to an alternative SSRI, to an alternative SSRI plus CBT, to venlafaxine, or to venlafaxine plus CBT. Youth who received combined CBT and a medication switch showed a higher response rate than a medication switch alone, particularly in the acute phase. No difference in response rate was noted between venlafaxine and a second SSRI. By 24-week follow-up, 39% achieved remission; remission rates were higher and occurred more rapidly for those who showed some response to treatment by week 12. Conversely, 19% of youth who responded by week 12 relapsed by week 24 (Emslie et al., 2010).

Nonsuicidal self-injurious behavior was a common behavior among youth with treatment-resistant depression and was predictive of future suicide attempts (Asarnow et al., 2011). One study examining predictors of self-harm adverse events revealed that although there were no main effects for treatment, those receiving venlafaxine who endorsed higher levels of suicidal ideation were more likely than those with lower levels of such thinking to engage in self-harm (Brent et al., 2009). Both suicidal and nonsuicidal self-harm occurred more often in youth prescribed benzodiazepines as an adjunctive treatment. Predictors of suicidal events included high levels of baseline suicidal ideation, family conflict, and substance use.

FDA Warning

Many are reluctant to consider antidepressants due to the potential link between SSRIs and suicidal behavior and the development of mania in youth (Mann et al., 2006). Concerns have become more pronounced in reaction to FDA warnings about the possibility of increased depressive symptoms and suicide risk for young persons on antidepressants. In October 2004, the FDA required that manufacturers inform consumers about the increased risk of suicidal thinking and behavior in youth treated with antidepressants via a boxed warning (black box) and Patient Education Guide. The FDA presented strategies for bolstering safeguards for children taking antidepressants and has a medication guide regarding the use of antidepressants in youth. Despite this, the FDA has not found that any antidepressants are contraindicated for pediatric use.

Although there were documented cases of increased suicidal ideation following the use of antidepressant medication, there were no completed suicides in studies involving adolescents and SSRIs (Leon et al., 2006; Moreno, Roche, & Greenhill, 2006). It remains unclear whether the black box warning has done more harm than good, and, indeed, it is concerning that it appears to be associated with significant reductions in aggregate rates of diagnosis and treatment of pediatric depression (Libby et al., 2007). Despite the presence of the black box warning, SSRI treatment, when properly monitored, remains a first-line pharmacological treatment for major depression in adolescents (Lovrin, 2009).

Other Biological Treatments

Electroconvulsive Therapy

There are limited data on the efficacy and optimal use of electroconvulsive therapy (ECT) with youth because of its controversial nature and infrequent use, despite minor side effects and mood disorder responsiveness (Shoirah & Hamoda, 2011; Walter & Rey, 2003). Practice parameters (American Academy of Child and Adolescent Psychiatry, 2004) recommend that ECT be used for adolescents with chronic, treatment-resistant depression when two or more medications have failed or when symptom severity may endanger the youth. Potential adverse effects include impaired memory and new learning, seizures, and procedure-related risks (American Academy of Child and Adolescent Psychiatry, 2004). Concern regarding ECT's impact on cognitive functions remains prominent, despite the lack of data to confirm such concerns (Cohen, Flament, Taieb, Thompson, & Basquin, 2000). Actually, ECT may improve auditory and verbal memory (Ghaziuddin, Dumas, & Hodges, 2011).

Extant studies support ECT for treatment-resistant adolescent depression (Ghaziuddin et al., 2011; Grover et al., 2013). Studies show a 60–100% response rate and indicate that ECT has comparable effectiveness for adolescents and adults (Bloch, Levcovitch, Bloch, Mendlovic, & Ratzoni, 2001). However, follow-up data do not show that ECT is more helpful than other interventions over time (Taieb et al., 2002). Despite general public concern, adolescent patients and parents find ECT helpful (Taieb et al., 2001).

Repetitive Transcranial Magnetic Stimulation

Another biological treatment garnering interest for severe depression is repetitive transcranial magnetic stimulation (rTMS). This treatment involves the noninvasive focal stimulation of brain cortex by high-intensity, fluctuating magnetic fields to generate eddy currents to depolarize neurons. It does not require anesthesia or induce seizure activity (Loo, McFarquhar, & Walter, 2006). There are little data on rTMS with adolescents (Quintana, 2005).

One small study with adolescents with treatment-resistant depression revealed lower levels of depression after rTMS (Bloch et al., 2008). Therapeutic gains have been maintained at 3-year follow-up (Mayer, Aviram, Walter, Levkovitz, & Bloch, 2012). Another small prospective open trial of adjunctive rTMS to SSRIs revealed that the intervention was well tolerated, safe, and associated with reductions in depression and suicidality (Wall et al., 2011).

It seems that rTMS is emerging as an effective and safe intervention (Croarkin, Wall, & Lee, 2011; Croarkin et al., 2010). However, until larger scale RCTs are conducted with follow-up, no definitive conclusions can be drawn.

PSYCHOSOCIAL TREATMENTS

Evidence-Based Descriptions and Categorizations

Consistent with the recommendations from the American Psychological Association's (2006) Presidential Task Force on Evidence-Based Practice in Psychology, interventions for youth with depression should be evidence based. This definition integrates the best available empirical evidence with clinical expertise in the context of the characteristics of the individual child/adolescent, the youth's culture, and preferences of all concerned parties.

Psychosocial Interventions for Elementary School Children

There are no well-established programs for children with depression. However, self-control therapy (SCT; Stark, Reynolds, & Kaslow, 1987) and the Penn Prevention Program/Penn Resiliency Program/Penn Enhancement Program/Penn Optimism Program (PPP/PRP/PEP/POP), which includes culturally relevant modifications (Cardemil, Reivich, Beevers, Seligman, & James, 2007; Gillham, Hamilton, Freres, Patton, & Gallop, 2006; Gillham, Reivich, et al., 2006; Gillham et al., 2007; Roberts, Kane, Thomson, Bishop, & Hart, 2003) are probably efficacious.

SCT is a school-based cognitive-behavior group intervention program that teaches self-management skills. It includes training in self-control, social skills, assertiveness, relaxation and imagery, and cognitive restructuring. It also can involve monthly family meetings that encourage parents to aid their children in incorporating their newly learned skills and to increase the number of positive family activities.

PPP/PRP/PEP/POP, a CBT approach, targets depressive symptoms among at-risk 10- to 15-year-olds in schools and primary care settings. Administered in a group format, it includes cognitive and social problem solving. It has been modified for females and youth from different cultural backgrounds. A meta-analysis revealed that participation in this program is associated with long-term reductions in depressive symptoms (Brunswasser, Gillham, & Kim, 2009). However, the treatment does not appear to be superior to other active treatments.

Other specific psychosocial interventions (Coping with Depression, Primary and Secondary Control Enhancement Training Program, Stress-Busters, Bereavement Group Intervention, Wisconsin Early Intervention, acceptance and commitment therapy [ACT], Assuring Depression Assessment and Proactive Treatment [ADAPT], ACTION, Taking Action, contextual emotion-regulation therapy), most of which are CBT or emotion-regulation focused, appear effective in reducing depressive symptoms relative to control conditions (Asarnow, Scott, & Mintz, 2002; Kovacs & Lopez-Duran, 2012; Stark et al., 2008; Stark et al., 2006; Weisz, Thurber, Sweeney, Proffitt, & LeGagnoux, 1997). Typically, these programs are prevention oriented for youth with elevated depressive symptoms and are administered in schools. Because little empirical attention has been paid to these protocols, or because the findings have yet to be published in peer-reviewed journals, these interventions are deemed experimental. Details with regard to both modality and theoretical orientation classification of psychosocial interventions for youth can be found elsewhere (David-Ferdon & Kaslow, 2008).

Psychosocial Interventions for Adolescents

No psychosocial intervention for adolescents with depression can be classified as well established (David-Ferdon & Kaslow, 2008). However, Coping with Depression— Adolescent (CWD-A; Clarke et al., 2001, 2002; Kaufman, Rohde, Seeley, Clarke, & Stice, 2005; Kovacs & Lopez-Duran, 2012; Rohde, Clarke, Mace, Jorgensen, & Seeley, 2004) and Interpersonal Psychotherapy for Adolescents (IPT-A; Mufson et al., 2004; Mufson, Weissman, Moreau, & Garfinkel, 1999) are probably efficacious (David-Ferdon & Kaslow, 2008).

CWD-A, shown effective in all but one trial, consists of 15–16 sessions of 45–120 minutes each and includes relaxation training, cognitive restructuring, pleasant activity scheduling, communication, and conflict-reduction techniques. Concurrent parent groups are incorporated into some protocols. CWD-A has informed the development of protocols by other investigatory teams (Asarnow et al., 2005; Clarke et al., 2005; March et al., 2004), with mixed outcomes. IPT-A, which includes 12 individual sessions and may incorporate weekly telephone contact between the therapist and the adolescent, has been found to be more efficacious than control conditions in two RCTs in ameliorating symptoms of depression and enhancing interpersonal functioning, and it is particularly successful for treating adolescents with depression with high levels of interpersonal conflict with parents, higher depressive severity, and comorbid anxiety. IPT-A encourages teenagers to link their difficulties to grief, role disputes, role transitions, interpersonal deficits, and single-parent families. It helps youth develop adaptive strategies for communication, affect expression, and social support system development and utilization.

A number of other specific psychosocial interventions already have been classified as experimental: Coping with Stress (CWS) program, attachment-based family therapy, Depression Treatment Programme, and Feeling Good have been found to be efficacious in reducing depressive symptoms relative to control conditions (Ackerson, Scogin, McKendree-Smith, & Lyman, 1998; Diamond, Siqueland, & Diamond, 2003; Wood, Harrington, & Moore, 1996). Some newer treatments also appear to meet this criterion, including a quality improvement intervention for adolescent depression in primary care clinics (Asarnow et al., 2005); Positive Thoughts and Actions (PTA), a group-based cognitive-behavioral preventative intervention (McCarty, Violette, Duong, Cruz, & McCauley, 2013); and SPARX, a computerized self-help intervention (Merry et al., 2012). Information about modality and theoretical orientation classification of these adolescent intervention programs can be found elsewhere (David-Ferdon & Kaslow, 2008).

PREVENTION PROGRAMS

This section highlights the literature on preventing depressive symptoms and disorders. Meta-analyses demonstrate that these programs are successful for 50–60% of cases under controlled conditions (Gladstone, Beardslee, & O'Connor, 2011). Developmentally oriented prevention programs that identify early risk factors are beneficial due to their attention to enhancing protective factors (Compas et al., 2011; Gladstone et al., 2011; Vitiello, 2011). Most efforts are CBT and interpersonal in nature (Sutton, 2007) and have been conducted in schools. Some school-based programs focus on at-risk youth, not defined by their depressive symptom status (Cutuli, Chaplin, Gillham, Reivich, & Seligman, 2006; Thompson, Eggert, & Herting, 2000), and have provided academic enhancement training, personal growth classes that integrate social support, and life skills training. Other efforts targeting at-risk youth incorporate the family (Compas et al., 2011; Gladstone et al., 2011), often with children of parents with depression (Beardslee, Gladstone, Wright, & Cooper, 2003; Clarke et al., 2001). These programs provide education about depressive disorders, stress identification, and emotion-regulation training provided by clinicians or via a lecture; cognitive-behavioral techniques and skills training; parent–child attachment-based work; and massage therapy.

Some studies incorporate universal interventions, delivered to all members of a population, whereas others use targeted or selective interventions delivered to a subgroup of high-risk youth. Some of the best studied universal programs include: the Beardslee Preventive Intervention Program for Depression (PIP), a family-based prevention program that has been adapted for low-income Latino families (Beardslee, Gladstone, & O'Conner, 2012; D'Angelo et al., 2009); Problem Solving for Life (PSFL), a school-based problem solving and cognitive restructuring program (Sheffield et al., 2006); Resourceful Adolescent Program (RAP), a CBT protocol that incorporates cognitive restructuring, problem solving, stress management, and accessing social support that can be conducted with or without family involvement (Merry, McDowell, Wild, Bir, & Cunliffe, 2004; Shochet & Ham, 2004); Penn Resiliency Program (PRP), a CBT program that targets cognitive and behavioral risk factors for children with depression (Brunswasser et al., 2009; Gladstone et al., 2011); and Project CATCH-IT, a family training program that combines CBT, behavioral activation, and interpersonal psychotherapy to enhance family resiliency (Gladstone et al., 2011). A meta-analysis revealed that targeted or selective programs are more effective than universal programs at postintervention and follow-up (Horowitz & Garber, 2006).

MEDIATORS, MODERATORS, AND PREDICTORS OF TREATMENT OUTCOME

Mediators and Moderators

Mediators refer to the question of what change processes underlie improvement. Treatment effects may be mediated by improvements in depressive symptoms and reductions in depressogenic thinking (Kaufman et al., 2005; Vitiello et al., 2006). There is a burgeoning literature on moderators, factors that interact with treatment in predicting outcome (Curry et al., 2006). Evidence supports the following moderating influences that improve outcome: female gender, fewer comorbid conditions, no history of nonsuicidal self-injurious behavior, higher family income, less severe depression, low hopelessness, fewer cognitive distortions, low childhood maltreatment, low family conflict, low maternal depression, parent involvement in treatment, and positive peer interactions (Asarnow et al., 2009; Clarke, DeBar, & Lewinsohn, 2003; Michael & Crowley, 2002; Sander & McCarty, 2005; Shamseddeen et al., 2011; Weisz et al., 2006).

Predictors

A number of variables are associated with more positive or negative treatment outcomes (Barbe, Bridge, Birmaher, Kolko, & Brent, 2004; Clarke et al., 2002; Cutuli et al., 2006; Gonzalez et al., 2012; Nilsen et al., 2013; Rohde, Seeley, Kaufman, Clarke, & Stice, 2006; Sander & McCarty, 2005; Young, Mufson, & Davies, 2006). Child and family factors include comorbidity, at-risk factors, neurobiology, attachment relationships, temperament, negative cognition, emotion regulation, pleasant events, childhood trauma, and parental depression (Barbe et al., 2004; Beardslee et al., 2012; Shamseddeen et al., 2011). Sociocultural predictors include life stress, diversity, family acculturation, peer relationships including victimization, economic burden, lower parental education, therapeutic alliance, and racial and cultural differences in depression treatment knowledge (Beardslee et al., 2012; Chandra et al., 2009; D'Angelo et al., 2009; Domino et al., 2009; Gibb, Stone, & Crossett, 2012; Lyon & Clarke, 2006; Shirk, Gudmundsen, Kaplinski, & McMakin, 2008). With regard to CBT factors, number of sessions and problem-solving and social skills training are associated with more positive outcomes (Kennard, Clarke, et al., 2009).

GUIDELINES FOR MANAGING DEPRESSION

Guidelines have been offered for managing depression in young people. Examples follow.

National Institute for Health and Clinical Excellence

The National Institute for Health and Clinical Excellence (NICE) in the United Kingdom (*www.nice.org.uk*) published guidelines for identifying and managing depression in young people in primary, community, and secondary care settings. The guidelines highlight conducting patient-centered care; taking into account child and family needs and preferences; engaging the child and family in decision making; communicating effectively; performing comprehensive assessments; coordinating care; addressing comorbid diagnoses and problems; and ascertaining the need for biopsychosocial interventions for other family members. A comprehensive, evidence-based approach that differs depending on the severity of the child's depression is delineated.

American Academy of Child and Adolescent Psychiatry Treatment Parameters

The American Academy of Child and Adolescent Psychiatry (1998) notes that a diagnosis of a depressive disorder should be made only after the completion of a culturally informed, comprehensive evaluation that involves multiple informants and a multimethod assessment. Treatment should be provided in the least restrictive environment. A treatment plan should identify biological and environmental factors, frequency of treatment sessions, and roles of the clinician(s). Efforts to promote successful therapy should be guided by creating a therapeutic alliance between the clinician, youth, and family. This effort can be enhanced by providing information to form a partnership with all involved and recognizing that the youth's depression affects all family members. Appropriate developmental considerations should be discussed. During acute treatment, psychotherapy (CBT, IPT, family therapy) may be effective for mild to moderate symptoms of depression. The guidelines recommend SSRIs for adolescents with depression in a fashion that is integrated with psychosocial interventions. To decrease the risk of relapse or recurrence, youth should continue to receive psychotherapy at least monthly and medication (if prescribed and shown effective) for at least 6–12 months. Subsequently, clinical judgment should be used with regard to maintenance therapy. It is recommended that adolescents who have experienced two to three episodes of MDD receive maintenance treatment for at least 1–3 years.

Texas Children's Medication Algorithm Project

Ten principles undergird the Texas Children's Medication Algorithm Project (Hughes et al., 2007). Stage 0 is diagnostic assessment and monitoring. Stage 1 is monotherapy with SSRIs. Stage 2 pertains to switching to an alternate SSRI but continuing with a monotherapy approach. Stage 3 includes switching from an SSRI to alternate antidepressant monotherapy.

FUTURE DIRECTIONS

Based on the extant empirical data and practice guidelines, the following recommendations can be offered for the assessment and treatment of depressed youth:

1. A biopsychosocial framework is valuable for conceptualizing depression and its treatment, and recently interventions with youth with depression have built on this model.

2. Interventions should be developmentally informed given etiological differences in depression in children versus adolescents with regard to genes and environment; differential risk factors for the onset of juvenile versus adult depression; variations across the lifespan in the manifestation of depression dependent on level of social, cognitive, emotional, and physiological development; and differential response to pharmacological and psychosocial treatments based on age.

3. Attention should be paid to gender in the future design and evaluation of interventions, given gender differences in rates of depression (that vary by age) and in symptom presentation. Biological, psychological, and social theories have been proposed to explain the gender gap and pertain to differences in the timing of the onset of puberty, hormonal changes, rates of negative childhood experiences and maltreatment, body image perceptions, health status, cognitive vulnerability, coping styles, stress levels and responses, interpersonal stress levels and orientations, socialization experiences, and sociocultural roles. There is some suggestion that there are differential treatment outcomes for males and females and that males and females may benefit differentially from different types of interventions.

4. Interventions need to take into account sociocultural variables and need to be developed and implemented in a culturally competent fashion. Although depression is evident in youth in all cultures, across ethnic and racial groups there may be differential prevalence rates, symptom presentations, and service utilization patterns. Furthermore, there is evidence for the value of culture-specific interventions for youth with depression and their families and the likelihood that such approaches facilitate treatment engagement. Interventions may be more effective for youth from some ethnic groups than from others, and interventions may be effective in some but not all cultures. Furthermore, evidence-based intervention protocols for youth with depression may be culturally transportable.

5. Future therapies that are strength-based and that enhance protective and resilience factors are likely to be effective and have good buy-in from all parties.

6. Screening in schools and physicians' offices can help identify youth with depression and youth at risk for depression. Screening is effective for reducing disease burden. Quality improvement programs in schools and primary care settings can enhance access to evidence-based intervention.

7. Prior to initiating treatment, a thorough diagnostic evaluation must be conducted, with attention to developmental considerations, co-occurring conditions, depression in other family members, family interaction patterns, school personnel feedback, and family conflict.

8. Recommendations for interventions with regard to modality and theoretical orientation should be guided by assessment findings, research data, and expert clinical consensus. Information on both pharmacological and nonpharmacological intervention options should be provided to youth with depression and their caregivers.

9. Treatment decisions should be made collaboratively with the assent/consent of the youth and his or her caregivers and should take into account family preferences, clinician judgment, and the aforementioned recommendations and information regarding treatment alternatives.

10. Treatments should target comorbid conditions, and if there are no evidence-based interventions for specific combinations of conditions, multiple evidence-based approaches may be needed, either concurrently or sequentially. Available interventions for comorbid conditions and prevention protocols for comorbid sets of symptoms or related disorders could serve as the basis for such decision making.

11. Interventions should emphasize treatment engagement and building a trusting therapeutic alliance.

12. Interventions, regardless of the nature of the program, modality, or theoretical approach, should target reducing risk factors and enhancing protective factors.

13. For elementary school children, some form of CBT should be considered separately or in conjunction with antidepressant medications. This treatment should include some or all of the following components: psychoeducation, affective education and mood monitoring, behavioral activation, cognitive restructuring, problem solving (including social problem solving), and coping skills training. It should also involve at minimum a parent education and training program. Ideally, concurrent family intervention would be provided.

14. For adolescents with depression, both CBT, as described above, and IPT may be useful. Again, some family involvement may be advantageous. These psychosocial interventions are likely to be most beneficial when combined with pharmacotherapy.

15. Based on the available evidence, prior to initiating an antidepressant trial, youth and their caregivers must be informed about the risk–benefit ratio of these medications and receive education about the need for close monitoring.

16. Youth with depression treated with antidepressants need close monitoring for worsening of their depressive symptoms, emergence of suicidality, manic-switching, and other indicators of psychological distress. These interventions must be accompanied by psychoeducation for youth with depression and their caregivers.

17. For youth with treatment-resistant depression, combined and alternative treatments should be considered, and second opinions and expert consultation should be obtained.

18. ECT may be indicated for severe and persistent depression, with or without psychotic features, in which symptoms are significantly disabling and life-threatening and when there has been a lack of adequate response to prior psychopharmacological and/or psychosocial interventions.

19. rTMS has begun garnering attention as an adjunctive treatment for adolescent depression, although it is not yet FDA approved for this population.

20. Most youth with depression will require some form of continuation therapy, and many will need maintenance treatment.

21. Prevention efforts may be most effective if they combine attention to cognitive-behavioral and interpersonal skills and include booster sessions.

REFERENCES

Ackerson, J., Scogin, F., McKendree-Smith, N., & Lyman, R. D. (1998). Cognitive bibliotherapy for mild and moderate adolescent depressive symptomatology. *Journal of Consulting and Clinical Psychology, 66,* 685–690.

American Academy of Child and Adolescent Psychiatry. (1998). Summary of the practice parameters for the assessment and treatment of children and adolescents with depressive disorders. *Journal of the American Academy of Child and Adolescent Psychiatry, 37,* 1234–1239.

American Academy of Child and Adolescent Psychiatry. (2004). Practice parameter for use of electroconvulsive therapy with adolescents. *Journal of the American Academy of Child and Adolescent Psychiatry, 43,* 1521–1539.

American Psychological Association. (2006). Evidence-based practice in psychology: APA Presidential Task Force on Evidence-Based Practice in Psychology. *American Psychologist, 61,* 271–285.

Asarnow, J. R., Emslie, G., Clarke, G. N., Wagner, K. D., Spirito, A., Vitiello, B., et al. (2009). Treatment of selective serotonin reuptake inhibitor-resistant depression in adolescents: Predictors and moderators of treatment response. *Journal of the American Academy of Child and Adolescent Psychiatry, 48,* 330–339.

Asarnow, J. R., Jaycox, L. H., Duan, N., LaBorde, A. P., Rea, M. M., Murray, P., et al. (2005). Effectiveness of a quality improvement intervention for adolescent depression in primary care clinics: A randomized controlled trial. *Journal of the American Medical Association, 293,* 311–319.

Asarnow, J. R., Porta, G., Spirito, A., Emslie, G. J., Clarke, G. N., Wagner, K. D., et al. (2011). Suicide attempts and nonsuicidal self-injury in the treatment of resistant depression in adolescents: Findings from the TORDIA study. *Journal of the American Academy of Child and Adolescent Psychiatry, 50,* 772–781.

Asarnow, J. R., Scott, C. V., & Mintz, J. (2002). A combined cognitive-behavioral family education intervention for depression in children: A treatment development study. *Cognitive Therapy and Research, 26,* 221–229.

Barbe, R. P., Bridge, J., Birmaher, B., Kolko, D., & Brent, D. A. (2004). Suicidality and its relationship to treatment outcome in depressed adolescents. *Suicide and Life-Threatening Behavior, 34,* 44–55.

Beardslee, W. R., Gladstone, T. R. G., & O'Conner, E. E. (2012). Developmental risk of depression: Experience matters. *Child and Adolescent Psychiatric Clinics of North America, 21,* 261–278.

Beardslee, W. R., Gladstone, T. R. G., Wright, E. J., & Cooper, A. B. (2003). A family-based approach to the prevention of depressive symptoms in children at risk: Evidence of parental and child change. *Pediatrics, 112,* 119–131.

Berard, R., Fong, R., Carpenter, D. J., Thomason, C., & Wilkinson, C. (2006). An international, multicenter, placebo-controlled trial of paroxetine in adolescents with major depressive disorder. *Journal of Child and Adolescent Psychopharmacology, 16,* 59–75.

Bloch, Y., Levcovitch, Y., Bloch, A. M., Mendlovic, S., & Ratzoni, G. (2001). Electroconvulsive therapy in adolescents: Similarities to and differences from adults. *Journal of the American Academy of Child and Adolescent Psychiatry, 40,* 1332–1336.

Bloch, Y., Nimrod, G., Hard, E., Beilter, G., Faivel, N., Ratzoni, G., et al. (2008). Repetitive transcranial magnetic stimulation of treatment of depression in adolescents: An open-label study. *Journal of ECT, 24,* 156–159.

Brent, D. A., Emslie, G., Clarke, G. N., Asarnow, J. R., Spirito, A., Ritz, L., et al. (2009). Predictors of spontaneous and systematically assessed suicidal adverse events in the Treatment of SSRI-Resistant Depression in Adolescents (TORDIA) Study. *American Journal of Psychiatry, 166,* 418–426.

Brent, D. A., Emslie, G. J., Clarke, G. N., Wagner, K. D., Asarnow, J. R., Keller, M., et al. (2008). Switching to another SSRI or to velafaxine with or without cognitive-behavioral therapy for adolescents with SSRI-resistant depression: The TORDIA randomized controlled trial. *Journal of the American Medical Association, 299*, 901–913.

Brunswasser, S. M., Gillham, J. E., & Kim, E. S. (2009). A meta-analytic review of the Penn Resiliency Program's effect on depressive symptoms. *Journal of Consulting and Clinical Psychology, 77*, 1042–1054.

Carandang, C., Jabbal, R., MacBride, A., & Elbe, D. (2011). A review of escitalopram and citalopram in child and adolescent depression. *Journal of the Canadian Academy of Child and Adolescent Psychiatry, 20*, 315–324.

Cardemil, E. V., Reivich, K. J., Beevers, C. G., Seligman, M. E. P., & James, J. (2007). The prevention of depressive symptoms in low-income, minority children: Two-year follow-up. *Behaviour Research and Therapy, 45*, 313–327.

Chandra, A., Scott, M. M., Jaycox, L. H., Meredith, L. S., Tanielian, T., & Burnam, A. (2009). Racial/ethnic differences in teen and parent perspectives toward depression treatment. *Journal of Adolescent Health, 44*, 546–553.

Cheung, A. H., Emslie, G. J., & Mayes, T. L. (2005). Review of the efficacy and safety of antidepressants in youth depression. *Journal of Child Psychology and Psychiatry, 46*, 735–754.

Cheung, A. H., Emslie, G. J., & Mayes, T. L. (2006). The use of antidepressants to treat depression in children and adolescents. *Canadian Medical Association Journal, 174*, 193–200.

Clarke, G. N., DeBar, L., Lynch, F., Powell, J., Gale, J., O'Connor, E., et al. (2005). A randomized effectiveness trial of brief cognitive-behavioral therapy for depressed adolescents receiving antidepressant medication. *Journal of the American Academy of Child and Adolescent Psychiatry, 44*, 888–898.

Clarke, G. N., DeBar, L. L., & Lewinsohn, P. M. (2003). Cognitive-behavioral group treatment for adolescent depression. In A. E. Kazdin & J. R. Weisz (Eds.), *Evidence-based psychotherapies for children and adolescents* (pp. 120–147). New York: Guilford Press.

Clarke, G. N., Hornbrook, M., Lynch, F., Polen, M., Gale, J., Beardslee, W. R., et al. (2001). A randomized trial of a group cognitive intervention for preventing depression in adolescent offspring of depressed parents. *Archives of General Psychiatry, 58*, 1127–1134.

Clarke, G. N., Hornbrook, M., Lynch, F., Polen, M., Gale, J., O'Connor, E., et al. (2002). Group cognitive-behavioral treatment for depressed adolescent offspring of depressed parents in a health maintenance organization. *Journal of the American Academy of Child and Adolescent Psychiatry, 41*, 305–313.

Cohen, D., Flament, M.-F., Taieb, O., Thompson, C., & Basquin, M. (2000). Electroconvulsive therapy in adolescence. *European Child and Adolescent Psychiatry, 9*, 1–6.

Compas, B. E., Forehand, R., Thigpen, J. C., Keller, G., Hardcastle, E. J., Cole, D. A., et al. (2011). Family group cognitive-behavioral preventive intervention for families of depressed parents: 18- and 24-month outcomes. *Journal of Consulting and Clinical Psychology, 79*, 488–499.

Cornelius, J. R., Bukstein, O. G., Salloum, I. M., Lynch, K., Pollock, N. K., Gershon, S., et al. (2001). Fluoxetine in adolescents with major depression and an alcohol use disorder. *Addictive Behaviors, 26*, 735–739.

Coyle, J. T., Pine, D. S., Charney, D. S., Lewis, L., Nemeroff, C. B., Carlson, G. A., et al. (2003). Depression and bipolar support alliance consensus statement on the unmet needs in diagnosis and treatment of mood disorders in children and adolescents. *Journal of the American Academy of Child and Adolescent Psychiatry, 42*, 1494–1503.

Croarkin, P. E., Wall, C. A., & Lee, J. (2011). Applications of transcranial magnetic stimulation (TMS) in child and adolescent psychiatry. *International Review of Psychiatry, 23*, 445–453.

Croarkin, P. E., Wall, C. A., McClintock, S. M., Kozel, F. A., Husain, M. M., & Sampson, S. M. (2010). The emerging role for rTMS in optimizing the treatment of adolescent depression. *Journal of ECT, 26*, 323–329.

Curry, J., Rohde, P., Simons, A., Silva, S., Vitiello, B., Kratochvil, C. J., et al. (2006). Predictors and moderators of acute outcome in the Treatment for Adolescents with Depression Study (TADS). *Journal of the American Academy of Child and Adolescent Psychiatry, 45*, 1427–1439.

Curry, J., Silva, S., Rohde, P., Ginsburg, G., Kratochvil, C. J., Simons, A., et al. (2011). Recovery and recurrence following treatment for adolescent major depression. *Archives of General Psychiatry, 68,* 263–270.

Cutuli, J. J., Chaplin, T. M., Gillham, J. E., Reivich, K., & Seligman, M. E. P. (2006). Preventing co-occurring depression symptoms in adolescents with conduct problems: The Penn Resiliency Program. *Annals of the New York Academy of Sciences, 1094,* 282–286.

Czaja, A., & Valuck, R. J. (2012). Off-label antidepressant use in children and adolescents compared with young adults: Extent and level of evidence. *Pharmacoepidemiology and Drug Safety, 21,* 997–1004.

D'Angelo, E. J., Llerena-Quinn, R., Shapiro, R., Colon, F., Rodriguez, P., Gallagher, K., et al. (2009). Adaptation of the preventive intervention program for depression for use with predominantly low-income Latino families. *Family Process, 48,* 269–291.

David-Ferdon, C., & Kaslow, N. J. (2008). Evidence-based psychosocial interventions for child and adolescent depression. *Journal of Clinical Child and Adolescent Psychology, 37,* 62–104.

Daviss, W. B., Bentivoglio, P., Racusin, R., Brown, K. M., Bostic, J. Q., & Wiley, L. (2001). Bupropion sustained release in adolescents with comorbid attention-deficit/hyperactivity disorder and depression. *Journal of the American Academy of Child and Adolescent Psychiatry, 40,* 307–314.

Delate, T., Gelenberg, A. J., Simmons, V. A., & Motheral, B. R. (2004). Trends in the use of antidepressants in a national sample of commercially insured pediatric patients, 1998–2002. *Psychiatric Services, 55,* 387–191.

Diamond, G. S., Siqueland, L., & Diamond, G. M. (2003). Attachment-based family therapy for depressed adolescents: Programmatic treatment development. *Clinical Child and Family Psychology Review, 6,* 107–127.

Domino, M. E., Foster, M., Vitiello, B., Kratochvil, C. J., Burns, B. J., Silva, S. G., et al. (2009). Relative cost-effectiveness of treatments for adolescent depression: 36-week results from the TADS randomized trial. *Journal of the American Academy of Child and Adolescent Psychiatry, 48,* 711–720.

Dubicka, B., Elvins, R., Roberts, C., Chick, G., WIlkinson, P., & Goodyer, I. M. (2010). Combined treatment with cognitive-behavioural therapy in adolescent depression: Meta-analysis. *British Journal of Psychiatry, 197,* 433–440.

Emslie, G. (2012). The psychopharmocology of adolescent depression. *Journal of Child and Adolescent Psychopharmacology, 22,* 2–4.

Emslie, G. J., Findling, R. L., Rynn, M., Marcus, R. N., Fernandes, L. A., D'Amico, M. F., et al. (2002). Efficacy and safety of nefazodone in the treatment of adolescents with major depressive disorder [Abstract]. *Journal of Child and Adolescent Psychopharmacology, 12,* 299.

Emslie, G. J., Findling, R. L., Yeung, P. P., Kunz, N. R., & Li, Y. (2007). Venlafaxine ER for the treatment of pediatric subjects with depression: Results of two placebo-controlled trials. *Journal of the American Academy of Child and Adolescent Psychiatry, 46,* 479–488.

Emslie, G. J., Heiligenstein, J. H., Hoog, S. L., Wagner, K. D., Findling, R. L., McCracken, J., et al. (2004). Fluoxetine treatment for prevention of relapse of depression in children and adolescents: A double-blind, placebo-controlled study. *Journal of the American Academy of Child and Adolescent Psychiatry, 43,* 1397–1405.

Emslie, G. J., Kratochvil, C. J., Vitiello, B., Silva, S., Mayes, T., McNulty, S., et al. (2006). Treatment for Adolescents with Depression Study (TADS): Safety results. *Journal of the American Academy of Child and Adolescent Psychiatry, 45,* 1440–1455.

Emslie, G. J., Mayes, T., Porta, G., Vitiello, B., Clarke, G. N., Wagner, K. D., et al. (2010). Treatment of Resistant Depression in Adolescents (TORDIA): Week 24 outcomes. *American Journal of Psychiatry, 167,* 782–791.

Emslie, G. J., Wagner, K. D., Kutcher, S., Krulewicz, S., Fong, R., Carpenter, D. J., et al. (2006). Paroxetine treatment in children and adolescents with major depressive disorder: A randomized, multicenter, double-blind, placebo-controlled trial. *Journal of the American Academy of Child and Adolescent Psychiatry, 45,* 709–719.

Ghaziuddin, N., Dumas, S., & Hodges, E. (2011). Use of continuation or maintenance electrocon-vulsive therapy in adolescents with severe treatment-resistant depression. *Journal of ECT, 27*, 168–174.

Gibb, B. E., Stone, L. B., & Crossett, S. E. (2012). Peer victimization and prospective changes in children's inferential styles. *Journal of Clinical Child and Adolescent Psychology, 41*, 561–569.

Gillham, J. E., Hamilton, J., Freres, D. R., Patton, K., & Gallop, R. (2006). Preventing depression among early adolescents in the primary care setting: A randomized controlled study of the Penn Resiliency Program. *Journal of Abnormal Child Psychology, 34*, 203–219.

Gillham, J. E., Reivich, K. J., Freres, D. R., Chaplin, T. M., Shatte, A. J., Samuels, B., et al. (2007). School-based prevention of depressive symptoms: A randomized controlled study of the effec-tiveness and specificity of the Penn Resiliency Program. *Journal of Consulting and Clinical Psychology, 75*, 9–19.

Gillham, J. E., Reivich, K., Freres, D. R., Lascher, M., Litzinger, S., Shatte, A. J., et al. (2006). School-based prevention of depression and anxiety symptoms in early adolescence: A pilot of a parent intervention component. *School Psychology Quarterly, 21*, 323–348.

Gladstone, T. R. G., Beardslee, W. R., & O'Connor, E. E. (2011). The prevention of adolescent depression. *Psychiatric Clinics of North America, 34*, 35–52.

Gonzalez, A., Boyle, M. H., Kyu, H. H., Georgiades, K., Duncan, L., & MacMillan, H. L. (2012). Childhood and family influences on depression, chronic physical conditions and their comor-bidity: Findings from the Ontario Child Health Study. *Journal of Psychiatric Research, 46*, 1475–1482.

Grover, S., Malhotra, S., Varma, S., Chakrabarti, S., Avasthi, A., & Mattoo, S. K. (2013). Elec-troconsulvie therapy in adolescents: A retrospective study from North India. *Journal of ECT, 29*(2), 122–126.

Horowitz, J. L., & Garber, J. (2006). The prevention of depressive symptoms in children and adolescents: A meta-analytic review. *Journal of Consulting and Clinical Psychology, 74*, 401–415.

Hughes, C. W., Emslie, G. J., Crismon, M. L., Posner, K., Birmaher, B., Ryan, N. D., et al. (2007). Texas Children's Medication Algorithm Project: Update from Texas Consensus Conference Panel on Medication Treatment of Childhood Major Depressive Disorder. *Journal of the American Academy of Child and Adolescent Psychiatry, 46*, 667–686.

Kaufman, N. K., Rohde, P., Seeley, J. R., Clarke, G., & Stice, E. (2005). Potential mediators of cognitive-behavioral therapy for adolescents with comorbid major depression and conduct disorder. *Journal of Consulting and Clinical Psychology, 73*, 38–46.

Kennard, B., Clarke, G. N., Weersing, V. R., Asarnow, J. R., Shamseddeen, W., Porta, G., et al. (2009). Effective components of TORDIA cognitive-behavioral therapy for adolescent depres-sion: Preliminary findings. *Journal of Consulting and Clinical Psychology, 77*, 1033–1041.

Kennard, B., Silva, S., Vitiello, B., Curry, J., Kratochvil, C. J., Simons, A., et al. (2006). Remis-sion and residual symptoms after short-term treatment in the Treatment of Adolescents with Depression Study (TADS). *Journal of the American Academy of Child and Adolescent Psy-chiatry, 45*, 1404–1411.

Kennard, B., Silva, S. G., Mayes, T., Rohde, P., Hughes, J. L., Vitiello, B., et al. (2009). Assess-ment of safety and long-term outcomes of initial treatment with placebo in TADS. *American Journal of Psychiatry, 166*, 337–344.

Kennard, B., Silva, S. G., Tonev, S., Rohde, P., Hughes, J. L., Vitiello, B., et al. (2009). Remission and recovery in the Treatment for Adolescents with Depression Study (TADS): Acute and long-term outcomes. *Journal of the American Academy of Child and Adolescent Psychiatry, 48*, 186–195.

Kovacs, M., & Lopez-Duran, N. (2012). Contextual emotion regulation therapy: A developmen-tally based intervention for pediatric depression. *Child and Adolescent Psychiatric Clinics of North America, 21*, 327–343.

Kratochvil, C. J., Emslie, G. J., Silva, S., McNulty, S., Walkup, J., Curry, J., et al. (2006). Acute time to response in the Treatment for Adolescents with Depression Study (TADS). *Journal of the American Academy of Child and Adolescent Psychiatry, 45*, 1412–1418.

Leon, A. C., Marzuk, P. M., Tardiff, K., Bucciarelli, A., Piper, T. M., & Galea, S. (2006). Antidepressants and youth suicide in New York City, 1999–2002. *Journal of the American Academy of Child and Adolescent Psychiatry, 45*, 1054–1058.

Libby, A. M., Brent, D. A., Morrato, E. H., Orton, H. D., Allen, R., & Valuck, R. J. (2007). Decline in treatment of pediatric depression after FDA advisory on risk of suicidality with SSRIs. *American Journal of Psychiatry, 164*, 884–891.

Loo, C., McFarquhar, T., & Walter, G. (2006). Transcranial magnetic stimulation in adolescent depression. *Australasian Psychiatry, 14*, 81–85.

Lovrin, M. (2009). Treatment of major depression in adolescents: Weighing the evidence of risk and benefit in light of black box warnings. *Journal of Child and Adolescent Psychiatric Nursing, 22*, 63–68.

Lynch, F. L., Dickerson, J. F., Clarke, G. N., Vitiello, B., Porta, G., Wagner, K. D., et al. (2011). Incremental cost-effectiveness of combined therapy vs. medication only for youth with selective serotonin reuptake inhibitor-resistant depression: Treatment of SSRI-Resistant Depression in Adolescent Trial finding. *Journal of the American Medical Association Psychiatry, 68*, 253–262.

Lyon, F. L., & Clarke, G. N. (2006). Estimating the economic burden of depression in children and adolescents. *American Journal of Preventive Medicine, 31*, 143–151.

Ma, J., Lee, K.-V., & Stafford, R. S. (2005). Depression treatment during outpatient visits by U.S. children and adolescents. *Journal of Adolescent Health, 37*, 434–442.

Mann, J. J., Graham, E., Baldessarini, R. J., Beardslee, W. R., Fawcett, J. A., Goodwin, F. K., et al. (2006). ACNP Task Force Report on SSRIs and suicidal behavior in youth. *Neuropsychopharmacology, 31*, 473–492.

March, J. S., Silva, S., Petrycki, S., Curry, J., Wells, K. C., Fairbank, J. A., et al. (2004). Fluoxetine, cognitive-behavioral therapy, and their combination for adolescents with depression: Treatment for Adolescents with Depression Study (TADS) randomized controlled trial. *Journal of the American Medical Association, 292*, 807–820.

March, J. S., Silva, S., Vitiello, B., & the TADS Team. (2006). The Treatment for Adolescents with Depression Study (TADS): Methods and message at 12 weeks. *Journal of the American Academy of Child and Adolescent Psychiatry, 45*, 1393–1403.

March, J. S., & Vitiello, B. (2009). Clinical messages from the Treatment for Adolescents with Depression Study (TADS). *American Journal of Psychiatry, 166*, 1118–1123.

Mayer, G., Aviram, S. B., Walter, G., Levkovitz, Y., & Bloch, Y. (2012). Long-term follow-up of adolescents with resistant depression treated with repetitive transcranial magnetic stimulation. *Journal of ECT, 28*, 84–86.

McCarty, C. A., Violette, H. D., Duong, M. T., Cruz, R. A., & McCauley, E. (2013). A randomized trial of the Positive Thoughts and Action program for depression among early adolescents. *Journal of Clinical Child and Adolescent Psychology, 42*(4), 554–563.

Melvin, G. A., Tonge, B. J., King, N. J., Heyne, D., Gordon, M. S., & Klimkeit, E. (2006). A comparison of cognitive-behavioral therapy, sertraline, and their combination for adolescent depression. *Journal of the American Academy of Child and Adolescent Psychiatry, 45*, 1151–1161.

Meredith, L. S., Stein, B. D., Paddock, S. M., Jaycox, L. H., Quinn, V. P., Chandra, A., et al. (2009). Perceived barriers to treatment for adolescent depression. *Medical Care, 47*, 677–685.

Merikangas, K. R., He, J.-P., Rapoport, J., Vitiello, B., & Olfson, M. (2013). Medication use in U.S. youth with mental disorders. *Journal of the American Medical Association Pediatrics, 167*, 141–148.

Merry, S., McDowell, H., Wild, C. J., Bir, J., & Cunliffe, R. (2004). A randomized placebo-controlled trial of a school-based depression prevention program. *Journal of the American Academy of Child and Adolescent Psychiatry, 43*, 538–547.

Merry, S. N., Stasiak, K., Shepherd, M., Frampton, C., Fleming, T. M., & Lucassen, M. F. G.

(2012). The effectiveness of SPARX, a computerised self-help intervention for adolescents seeking help for depression: Randomised controlled non–inferiority trial. *BMJ, 344*.

Michael, K. D., & Crowley, S. L. (2002). How effective are treatments for child and adolescent depression?: A meta-analytic review. *Clinical Psychology Review, 22*, 247–269.

Moreno, C., Roche, A. M., & Greenhill, L. L. (2006). Pharmacotherapy of child and adolescent depression. *Child and Adolescent Psychiatric Clinics of North America, 15*, 977–998.

Mufson, L. H., Dorta, K. P., Wickramaratne, P., Nomura, Y., Olfson, M., & Weissman, M. M. (2004). A randomized effectiveness trial of interpersonal psychotherapy for depressed adolescents. *Archives of General Psychiatry, 61*, 577–584.

Mufson, L. H., Weissman, M. M., Moreau, D., & Garfinkel, R. (1999). Efficacy of interpersonal psychotherapy for depressed adolescents. *Archives of General Psychiatry, 56*, 573–579.

Nilsen, T. S., Eisemann, M., & Kvernmo, S. (2013). Predictors and moderators of outcome in child and adolescent anxiety and depression: A systematic review of psychological treatment studies. *European Child and Adolescent Psychiatry, 22*, 69–87.

Quintana, H. (2005). Transcranial magnetic stimulation in persons younger than the age of 18. *Journal of ECT, 21*, 88–95.

Roberts, C., Kane, R., Thomson, H., Bishop, B., & Hart, B. (2003). The prevention of depressive symptoms in rural school children: A randomized controlled trial. *Journal of Consulting and Clinical Psychology, 71*, 622–628.

Rohde, P., Clarke, G., Mace, D. E., Jorgensen, J. S., & Seeley, J. R. (2004). An efficacy/effectiveness study of cognitive-behavioral treatment for adolescents with comorbid major depression and conduct disorder. *Journal of the American Academy of Child and Adolescent Psychiatry, 43*, 660–668.

Rohde, P., Seeley, J. R., Kaufman, N. K., Clarke, G. N., & Stice, E. (2006). Predicting time to recovery among depressed adolescents treated in two psychosocial group interventions. *Journal of Consulting and Clinical Psychology, 74*, 80–88.

Ryan, N. D. (2005). Treatment of depression in children and adolescents. *Lancet, 366*, 933–940.

Sander, J. B., & McCarty, C. A. (2005). Youth depression in the family context: Familial risk factors and models of treatment. *Clinical Child and Family Psychology Review, 8*, 203–219.

Shamseddeen, W., Asarnow, J. R., Clarke, G. N., Vitiello, B., Wagner, K. D., Birmaher, B., et al. (2011). Impact of physical and sexual abuse on treatment response in the Treatment of Resistant Depression in Adolescent Study (TORDIA). *Journal of the American Academy of Child and Adolescent Psychiatry, 50*, 293–301.

Sheffield, J. K., Spence, S. H., Rapee, R. M., Kowalenko, N., Wignall, A., Davis, A., et al. (2006). Evaluation of universal, indicated, and combined cognitive-behavioral approaches to the prevention of depression in adolescents. *Journal of Consulting and Clinical Psychology, 74*, 66–79.

Shirk, S. R., Gudmundsen, G., Kaplinski, H. C., & McMakin, D. L. (2008). Alliance and outcome in cognitive-behavioral therapy for adolescent depression. *Journal of Clinical Child and Adolescent Psychology, 37*, 631–639.

Shochet, I. M., & Ham, D. (2004). Universal school-based approaches to preventing adolescent depression: Past findings and future directions of the Resourceful Adolescent Program. *International Journal of Mental Health Promotion, 6*, 17–25.

Shoirah, H., & Hamoda, H. M. (2011). Electroconvulsive therapy in children and adolescents. *Expert Review of Neurotherapeutics, 11*, 127–137.

Spirito, A., Esposito-Smythers, C., Wolff, J., & Uhl, K. (2011). Cognitive-behavioral therapy for adolescent depression and suicidality. *Child and Adolescent Psychiatric Clinics of North America, 20*, 191–204.

Stark, K. D., Hargrave, J., Hersh, B., Greenberg, M., Herren, J., & Fisher, M. (2008). Treatment of childhood depression: The ACTION treatment program. In J. R. Z. Abela & B. L. Hankin (Eds.), *Handbook of depression in children and adolescents* (pp. 224–249). New York: Guilford Press.

Stark, K. D., Hargrave, J., Sander, J., Schnoebelen, S., Simpson, J., & Molnar, J. (2006). Treatment of childhood depression: The ACTION treatment program. In P. C. Kendall (Ed.), *Child and adolescent therapy: Cognitive-behavioral procedures* (3rd ed., pp. 169–216). New York: Guilford Press.

Stark, K. D., Reynolds, W. M., & Kaslow, N. J. (1987). A comparison of the relative efficacy of self-control therapy and behavior problem-solving therapy for depression in children. *Journal of Abnormal Child Psychology, 15*, 91–113.

Sutton, J. M. (2007). Prevention of depression in youth: A qualitative review and future suggestions. *Clinical Psychology Review, 27*, 552–571.

Taieb, O., Flament, M.-F., Chevret, S., Jeammet, P., Allilaire, J.-F., Mazet, P., et al. (2002). Clinical relevance of electroconvulsive therapy (ECT) in adolescents with severe mood disorder: Evidence from a follow-up study. *European Psychiatry, 17*, 206–212.

Taieb, O., Flament, M.-F., Corcos, M., Jeammet, P., Basquin, M., Mazet, P., et al. (2001). Electroconvulsive therapy in adolescents with mood disorder: Patients' and parents' attitudes. *Psychiatry Research, 104*, 183–190.

Tao, R., Emslie, G., & Mayes, T. (2010). Pharmacotherapy for pediatric major depression. *Psychiatric Annals, 40*, 192–202.

Thompson, E. A., Eggert, L. L., & Herting, J. R. (2000). Mediating effects of an indicated prevention program for reducing youth depression and suicide risk behaviors. *Suicide and Life-Threatening Behavior, 30*, 252–271.

Treatment for Adolescents with Depression Study Team. (2003). Treatment for Adolescents with Depression Study (TADS): Rationale, design, and methods. *Journal of the American Academy of Child and Adolescent Psychiatry, 42*, 531–542.

Treatment for Adolescents with Depression Study Team. (2005). The Treatment for Adolescents with Depression Study (TADS): Demographic and clinical characteristics. *Journal of the American Academy of Child and Adolescent Psychiatry, 44*, 28–40.

Varley, C. K. (2006). Treating depression in children and adolescents: What options now? *CNS Drugs, 20*, 1–13.

Vitiello, B. (2011). Prevention and treatment of child and adolescent depression: Challenges and opportunities. *Epidemiology and Psychiatric Services, 20*, 37–43.

Vitiello, B., Rohde, P., Silva, S., Wells, K. C., Casat, C., Waslick, B. D., et al. (2006). Functioning and quality of life in the Treatment for Adolescents with Depression Study (TADS). *Journal of the American Academy of Child and Adolescent Psychiatry, 45*, 1419–1426.

Vitiello, B., Silva, S., Rohde, P., Kratochvil, C. J., Kennard, B., Reinecke, M., et al. (2009). Suicidal events in the Treatment for Adolescents with Depression Study (TADS). *Journal of Clinical Psychiatry, 70*, 741–747.

von Knorring, A., Olsson, G. I., Thomsen, P. H., Lemming, O. M., & Hulten, A. (2006). A randomized, double-blind, placebo-controlled study of citalopram in adolescents with major depressive disorder. *Journal of Clinical Psychopharmacology, 26*, 311–315.

Wagner, K. D., Ambrosini, P., Rynn, M., Wohlberg, C., Yang, R., Greenbaum, M. S., et al. (2003). Efficacy of sertraline in the treatment of children and adolescents with major depressive disorder: Two randomized controlled trials. *Journal of the American Medical Association, 290*, 1033–1041.

Wagner, K. D., Jonas, J., Findling, R. L., Ventura, D., & Saikali, K. (2006). A double-blind, randomized, placebo-controlled trial of escitalopram in the treatment of pediatric depression. *Journal of the American Academy of Child and Adolescent Psychiatry, 45*, 280–288.

Wagner, K. D., Robb, A. S., Findling, R. L., Jin, J., Gutierrez, M. M., & Heydorn, W. E. (2004). A randomized, placebo-controlled trial of citalopram for the treatment of major depression in children and adolescents. *American Journal of Psychiatry, 161*, 1079–1083.

Wall, C. A., Croarkin, P. E., Sim, L. A., Husain, M. M., Janicak, P. G., Kozel, F. A., et al. (2011). Adjunctive use of repetitive transcranial magnetic stimulation in depressed adolescents: A prospective pilot study. *Journal of Clinical Psychiatry, 72*, 1263–1269.

Walter, G., & Rey, J. M. (2003). Has the practice and outcome of ECT in adolescents changed?: Findings from a whole-population study. *Journal of ECT, 19*, 84–87.

Weisz, J. R., McCarty, C. A., & Valeri, S. M. (2006). Effects of psychotherapy for depression in children and adolescents: A meta-analysis. *Psychological Bulletin, 132*, 132–149.

Weisz, J. R., Thurber, C., Sweeney, L., Proffitt, V., & LeGagnoux, G. (1997). Brief treatment of mild to moderate child depression using primary and secondary control enhancement training. *Journal of Consulting and Clinical Psychology, 65*, 703–707.

Whittington, C. J., Kendall, T., Fonagy, P., Cottrell, D., Cotgrove, A., & Boddington, E. (2004). Selective serotonin reuptake inhibitors in childhood depression: Systematic review of published versus unpublished data. *Lancet, 363*, 1341–1345.

Wood, A., Harrington, R., & Moore, A. (1996). Controlled trial of a brief cognitive-behavioural intervention in adolescent patients with depressive disorders. *Journal of Child Psychology and Psychiatry, 37*, 737–746.

Young, J. F., Mufson, L., & Davies, M. (2006). Impact of comorbid anxiety in an effectiveness study of interpersonal psychotherapy for depressed adolescents. *Journal of the American Academy of Child and Adolescent Psychiatry, 45*, 904–912.

Closing Comments
and Future Directions

CONSTANCE L. HAMMEN *and* IAN H. GOTLIB

With the publication of the third edition of this *Handbook*, it is apparent that the extensive and energetic engagement of talented investigators in the depression field continues unabated. The advances in the field since the second edition are ably described in the chapters; this final segment is intended to reflect briefly on some of these accomplishments and on the challenges that lie ahead. In addition to the empirical content of each chapter, identifying the current state of the topic, all of the chapters include penetrating observations not only about content gaps but also about methodological deficiencies and conceptual limitations to be addressed in the next wave of depression research. The challenges are daunting, including no less than what one author expressed as "recursive feedback loops that transcend levels of analysis."

DESCRIPTIVE ASPECTS OF DEPRESSION

The opening section consists of eight chapters that cover epidemiological and clinical features, including depression and medical illness, as well as assessment and methodological issues. Four of the chapters are new topics for the *Handbook*, discussing features of bipolar disorder, chronicity of depression, depression–anxiety comorbidity, and emotional functioning in depression.

Several chapters in previous editions of this *Handbook* noted the problems of diagnostic heterogeneity and comorbidity and the questionable validity and utility for many purposes of the traditional diagnostic categories of depression. Not surprisingly, therefore, as this volume arrives on the scene shortly after the Research Domain Criteria (RDoC) mandate of the National Institute of Mental Health, authors of many of the chapters championed new approaches to the measurement and conceptualization of depressive phenomena in research based on dimensional, transdiagnostic, and specific relevant facets, as well as course features. These approaches should help to refine depression-relevant phenotypes and thereby sharpen and integrate findings across multiple focuses of investigation and identify factors that are common to emotional disorders but specific to depression. These chapters have also noted the need for improved assessments of depressive phenomena, including improved considerations of the severity, chronicity, and functional debility of depressive disorders, and for methods of capturing the experience and expression of depressive phenomena to reflect sociocultural diversity, in addition to their expression in special populations such as the medically ill, older adults, and children. Acknowledging the limitations of researchers' dependence on diagnostic categories and abandoning the underlying "uniformity myth" should lead to significant paradigm shifts in how depressive phenomena are conceptualized and studied. It is intriguing to speculate about what the next generation of research will yield—and, of course, whether such shifts will lead to significant advances in understanding mechanisms of depressive disorders and developing more effective treatments and preventive interventions.

It is also likely that some of our fundamental assumptions about the nature and assessments of bipolar disorder will change as the limitations of the Kraepelinian approach are challenged by growing bodies of research. Similarly, the recognition of the pervasive impact of depression on medical disorders presents new challenges and opportunities as investigators explore not only the consequences of depression on illness but also its etiological significance in specific disorders and its impact on health behaviors and outcomes. As public attention focuses increasingly critically on health care access and cost containment, we believe that depression research has much to offer in understanding and ameliorating the course of common medical disorders and much to contribute to discoveries of ways in which specific disease processes such as inflammation are related to mechanisms of depression.

Several chapters in the opening section—and throughout the volume—also note the increasing use of new technologies for measuring depressive phenomena, whether through Internet applications, novel experimental paradigms, or ecological momentary assessments, for example. Innovations in methods—as well as in conceptualizations—are always necessary to the vitality of psychopathology research.

VULNERABILITY, RISK, AND MODELS OF DEPRESSION

This section of the book contains nine chapters discussing genetic, neurobiological, developmental, and psychosocial approaches to depression vulnerability, including family, cognitive, interpersonal, and environmental perspectives, as well as a chapter on risk factors for bipolar disorders. These chapters represent topics in which researchers continue to be highly active, particularly in those areas reflecting conceptual, empirical, and methodological advances in biological aspects of depression and integration across genetic, biological, environmental, and developmental levels of analysis. Each of the chapters notes significant increases in recent years in our knowledge of how these diverse ingredients contribute to depressive outcomes.

Advances in genetic studies of depression, paralleling advances in the genetics of other illnesses and psychopathological conditions, reflect an explosion of new methodologies and research designs. In contrast to older models of genetic effects seeking the "gene for" particular psychological disorders, there is acceptance of the reality of small effects of multiple genes, necessitating very large sample sizes. In this context, genomewide association studies are now common but often yield disappointingly low levels of significant loci identification and replication. In addition to acknowledging methodological limitations, including sample sizes and heterogeneity of the depression phenotype, scientists have increasingly come to accept the conceptualization that many genetic factors potentially relevant to depressive (emotional) disorders may have effects that are dependent on environmental and developmental experiences. Indeed, the interplay between genetic and environmental factors is recognized as vastly complex because such factors are not independent of each other. Such realities present enormous challenges to future research, along with the need for matching the quality of measurement of environmental and developmental factors with that of measurement of molecular genetic factors. Increasingly, also, recent research has underscored the importance of linkage of genetic factors with mechanisms of neurobiological effects, as evidenced by growing fields of imaging genomics, pharmacogenetics, social genomics, epigenetics, and the like.

The explosion of genetic research in psychopathology clearly has been paralleled by neuroscience research, commonly featuring neuroimaging methods. Collectively, this work has contributed enormously to our understanding of the brain generally, and depression specifically. New worlds have opened up at different levels, from systems neuroscience down to intracellular processes. Unfortunately, some of the excitement of new developments and discoveries has been accompanied by a tendency toward reductionism that many would argue is not only erroneous but also misleading, if not destructive (e.g., Miller, 2010). Several of the authors in this edition of the *Handbook* have specifically noted that the complexities are enormous and that depressive disorders (and many psychological constructs) cannot be reduced to fundamental biological processes. Healthy humility is in order, and improving the conceptualization and measurement of developmental and environmental factors that influence biological mechanisms must be a priority in advancing the field of depression.

Several of the "nonbiological" chapters in this section, covering childhood exposure to adversity, stress, cognition, parental depression, and interpersonal aspects of depression, report noteworthy advances in their areas—in both content and methodologies. Although representing some of the longest running approaches to the study of depression risk factors, these topics remain active and innovative. Across these topics, advances in integrative research combining psychosocial, developmental, and biological approaches are the new standard. Nevertheless, in virtually all of the chapters, authors emphasize the need for even more empirical studies of integrative models and urge further study of the interactive and dynamic associations among variables over time. Several authors have acknowledged or called for translational applications in which intermediate phenotypes or specific facets of depressive phenomena, rather than diagnostic categories, are studied. Authors also noted the need for further elaboration and development of interventions based on the accumulated knowledge of effects of early adversity exposure, cognition, interpersonal dysfunction, stress sensitization, and high-risk status. The research represented by these chapters also supports the continuing need for conceptual, empirical, and methodological leadership in representing the environmental, developmental, and transactional perspectives in the RDoC approach.

The chapter on risk factors in bipolar disorder acknowledges the relatively "emerging" research efforts by behavioral scientists to advance our understanding in this area. Issues demanding attention are not dissimilar to those of the more mature unipolar depression field but are nonetheless challenging due to ongoing unresolved questions about core phenomena and diagnosis and to the absence of well-established etiological models. Psychologists have key roles to play and potentially much to add to the future direction of this research field.

DEPRESSION IN SPECIFIC POPULATIONS

The seven chapters in this section of the *Handbook* are a dramatic reminder of the heterogeneity of depression—how its occurrence, features, and manifestations, and even causal and treatment implications, vary considerably by gender, age, and culture. Consistent with most of the chapters throughout the book, this set of chapters also notes the need for complex, integrative research examining the influence and interactions (transactions) among many relevant variables.

Gender differences in depression are virtually universal, as is being demonstrated increasingly in international studies—despite enormous variation in the cultural and environmental circumstances of women's lives. Considerable research has been conducted examining these factors, and investigators now commonly analyze, report, and/or control for gender differences in aspects of depression. Nevertheless, many issues remain to be resolved, including the emergence of gender differences in adolescence and the apparent differences in first onset but not recurrence of depression. Along with the development of new paradigms in psychopathology, such as gene–environment interactions, a focus on intermediate phenotypes, and epigenetics, it will be important in future work to continue to explore and report gender differences in these constructs and models.

Cultural differences in the expression of and attributions about the meaning and causes of depression have become topics of increased research focus over recent years. Such studies not only contribute to expanding our conceptualizations of depression but also have practical implications for developing and matching individuals to culturally accepted interventions. Intriguing new perspectives that integrate culture, mind, and brain will promote deeper understanding of distress phenomena and must find their way into RDoC-based epistemological frameworks. Research on cultural and ethnic differences in depression phenomena have had, and will continue to have, an important role in developing applications of culturally competent clinical psychology.

Three separate chapters presented research on depression in children, adolescents, and older adults. We chose to include distinct chapters on these topics both because of the enormous amount of research conducted over the past few years and because of emerging evidence of the significant differences among children, adolescents, and older adults in clinical features and course, as well as in likely risk factors and etiological processes. Research findings support the premise that first-onset depressions in each of these age groups have different etiological and course implications. Research on depression in children no longer mostly reflects downward extensions of adult models; instead, it attempts to explore depression in terms of developmental processes and challenges, including temperament, stress reactivity and emotion-regulation processes, and pubertal events. Although the full syndrome of depression is rare in children, refinements in assessment and detection of possible endophenotypic expressions may help to clarify the course and etiology. Adolescent depression is arguably the prototypical form of depression, given that a large proportion of adults with depression experienced their first episode in the teenage decade. The intriguing questions of emergence of gender differences and the high rates of depression in youth continue to challenge the field. The need for multivariate, transactional models that include developmentally salient factors and mechanisms is clearly articulated in several chapters and presents a challenging, if not daunting, task. The issue of depression in older adults has stimulated an increasing amount of attention, given the likelihood of its unique features and its implications for quality of life and public health considerations. Increasingly, depression in older adults is recognized as a potential early warning sign of dementing disorders, as a contributor to ill health, and as detrimental to effective functioning in both individuals and their families. Because many early epidemiological studies omitted the oldest members of the population and many diagnostic and developmental issues (and even biased perceptions of older adults) obscured the detection of depression, the increased research focus on depression in older individuals in recent years is a welcome addition.

The chapter on depression in couples and families reflects several key issues: the impairing consequences of depression and the detrimental effects on functioning in important roles; the importance of environmental context as a moderator and mediator of risk factors for depression; unique and similar relationship factors in unipolar and bipolar disorders. Although depression may be variously characterized as a mood disorder, as a disorder of negative cognition, or as a disorder of emotion regulation, it is most decidedly an interpersonal disorder: Relationships may play a central role in contributing to, or protecting from, depression. It is also an interpersonal disorder in the sense that those in close relationships with the individual suffering from depression are also affected; the transactions among members of the relationship serve to alter the course of depression for worse or better. Increasingly, research with couples or families with a member with bipolar disorder is reflecting similar patterns. Intergenerational transmission of depression associated with family processes represents a potentially modifiable risk factor greatly in need of intervention. The chapters on depression in children, adolescents, older adults, and couples also remind us of the continuing and widespread relevance of two considerations: the specificity of effects to depression and developmental perspectives requiring analyses of multiple factors, with transactional and interaction processes leading to different levels of adaptive functioning, unfolding over time.

Suicidal individuals are also a special population, closely but not exclusively entwined with depressive disorders. This is depression at its most lethal and tragic. Increasingly recognized new populations of the vulnerable capture attention and present research opportunities—military personnel, self-harming teens, dispirited older adults. Research continues to promote refinements in definitions of suicidality and prediction of suicidal behavior—but with continuing challenges in saving lives and well-being through identification and treatment and effective prevention. These tasks are made even more challenging with increasingly culturally and ethnically diverse populations.

PREVENTION AND TREATMENT OF DEPRESSION

The six chapters in this final section of the *Handbook* represent the diverse forms of evidence-based treatment and prevention of depression in adults and children. Because depression is so prevalent, and because its treatment with medication or psychotherapy has largely set the standards for "success" in treatment research, there is an enormous body of research that continues to contribute to refinements in interventions, research designs, outcomes assessment, and dissemination. It cannot be said that there are substantial new developments overall in treatment in recent years; established treatment modalities continue to show solid results for many patients with depression, but with evidence of relapse and recurrence for a good many individuals. Virtually all of the chapters in the treatment section highlight the need to address issues of wider dissemination of effective treatments, including novel methods using Internet and telephone communications, and for adaptations of effective treatments to reach and meet the needs of ethnically and economically disadvantaged populations. Many of these chapters also supplement their presentations of the empirical basis of treatment and preventive interventions with therapist guidelines and recommendations useful for individual practitioners.

Despite its intrinsic appeal, the ideal of preventing major depression has not been fully realized. However, the authors of the prevention chapters argue for the likelihood that 50% of depressive episodes might be prevented in higher risk groups with improved methodologies of design and measurement, optimization of promising methods, and increasing the focus on risk populations, such as women with perinatal depression, offspring of mothers with depression, and those with previous depression.

Pharmacotherapy and other somatic treatments for unipolar depression continue to be a primary approach to intervention. It is noteworthy, however, that there have been few new antidepressant medications in recent years and no improvements in success rates for remission and prevention of recurrence. Medication treatments for special populations, such as pregnant women, children, and older adults, require continued research on issues of safety and efficacy. New biological treatment prospects that stimulate excitement and promise future research include the use of the drug ketamine, identifying possible genetic predictors of antidepressant treatments, and new neuromodulatory methods for treating severe depression that alter local neural conduction, such as transcranial magnetic stimulation and others.

Empirically supported psychotherapies for depression for adults, children, couples, and families have proliferated over the past three decades, as documented in chapters covering cognitive, behavioral, and marital/family/interpersonal approaches. As noted earlier, treatment researchers are mindful of gaps in dissemination, barriers to treatment among the disadvantaged, and the need for culturally sensitive adaptations of established empirically supported treatments. Most also endorse additional studies focused on helping to understand the mechanisms by which change may occur and to identify characteristics of patients who do less well so that modifications may be developed to improve outcomes among such groups.

Recent studies indicate that cognitive-behavioral therapy (CBT) and behavioral activation are as efficacious as pharmacotherapy even for severe depression, with some possible advantage in prevention of recurrence. Behavioral treatments, including behavioral activation, are not only efficacious but might also have some advantages in future dissemination, requiring less rigorous training and possibly greater client acceptance and ease of application. Family and couple therapies may specifically address the interpersonal discord and distress that are so central to the experience of depressive disorders, and one chapter notes the centrality of a focus on reducing interpersonal "stress generation."

The chapter on treatments for bipolar disorder attests to the importance of adding psychosocial interventions as options to the traditional pharmacotherapy for patients with bipolar disorder. Medication treatments alone have not proven to be sufficient; although they are critically important, especially for treatment and prevention of manias, many patients remain substantially depressed, symptomatic, and impaired. Growing recognition of bipolar disorder in children and adolescents has further highlighted the limitations of medication treatment alone, especially in view of dysfunctional family communication and relationship quality that affect youth with bipolar disorder and the course of their illness. The chapter also highlights gaps in research on the treatments needed for children and adolescents at risk for bipolar disorder or who display early symptoms—research with both the practical goal of helping such youth and their families and the conceptual goal of addressing the issue of whether early intervention may alter (improve) the course of bipolar disorder.

The contributors to this volume are to be commended for their chapters and for their own research that has provided many of the advances and much of the vitality of this field in recent years. We believe that these chapters will help to inspire and inform both emerging scholars and established scientists and practitioners to continue their work illuminating the many dark corners of this field, serving both the scientific and the practical aims of understanding and ameliorating the debilitating impact of depression on the lives of countless sufferers.

REFERENCE

Miller, G. A. (2010). Mistreating psychology in the Decades of the Brain. *Psychological Science, 5*, 716–743.

Author Index

Subject Index

Page numbers followed by *f* indicate figure, *t* indicate table